Perioperative Pain Management

Alaa Abd-Elsayed · Kristopher Schroeder
Editors

Perioperative Pain Management

A Clinical Guide

Springer

Editors
Alaa Abd-Elsayed
Department of Anesthesiology
University of Wisconsin
Madison, WI, USA

Kristopher Schroeder
Department of Anesthesiology
University of Wisconsin
Madison, WI, USA

ISBN 978-3-031-67647-5 ISBN 978-3-031-67648-2 (eBook)
https://doi.org/10.1007/978-3-031-67648-2

This Springer imprint is published by the registered company Springer Nature Switzerland AG
The registered company address is: Gewerbestrasse 11, 6330 Cham, Switzerland

To my two beautiful children Maro and George
To all patients in pain
To all authors who contributed to this book

Alaa Abd-Elsayed

Each of the authors of this text sacrificed significant pieces of themselves and their time to create something that will benefit their colleagues and patients. Our families and social networks share in this sacrifice as we spend time away from them seeking to create a product that will resonate and provide substantial clinical benefit. To all those impacted—thank you! Your patience, love, and support remain critical to each of us as we strive to balance clinical, academic, and home responsibilities. Carrie, Cora, Evie, and Rose—this is my opportunity to say thank you and I love you!

Kristopher Schroeder

Preface

Perioperative pain management was, at one time, existed in a real of simplicity that was simultaneously woefully inadequate. Patients were subjected to extensive surgical procedures with scant regard for limiting the size of incisions, and pain management was provided mostly by opioid analgesics. Forward-thinking physicians might consider broadening pain management with acetaminophen or a non-steroidal anti-inflammatory agent but, in many cases, patients remained fasted and these agents were therefore infrequently viable options. Regional anesthesia was practiced by a select group of wizards facile in the palpation of opaque bony or muscular landmarks and reliant on pops, clicks, and subtle changes in resistance to accurately site local anesthetics near a limited number of analgesic targets. Patients subjected to these regimens, frequently required prolonged hospitalizations, and often realized chronic pain that impacted their ability to return to full functional status and enjoy a reasonable quality of life.

In the background, the medical profession was misled and inadvertently harmed itself through prescribing outpatient opioids at alarming rates and manufacturing patients with significant tolerance to those opioid receptor agonists that were the cornerstone of postoperative pain management. Recently, in an effort to mend those patients so negatively impacted by our collective opioid prescribing habits, partial opioid receptor agonists or full antagonists are frequently prescribed and these agents effectively mute the postoperative analgesic efficacy of our traditional opioid stalwarts. Our patients have become frustrated by our lack of success with postoperative analgesia and our healthcare colleagues share in this frustration. Too frequently, patients will be de-humanized and labeled as "chronic painers" by colleagues frustrated and exhausted by our collective failed efforts at managing these patients.

Fortunately, this is a problem that is not without solutions and collaborative efforts to mitigate surgical insults, manage pain, and recognize the patient's critical role in analgesic management have started to move the needle and make an impactful difference in the postoperative recovery of our patients. Our surgeons have worked diligently to limit the scope of their surgical procedures and now laparoscopic and robotic procedures can substantially diminish the extent of surgical wounds and dramatically hasten recovery. In addition, enhanced recovery protocols have ushered in an era of reduced perioperative inflammation and dramatically decreased the impact of surgery on postoperative functional recovery. Even our analgesic armamentarium has been substantially bolstered as we now have intravenous preparations of most drugs and an expanded array of medications that impact pain at a diverse array of receptors. Regional anesthesia, once the domain of the wizard, has been brought down from Mount Olympus, and improvements in ultrasound technology and training have allowed for an expanded pool of healthcare professionals trained to delivery effective regional anesthesia. In addition, these same advancements in ultrasound imaging have ushered in an era of anatomical exploration, and novel analgesic targets have emerged that provide targeted regional anesthesia in areas previously spared by traditional techniques. Finally, the traditional walls between "acute" and "chronic" pain have started to erode as clinicians have increasingly recognized the blurred boundaries between these two practices.

In conjunction with these advances in technology, there has been a collective recognition of the benefits to be realized through collaboration and thoughtful perioperative planning. Anesthesia preoperative clinics, interventional pain physicians, psychiatrist, primary care providers, physical therapists, and surgical team members all play vital roles in ensuring that patients are optimized for surgery and that the patient is an engaged member of the team. The ease of communication and collaboration among these groups has never been more accessible, ensuring that all available analgesic modalities are mobilized for patients facing challenging pain management scenarios.

We are all simultaneously fortunate that the present and near future offer tantalizing options for improved and extended analgesia. Extended-release local anesthetic preparations, cryoneurolysis, and peripheral nerve stimulation are but a few of the technologies and approaches that each of us may soon offer to our patients. Beyond these technologies, an enhanced recognition of the benefits to be realized through collegial collaboration remains an important consideration when treating challenging patients that may offer the promise of improved clinician wellbeing through strengthened supportive networks.

Undoubtedly, this work is challenging and occasionally unrewarding. However, the impact that might be realized through improvements in patient care and a diminished community opioid burden make the effort more than worthwhile.

Madison, USA

Alaa Abd-Elsayed, MD, MBA, MPH, CPE, FASA
Kristopher Schroeder, MD, FASA

Contents

Closing Remarks

Introduction

Perioperative Pain Management-Introduction

David L. Snyder, Girgis Girgis, and Alaa Abd-Elsayed

Abstract A greater understanding of acute and chronic pain is vital to creating a safe and effective perioperative pain management plan for surgical patients. Expedited recovery after surgery (ERAS) protocols aimed at improving perioperatively pain control help facilitate early postoperative ambulation and rehabilitation for patients. This is of great interest to patients who experience less postoperative complications and to hospitals who seek high patient satisfaction scores and shorter length of stay times. The perioperative team has many techniques at their disposal to provide patients with these benefits: medications which target various pain receptors, minimally invasive procedures which utilize image-guidance to maximize effectiveness and reduce risk, and tailored care to address the biopsychosocial profile of the individual patients.

Keywords Perioperative pain · Analgesia · Anesthesiology · Pain management · Regional anesthesia · Opioids · Multimodal pain control · Biopsychosocial pain model

Perioperative pain management is an important aspect of surgical care for healthcare professionals and patients alike. Understanding the pathophysiology, psychosociology and pharmacology of pain is essential to devising an appropriate plan for pain prevention and/or treatment of pain in the perioperative setting. This book aims to comprehensively outline and evaluate the current understanding of perioperative pain and the various tools which the medical community has available to address it.

But first we must examine why effective perioperative pain control matters. Poor perioperative pain control can obviously lead to acute patient suffering but has other important short and long term physiologic and psychological consequences [1]. The

D. L. Snyder · G. Girgis
Pain Management, Cleveland Clinic, Cleveland, OH, USA
e-mail: GirgisG@ccf.org

A. Abd-Elsayed (✉)
Anesthesiology, University of Wisconsin, Madison, WI, USA
e-mail: alaaawny@hotmail.com

A. Abd-Elsayed and K. Schroeder (eds.), *Perioperative Pain Management*,
https://doi.org/10.1007/978-3-031-67648-2_1

postoperative period carries the highest risk of complications as patients recover from surgery. The role that pain plays in increasing that risk and exacerbating those potential problems is becoming better defined. One example of this is the clear benefit seen in patients recovering from joint replacement surgery where anesthetic techniques focused on improved pain management help facilitate early postoperative ambulation and rehabilitation which leads to decreased postoperative complications and shorter length of stay [2].

The clearest example of this is seen with the increased utilization of regional anesthetic techniques. Peripheral nerve, epidural, and spinal blocks are the mainstays of regional anesthesia. Their use can provide better pain control than intravenous narcotics, promote early recovery of bowel function and easier breathing from less splinting due to pain, require less need for systemic pain medications (including opioids) and therefore less systemic adverse effects, and allow for easier and earlier participation in physical therapy [3]. While regional anesthesia techniques come with their own risks, in general they can be implemented safely and effectively in the perioperative arena at hospitals and ambulatory surgery centers, in the emergency department and the intensive care unit. This book will discuss the vast role that regional anesthesia can play in perioperative pain control.

An undeniable fact of medicine is that so many of the driving forces behind what we do are determined by financial feasibility, and perioperative pain management is no exception. Shorter length of stay times are not only important to healthcare facilities but also to patients who are eager to be home with their loved ones to continue their recovery and rehabilitation. Effective perioperative pain management is one of the major facilitators of this and lies at the core of their shared goal of hospitals and patients. Enhanced recovery after surgery (ERAS) protocols have helped to improve perioperative pain management through advanced planning and implementing multimodal analgesia (MMA) leading to shorter length of stay and overall direct and indirect reduction of healthcare cost to the patient and general population [4]. Proper and effective perioperative pain control adds tremendous value to the overall health system.

One cannot talk about pain, especially in the United States, without mentioning opioids and the opioid epidemic. According to the Center for Disease Control (CDC), the deaths related to opioid overdose in the United States was the highest in history in 2021, with more than 80,000 deaths attributed [5]. Our role in in this cannot be ignored; when we dive deeper into the statistics, we find that prescription opioid-involved death rates continue to rise (increased 17% from 2019 to 2020) [6]. Even though care is shifting away from indiscriminate opioid prescribing for postoperative pain as part of a larger movement towards more restrictive opioid distribution, this book will delve into various opioids and their safe utility in the perioperative setting [7]. Furthermore, this book will elucidate various perioperative pain control techniques that can help decrease opioid consumption as part of a movement towards more responsible opioid stewardship in anesthesiology and the larger medical community [8].

Patient satisfaction after surgery is largely determined by the effectiveness of their pain management. A review of studies looking at patient satisfaction ubiquitously site pain as a significant factor in a patient's interpretation of the quality of care they receive [9]. Furthermore, the perception of showing concern for patient's pain by physicians and nurses was associated with greater patient satisfaction [10]. At the heart of managing emotional and physical symptoms in the perioperative setting is acknowledging and addressing pain effectively. We will discuss how to best manage pain in the perioperative setting to maximize effectiveness and therefore patient satisfaction.

The following chapters will examine the various mechanisms of pain including the transition from acute to chronic pain, as well as the various influences on pain including genetics and patient history. As mentioned above, we delve into the controversial topic of opioids and the role they play in perioperative setting with specific attention to pharmacology and clinical application of specific opioids. We also aim to highlight non-opioid, systemic pain medications as well as more advanced, interventional techniques and technologies such as regional anesthesia, catheters, stimulators, and ablations. As a result of the above, we wish to dissect the role of the inpatient pain service as leaders on the perioperative team in the clinic, post-anesthesia care unit, and wards. This book will also look at the various populations and their distinct pain considerations including LGBTQIA, prisoners, children, patients with sickle cell disease, non-English speakers, critical care patients in the intensive care unit, patients with significant psychiatric disease, patients with history of substance abuse, and patients who are terminally ill and/or are on the palliative care service. We will also give attention to specific surgical subspecialties because patients who undergo spine, cardiac, breast, or obstetric and gynecologic surgeries have distinct needs. Finally, we will look ahead in perioperative pain to give our analysis on what perioperative pain management may look like in the near future.

References

1. Peters ML, Sommer M, van Kleef M, Marcus MA. Predictors of physical and emotional recovery 6 and 12 months after surgery. Br J Surg. 2010;97(10):1518–27. https://doi.org/10.1002/bjs.7152. PMID: 20737463.
2. Zhu S, Qian W, Jiang C, Ye C, Chen X. Enhanced recovery after surgery for hip and knee arthroplasty: a systematic review and meta-analysis. Postgrad Med J. 2017;93(1106):736–42. https://doi.org/10.1136/postgradmedj-2017-134991.
3. American Society of Regional Anesthesia (ASRA)—Risks and benefits of regional anesthesia. https://www.asra.com/patient-information/regional-anesthesia/risks-and-benefits. Accessed 15 April 2023.
4. Dong Y, Zhang Y, Jin C. Comprehensive economic evaluation of enhanced recovery after surgery in hepatectomy. Int J Equity Health. 2021;20(1):245. https://doi.org/10.1186/s12939-021-01583-3.
5. CDC—National Center for Health Statistics, U.S. Overdose Deaths In 2021 Increased Half as Much as in 2020 – But Are Still Up 15%. https://www.cdc.gov/nchs/pressroom/nchs_press_releases/2022/202205.htm. Accessed 20 March 2023.

6. CDC—Injury prevention and control, understanding the opioid overdose epidemic. https://www.cdc.gov/opioids/basics/epidemic.html. Accessed 20 March 2023.
7. Klueh MP, Sloss KR, Dossett LA, Englesbe MJ, Waljee JF, Brummett CM, Lagisetty PA, Lee JS. Postoperative opioid prescribing is not my job: A qualitative analysis of care transitions. Surgery. 2019;166(5):744–751. https://doi.org/10.1016/j.surg.2019.05.033. Epub 2019 Jul 11. PMID: 31303324; PMCID: PMC7068723.
8. Hyland SJ, Brockhaus KK, Vincent WR, Spence NZ, Lucki MM, Howkins MJ, Cleary RK. Perioperative pain management and opioid stewardship: a practical guide. Healthcare (Basel). 2021;9(3):333. https://doi.org/10.3390/healthcare9030333.
9. Trinh LN, Fortier MA, Kain ZN. Primer on adult patient satisfaction in perioperative settings. Perioper Med (Lond). 2019;8:11. https://doi.org/10.1186/s13741-019-0122-2.
10. Jamison RN, Ross MJ, Hoopman P, Griffin F, Levy J, Daly M, Schaffer JL. Assessment of postoperative pain management: patient satisfaction and perceived helpfulness. Clin J Pain. 1997;13(3):229–36. https://doi.org/10.1097/00002508-199709000-00008.

Foundations

General Principles of Perioperative Pain Management

Tyler Speaks, Margeaux Epner, Sandra Chavez-Carmona, James Kim, and Anthony T. Machi

Abstract Perioperative pain management is founded on the science and understanding of acute pain. The analgesic process begins with a preoperative evaluation that focuses on screening and making strategic assessments to individualize pain therapy. This information is inserted into a multimodal analgesia framework, with or without the aid of standardized protocols, such as Enhanced Recovery Protocols, and used as a basis to inform and educate patients on planned therapeutics and expected analgesic outcomes. The framework is then utilized to craft a pain management strategy that is patient and pain mechanism-specific and employs pharmacologic therapies, nonpharmacologic therapies, and interventional therapies that mitigate pain and the physiologic stresses of surgery. Frequent assessment and reassessment are used to fine-tune therapy and assist the patient in mitigating pain and helping them progress along their goals for functional recovery.

Keywords Perioperative pain management · Pain pathway · Pain assessment · Multimodal analgesia · Enhanced Recovery after Surgery (ERAS) · Interventional acute pain management · Regional analgesia

---

T. Speaks · M. Epner · S. Chavez-Carmona · J. Kim · A. T. Machi (✉)
Anesthesiology and Pain Management, University of Texas Southwestern, Dallas, TX, USA
e-mail: anthony.machi@utsouthwestern.edu

T. Speaks
e-mail: tyler.speaks@utsouthwestern.edu

M. Epner
e-mail: margeaux.epner@utsouthwestern.edu

S. Chavez-Carmona
e-mail: sandra.chavez-carmona@utsouthwestern.edu

J. Kim
e-mail: james.kim2@utsouthwestern.edu

A. Abd-Elsayed and K. Schroeder (eds.), *Perioperative Pain Management*,
https://doi.org/10.1007/978-3-031-67648-2_2

1 Introduction

Descriptions of perioperative pain management can be traced as far back as ancient Egyptian civilizations [1]. The ancient Greeks advanced the theories of perioperative pain management with basic ideas of the nervous system, sensory experience and perception of pain. Over the ensuing millennia, modest, incremental advances were made with the discovery of analgesic medications, such as opium, therapeutic modalities, such as heat and cold applications, and even electricity via the electrogenic torpedo fish. Nonetheless, perioperative analgesia remained rudimentary until the Scientific Revolution of the eighteenth and nineteenth centuries heralded new theories, techniques, tools, and medications that modernized the practice of pain management into a field recognizable as today's practices. A key step was the development of the specificity theory proposed by Descartes and refined by Schiff in 1858, which postulated a basic concept of pain pathways [1]. Further work by Bliz, Goldschieder and von Frey in the late nineteenth century distinguished fundamental aspects of the nervous system including separate receptors for pain, touch, warmth and cold. This may be viewed as the nascent basis for the development of multimodal analgesia.

The nineteenth century witnessed two key areas for development of perioperative analgesia: the discovery of applications and techniques for local anesthetics and harnessing the powers of opioids. The next 100 years would see perioperative pain management focus largely on those two aspects. The many great wars of the nineteenth and twentieth centuries, and in particular World War I and II, provided stimulus for further developments due to the magnitude of traumas, ensuing surgeries, and exigencies of war. For the use of local anesthetics, development of three key features were necessary for clinical use: the syringe, the needle, and a local anesthetic drug. The oldest of these three is the local anesthetic drug, the first being cocaine. Derived from the plant Erythroxylum coca, which was known to the peoples of Central and South America for thousands of years, it was first recognized for its pain relieving properties by a Westerner and Jesuit priest, Bernabé Cobo in 1653 [2]. Its medicinal application was limited until the mid-nineteenth century when incremental improvements were made toward creating a hollow bore needle, connecting that needle to a syringe for medicinal application, and isolating the cocaine alkaloid from the coca plant [3]. However, it was not until the Viennese ophthalmologist, Karl Koller, discovered the utility of cocaine as a topical local anesthetic in 1884 that Western medicine found a substrate to utilize for regional anesthesia. Soon thereafter, various physicians broadened the application of local anesthesia to local infiltration, neuraxial blockade, and peripheral nerve blockade. The various toxicities and limitations of cocaine were also recognized, and chemists embarked on identifying and creating novel chemicals to serve as local anesthetics that would be safer and have more desirable characteristics of faster onset, longer duration, and specificity of neuronal blockade.

In parallel to the development of local anesthetics, the history of opioids dates to ancient civilizations with some of the earliest reference to medicinal properties of opioids associated with ancient Sumeria at the end of the third millennia BCE [4]. In the ensuing centuries, opium spread across civilizations and throughout the world. It was used as an analgesic, particularly in Arabic, Indian and Chinese medicinal traditions, and it was also used as a drug of abuse, notably in China in the seventeenth and eighteenth centuries. However, specific reference to perioperative application remained sparse. In 1806, morphine was isolated by Sertürner, and codeine was identified a few years later [4]. Like local anesthetics, medicinal use remained limited by the ability to deliver it until the mid-nineteenth century with the invention of the hollow bore needle and glass syringe. From there, perioperative usage developed, and investigators sought to develop opioids with greater potency and safety profiles. In the process, thebaine and the semi-synthetic opioids hydrocodone, hydromorphone, oxycodone, and diacetylmorphine (heroin) were identified. The constraint of opium supply due to World War II spurred on the development of synthetic opioids, such as meperidine and methadone [5, 6].

Despite the developments of new medications and refined methods of delivery, the strategy of perioperative analgesia centering around local anesthetic administration and opioids remained unchanged until the second half of the twentieth century. During this time, many investigations were conducted regarding the mechanisms of analgesia related to local anesthetics, opioids, other medications, and techniques. A seminal event in pain management history occurred in 1965 when Melzack and Wall developed and published the gate control theory which related the impact of ascending and descending modulation systems on neural impulse propagation, providing a marked impact on the understanding of pain mechanisms. While initially most impactful in the realm of chronic pain management in the immediate decades, the concept began to find new application in the perioperative setting in the twenty-first century. Also in the second half of the twentieth century, the investigations in the mechanisms of pain and pain pathways led to the conceptual framework of multimodal analgesia by the Danish surgeon Henrik Kehlet [7]. This approach refers to the use of more than one analgesic medicine or technique to leverage additive or synergistic analgesic effects while minimizing adverse effects. It is with this background that we apply a current theory for perioperative pain management.

2 Contemporary Principles of Perioperative Pain Management

The analgesic process begins with a preoperative evaluation that defines the individual's pain experience and conducts a strategic assessment while considering the following questions:

1. How much pain is anticipated from the surgery? What is the expected duration of pain? What is the location of pain?
2. What are the specific post-operative functional goals to facilitate?

3. How is the pain anticipated to affect the patient, and what physiologic challenges may arise directly or indirectly because of it?
4. Will the patient be ambulatory or hospitalized following surgery?
5. Can regional anesthesia be utilized?
6. Does the patient have specific baseline pain modifying considerations, such as:
    a. Advanced age
    b. Mental health disorder: anxiety, depression, substance use, PTSD
    c. History of pain: chronic, neuropathic, nociplastic
    d. Opioid tolerance or central sensitization
    e. Pain catastrophizing
7. Are there any contraindications to any specific treatments or techniques? [8–10].

Following the initial evaluation, education should be provided to the patient and caregivers regarding goals of care, treatment options and coordination made with the anesthesia professional or team, surgeon, and any consultants, if necessary. Analgesic elements then begin prior to surgery with multimodal analgesia delivered via oral medication and regional analgesia, continued intraoperatively with intravenous medications and the application of local anesthetics via local infiltration, peripheral blockade or neuraxial blockade and continued in the postoperative period with multimodal analgesia by all suitable means to provide the most comfort while incurring the least side effects and permitting the patient to engage in rehabilitation as soon as possible. Newer long-lasting analgesic modalities, such as cryoneurolysis or percutaneous peripheral nerve stimulation, may play important roles for longer duration perioperative pain management in the future. Throughout the treatment period, validated tools for assessment should be utilized and documented to track responses to treatment and guide when adjustment of the regimen is necessary in relation to adequacy of relief.

The cornerstones of this approach are the rational selection of pharmacological agents and the strategic use of peripheral and central neural blockade. Because perioperative pain results from a variety of mechanisms, including nociception, inflammation, nerve injury, peripheral and central sensitization, transcriptional and post-transcriptional dysregulation, augmented facilitation, structural organization and disinhibition, multimodal analgesia provides an approach capable of addressing these distinct analgesic requirements of the perioperative patient [11, 12]. Specific medications and techniques that are recommended will be reviewed.

3 Types of Pain

The current International Association for the Study of Pain (IASP) definition of pain is "an unpleasant sensory and emotional experience associated with, or resembling that associated with, actual or potential tissue damage" [13]. According to the American Society of Anesthesiologists, acute pain in the perioperative setting is defined as pain that is "present in a surgical patient after a procedure" and is "the result of trauma from the procedure or procedure related complications" [14]. Acute pain occurs when an insult to tissue causes nociceptive neuronal firing in peripheral nerves that is transmitted to the dorsal horn of the spinal cord and up to the brain. The trauma leads to a local inflammatory response and release of immune cell mediators. Recurrent release of these mediators typically resolves within days to weeks. Pain, especially in the perioperative period, is coupled with a stress response. The stress response to pain, when combined with the stress response from surgery itself, can further promote the proinflammatory state, decrease the immune response, and predispose the patient to a higher risk of chronic pain after surgery. Several patient and surgical factors increase the risk of developing chronic pain, and it is imperative that perioperative pain be treated adequately to minimize this evolution.

Chronic pain has been described as pain that persists beyond the normal expected time of healing [15]. According to the American Society of Anesthesiologists, "Chronic pain is defined as pain of any etiology not directly related to neoplastic involvement, associated with a chronic medical condition or extending in duration beyond the expected temporal boundary of tissue injury and normal healing, and adversely affecting the function or well-being of the individual" [14]. In the perioperative period, acute post-operative pain may persist, and it is described as chronic postsurgical pain (CPSP) if it is specifically a pain that has developed or increased in intensity after a surgical procedure or tissue injury and persists beyond the healing process beyond 3 months from the time of surgery [16]. The incidence of CPSP varies greatly depending on the type of surgery (5–85%) with many studies indicating 10–20% of all patients who undergo surgery will have persistent chronic pain that limits functionality after surgery [17].

Chronic postsurgical pain is frequently associated with effects on mood and sleep, often causing disruption to quality of life. Mood disorders (i.e., anxiety, depression, and PTSD) and poor social support, which are frequently associated with chronic pain, predispose individuals to developing chronic pain. Several predictive factors of developing chronic pain can be used to identify higher risk individuals to prevent CPSP. These risk factors include younger adults, high BMI, lower educational level, smokers, more medical comorbidities, prior disability, longer surgery time, more surgical complications, depression, and anxiety [18]. Additionally, specific surgeries are more frequently associated with post-operative chronic pain, and these include amputation, thoracotomy, and mastectomy [17].

Several animal models have been used to hypothesize the mechanisms by which chronic pain changes our central nervous system. Acute injury and chronic inflammation are thought to cause changes in gene expression in the spinal cord and cerebral cortex. This tissue damage and inflammation can form pathological changes to the peripheral and central nervous system, resulting in nociceptive hypersensitivity [19]. Neuronal changes and remodeling can lead to sensitization, which can progress to hyperalgesia and allodynia [20]. In time, gene expression plays a role in spinal and supraspinal areas which are distant from the initial inciting lesion [19]. Beyond changes in primary DNA sequencing, there is evidence of the roles of DNA methylation, histone modification, and expression of mRNAs in the continuation of pain.

In contrast to postsurgical pain, neuropathic pain is that which stems from pathology of the nervous system itself [21]. Neuropathic pain is one of the leading causes of chronic pain across the world and is only becoming increasingly prevalent. Approximately 15–25% of chronic pain is neuropathic [22]. Diabetes (diabetic neuropathy), infection (herpes zoster), nerve compression, nerve trauma, and autoimmune disease (multiple sclerosis) are some examples of different types of neuropathic pain. Compared with nociceptive pain, neuropathic pain is typically associated with more numbness, allodynia, and neurological findings. Neuropathic pain is often described as shooting and tingling, whereas nociceptive pain is more commonly described as aching, stabbing, and throbbing. In the perioperative period, neuropathic pain is important to consider for pain management. Preoperative neuropathic pain can lead to worse pain in the post-operative period through central sensitization [23–25]. CPSP commonly manifests from neuropathic pain either worsened by or originating from the surgery. Intraoperative nerve damage or impaired pain modulation may lead to chronic neuropathic pain. Management and prevention of CPSP involves perioperative prophylactic strategies and the adequate treatment of chronic neuropathic pain [26].

4 Neurophysiology of Pain

In order to manage perioperative pain, a basic understanding of the pain system is necessary. Pain has four major elements of signal processing: transduction, transmission, modulation, and perception [27]. The pathway starts at the peripheral nociceptive receptors located throughout the body and terminates at the cerebral somatosensory cortex. Each element provides an avenue to intervene on the pain signal, and therefore, an opportunity to modify the pain experience.

5 Transduction

Transduction refers to the activation of primary afferent nociceptive receptors by mechanical (e.g., pressure, stretching), chemical (e.g., prostaglandins, histamine), or thermal stimuli [27]. When activated by a noxious stimulus, nociceptors generate electrical impulses that travel via the peripheral nerves to the spinal cord and then ascend to the brain. Nociceptors are found throughout the body, including the skin, muscles, joints, and internal organs. There are no nociceptors found in the CNS [28, 29].

Nociceptors are comprised of two major classes of afferent free nerve endings: Aδ fibers and c-fibers [30]. Aδ fibers are medium diameter, thinly myelinated afferents that transmit acute, well-localized, fast pain signals. Aδ fibers play an important role in alerting the body of impending tissue damage and in initiating protective reflexes, such as withdrawal from noxious stimuli. In contrast to Aδ fibers, c-fibers are smaller diameter, unmyelinated afferents that are responsible for dull, poorly localized, slow pain signals. A common example of these nociceptors is displayed by a stubbed toe which leads to an initial, sharp pain transmitted by Aδ fibers, followed by a dull, throbbing pain elicited by c-fiber nerve endings.

By targeting the first step of pain processing—activation of mechanical, thermal, and chemical stimuli—pain can be inhibited or modified. For example, there are several factors released from damaged tissues that activate nociceptors and initiate the pain signaling process. Extreme temperature, force and tissue destruction activate nociceptors directly and indirectly via inflammatory chemicals such as prostaglandins, histamine, bradykinin, and substance-P [30]. NSAID's, such as ibuprofen or naproxen, block the production of prostaglandins, thereby providing a means to inhibit transduction and reduce pain.

6 Transmission

Once nociceptors are activated by noxious stimuli and an action potential is generated, the impulse is transmitted from the periphery to the central nervous system through first, second and third-order neurons [27]. The first-order neuron starts with transduction at nociceptors and ends with a synapse at the dorsal horn of the spinal cord. The second-order neuron begins at the dorsal horn and ends at the thalamus. Finally, the third-order neuron travels from the thalamus to the somatosensory cortex. This process involves interplay between the nervous system, neurotransmitters and other signaling molecules.

The ability to generate action potentials underlies the pain signal pathway. Noxious stimuli activate nociceptors causing voltage-gated sodium channels to open which lead to an influx of sodium that is then propagated along the nerve [31]. Local anesthetics block nerve impulse transmission by blocking voltage-gated sodium channels. Regional blocks are an invaluable tool to manage perioperative pain in the setting of a wide variety of surgeries.

7 Modulation

Modulation involves the alteration of afferent pain propagation along the neural pathway [27, 31]. The dorsal horn of the spinal cord is the site where many receptors, such as NMDA and neurokinin, affect action potential propagation. Many inhibitory neurotransmitters, including endorphins, glycine, and GABA, work at these sites [11]. In contrast, augmentation of pain can also result via neurotransmitters like glutamate, substance-P, calcitonin gene-related peptide, and aspartate [31]. Additionally, the modulation process can lead to neuroplasticity resulting in hyperalgesia, making subsequent pain more difficult to manage.

8 Perception

The culmination of the pain propagation system is the integration of signals from the somatosensory and limbic cortices to produce pain perception [32].This is how the brain interprets and responds to signals indicating tissue injury or potential harm. Pain is both a sensory and emotional experience. Emotional factors, such as previous experiences, anxiety, and fear, all play a role in the perception of pain.

There are many ways to target the perception of pain in the perioperative setting, and pain is a result of intricate peripheral and central processes. By understanding how pain signals are transmitted and processed, clinicians may select from among the available tools to administer effective perioperative pain management.

9 Pain Assessment

Reliable assessments of pain are essential for perioperative pain management. Pain is a multi-dimensional subjective experience dictated by the character and intensity of the pain, the patient's emotional state, and many other variables. These factors make it difficult to measure pain objectively. Patient self-report using their own pain vocabulary, when cognitively and physically able, is the best way to measure changes in pain character and intensity over time [33]. Self-reporting scales are useful in simplifying and standardizing pain data. The Numerical Rating Scale (NRS) and Visual Analog Scale (VAS) are viewed as the gold standard methods for assessing pain; however, there are other pain assessment scales that incorporate non-verbal cues when a patient is unable to self-report [34]. These include the Adult Non-Verbal Pain Scale (NVPS), Behavioral Pain Scale (BPS), and Pain Assessment in Advanced Dementia Scale (PAINAD), among others. Overall, these tools are best for measuring changes in acute pain and are less helpful for measuring pain in absolute terms or in comparing the pain for two different individuals' experiences.

The NRS and VAS scales focus on pain intensity, as intensity is typically the distinguishing dimension of acute pain for acute treatment. In the NRS assessment, patients are asked to choose a number between 0 (no pain) and 10 (worst possible pain) [35]. It is a simple and quick tool that can easily be administered verbally, over the phone or through surveys. The VAS is similar but consists of a straight line upon which a scale is constructed ranging from 0 to 100 and which can be marked anywhere along its continuous spectrum. In one study, NRS, VAS, and Brief Pain Inventory (BPI-PS) were compared, and the results did not show a significant difference in validity or effectiveness among the three scales [36]. Similarly, another study showed that there was no significant difference between the reliability of the VAS and NRS

[37]. Overall, these self-reporting scales are reliable and interchangeable; however, they lack objectivity and are still poor measurements of pain.

Two of the most widely used pain scales for patients who are unable to self-report pain are the Adult Non-Verbal Pain Scale (NVPS) and the Behavioral Pain Scale (BPS). These tools, along with all the other non-verbal pain assessment tools, are useful for patients with dementia, who are non-verbal, or who have intellectual impairment. The BPS assesses critically-ill patients who are sedated and intubated. Patients are given a score which is comprised of the sum of 3 categories: Facial Expressions, Movements of Upper Limbs, and Compliance with Mechanical Ventilation. The NVPS consists of five categories scored 0–2: Facial expression, Activity level, Guarding, Physiology (vital signs), and Respiratory status [38]. Unfortunately, none of these non-verbal pain assessment scales are particularly reliable. It can be nearly impossible to distinguish between pain and emotional distress or determine a patient's pain intensity. The inability for us to objectively measure pain, especially in those who are unable to self-report, can often lead to undertreatment of pain.

10 Treatment of Perioperative Pain

An individual's experience of pain is a complex and subjective issue, which has physical, emotional, and existential implications. A physician's understanding of pain must incorporate an understanding of the physiological origin of the sensation, and a method of assessing and anticipating an individual's need for pain treatment. The final common pathway, however, lies in the treatment of pain. Improper treatment of perioperative pain can lead to poor patient satisfaction and chronic pain, as well as numerous objective complications such as delayed mobility and cardiopulmonary morbidity [39–41]. The aim of this section is to briefly introduce several common, contemporary methods for the treatment of perioperative pain, and how their use can assist the physician and patient as part of a broader pain control toolbox that can be adjusted for an individual and procedure-specific clinical situation.

11 Local Anesthetics

Local anesthetics are a class of drugs that reversibly block voltage-gated sodium ion channels in nerves, reducing the transmission of an action potential [42]. Local anesthetics have a long and diverse history in anesthesia and pain management, and the permutations of their application regarding site, injection technique, drug choice, dose and use of adjuncts are vast. Depending on the nerves blocked by the local anesthetic, the effect may be the elimination of painful sensation, temperature, touch, or motor blockade. These drugs are often administered directly at the surgical site, surrounding peripheral nerves or nerve plexuses of the upper and lower extremities, in fascial planes where nerves travel, or the epidural and intrathecal spaces. The utility of local anesthesia is that it provides safe, exquisite pain control, and can serve as a sole anesthetic, adjunct to general anesthesia, or be used for post-operative pain control.

Intravenous (IV) administration of lidocaine in the perioperative period is the only common non-regional analgesia use of a local anesthetic to reduce surgical pain [43]. Evidence from meta-analysis suggests it yields a small reduction in pain scores in the immediate postoperative period, and its use may be more beneficial as an intraoperative adjunct in large abdominal and spine surgeries, particularly in patients who are not candidates for neuraxial anesthesia [44, 45].

Local and regional analgesia involve injection of local anesthetic at the surgical site, or along the afferent pathway of pain transmission, which can involve a single peripheral nerve, fascial planes containing peripheral nerves, a nerve plexus, or near nerve roots exiting the spinal cord. Injection can be performed as a single injection or placement of an indwelling catheter. Regional analgesia has become a mainstay of multimodal and opioid-sparing perioperative pain control [8, 46, 47]. The diverse individual applications are beyond the scope of this section, but a large body of evidence suggests safety and efficacy behind techniques used for pain management in orthopedic, thoracic, and large abdominal surgeries [48, 49]. In addition to superior pain control compared to IV pharmacotherapy alone, regional blocks lead to a reduction in postoperative opioid use, reduced pulmonary complications, earlier discharge, and may decrease the risk of postoperative cognitive decline. Thus, in addition to their role as an adjunct to multimodal pain management, they may serve as a useful option for providing anesthesia in patients too fragile to undergo general anesthesia [50–53]. Local anesthetic is also commonly deposited into the epidural and/or intrathecal space for perioperative pain control. Epidural analgesia is a cornerstone technique for analgesia in major open surgeries of the chest, abdomen and pelvis associated with severe pain, with evidence showing epidurals are associated with superior pain control over systemic opioid administration alone [49, 54–56]. Aside from reduced opioid use, benefits include reduced cardiac and pulmonary complications and decreased ileus.

12 Non-opioid Pharmacologic Therapies

Multiple physiologic mechanisms and receptors are responsible for the production and processing of surgical pain phenomena. Thus, it makes sense that targeting multiple receptors with different analgesics will be more effective than monotherapy. This is the basis for multimodal analgesia, wherein more than one pharmacologic class of analgesic targets different receptors in order to improve analgesia and reduce class-specific side effects [7]. Several common drugs and their role in the perioperative pain regimen are introduced below.

Acetaminophen is a common and effective first-line analgesic. It is safe, affordable, widely available, and often used to treat mild to moderate pain and fever [8, 57, 58]. Acetaminophen in the perioperative setting is commonly used preoperatively in the oral form, as well as intravenously in patients not tolerating oral medication. Acetaminophen is most useful as a scheduled analgesic, in combination with other drugs such as nonsteroidal anti-inflammatory drugs, where it has a synergistic and opioid sparing effect [59, 60].

Nonsteroidal anti-inflammatory drugs (NSAIDs) are a diverse group of medications that exert analgesic and anti-inflammatory effects through inhibition of the COX-1 and COX-2 enzymes. Like acetaminophen, these drugs are affordable, and available in multiple formulations. Their role in perioperative pain treatment has been widely studied. They are effective for treating pain, reducing pain with movement and are most effective when scheduled [61–63]. Providers must be aware of potential side effects such as platelet inhibition, renal impairment and additional risks when used for prolonged periods of time.

Glucocorticoids are another widely used class of drugs that decrease inflammation. They are frequently used in the perioperative setting to decrease nausea and vomiting, but there is also evidence that suggests a marked reduction in pain by decreasing the inflammatory response to surgery [64, 65]. Single dose intravenous dexamethasone is an effective component of an analgesic regimen, but providers must always be aware of the potential side effects of increased blood glucose levels, fluid retention, mood changes and other side effects if given more frequently [66].

Ketamine is a NMDA receptor antagonist with actions at numerous additional sites involved in transmission and processing of painful stimuli. Depending on the dose, ketamine is used as a dissociative anesthetic, an anesthetic adjunct, or in anti-nociceptive pain therapy [67]. Research suggests improved analgesia and decreased opioid consumption with perioperative ketamine administration in certain patient populations. Ketamine is particularly useful in opioid-tolerant patients to reduce hyperalgesia by decreasing neuronal excitability and the transmission of pain impulses [68].

Gabapentin and pregabalin are structurally related to the neurotransmitter γ-aminobutyric acid and are commonly used anticonvulsants that modulate voltage-gated calcium channels in the central nervous system [69]. Gabapentinoids are often used for treatment of neuropathic pain, and much recent work has been devoted to understanding their role in acute perioperative pain. Studies suggest a modest reduction in pain scores and opioid-sparing effects in specific populations, though use must be balanced against common side effects of dizziness, sedation and potentiation of respiratory depression [70]. Due to these side effects, perioperative use should be limited to patients and scenarios at risk for the effects of neuropathic pain [71].

Dexmedetomidine is a selective α_2 receptor agonist that is used in the perioperative and intensive care setting for sedation, and as an anesthetic adjunct. Some evidence supports dexmedetomidine as a modest analgesic adjunct that reduces pain scores and has opioid-sparing effects [72, 73]. Despite a lack of respiratory depression, it must be administered with caution due to the sedating effects, as well as hypotension and bradycardia.

Magnesium is a common intracellular ion that also acts as a NMDA antagonist. A meta-analysis suggested a modest pain-reduction and opioid-sparing effect from magnesium administration, though further research is needed to determine optimal timing and dosage for its use in the perioperative setting [74].

13 Opioid and Opiate Therapies

Opioids and their synthetic derivatives have a long and well-studied history in the treatment of pain. Long-considered the standard for pain management due to their effectiveness in relieving acute pain, their central role is now under increasing scrutiny due to the numerous harmful side-effects and the ineffectiveness of a unilateral approach [75, 76]. Opioid receptors are g-protein coupled receptors that are diffusely present throughout the nervous system and body, thus the effects from these drugs are widespread [77]. The most dangerous is respiratory depression, but the most common are nausea, pruritis and constipation [78]. In addition to physiologic side effects, opioids rapidly produce tolerance and can lead to dependence, which is a growing international concern [79, 80].

Opioids are administered in a variety of ways, but the most common perioperative routes are oral, intravenous, and neuraxial, with short, intermediate, and long-acting variations available [81]. Fentanyl, morphine and hydromorphone are administered IV in the operating and recovery rooms, with transition to longer acting oral medication when appropriate. Patient controlled analgesia (PCA) allows the conscious patient to self-bolus medication, resulting in improved patient satisfaction and decreased nursing demand, but with no reduction in total opioid use or hospital length of stay [82]. Despite their powerful role in suppressing acute pain, it is recognized that opioids should be used at the minimum effective dose for the shortest duration possible [83].

14 Non-pharmacologic Therapies

Pharmacologic agents and regional anesthetic techniques are the backbone of perioperative pain management, but the practitioner should be aware of the physical and behavioral interventions that may also be helpful. These techniques can assist with specific scenarios, though evidence is generally weak and still emerging [8]. Transcutaneous electrical nerve stimulation (TENS) involves generation of non-painful electrical current across the skin that activates a neural inhibitory network, causing analgesia [84, 85]. The use of acupuncture for pain management is on the rise, but requires a highly experienced practitioner [86–88]. Modulation of central processing and the subjective nature of pain is the goal of behavioral and psychological interventions. Cognitive-behavioral therapy and biofeedback may adjust the central perception of pain, increase a patient's ability to deal with pain, and improve patient coping [89, 90].

15 Treatment Summary

The most effective management of perioperative pain involves patient and surgery specific targeting of the diverse mechanisms and receptors involved in producing painful stimulations. The above therapies are most beneficial as part of a large toolbox used by the perioperative physician to improve patient comfort while minimizing pharmacologic side effects [12]. Further sections will address these and additional treatment modalities and their supporting evidence in greater detail.

16 Role of Pain Management in ERAS

The primary goals of an enhanced recovery protocol are to achieve the highest quality results and fastest recovery for patients after surgery to lead them to optimal health outcomes. Optimal perioperative pain management is a fundamental feature of enhanced recovery protocols. The idea for Enhanced Recovery After Surgery® was developed by a group of academic surgeons in Europe in 2001 who aimed to shift the focus of recovery from a singular goal of speed popularized by "fast-track surgery" in the 1990s to quality of recovery [91]. The enhanced recovery concepts leveraged multi-disciplinary teamwork, evidence-based guidelines and continuous cycles of audit and refinement [92–94]. From the outset the group aimed to modify the endocrine and metabolic response by addressing nutrition, inflammation, protein metabolism and analgesia, while also revealing to the surgical community how complete perioperative care rather than surgical technique alone determined post-surgical outcomes [95]. The group formed the ERAS Society in 2010, and they published the first protocols addressing colorectal surgery and pancreaticoduodenectomy in 2012. Their ideas spread to many other types of surgery and led to the creation of protocols both by society members and by other professionals [96–100]. As the groups developed comprehensive protocols to achieve these goals, optimizing analgesia featured prominently.

While published protocols such as those developed by the ERAS Society are a good starting point, forming a pathway involves many components beyond the concerns of pain management [101, 102]. The first step is forming a multidisciplinary team that includes surgeons, anesthesiologists, nurses, and may include other stakeholders, such as physical therapists, occupational therapists and care coordinators. This team will then set goals and priorities, review existing evidence-based guidelines and literature, identify concerns for design and implementation and identify existing resources. The next step is creating a pathway that is service and institution specific that meets the core tenets of enhanced recovery protocols, including comprehensive analgesia, the return to homeostasis, early mobilization, restoration of postoperative alimentation and early discharge from the hospital. Following this, support must be garnered from leadership and additional stakeholders and users must be educated. The protocol and corresponding pathway may then be implemented for patient care and systems created to collect data, audit, and analyze protocol elements and patient outcomes. Data collection and cyclical review and revision are crucial to the success of enhanced recovery programs.

17 Emerging Therapies

New and emerging therapies create opportunities to optimize perioperative analgesia. There are two broad areas of novelty to enhance perioperative analgesia. The first are therapies that target specific nerves to achieve a longer duration of analgesia compared to single injection or continuous perineural blocks using local anesthetics, such as peripheral nerve stimulation and cryoneurolysis. The second are various emerging pharmacologic agents that improve on existing drugs, such as opioids with potentially less adverse effects (Oliceridine), TRPV1 agonists with potentially more favorable pharmacokinetics than capsaicin, extended-release local anesthetic formulations (bupivacaine/meloxicam, SABER-Bupivacaine, INL-001), and adjuvants that may increase the duration of action of local anesthetics (tetrodotoxin and neosaxitoxin).

18 Peripheral Nerve Stimulation

Peripheral nerve stimulation (PNS) is an emerging field in adjunctive perioperative analgesic therapies [103]. As a temporary but semi-long duration analgesic technique, PNS may serve as a useful modality in both acute and chronic pain management. The approach to the targeted nerves is like that of peripheral nerve blocks, which allows for PNS placement in any location commonly used for peripheral nerve blocks [104]. Ideally, the PNS lead should be placed at a slight distance to a nerve (0.5–1.5 cm), which allows for optimal selective fiber stimulation, and studies have shown that many nerves are acceptable targets, including the femoral nerve, sciatic nerve, sural nerve, peroneal nerve, tibial nerve, brachial plexus, suprascapular nerve, radial nerve, median nerve, ulnar nerve, greater occipital nerve and medial branch nerves of the dorsal rami of the lumbar spine [104–106].

The most widely accepted theory to explain the analgesic effects of PNS is Melzack and Wall's "gate control theory" [107]. These two authors described in 1965 how exposing large, myelinated, afferent peripheral nerve fibers to an electrical current results in pain signal conduction impedance within the spinal cord of small-diameter pain fibers. Shortly after, they hypothesized that stimulating primary afferent neurons could produce analgesia, eventually leading to the off-label use of commercially available stimulators for peripheral nerves [103]. The clinical application of PNS remained limited until the last ten years when PNS specific devices were designed to improve their utility and function. PNS also activates and modulates the central nervous system at subcortical and cortical areas in ways that may impact the processing of pain [108].

There is a wide range of indications for PNS, namely conditions resulting in pain in the distribution of a single nerve or single group of nerves [109]. There are very few contraindications for PNS. Absolute contraindications include allergy to any component of the stimulator and patient refusal, while relative contraindications include coagulopathy and local infection near the access site. Placing a PNS involves using sterile technique and an ultrasound machine. Like a peripheral nerve block, the targeted nerve is identified using ultrasound-guidance, and a monopolar needle is inserted roughly 0.5–1.5 cm from the nerve. An electrical stimulator is attached to the needle to deliver a test stimulation with the goal of localized stimulation without muscle contractions or discomfort. Uncomfortable local sensations may be due to superficial needle placement, while muscle contractions or distal extremity discomfort may be due to deep needle placement. Once localized stimulation without muscle contractions or discomfort is achieved, the monopolar needle is withdrawn, and the stimulator lead is placed through the introducer needle in the same location. The introducer needle is then withdrawn, the lead is attached to a stimulator, and the surface electrode is placed on the ipsilateral limb. Appropriate lead placement results in comfortable sensations in the desired dermatomal distribution without muscle contractions. Once proper lead placement is confirmed, it is secured in place with a sterile dressing. Although complication rates and risks are very low, some include pain during the procedure, infection, allergic dermatitis, stimulation intolerance, and hematoma formation. The most common complication is lead migration, which is more common with chronic stimulators. The helical shape of the lead may help decrease the incidence of fracture, migration, and risk of infection to much less than 0.1% when left in for up to 60 days [104].

The use of PNS provides regional anesthesia without the systemic effects of most pain medications. Also, PNS may be left in longer (up to 60 days) than perineural catheters with local anesthetic while also potentially sparing motor blockade. PNS for analgesia could significantly change the practice of regional anesthesia and perioperative pain medicine by impacting patient satisfaction, pain control, and quality of life. The idea of minimizing, or even replacing opioids with PNS in the setting of the current opioid crisis makes this emerging modality an excellent and desirable option to achieve analgesia when used concurrently with other multimodal agents and techniques.

19 Cryoneurolysis

Cryoanalgesia is the use of cold temperature to treat pain. Though known by ancient civilizations, such as the Egyptians and Greeks, the clinical application remained crude until the first closed cryoprobe apparatus was described in 1961 [104]. Following this, more modern probes called cannulas, were invented. A cannula for cyroanalgesia is a tube within a tube that conveys a gas at high pressures (600–800 psi) down its shaft through a small annulus (0.002 mm), and into a low-pressure closed end before the gas is vented back up the shaft of the probe in a retrograde direction. The decrease in pressure at the tip results in a corresponding volume expansion, leading to a decrease in temperature due to the Joule–Thomson effect. This drop in temperature results in an ice-ball formation around the tip of the probe, which induces neuronal injury around the affected region. The target temperature is between −20 and −100 °C, which is why nitrous oxide or carbon dioxide are the two most frequently used gases for cryoneurolysis. With boiling points of −88 and −78 °C, nitrous oxide and carbon dioxide become solid once temperatures fall below these levels, inherently limiting their cooling process to within a safe and therapeutic range [110].

After cryoneurolysis, axons re-grow distally at a rate of 1–2 mm/day from the initial point of treatment, which most likely explains its prolonged duration of action. Analgesia may last for weeks or months with a single treatment, with high variability based on the distance from the point of cryoneurolysis to the terminal nerve branches innervating the affected tissue [104]. Due to the unpredictable duration of hypesthesia, motor weakness, and loss of proprioception, the use of cryoneurolysis may be limited in the treatment of acute pain. However, in situations where these limitations are acceptable, cryoneurolysis may be a promising technique that offers analgesia orders of magnitude beyond the duration of action provided by local anesthetics [111]. Benefits of cryoneurolysis have been shown in the application of surgically exposed intercostal nerves during thoracotomy, intraoperative application in the setting of inguinal herniorrhaphy, repeated debridement of burns, severe pain from traumatic rib fractures, limb or digit amputations of either the upper or lower extremity, and pain after total knee or shoulder arthroplasty [112, 113]. Initially, anatomic landmarks and/or nerve stimulation were used to guide probe insertion, but these techniques were soon supplemented and replaced with imaging modalities, particularly, fluoroscopy and ultrasound. Ultrasound-guided percutaneous cryoneurolysis is a procedure that can be performed in an outpatient setting without sedation, giving rise to a more accessible treatment plan for chronic pain. This technique is nearly identical to that of a single injection peripheral nerve block. Instead of injecting local anesthetic, the probe is inserted adjacent to the target nerve and the ice ball that forms at the tip envelopes it. Relative contraindications to percutaneous cryoneurolysis include local/systemic infection, anticoagulation, bleeding diathesis, and immunosuppression. Specific contraindications to cryoneurolysis include cold urticaria, Raynaud's disease, cryofibrinogenemia, cryoglobulinemia, and paroxysmal cold hemoglobinuria.

Risks of cryoneurolysis include pain during and after the procedure, superficial bruising, and transient or permanent alopecia or changes in hair pigmentation if the ice ball involves the skin. Of note, due to a continuous flow of warm blood, large blood vessels have been shown to tolerate the cold temperatures and demonstrate a low risk of complications such as vessel rupture, coagulation, or thrombosis [104]. A few RCTs demonstrated an increased incidence of neuropathic pain 3–6 months after open thoracotomy with surgically applied cryoneurolysis, but the majority of

RCTs have not reported similar data [114, 115]. The variability in data may be due to the differing techniques of exposing the target nerves intraoperatively among surgeons prior to applying cryoneurolysis under direct visualization. Like the double crush phenomenon, it is hypothesized that the physical manipulation of the target nerve results in an afferent barrage, leading to central sensitization such that when axonal regeneration occurs after injury, the fiber activity is perceived as dysesthetic [116]. By eliminating the need of intraoperative nerve manipulation, ultrasound-guided cryoneurolysis has demonstrated no incidence of neuropathic pain thus far, but caution is still warranted because the number of patients who underwent ultrasound-guided percutaneous cryoneurolysis is currently far fewer than those who received intraoperative application under direct visualization [104, 117].

Cryoneurolysis is a promising, emerging therapy that could potentially provide a safe, effective, and non-pharmacological therapeutic option for perioperative pain. The shift from current pain treatments that may have limited efficacy or potential risks to multimodal treatment plans that incorporate non-pharmacologic modalities makes cryoneurolysis a promising, emerging therapy that provides immediate, localized, and long-lasting analgesia.

20 Oliceridine—Biased Ligand

Conventional opioids exert their analgesic effects by activating the μ-opioid receptor and its downstream G-protein signaling pathway [118]. Unfortunately, the activated μ-opioid receptor also stimulates an alternative pathway mediated by β-arrestin, which has been associated with opioid-induced respiratory depression, gastrointestinal effects, and attenuation of analgesia. This information directed the novel idea of creating an agent that preferentially activates the G-protein pathway while minimizing the adverse effects mediated by β-arrestin seen with conventional opioids. Oliceridine (brand name Olinvyk), is the first drug in this new class of opioids called biased ligands. Unlike conventional opioids, oliceridine has been shown in vitro to induce only 14% of β-arrestin signaling activity compared to morphine [119]. An Oliceridine dose of 1 mg is equipotent to 5 mg of intravenous morphine. The time of onset of analgesia occurs rapidly within 1–2 minutes, peaks at 6–12 minutes, and lasts for 1–3 hours [118].

Several randomized controlled Phase III studies comparing oliceridine with morphine showed significantly higher treatment response rates, shorter time to meaningful pain relief (12 versus 30 minutes), and non-inferior analgesia in the oliceridine groups. One study showed a dose-dependent decrease in the incidence of respiratory events across all oliceridine regimens, though the highest dose of oliceridine was not much different from morphine [120]. In another study, the oliceridine groups were not associated with a significantly different respiratory safety burden than the placebo group [121]. In the same studies, gastrointestinal adverse effects increased in a dose-dependent manner, but the odds of requiring rescue antiemetics were significantly lower with all oliceridine regimens than morphine.

Although Phase I and II studies suggested that oliceridine may be associated with a lower risk of opioid-induced respiratory depression and adverse gastrointestinal side effects compared to morphine, the modest differences or lack of differences in subsequent Phase III clinical trials suggest that further prospective studies evaluating these safety parameters as their primary outcomes are needed [118]. With future studies, biased ligands like oliceridine may play an important and favorable pharmacological role in the multimodal analgesic pathway while minimizing adverse effects seen with conventional opioids.

21 Transient Receptor Potential Vanilloid 1 Channel Agonists

The Transient Receptor Potential Vanilloid 1 (TRPV1) ion channel is a polymodal protein with functions linked to the generation of pain. These ion channels are mainly expressed in all sensory ganglia and smaller-diameter neurons, such as sensory-C and Aδ [122]. TRPV1 receptors are activated by mediators of noxious stimuli and up-regulated in chronic pain states, increasing the perception of pain. TRPV1 agonists, like capsaicin, activate and depolarize TRPV1 receptors, leading to an initial burning sensation from the nerve stimulation, but eventual desensitization and analgesia once the receptors are completely depolarized [123]. Multiple molecules have been identified that have similar agonist effects as capsaicin but with more favorable pharmacokinetics [124]. One such molecule, vocacapsaicin, is a water-soluble prodrug that rapidly converts to capsaicin and has shown promise in a pilot study [125]. Various TRPV1 agonists with more favorable pharmacodynamics than capsaicin may play an important role in the setting of perioperative pain management. When we think of multimodal analgesia and all the implicated receptors and pathways associated with pain, TRPV1 is yet another target that should be considered, making these various emerging TRPV1 agonists important medications to study.

22 Extended-Release Local Anesthetic Formulations

Extended-release bupivacaine is a newer technique for administering local anesthetic over a longer period, allowing for an increased duration of action. Liposomal bupivacaine (Exparel), the most widely used and clinically relevant long-acting local anesthetic, uses a multivesicular liposomal delivery system that releases bupivacaine in a steady, controlled fashion. In recent years, other extended-release formulations have been developed, including bupivacaine/meloxicam (Zynrelef), SABER-Bupivacaine (Posimir), and INL-001 (Xaracoll).

Bupivacaine/meloxicam (HTX-011) is an extended-release local anesthetic that consists of a combination of bupivacaine and meloxicam [126]. Meloxicam is added in the attempt to decrease local inflammation and decrease local environment acidification, thereby improving the pH balance for bupivacaine, resulting in enhanced effectiveness. Bupivacaine/meloxicam is encapsulated in a polymer that hydrolyzes slowly, releasing bupivacaine and meloxicam at a gradual and sustained rate, with analgesic effects lasting for up to 72 hour. Due to its high viscosity, HTX-011 is a formulation that cannot be injected perineurally, but instead, it is designed for the surgical team to apply it on the surgical site prior to final closure. While it has been shown to be more effective than placebo and plain bupivacaine, it is not yet known if it is more effective than liposomal bupivacaine [127].

Like other extended-release local anesthetics, SABER-bupivacaine is a depot formulation of slowly released bupivacaine. In contrast to other formulations, SABER-bupivacaine is a polymer that uses a sucrose acetate isobutyrate 66% in benzyl alcohol 22% to deliver the active component, bupivacaine 12%. This compound was also designed for surgical infiltration and allows for slow release of bupivacaine over several days following injection; however, the benzyl alcohol component prevents the perineural use of SABER-bupivacaine [128]. While it has had a positive phase 3 clinical trial, other trials of effectiveness have been negative [129]. It received a narrow FDA approval in 2021 for shoulder analgesia for subacromial decompression surgery with administration into the subacromial space under direct arthroscopic visualization [130].

The final extended-release local anesthetic formulation is INL-001 (Xaracoll), which is a biodegradable resorbable collagen matrix impregnated with bupivacaine. It is designed for direct deposit in the surgical site, providing extended delivery of local anesthetic directly at the site. With few studies yet to support its efficacy, it has only been FDA-approved for placement into the surgical site following open inguinal hernia repair [131].

23 Local Anesthetic Adjuvants

The ability to prolong the duration of action of local anesthetics has long been a topic of great interest in the field of regional anesthesia. Various efforts to accomplish this goal include the use of additives to local anesthetic. The most commonly used additives currently include epinephrine, dexamethasone, buprenorphine, clonidine, and dexmedetomidine. Other additives currently being studied include sodium channel toxins, like tetrodotoxin and neosaxitoxin.

Tetrodotoxin is a naturally occurring reversible sodium channel toxin derived from pufferfish and shellfish that has been shown to block conduction of isolated nerves. In preliminary animal studies, tetrodotoxin significantly prolonged block duration when used with bupivacaine [132, 133]. Neosaxitoxin, found in pufferfish and other shellfish, is a more potent reversible sodium channel toxin that preferentially targets sodium channels in the periphery compared to the myocardium. Combined with bupivacaine, neosaxitoxin demonstrates a prolonged duration of effect compared to bupivacaine, neosaxitoxin, and placebo independently [134, 135]. Sodium channel toxins are still investigational but hold promise to extend the duration of action of local anesthetics to better match the needs of patients undergoing surgery associated with moderate to severe pain of longer duration.

24 Summary

Perioperative pain management is a dynamic field with many emerging therapies aimed to improve analgesia and overall patient care. The quest for safe, effective, and longer-acting therapies to improve pain control while minimizing the adverse effects of traditional therapies continues. With more research in these emerging therapies, the road to improvement looks very promising. While that search continues, we utilize a solid framework of pain management strategy in patient and pain mechanism-specific multimodal analgesia that employs pharmacologic and interventional therapies that mitigate pain and the physiologic stresses of surgery.

25 Key Takeaways of Chapter

Perioperative pain management attempts to mitigate post-surgical pain and help patients supersede the challenges and stressors of surgery.

Non-opioid pain medications of different classes with relevant regional anesthesia or local anesthetic infiltration provide a foundation of analgesia upon which judicial use of opioids can be added as needed to provide post-surgical pain control while decreasing opioid-related adverse events.

Interventional acute pain management techniques are effective modalities for patients undergoing surgeries associated with severe and moderately-severe pain.

Enhanced recovery protocols aim to decrease physiologic stress, restore homeostasis, and lead patients to faster recovery and optimal quality outcomes.

References

1. Parris WCV, Johnson BW. 1—The history of pain medicine. In: Benzon HT, Rathmell JP, Wu CL, Turk DC, Argoff CE, Hurley RW, editors. Practical management of pain. 5th ed. Philadelphia: Mosby; 2014. p. 3- 12.e1.
2. Naranjo P. Social function of coca in pre-Columbian American. J Ethnopharmacol. 1981;3(2–3):161–72.
3. Chuan A, Harrop-Griffiths W. The history of local anesthesia. In: Hadzic A, editor. Hadzic's textbook of regional anesthesia and acute pain management, 2e. New York, NY: McGraw-Hill Education; 2017.
4. Brownstein MJ. A brief history of opiates, opioid peptides, and opioid receptors. Proc Natl Acad Sci USA. 1993;90(12):5391–3.

5. Batterman RC, Himmelsbach CK. Demerol—a new synthetic analgesic: a review of its present status and comparison with morphine. J Am Med Assoc. 1943;122(4):222–6.
6. Scott CC, Chen KK. The action of 1,1-diphenyl-1 (dimethylaminoisopropyl) butanone-2, a potent analgesic agent. J Pharmacol Exp Ther. 1946;87:63–71.
7. Kehlet H, Dahl JB. The value of "multimodal" or "balanced analgesia" in postoperative pain treatment. Anesth Analg. 1993;77(5):1048–56.
8. Chou R, Gordon DB, de Leon-Casasola OA, Rosenberg JM, Bickler S, Brennan T, et al. Management of postoperative pain: a clinical practice guideline from the American pain society, the American society of regional anesthesia and pain medicine, and the American society of anesthesiologists' committee on regional anesthesia, executive committee, and administrative council. J Pain: Offic J Am Pain Soc. 2016;17(2):131–57.
9. Mariano ER, Dickerson DM, Szokol JW, Harned M, Mueller JT, Philip BK, et al. A multi-society organizational consensus process to define guiding principles for acute perioperative pain management. Reg Anesth Pain Med. 2022;47(2):118–27.
10. Shah S, Schwenk ES, Sondekoppam RV, Clarke H, Zakowski M, Rzasa-Lynn RS, et al. ASRA pain medicine consensus guidelines on the management of the perioperative patient on cannabis and cannabinoids. Reg Anesth Pain Med. 2023;48(3):97–117.
11. Woolf CJ. Pain: moving from symptom control toward mechanism-specific pharmacologic management. Ann Intern Med. 2004;140(6):441–51.
12. Memtsoudis SG, Poeran J, Zubizarreta N, Cozowicz C, Morwald EE, Mariano ER, et al. Association of multimodal pain management strategies with perioperative outcomes and resource utilization: a population-based study. Anesthesiology. 2018;128(5):891–902.
13. Raja SN, Carr DB, Cohen M, Finnerup NB, Flor H, Gibson S, et al. The revised international association for the study of pain definition of pain: concepts, challenges, and compromises. Pain. 2020;161(9):1976–82.
14. Practice guidelines for acute pain management in the perioperative setting: an updated report by the American Society of Anesthesiologists Task Force on Acute Pain Management. Anesthesiology. 2012;116(2):248–73.
15. Treede R-D, Rief W, Barke A, Aziz Q, Bennett MI, Benoliel R, et al. A classification of chronic pain for ICD-11. Pain. 2015;156(6):1003–7.
16. Schug SA, Lavand'homme P, Barke A, Korwisi B, Rief W, Treede RD. The IASP classification of chronic pain for ICD-11: chronic postsurgical or posttraumatic pain. Pain. 2019;160(1):45–52.
17. Richebé P, Capdevila X, Rivat C. Persistent postsurgical pain: pathophysiology and preventative pharmacologic considerations. Anesthesiology. 2018;129(3):590–607.
18. Glare P, Aubrey KR, Myles PS. Transition from acute to chronic pain after surgery. Lancet (London, England). 2019;393(10180):1537–46.
19. Descalzi G, Ikegami D, Ushijima T, Nestler EJ, Zachariou V, Narita M. Epigenetic mechanisms of chronic pain. Trends Neurosci. 2015;38(4):237–46.
20. Carr DB, Goudas LC. Acute pain. The Lancet. 1999;353(9169):2051–8.
21. Campbell JN, Meyer RA. Mechanisms of neuropathic pain. Neuron. 2006;52(1):77–92.
22. Cohen SP, Vase L, Hooten WM. Chronic pain: an update on burden, best practices, and new advances. The Lancet. 2021;397(10289):2082–97.
23. Wluka AE, Yan MK, Lim KY, Hussain SM, Cicuttini FM. Does preoperative neuropathic-like pain and central sensitisation affect the post-operative outcome of knee joint replacement for osteoarthritis? a systematic review and meta analysis. Osteoarthritis Cartil. 2020;28(11):1403–11.
24. Nagata K, Tozawa K, Miyahara J, Ito Y, Nakamoto H, Nakajima K, et al. Association between preoperative neuropathic pain and patient reported outcome measures after cervical spinal cord decompression surgery. Global Spine J. 2022:21925682221109560.
25. Kurien T, Arendt-Nielsen L, Petersen KK, Graven-Nielsen T, Scammell BE. Preoperative neuropathic pain-like symptoms and central pain mechanisms in knee osteoarthritis predicts poor outcome 6 months after total knee replacement surgery. J Pain. 2018;19(11):1329–41.

26. Vergne-Salle P. Management of neuropathic pain after knee surgery. Joint Bone Spine. 2016;83(6):657–63.
27. Westlund K. Pain pathways: peripheral, spinal, ascending, descending pathways. Practical Management of Pain: Elsevier; 2014. p. 87–112.
28. Chen J, Kandle PF, Murray IV, Fitzgerald LA, Sehdev JS. Physiology, Pain. StatPearls. Treasure Island (FL): StatPearls Publishing Copyright © 2023, StatPearls Publishing LLC.; 2023.
29. Messlinger K. Functional morphology of nociceptive and other fine sensory endings (free nerve endings) in different tissues. Prog Brain Res. 1996;113:273–98.
30. Basbaum AI, Bautista DM, Scherrer G, Julius D. Cellular and molecular mechanisms of pain. Cell. 2009;139(2):267–84.
31. Yaksh TL. 9—a review of pain-processing pharmacology. In: Benzon HT, Rathmell JP, Wu CL, Turk DC, Argoff CE, Hurley RW, editors. Practical management of pain. 5th ed. Philadelphia: Mosby; 2014. p. 99–112.
32. Casey KL, Tran TD. Chapter 12 Cortical mechanisms mediating acute and chronic pain in humans. Handb Clin Neurol. 2006;81:159-iii.
33. Gordon DB. Acute pain assessment tools: let us move beyond simple pain ratings. Curr Opin Anesthesiol. 2015;28(5):565–9.
34. Breivik H, Borchgrevink PC, Allen SM, Rosseland LA, Romundstad L, Hals EK, et al. Assessment of pain. Br J Anaesth. 2008;101(1):17–24.
35. Haefeli M, Elfering A. Pain assessment. Eur Spine J. 2006;15(1):S17–24.
36. Chiarotto A, Maxwell LJ, Ostelo RW, Boers M, Tugwell P, Terwee CB. Measurement properties of visual analogue scale, numeric rating scale, and pain severity subscale of the brief pain inventory in patients with low back pain: a systematic review. J Pain: Offic J Am Pain Soc. 2019;20(3):245–63.
37. Shafshak TS, Elnemr R. The visual analogue scale versus numerical rating scale in measuring pain severity and predicting disability in low back pain. J Clin Rheumatol. 2021;27(7):282–5.
38. McGuire DB, Kaiser KS, Haisfield-Wolfe ME, Iyamu F. Pain assessment in noncommunicative adult palliative care patients. Nurs Clin North Am. 2016;51(3):397–431.
39. Aalberg JJ, Kimball MD, McIntire TR, McCullen GM. Long-term outcomes of persistent post-operative opioid use: a retrospective cohort study. Ann Surg. 2022.
40. Joshi GP, Kehlet H. Guidelines for perioperative pain management: need for re-evaluation. Br J Anaesth. 2017;119(4):703–6.
41. Lovich-Sapola J, Smith CE, Brandt CP. Postoperative pain control. Surg Clin North Am. 2015;95(2):301–18.
42. Butterworth JFt, Strichartz GR. Molecular mechanisms of local anesthesia: a review. Anesthesiology. 1990;72(4):711–34.
43. Dunn LK, Durieux ME. Perioperative use of intravenous lidocaine. Anesthesiology. 2017;126(4):729–37.
44. Terkawi AS, Tsang S, Kazemi A, Morton S, Luo R, Sanders DT, et al. A clinical comparison of intravenous and epidural local anesthetic for major abdominal surgery. Reg Anesth Pain Med. 2016;41(1):28–36.
45. Weibel S, Jelting Y, Pace NL, Helf A, Eberhart LH, Hahnenkamp K, et al. Continuous intravenous perioperative lidocaine infusion for postoperative pain and recovery in adults. Cochr Database Systemat Rev. 2018;6:Cd009642.
46. Boezaart AP, Wright TW. Rational use and pitfalls of regional anesthesia for orthopedic surgery. Tech Orthopaed. 2017;32(4).
47. Joshi G, Gandhi K, Shah N, Gadsden J, Corman SL. Peripheral nerve blocks in the management of postoperative pain: challenges and opportunities. J Clin Anesth. 2016;35:524–9.
48. Memtsoudis SG, Cozowicz C, Bekeris J, Bekere D, Liu J, Soffin EM, et al. Peripheral nerve block anesthesia/analgesia for patients undergoing primary hip and knee arthroplasty: recommendations from the International Consensus on Anesthesia-Related Outcomes after Surgery (ICAROS) group based on a systematic review and meta-analysis of current literature. Reg Anesth Pain Med. 2021;46(11):971–85.

49. Popping DM, Elia N, Van Aken HK, Marret E, Schug SA, Kranke P, et al. Impact of epidural analgesia on mortality and morbidity after surgery: systematic review and meta-analysis of randomized controlled trials. Ann Surg. 2014;259(6):1056–67.
50. Saied NN, Helwani MA, Weavind LM, Shi Y, Shotwell MS, Pandharipande PP. Effect of anaesthesia type on postoperative mortality and morbidities: a matched analysis of the NSQIP database. Br J Anaesthes. 2017;118(1):105–11.
51. Neuman MD, Feng R, Carson JL, Gaskins LJ, Dillane D, Sessler DI, et al. Spinal anesthesia or general anesthesia for hip surgery in older adults. N Engl J Med. 2021;385(22):2025–35.
52. Lim JA, Seo Y, Choi EJ, Kwak SG, Ryu T, Lee JH, et al. Impact of regional anesthesia on outcomes of geriatric patients undergoing lower extremity revascularization: a propensity score-matched cohort study. Medicine. 2022;101(52): e32597.
53. Memtsoudis SG, Sun X, Chiu YL, Stundner O, Liu SS, Banerjee S, et al. Perioperative comparative effectiveness of anesthetic technique in orthopedic patients. Anesthesiology. 2013;118(5):1046–58.
54. Guay J, Kopp S. Epidural pain relief versus systemic opioid-based pain relief for abdominal aortic surgery. Cochr Database Systemat Rev. 2016;2016(1):Cd005059.
55. Lee GC, Fong ZV, Ferrone CR, Thayer SP, Warshaw AL, Lillemoe KD, et al. High performing whipple patients: factors associated with short length of stay after open pancreaticoduodenectomy. J Gastrointest Surg: Offic J Soc Surg Aliment Tract. 2014;18(10):1760–9.
56. Wu CL, Cohen SR, Richman JM, Rowlingson AJ, Courpas GE, Cheung K, et al. Efficacy of postoperative patient-controlled and continuous infusion epidural analgesia versus intravenous patient-controlled analgesia with opioids: a meta-analysis. Anesthesiology. 2005;103(5):1079–88; quiz 109–10.
57. Toms L, McQuay HJ, Derry S, Moore RA. Single dose oral paracetamol (acetaminophen) for postoperative pain in adults. Cochr Database Systemat Rev. 2008(4):Cd004602.
58. De Oliveira GS, Jr., Castro-Alves LJ, McCarthy RJ. Single-dose systemic acetaminophen to prevent postoperative pain: a meta-analysis of randomized controlled trials. Clinic J Pain. 2015;31(1):86–93.
59. Oscier CD, Milner QJ. Peri-operative use of paracetamol. Anaesthesia. 2009;64(1):65–72.
60. Wick EC, Grant MC, Wu CL. Postoperative multimodal analgesia pain management with nonopioid analgesics and techniques: a review. JAMA Surg. 2017;152(7):691–7.
61. Moore RA, Derry S, Aldington D, Wiffen PJ. Single dose oral analgesics for acute postoperative pain in adults—an overview of Cochrane reviews. The Cochrane database of systematic reviews. 2015(9):Cd008659.
62. McNicol ED, Ferguson MC, Schumann R. Single-dose intravenous ketorolac for acute postoperative pain in adults. Cochr Database Systemat Rev. 2021;5(5):Cd013263.
63. Thybo KH, Hägi-Pedersen D, Dahl JB, Wetterslev J, Nersesjan M, Jakobsen JC, et al. Effect of combination of paracetamol (Acetaminophen) and ibuprofen vs either alone on patient-controlled morphine consumption in the first 24 hours after total hip arthroplasty: the pansaid randomized clinical trial. JAMA. 2019;321(6):562–71.
64. De Oliveira GS, Jr., Almeida MD, Benzon HT, McCarthy RJ. Perioperative single dose systemic dexamethasone for postoperative pain: a meta-analysis of randomized controlled trials. Anesthesiology. 2011;115(3):575–88.
65. Turan A, Sessler DI. Steroids to ameliorate postoperative pain. Anesthesiology. 2011;115(3):457–9.
66. Waldron NH, Jones CA, Gan TJ, Allen TK, Habib AS. Impact of perioperative dexamethasone on postoperative analgesia and side-effects: systematic review and meta-analysis. Br J Anaesth. 2013;110(2):191–200.
67. Schwenk ES, Viscusi ER, Buvanendran A, Hurley RW, Wasan AD, Narouze S, et al. Consensus guidelines on the use of intravenous ketamine infusions for acute pain management from the American society of regional anesthesia and pain medicine, the American academy of pain medicine, and the American society of anesthesiologists. Reg Anesth Pain Med. 2018;43(5):456–66.

68. Brinck EC, Tiippana E, Heesen M, Bell RF, Straube S, Moore RA, et al. Perioperative intravenous ketamine for acute postoperative pain in adults. Cochr Database Systemat Rev. 2018;12:Cd012033.
69. Schmidt PC, Ruchelli G, Mackey SC, Carroll IR. Perioperative gabapentinoids: choice of agent, dose, timing, and effects on chronic postsurgical pain. Anesthesiology. 2013;119(5):1215–21.
70. Verret M, Lauzier F, Zarychanski R, Perron C, Savard X, Pinard AM, et al. Perioperative use of gabapentinoids for the management of postoperative acute pain: a systematic review and meta-analysis. Anesthesiology. 2020;133(2):265–79.
71. Kharasch ED, Clark JD, Kheterpal S. Perioperative gabapentinoids: deflating the bubble. Anesthesiology. 2020;133(2):251–4.
72. Blaudszun G, Lysakowski C, Elia N, Tramer MR. Effect of perioperative systemic alpha2 agonists on postoperative morphine consumption and pain intensity: systematic review and meta-analysis of randomized controlled trials. Anesthesiology. 2012;116(6):1312–22.
73. Jessen Lundorf L, Korvenius Nedergaard H, Moller AM. Perioperative dexmedetomidine for acute pain after abdominal surgery in adults. Cochrane Database Systemat Rev. 2016;2:Cd010358.
74. De Oliveira GS, Jr., Castro-Alves LJ, Khan JH, McCarthy RJ. Perioperative systemic magnesium to minimize postoperative pain: a meta-analysis of randomized controlled trials. Anesthesiology. 2013;119(1):178–90.
75. Meldrum ML. A capsule history of pain management. JAMA. 2003;290(18):2470–5.
76. Yaster M, Benzon HT, Anderson TA. "Houston, We Have a Problem!": the role of the anesthesiologist in the current opioid epidemic. Anesth Analg. 2017;125(5):1429–31.
77. Stein C. Opioids, sensory systems and chronic pain. Eur J Pharmacol. 2013;716(1):179–87.
78. Benyamin R, Trescot AM, Datta S, Buenaventura R, Adlaka R, Sehgal N, et al. Opioid complications and side effects. Pain Physic. 2008;11(2 Suppl):S105–20.
79. Larach DB, Hah JM, Brummett CM. Perioperative opioids, the opioid crisis, and the anesthesiologist. Anesthesiology. 2022;136(4):594–608.
80. Colvin LA, Bull F, Hales TG. Perioperative opioid analgesia-when is enough too much? A review of opioid-induced tolerance and hyperalgesia. Lancet (London, England). 2019;393(10180):1558–68.
81. Shanthanna H, Ladha KS, Kehlet H, Joshi GP. Perioperative opioid administration: a critical review of opioid-free versus opioid-sparing approaches. Anesthesiology. 2021;134(4):645–59.
82. McNicol ED, Ferguson MC, Hudcova J. Patient controlled opioid analgesia versus non-patient controlled opioid analgesia for postoperative pain. Cochr Database Systemat Rev. 2015;2015(6):Cd003348.
83. Kharasch ED, Brunt LM. Perioperative opioids and public health. Anesthesiology. 2016;124(4):960–5.
84. Vance CG, Dailey DL, Rakel BA, Sluka KA. Using TENS for pain control: the state of the evidence. Pain Manag. 2014;4(3):197–209.
85. Johnson MI, Paley CA, Jones G, Mulvey MR, Wittkopf PG. Efficacy and safety of transcutaneous electrical nerve stimulation (TENS) for acute and chronic pain in adults: a systematic review and meta-analysis of 381 studies (the meta-TENS study). BMJ Open. 2022;12(2): e051073.
86. Acar HV. Acupuncture and related techniques during perioperative period: a literature review. Complement Ther Med. 2016;29:48–55.
87. Shah S, Godhardt L, Spofford C. Acupuncture and postoperative pain reduction. Curr Pain Headache Rep. 2022;26(6):453–8.
88. Cheng SI, Kelleher DC, DeMeo D, Zhong H, Birch G, Ast MP. Intraoperative acupuncture as part of a multimodal analgesic regimen to reduce opioid usage after total knee arthroplasty: a prospective cohort trial. Med Acupunct. 2022;34(1):49–57.
89. Zgierska AE, Burzinski CA, Cox J, Kloke J, Stegner A, Cook DB, et al. Mindfulness meditation and cognitive behavioral therapy intervention reduces pain severity and sensitivity in

opioid-treated chronic low back pain: pilot findings from a randomized controlled trial. Pain medicine (Malden, Mass). 2016;17(10):1865–81.
90. McClintock AS, McCarrick SM, Garland EL, Zeidan F, Zgierska AE. Brief mindfulness-based interventions for acute and chronic pain: a systematic review. J Altern Complement Med. 2019;25(3):265–78.
91. Ljungqvist O, Scott M, Fearon KC. Enhanced recovery after surgery: a review enhanced recovery after surgery enhanced recovery after surgery. JAMA Surg. 2017;152(3):292–8.
92. Bardram L, Funch-Jensen P, Jensen P, Crawford ME, Kehlet H. Recovery after laparoscopic colonic surgery with epidural analgesia, and early oral nutrition and mobilisation. Lancet (London, England). 1995;345(8952):763–4.
93. Kehlet H, Mogensen T. Hospital stay of 2 days after open sigmoidectomy with a multimodal rehabilitation programme. Br J Surg. 1999;86(2):227–30.
94. Lassen K, Soop M, Nygren J, Cox PBW, Hendry PO, Spies C, et al. Consensus review of optimal perioperative care in colorectal surgery: enhanced recovery after surgery (eras) group recommendations. Arch Surg. 2009;144(10):961–9.
95. Nygren J, Hausel J, Kehlet H, Revhaug A, Lassen K, Dejong C, et al. A comparison in five European Centres of case mix, clinical management and outcomes following either conventional or fast-track perioperative care in colorectal surgery. Clin Nutr. 2005;24(3):455–61.
96. Wainwright T, Middleton R. An orthopaedic enhanced recovery pathway. Curr Anaesth Crit Care. 2010;21(3):114–20.
97. Wainwright TW, Immins T, Middleton RG. Enhanced recovery after surgery (ERAS) and its applicability for major spine surgery. Best Pract Res Clin Anaesthesiol. 2016;30(1):91–102.
98. Wainwright TW, Gill M, McDonald DA, Middleton RG, Reed M, Sahota O, et al. Consensus statement for perioperative care in total hip replacement and total knee replacement surgery: enhanced Recovery After Surgery (ERAS(®)) Society recommendations. Acta Orthop. 2020;91(1):3–19.
99. Soffin EM, YaDeau JT. Enhanced recovery after surgery for primary hip and knee arthroplasty: a review of the evidence. Br J Anaesthesia. 2016;117(suppl 3):iii62–72.
100. Kopp SL, Børglum J, Buvanendran A, Horlocker TT, Ilfeld BM, Memtsoudis SG, et al. Anesthesia and analgesia practice pathway options for total knee arthroplasty: an evidence-based review by the American and European societies of regional anesthesia and pain medicine. Reg Anesth Pain Med. 2017;42(6):683–97.
101. Brindle M, Nelson G, Lobo DN, Ljungqvist O, Gustafsson UO. Recommendations from the ERAS® Society for standards for the development of enhanced recovery after surgery guidelines. BJS Open. 2020;4(1):157–63.
102. Lam JY, Howlett A, McLuckie D, Stephen LM, Else SDN, Jones A, et al. Developing implementation strategies to adopt Enhanced Recovery After Surgery (ERAS®) guidelines. BJS Open. 2021;5(2).
103. Ilfeld BM, Grant SA, Gilmore CA, Chae J, Wilson RD, Wongsarnpigoon A, et al. Neurostimulation for postsurgical analgesia: a novel system enabling ultrasound-guided percutaneous peripheral nerve stimulation. Pain Pract: Offic J World Inst Pain. 2017;17(7):892–901.
104. Ilfeld BM, Finneran JJ, IV. Cryoneurolysis and percutaneous peripheral nerve stimulation to treat acute pain: a narrative review. Anesthesiology. 2020.
105. Deer TR, Eldabe S, Falowski SM, Huntoon MA, Staats PS, Cassar IR, et al. Peripherally induced reconditioning of the central nervous system: a proposed mechanistic theory for sustained relief of chronic pain with percutaneous peripheral nerve stimulation. J Pain Res. 2021;14:721–36.
106. Gabriel RA, Ilfeld BM. Acute postoperative pain management with percutaneous peripheral nerve stimulation: the SPRINT neuromodulation system. Expert Rev Med Dev. 2021;18(2):145–50.
107. Melzack R, Wall PD. Pain mechanisms: a new theory. Science. 1965;150(3699):971–9.
108. Strand NH, D'Souza R, Wie C, Covington S, Maita M, Freeman J, et al. Mechanism of action of peripheral nerve stimulation. Curr Pain Headache Rep. 2021;25(7):47.

109. Knotkova H, Hamani C, Sivanesan E, Le Beuffe MFE, Moon JY, Cohen SP, et al. Neuromodulation for chronic pain. Lancet (London, England). 2021;397(10289):2111–24.
110. Trescot AM. Cryoanalgesia in interventional pain management. Pain Physic. 2003;6(3):345–60.
111. Ilfeld BM, Gabriel RA, Trescot AM. Ultrasound-guided percutaneous cryoneurolysis for treatment of acute pain: could cryoanalgesia replace continuous peripheral nerve blocks? Br J Anaesth. 2017;119(4):703–6.
112. Khanbhai M, Yap KH, Mohamed S, Dunning J. Is cryoanalgesia effective for post-thoracotomy pain? Interact Cardiovasc Thorac Surg. 2014;18(2):202–9.
113. Wood GJ, Lloyd JW, Bullingham RE, Britton BJ, Finch DR. Postoperative analgesia for day-case herniorrhaphy patients. A comparison of cryoanalgesia, paravertebral blockade and oral analgesia. Anaesthesia. 1981;36(6):603–10.
114. Ju H, Feng Y, Yang BX, Wang J. Comparison of epidural analgesia and intercostal nerve cryoanalgesia for post-thoracotomy pain control. Euro J Pain (London, England). 2008;12(3):378–84.
115. Mustola ST, Lempinen J, Saimanen E, Vilkko P. Efficacy of thoracic epidural analgesia with or without intercostal nerve cryoanalgesia for postthoracotomy pain. Ann Thorac Surg. 2011;91(3):869–73.
116. DeLeo JA, Coombs DW, Willenbring S, Colburn RW, Fromm C, Wagner R, et al. Characterization of a neuropathic pain model: sciatic cryoneurolysis in the rat. Pain. 1994;56(1):9–16.
117. Bittman RW, Peters GL, Newsome JM, Friedberg EB, Mitchell JW, Knight JM, et al. Percutaneous image-guided cryoneurolysis. AJR Am J Roentgenol. 2018;210(2):454–65.
118. Tan HS, Habib AS. Oliceridine: a novel drug for the management of moderate to severe acute pain—a review of current evidence. J Pain Res. 2021;14:969–79.
119. DeWire SM, Yamashita DS, Rominger DH, Liu G, Cowan CL, Graczyk TM, et al. A G Protein-Biased Ligand at the <em>μ</em>-opioid receptor is potently analgesic with reduced gastrointestinal and respiratory dysfunction compared with morphine. J Pharmacol Exp Ther. 2013;344(3):708–17.
120. Viscusi ER, Skobieranda F, Soergel DG, Cook E, Burt DA, Singla N. APOLLO-1: a randomized placebo and active-controlled phase III study investigating oliceridine (TRV130), a G protein-biased ligand at the micro-opioid receptor, for management of moderate-to-severe acute pain following bunionectomy. J Pain Res. 2019;12:927–43.
121. Singla NK, Skobieranda F, Soergel DG, Salamea M, Burt DA, Demitrack MA, et al. APOLLO-2: A randomized, placebo and active-controlled phase III Study Investigating Oliceridine (TRV130), a G protein-biased ligand at the μ-opioid receptor, for management of moderate to severe acute pain following abdominoplasty. Pain Pract: Offic J World Inst Pain. 2019;19(7):715–31.
122. Jara-Oseguera A, Simon SA, Rosenbaum T. TRPV1: on the road to pain relief. Curr Mol Pharmacol. 2008;1(3):255–69.
123. Hartrick CT, Pestano C, Carlson N, Hartrick S. Capsaicin instillation for postoperative pain following total knee arthroplasty: a preliminary report of a randomized, double-blind, parallel-group, placebo-controlled, multicentre trial. Clin Drug Investig. 2011;31(12):877–82.
124. Duarte Y, Cáceres J, Sepúlveda RV, Arriagada D, Olivares P, Díaz-Franulic I, et al. Novel TRPV1 channel agonists with faster and more potent analgesic properties than capsaicin. Front Pharmacol. 2020;11:1040.
125. Teichman S, Garza J, Kleinman M, Solomon B, Stelmack V, Leiman D, et al. Pilot study of vocacapsaicin for treatment of pain after open laparotomy. J Am Coll Surg. 2022;235(5):S23.
126. Kaye AD, Edinoff AN, Yan JY, Kaye AJ, Alvarado MA, Pham AD, et al. Novel local anesthetics in clinical practice: pharmacologic considerations and potential roles for the future. Anesth Pain Med. 2022;12(1): e123112.
127. Viscusi E, Gimbel JS, Pollack RA, Hu J, Lee G-C. HTX-011 reduced pain intensity and opioid consumption versus bupivacaine HCl in bunionectomy: phase III results from the randomized EPOCH 1 study. Reg Anesth Pain Med. 2019;44(7):700–6.
128. Taylor A, McLeod G. Basic pharmacology of local anaesthetics. BJA Educ. 2020;20(2):34–41.

129. Ekelund A, Peredistijs A, Grohs J, Meisner J, Verity N, Rasmussen S. SABER-Bupivacaine reduces postoperative pain and opioid consumption after arthroscopic subacromial decompression: a randomized, placebo-controlled trial. J Am Acad Orthop Surg Glob Res Rev. 2022;6(5).
130. Gasteiger L, Kirchmair L, Hoerner E, Stundner O, Hollmann MW. Peripheral regional anesthesia using local anesthetics: old wine in new bottles? J Clin Med. 2023;12(4):1541.
131. Velanovich V, Rider P, Deck K, Minkowitz HS, Leiman D, Jones N, et al. Safety and efficacy of bupivacaine hcl collagen-matrix implant (INL-001) in open inguinal hernia repair: results from two randomized controlled trials. Adv Ther. 2019;36(1):200–16.
132. Kohane Daniel S, Yieh J, Lu NuT, Langer R, Strichartz Gary R, Berde CB. A re-examination of tetrodotoxin for prolonged duration local anesthesia. Anesthesiology. 1998;89(1):119–31.
133. Kohane DS, Lu NT, Gökgöl-Kline AC, Shubina M, Kuang Y, Hall S, et al. The local anesthetic properties and toxicity of saxitonin homologues for rat sciatic nerve block in vivo. Reg Anesth Pain Med. 2000;25(1):52–9.
134. Rodriguez-Navarro AJ, Berde CB, Wiedmaier G, Mercado A, Garcia C, Iglesias V, et al. Comparison of neosaxitoxin versus bupivacaine via port infiltration for postoperative analgesia following laparoscopic cholecystectomy: a randomized, double-blind trial. Reg Anesth Pain Med. 2011;36(2):103–9.
135. Lobo K, Donado C, Cornelissen L, Kim J, Ortiz R, Peake RW, et al. A phase 1, dose-escalation, double-blind, block-randomized, controlled trial of safety and efficacy of neosaxitoxin alone and in combination with 0.2% bupivacaine, with and without epinephrine, for cutaneous anesthesia. Anesthesiology. 2015;123(4):873–85.

Patient/Surgical Risk Factors for Chronic Pain and Opioid Dependency

Whitney Carter, Chelsea-Ann Patry, Andrew Mendelson, and Lynn Kohan

Abstract Post operative pain is a primary concern for patients undergoing surgery. Acute post-surgical pain can lead to the development of chronic post-surgical pain. While opioids were, at one point, overwhelmingly and exclusively utilized in the treatment of acute pain, it is now recognized that exposure to opioids may increase the risk of opioid dependence and opioid use disorder. Multimodal analgesia now represents the mainstay of analgesic treatment that seems to address acute surgical pain, chronic post-surgical pain, and minimize the development of opioid dependence. In this chapter, we discuss development risk factors, prevention strategies, and the treatment of chronic postsurgical pain while considering how pain management interventions might decrease the risk of opioid dependence/opioid use disorder.

Keywords Chronic post-surgical pain · Opioid dependence · Opioid use disorder

1 Introduction

It is estimated that approximately 15 million patients undergo surgeries each year in the United States (U.S) [1]. Health care costs associated with surgeries continue to rise; accounting for 40% of total health care expenditures [2]. A national survey reports that "pain after surgery" is most frequently listed by patients as their primary

W. Carter · C.-A. Patry · A. Mendelson · L. Kohan (✉)
Department of Anesthesiology, University of Virginia School of Medicine, Charlottesville, VA, USA
e-mail: LRK9G@UVAHealth.org; lrk9g@hscmail.mcc.virginia.edu

University of Virginia Hospital, Charlottesville, VA, USA

W. Carter
e-mail: QHM7QR@UVAHealth.org

C.-A. Patry
e-mail: CAP6Q@UVAHealth.org

A. Mendelson
e-mail: HAV4PM@UVAHealth.org

A. Abd-Elsayed and K. Schroeder (eds.), *Perioperative Pain Management*,
https://doi.org/10.1007/978-3-031-67648-2_3

concern when undergoing a surgical procedure [3]. Additionally, patients often report moderate to severe pain following surgery resulting in decreased functional status and delayed hospital discharge [4]. Opioids have traditionally been the primary analgesic for post operative pain [5, 6]. While potentially effective analgesics, opioids are associated with numerous risks including respiratory depression, hyperalgesia, tolerance, and the development of persistent long term opioid use or opioid use disorder [7, 8]. The Centers for Disease Control (CDC) Guidelines on opioids helped to curtail excessive prescribing for chronic pain but offered limited guidance for those patients seeking analgesia in the perioperative period [9, 10]. As a potential corollary, there continues to be large variation in post-operative opioid prescribing, often to excess, regardless of the extent of the surgery [11, 12]. Studies suggest persistent post-surgical opioid use (6–10%) can develop even after short exposure to opioids [13, 14]. Opioid use disorder (OUD) may also be a consequence after even short term exposure, with a prevalence of approximately 1–5% following surgery [15, 16]. While clinicians may have concerns regarding patient satisfaction if opioids are limited post operatively, studies suggest similar clinical and patient reported outcomes whether they were prescribed opioids or not [17]. Additionally, it has been demonstrated that patients frequently stop taking opioids prior to the resolution of post-surgical pain, thus high doses and long durations of opioids may not be necessary following surgery [18, 19]. Limiting opioid prescribing may help to decrease the risk of long-term opioid use as well as the development of OUD. Anesthesiologists, surgeons, and other healthcare professionals all play a key role in recognizing risk factors for the development of chronic post-surgical pain (CPSP), long-term opioid therapy (LTOT), and OUD.

2 Chronic Post-surgical Pain

Chronic post-surgical pain (CPSP) is pain that develops or increases in intensity after a surgical procedure or injury and persists for at least 3 months following the surgery and typical healing process. Other causes of pain, whether it be infection, malignancy, or a pre-existing condition, need to be ruled out [20]. The location of the pain is important for a CPSP diagnosis; the pain is located at the surgical site or the area of injury, it affects the nerves that innervate the surgical area, or it is related to the dermatomes in the area of injury. Additionally, it is important to distinguish whether the tissue trauma develops from a controlled procedure (surgery) or uncontrolled damage (accidental traumas) [20]. Although the exact mechanism of CPSP is not known, the development of CPSP is thought to be related to immune and inflammatory responses to trauma [20]. The pathophysiology involves both peripheral and central sensitization and symptoms typically include hyperalgesia, allodynia, and dysesthesia [19]. Approximately 35–57% of patients with CPSP demonstrate signs of neuropathic pain, but it appears that visceral, inflammatory, and neuroplastic pain might also play a role depending on the surgical procedure [20].

CPSP is unfortunately a common complication after surgery and while it can negatively impact quality of life and activities of daily living, it also results in an economic and healthcare resource utilization burden. While the exact incidence of CPSP is unknown, studies have reported it to be approximately 11.8% at 12 months [21]. This figure varies with the type of surgery as a higher incidence of CPSP was noted among patients undergoing orthopedic surgeries [21].

3 CPSP Risk Factors

While predicting the development of CPSP is extremely difficult, there appears to be a number of modifiable and non-modifiable risk factors. Severe preoperative and acute surgical pain appear to positively correlate with the development of CPSP [22]. Psychological factors are also predictors of CPSP with anxiety, catastrophizing and depression the most likely linked [23]. Younger age, higher BMI and female sex have been reported to increase the risk of CPSP [20]. Surgical technique can also influence the development of CPSP; laparoscopic approaches have been shown to decrease the development of CPSP for cholecystectomy and herniorrhaphy [24, 25]. Orthopedic surgeries have also been shown to have a higher incidence of CPSP development [21].

4 CPSP Prevention/CPSP Treatment

CPSP is a complex and unwanted adverse condition occurring after surgical procedures that leads to functional limitations and psychological trauma for patients [26]. Thus, the importance of developing preventive measures becomes imminent. Prevention of CPSP can vary from limiting nerve injury via modifying surgical techniques, utilizing local/regional anesthetics, and implementing ketamine IV treatments [27]. While managing CPSP, physicians can utilize pharmacologic treatments like topicals, NSAIDS, acetaminophen, antidepressants, corticosteroids, regional/local anesthesia, anticonvulsants, NMDA antagonist, and opioids [28].

Modification of Surgical Technique

One of the risks of CPSP occurring in patients is related to the extent of nerve and tissue injury during surgical procedures. Modifying surgical techniques is one possible way to help prevent the occurrence of chronic pain in post-operative settings [26]. A prospective, multicentric study by Alfieri demonstrated that the lack of nerve identification in the setting of hernioplasty was significantly correlated with the development of chronic pain [29]. In this study, surgeons were asked to report whether or not each nerve had been identified and preserved or divided and the primary endpoint of the study then sought to determine the presence of moderate and severe chronic pain at 6 months and 1 year post-op [29]. Statistical analysis demonstrated that patients in whom all nerves were identified had a significantly diminished risk of developing moderate to severe chronic pain compared to patients with only 1 or 2 nerves identified or patients whose nerves were not identified during surgery [29]. Thus the identification and preservation of nerves during open inguinal hernia repair reduced chronic groin pain.

Local/Regional Anesthesia

Local anesthetics aim to suppress and prevent sensitization with the goal of reducing pain and analgesic requirements in acute and chronic pain settings [30]. Perioperative lidocaine may suppress many pathways that are known to contribute to persistent post-surgical pain [31]. Local anesthetics have potent anti-inflammatory properties and have been found to reduce circulating levels of IL-1, IL-6, and TNF-alpha [32]. Local anesthetics have also demonstrated NMDA receptor antagonism in ex-vivo human models [33]. In addition, lidocaine reduces peripheral nociceptive input via blockade of sodium channels as well as other peripheral signal transduction pathways [34]. Local anesthetics are an important adjunct used to decrease pain, opioid consumptions and opioid-related adverse effects [30] and have been found to provide analgesia in the setting of acute and chronic pain [35, 36].

Multiple independent studies have sought to determine the effect of several different local anesthetic administration regimens on the development of CPSP. Patients who underwent breast cancer surgery receiving IV lidocaine demonstrated a lower incidence of CPSP 3 months following surgery [37]. A randomized, double blind, parallel-group, placebo- controlled study by Albi-Feldzer et al. looked at 236 patients scheduled for breast cancer surgery who were randomized to receive ropivacaine or placebo infiltration to the wound [38]. It was found that ropivacaine infiltration significantly decreased immediate post-operative pain for the first 90 min but did not decrease chronic pain at 3, 6, or 12 months postoperatively [38]. Additionally, 40 patients with ischemic heart disease scheduled for elective CABG were prospectively randomized to receive either general anesthesia or thoracic epidural anesthesia to evaluate the effects on postoperative pain [39]. The differences in pain scores were decreased at rest during 6, 12 and 24 hours in the thoracic epidural anesthesia group. Pain scores among the epidural group continued to remain decreased at one-month follow-up [39].

A recent systematic review of perioperative lidocaine infusion efficacy that included 420 patients in 6 trials found a reduction in the development of CPSP, however no significant differences were found on the McGill Pain Questionnaire [31]. Furthermore, clear data on systematic safety is lacking [31]. In conclusion, lidocaine infusions may offer some benefit in the prevention of CPSP, however more information on efficacy and safety is warranted. Wound infiltration data related to the prevention of CPSP is similarly lacking but the safety profile of this practice makes it something generally worth considering if other regional anesthesia techniques are contraindicated.

Regional anesthesia including peripheral nerve blocks and neuraxial anesthesia have been investigated in the prevention of CPSP. Peripheral nerve blocks may reduce neuronal inflammation and glial cell activation resulting in decreased CPSP [28]. However, results have been somewhat inconsistent. At least one study suggests the relationship between peripheral nerve blocks and reduced CPSP may depend on the type of block and that some blocks may even increase the risk of CPSP [40]. Other studies suggest that while peripheral nerve blocks result in short term reduction of postoperative pain, the long term impact is less substantial. Ilfield et al. found that the use of peripheral nerve blocks (PNB) helped to reduce the occurrence of phantom limb pain up to 4 weeks post-surgery but had no impact at 12 weeks when compared to placebo [41].

The evidence for neuraxial anesthesia is also mixed. Richebé et al. found that epidural analgesia reduced the incidence of CPSP at 1 year in thoracotomy, abdominal surgery, and breast surgery, however the optimal dosing and duration needed was unclear and there was no reduction in opioid use found [28]. A recent Cochrane review reported that epidural analgesia resulted in reduced CPSP after thoracotomy [42]. In addition, a recent meta-analysis found low quality evidence that pre-emptive epidural analgesia reduced chronic pain after thoracotomy [43].

Unfortunately, the use of paravertebral blocks did not show a beneficial impact on the prevention of CPSP. A large multicenter international study found no difference in CPSP assessed at 6 and 12 months in 2108 women with breast cancer who received paravertebral block plus propofol versus general anesthesia and opioids [44].

Overall, the evidence for the use of epidural anesthesia is moderate for the prevention of CPSP, while the evidence for the use of PNBs is unknown, with limited to no evidence for the use of paravertebral nerve blocks in the prevention of CPSP [41].

Ketamine

Ketamine is a N-methyl-D-aspartate (NMDA) receptor antagonist that has shown to have anesthesia, analgesic, anti-hyperalgesic, and also anti-inflammatory properties [45]. NMDA receptors are important for understanding the pathophysiology of central sensitization after surgery and blocking this receptor has been shown to prevent the development and reduce both acute postoperative pain intensity and opioid consumption [45]. Ketamine can be administered intranasally, orally, subcutaneously, intravenously and epidurally in a perioperative setting [46].

A recent randomized, blinded clinical trial examined if intra-operative low-dose ketamine would reduce postoperative opioid consumption and acute pain in 147 patients that underwent lumbar fusion surgery when compared to a placebo group. In this study, perioperative ketamine administration was associated with a significant decrease in morphine consumption at 0–24 hours following surgery [47]. Additionally, six months post-operatively, patients in the ketamine group reported significantly more improvement of their back pain compared to the placebo group, improvement in ambulation was noted as well [47]. A 2014 meta-analysis reported a reduction in CPSP symptoms at 3 and 6 months after surgery when intravenous ketamine was administered. However, significant variability in timing and dosing of ketamine resulted in the authors being unable to provide an optimal regimen [46]. Additionally, Kang et al. found a reduction in CPSP at 3 months after breast surgery in patients receiving ketamine but the clinical importance was minimal [48].

In conclusion, ketamine may reduce the incidence of CPSP but the overall strength of evidence is low [48].

Non-steroidal Anti-inflammatory Drugs (NSAIDs) and Acetaminophen

NSAIDs are potent anti-inflammatory agents that prevent prostaglandin synthesis by inhibiting cyclooxygenase enzymes. While acetaminophen also inhibits cyclooxygenase enzymes, its therapeutic mechanism remains unknown [49]. While there is strong evidence that both NSAIDs and Acetaminophen are effective for acute post-surgical pain, there is minimal evidence to support the use of NSAIDs and Acetaminophen in the prevention of CPSP [30]. Multiple prospective studies have shown NSAIDs have little or no effect on the development on CPSP [50, 51].

Antidepressants

Tricyclic antidepressants and selective serotonin-norepinephrine reuptake inhibitors are becoming a common treatment for chronic pain, especially since these medications are effective in reducing neuropathic pain and depression [26]. 150 patients who were scheduled for a partial or radical mastectomy with axillary dissection were involved in a randomized, double-blind study. The study consisted of the patients falling into three groups taking either venlafaxine, gabapentin, or placebo medication for 10 days starting the night before their operation. Results suggest that venlafaxine or gabapentin have an equipotent effect in reducing analgesic requirements [52]. Venlafaxine was found to significantly reduce the incidence of post-mastectomy pain syndrome 6 months in women having breast cancer surgery [52].

A systematic review across fifteen studies (total of 985 participants) evaluated the efficacy of antidepressants at reducing post-operative pain. Unfortunately, the evidence currently does not support the clinical use of antidepressants beyond controlled investigations for the treatment of acute, or prevention of chronic, post-operative pain [53]. However, there are multiple positive trials suggesting potential benefits associated with antidepressant administration and additional future studies should seek to replicate these findings [53].

Anticonvulsants (Gabapentinoids)

Gabapentinoids such as gabapentin and pregabalin are commonly used in treatment of CPSP as there is frequently a neuropathic component [28]. Gabapentinoids bind to the α-2δ subunit of presynaptic voltage-gated calcium channels which blocks the release of excitatory neurotransmitters from activating pain-transmitting neurons [54]. A study conducted on patients who underwent single-level lumbar discectomy showed that patients who received gabapentin 300 mg had significantly lower VAS score at all time points and they consumed less fentanyl. Patients who received gabapentin 600, 900, 1200 mg had lower VAS scores at all the time points than patients who received gabapentin 300 mg [55]. Other recent studies have demonstrated that gabapentinoids may have minimal effect on length of postoperative pain but are associated with a decreased duration of postoperative opioid use [18]. Additional studies are needed to determine the appropriate use of gabapentinoids as a CPSP prevention modality [18].

5 Opioid Dependence and OUD Background

OUD is a treatable disease that affects nearly 16 million patients worldwide and over 6 million Americans [56, 57]. OUD is defined as a problematic use of opioids resulting in clinically significant distress or impairment [58]. The diagnosis spans a continuum from mild, moderate, to severe including opioid dependence in the mild subset and addiction in the severe subset [58].

The following criteria are required for diagnosis of OUD.

1. Opioid are taken in larger amounts or over a longer period of time than was intended.
2. There is a persistent desire or unsuccessful efforts to cut down or control opioid use.
3. A great deal of time is spent in activities necessary to obtain the opioid, use the opioid, or recover from its effects.
4. Craving, or a strong desire or urge to use opioids.
5. Recurrent opioid use resulting in a failure to fulfill major role obligations at work, school, or home.
6. Continued opioid use despite having persistent or recurrent social or interpersonal problems caused or exacerbated by the effects of opioids.
7. Important social, occupational, or recreational activities are given up or reduced because of opioid use.

8. Recurrent opioid use in situations in which it is physically hazardous.
9. Continued opioid use despite knowledge of having a persistent or recurrent physical or psychological problem that is likely to have been caused or exacerbated by the substance.
10. Tolerance, as defined by either of the following:
    a. A need for markedly increased amounts of opioids to achieve intoxication or desired effect.
    b. A markedly diminished effect with continued use of the same amount of an opioid.

Note: This criterion is not considered to be met for those taking opioids solely under appropriate medical supervision.

11. Withdrawal, as manifested by either of the following:
    a. The characteristic opioid withdrawal syndrome (refer to Criteria A and B of the criteria set for opioid withdrawal, pp. 547–548).
    b. Opioids (or a closely related substance) are taken to relieve or avoid withdrawal symptoms.

Note: This criterion is not considered to be met for those individuals taking opioids solely under appropriate medical supervision.

Opioid use disorder can be classified by severity according to the number of criteria met: Mild (2–3 criteria); Moderate (4–5 criteria); Severe (6 or greater criteria). Note: Criteria from *American Psychiatric Association (2013). Diagnostic and Statistical Manual of Mental Disorders,* Fifth Edition. Washington, DC, American Psychiatric Association page 541 [58].

OUD does not discriminate, impacting all races, ethnicities, and economic groups [59]. While OUD is similar to other substance use disorders, it is unique in the short lead time (4–8 weeks) to physical dependence [60]. The intrinsic properties of opioid receptors and downward impact on dopamine pathways, leads to higher levels of positive reinforcement than most other substances. Additionally, the negative symptoms of opioid withdrawal, including chills, diaphoresis, nausea and vomiting, and intense cravings further reinforce the need to continue opioid use [60].

6 Opioid Dependence Risk Factors

While persistent opioid use after surgery may be the result of continued postoperative surgical pain, it may also represent non-pain etiologies including emotional suffering, the development of opioid dependence, or the development of an OUD. Some studies suggest persistent use of opioids following TKA despite improvement in joint pain suggesting the possible development of misuse [10]. The etiology for opioid dependence and OUD is multifactorial, including both genetic, psychologic, pharmacologic, and environmental factors.

Risk factors for the development of persistent post-surgical opioid use include younger age, sleep disturbance, tobacco use, history of past opioid use (including remote), mood disorders, history of chronic pain, and history of a substance use disorder [14].

Exposure to opioids is also a known pharmacological risk factor. Even short exposure to opioids has been associated with tolerance and hyperalgesia. High intraoperative doses of opioids have been found to contribute to higher levels of postoperative pain and higher amounts of morphine milliequivalents (MME) [61–64]. Each day of prescription opioid use can increase the risk of LTOT, with chronic opioid use occurring in as little as 5 days [64] in opioid naive patients [15].

Preoperative Assessment

All patients should be screened for OUD preoperatively. Early identification of patients with OUD can enable improved coordination of care and patient education. Validated screening tools include National Institutes on Drug Abuse (NIDA) quick screen, Drug Abuse Screening Tool (DAST-10), and Screening, Brief Interventions, Referral to Treatment (SBIRT) [65]. Additionally, obtaining a personal or family history of OUD, SUD, or untreated mental illness is advised [65, 66]. Furthermore, attention to signs of withdrawal, including nausea/vomiting, diarrhea, lacrimation, rhinorrhea, diaphoresis, shivering, piloerection, yawning, sneezing, restlessness, and tremor are warranted [67]. When assessing a patient for OUD, it is important to use non-stigmatizing language and to set realistic expectations for pain control.

7 Opioid Dependence Prevention

Despite the development of minimally invasive surgeries and new non-opioid medications, 80% of patients worldwide who undergo surgery receive opioids for postoperative pain relief [68]. Therefore, the reduction of opioid overuse is of utmost importance. During the perioperative period it is important to minimize opioids while also providing adequate analgesia. This can be accomplished in a variety of ways. One way is using multimodal analgesics; a regimen consisting of opioid, non-opioid medications and nonpharmacologic methods should be employed. A combination of anti-inflammatory (NSAID), gabapentin, acetaminophen, dexmedetomidine, and weak opioids can provide adequate analgesia without significant adverse effects [68]. The use of Enhanced Recovery after Surgery (ERAS) protocols are essential to creating multimodal analgesia regiments. One study of more than 600 patients managed with an ERAS protocol showed a 72% reduction in median opioid consumption and 16% of these patients were opioid-free from admission to the third postoperative day [69]. When appropriate, neuraxial or regional anesthesia techniques can be used for pain control to further decrease opioid use. Multiple studies have demonstrated the significant benefits of using regional anesthesia for various surgical procedures including total knee arthroplasty, hepatectomy, colectomy [68]. Furthermore, it is also recommended to discharge patients on a multimodal analgesic regimen with the minimal amount of opiates needed to decrease overall opiate use and opiate-related side effects [70].

8 OUD/Treatment

Multifactorial care is the mainstay of OUD treatment, including behavioral and pharmacological therapies. Nonpharmacological therapies to treat OUD include: cognitive behavioral therapy (CBT), contingency management, and group therapy. Currently, there are 3 Federal Drug Administration medications, methadone, buprenorphine, and naltrexone, for the treatment of OUD (MOUD). MOUD has been found to improve outcomes, decrease morbidity and mortality, and increase retention in treatment [71]. Despite the evidence for MOUD, access to these medications continues to be limited [72]. The pharmacologic profiles and dosing for all three MOUD differ and are reviewed in Table 1. Prior to 2023, it was required that physicians prescribing suboxone for OUD obtain an X-waiver, however with the passage of the 2023 Consolidated Appropriations Act (P.L. 117–328) [73], signed into law on Dec. 29, 2022, the requirement has since been lifted. The act amended the Controlled Substances Act to eliminate the requirement for qualified practitioners to first obtain a special x waiver to prescribe medications such as BUP for the treatment of opioid use disorder (OUD).

It is important for patients currently prescribed MOUD and scheduled for upcoming surgery be evaluated preoperatively. Part of the preoperative assessment includes coordinating care between the surgical, anesthesiology, and outpatient treatment teams as well as with the patient. If the patient is prescribed either a full mu-agonist (methadone) or partial mu-agonist (buprenorphine) it is recommended to continue these medications during the perioperative period [67]. Unlike full mu-agonist or partial mu-agonist, which are routinely continued perioperatively, patients prescribed mu-antagonist (naltrexone) need to have the medication discontinued prior to surgery when opioids are anticipated to be needed. If patients receive monthly injectable naltrexone, XR-NXT, it is recommended elective surgery be delayed 28 days following the last administration [74]. Oral naltrexone is recommended to be discontinued 48–72 hour prior to surgery [75]. Regardless of what the patient is prescribed for OUD, it is encouraged that the perioperative plan is individualized to the patient and multimodal analgesics are employed during the perioperative period; opioids, non-opioid medications and nonpharmacologic methods.

Table 1 Comparison of the 3 FDA-approved medications for OUD treatment [66]

	Methadone	Buprenorphine	Naltrexone
Mechanism of action	Full agonist at mu-opioid receptor	Partial agonist at mu-opioid receptor	Antagonist at mu-opioid receptor
Dosing average range	• 80–100 mg PO daily	• 4–24 mg SL/PO daily	• 380 mg IM Depot injection • 50 mg PO daily
Setting	• Licensed outpatient treatment program (OTP)	• Any medical setting • X-waiver no longer required as of 2023	• Any medical setting
Advantages	• Care provided in highly structured supervised setting with built in resources • Use in co-morbid pain management • Low diversion	• Care provided in a variety of outpatient models; less structured then OTP • Lower risk of overdose • Use in co-morbid pain management • Dosing flexibility	• Low diversion • Not an opioid • Improved compliance • No physical dependence • Verifiable dosing • Less stigma
Disadvantages	• Caution with QTc prolongation • Adverse Effects: May increase LFTs, constipation and other opioid-related side effects • Caution with increased overdose risk • Withdrawal with abrupt cessation	• Diversion possible • Adverse Effects: Constipation and other opioid-related side effects • Withdrawal with abrupt cessation	• Cannot be used for comorbid pain management • Adverse Effects: Flu like symptoms at first injection • Requires ~10-day opioid free period prior to initiation to avoid precipitated withdrawal

9 Conclusion

CPSP and opioid dependence continues to be an issue affecting patients following surgery. Although the mechanism behind CPSP development is not fully understood, it is important to employ multimodal analgesics; opioids, non-opioid medications and nonpharmacologic methods, when applicable. Prior to surgery, all patients should be screened for opioid use disorder as there are additional analgesic techniques and medications that can be used throughout the perioperative period to further benefit these patients.

Key Takeaways

1. CPSP is pain that develops or increases in intensity after a surgical procedure or injury and persists for at least 3 months following the surgery and typical healing

process. Prevention of CPSP can vary from using minimally invasive surgical technique, utilizing local/regional anesthetics, and ketamine IV treatments.
2. Limiting opioid prescribing may help to decrease the risk of long-term opioid use as well as the development of OUD.
3. It is encouraged that the perioperative analgesic plan is individualized to the patient and that multimodal analgesics are employed during the perioperative period; opioids, non-opioid medications as well as nonpharmacologic methods.

References

1. Cullen KA, Hall MJ, Golosinskiy A. Ambulatory surgery in the United States, 2006. Natl Health Stat Rep. 2009;11:1–25.
2. Russo A, Elixhauser A, Steiner C, Wier L. Hospital-based ambulatory surgery, 2007. In: Statistical brief #86. 200AD.
3. Apfelbaum JL, Chen C, Mehta SS, Gan ATJ. Postoperative pain experience: results from a national survey suggest postoperative pain continues to be undermanaged. Anesth Analg. [Internet]. 2003;97(2):534–40. https://doi.org/10.1213/01.ane.0000068822.10113.9e
4. Clarke H, Soneji N, Ko DT, Yun L, Wijeysundera DN. Rates and risk factors for prolonged opioid use after major surgery: population based cohort study. BMJ [Internet]. 2014;348(feb11 3):g1251–g1251. https://doi.org/10.1136/bmj.g1251
5. Strassels SA, McNicol E, Suleman R. Postoperative pain management: a practical review, part 2. Am J Health Syst Pharm [Internet]. 2005;62(19):2019–25. https://doi.org/10.2146/ajhp040490.p2
6. Duas F. After surgery in Germany, I wanted Vicodin, not herbal tea. The New York times [Internet]. Available from: https://www.nytimes.com/2018/01/27/opinion/sunday/surgery-germamny-vicodin.html[(2018). Accessed 6 Mar 2023.
7. Alam A, Gomes T, Zheng H, Mamdani MM, Juurlink DN, Bell CM. Long-term analgesic use after low-risk surgery: a retrospective cohort study: a retrospective cohort study. Arch Intern Med [Internet]. 2012;172(5):425–30. https://doi.org/10.1001/archinternmed.2011.1827
8. Mercadante S, Arcuri E, Santoni A. Opioid-induced tolerance and hyperalgesia. CNS Drugs [Internet]. 2019;33(10):943–55. https://doi.org/10.1007/s40263-019-00660-0
9. U.S. Opioid Dispensing Rate Maps I Drug Overdose I CDC Injury Center. Available at: https://www.cdc.gov/drugoverdose/rxrate-maps/index.html. Accessed 4 Dec 4 2022.
10. Goesling J, Moser SE, Zaidi B, et al. Trends and predictors of opioid use after total knee and total hip arthroplasty. Pain. 2016;157(6):1259–1265. https://doi.org/10.1097/j.pain.0000000000000516
11. Hill MV, McMahon ML, Stucke RS, Barth RJ Jr. Wide variation and excessive dosage of opioid prescriptions for common general surgical procedures. Ann Surg. 2016. https://doi.org/10.1097/sla.0000000000001993
12. Waljee JF, Zhong L, Hou H, Sears E, Brummett C, Chung KC. The use of opioid analgesics following common upper extremity surgical procedures: a national, population-based study. Plast Reconstr Surg. 2016;137(2):355e–364e. https://doi.org/10.1097/01.prs.0000475788.52446.7b
13. Brummett CM, Waljee J, Goesling J, et al. New persistent opioid use after major and minor surgery in U.S. adults. JAMA Surg. 2017;152(6):el70504. https://doi.org/10.1001/jamasurg.2017.0504
14. Larach DB, Hah JM, Brummett CM. Perioperative opioids, the opioid crisis, and the anesthesiologist. Anesthesiology. 2022;136(4):594–608. https://doi.org/10.1097/ALN.0000000000004109. PMID: 35108351; PMCID: PMC8904272

15. Higgins C, Smith BH, Matthews K. Incidence of iatrogenic opioid dependence or abuse in patients with pain who were exposed to opioid analgesic therapy: a systematic review and meta-analysis. Br J Anaesth. 2018;120:1335–44. https://doi.org/10.1016/j.bja.2018.03.009
16. Brat GA, Agniel D, Beam A, et al. Postsurgical prescriptions for opioid naive patients and association with overdose and misuse: retrospective cohort study. BMJ 2018;360:j5790. https://doi.org/10.1136/bmj.j5790
17. Howard R[*,†], Brown CS[*,†], Lai YL[*,‡], Gunaseelan V[‡,§], Chua KP, Brummett C[‡,§], Englesbe M[*,‡], Waljee J[*,‡], Bicket MC[‡,§]. The association of postoperative opioid prescriptions with patient outcomes. Annal Surg 276(6):p e1076–e1082. https://journals.lww.com/annalsofsurgery/Abstract/2022/12000/The_Association_of_Postoperative_Opioid.77.aspx
18. Hah J, Mackey SC, Schmidt P, McCue R, Humphreys K, Trafton J, Efron B, Clay D, Sharifzadeh Y, Ruchelli G, Goodman S, Huddleston J, Maloney WJ, Dirbas FM, Shrager J, Costouros JG, Curtin C, Carroll I. Effect of perioperative gabapentin on postoperative pain resolution and opioid cessation in a mixed surgical cohort: a randomized clinical trial. JAMA Surg. 2018;153(4):303–311. https://doi.org/10.1001/jamasurg.2017.4915. Erratum in: JAMA Surg. 2018;153(4):396. Erratum in: JAMA Surg. 2022;157(6):553. PMID: 29238824; PMCID: PMC5933381. https://doi.org/10.1001/jamasurg.2017.4915
19. Hah JM, Hilmoe H, Schmidt P, McCue R, Trafton J, Clay D, Sharifzadeh Y, Ruchelli G, Hernandez Boussard T, Goodman S, Huddleston J, Maloney WJ, Dirbas FM, Shrager J, Costouros JG, Curtin C, Mackey SC, Carroll I. Preoperative factors associated with remote postoperative pain resolution and opioid cessation in a mixed surgical cohort: post hoc analysis of a perioperative gabapentin trial. J Pain Res. 2020;13:2959–70. https://doi.org/10.2147/JPR.S269370.
20. Rosenberger DC, Pogatzki-Zahn EM. Chronic post-surgical pain—update on incidence, risk factors and preventive treatment options. BJA Educ. 2022. https://doi.org/10.1016/j.bjae.2021.11.008.
21. Fletcher D, Stamer UM, Pogatzki-Zahn E, Zaslansky R, Tanase NV, Perruchoud C, Kranke P, Komann M, Lehman T, Meissner W. Chronic postsurgical pain in Europe. Eur J Anaesthesiol. 2015;32(10):725–34. https://doi.org/10.1097/eja.0000000000000319.
22. Kehlet H, Jensen TS, Woolf CJ. Persistent postsurgical pain: risk factors and prevention. The Lancet. 2006;367(9522):1618–25. https://doi.org/10.1016/s0140-6736(06)68700-x.
23. Giusti EM, Lacerenza M, Manzoni GM, Castelnuovo G. Psychological and psychosocial predictors of chronic postsurgical pain: a systematic review and meta-analysis. Pain. 2021;162(1):10–30. https://doi.org/10.1097/j.pain.0000000000001999.
24. Callesen T, Kehlet H. Postherniorrhaphy pain. Anesthesiol. 1997;87(5):1219–30. https://doi.org/10.1097/00000542-199711000-00027.
25. Stiff G, Rhodes M, Kelly A, Telford K, Armstrong CP, Rees BI. Long-term pain: less common after laparoscopic than open cholecystectomy. Br J Surg. 1994;81(9):1368–70. https://doi.org/10.1002/bjs.1800810939.
26. Thapa P, Euasobhon P. Chronic postsurgical pain: current evidence for prevention and management. Korean J Pain. 2018;31(3):155. https://doi.org/10.3344/kjp.2018.31.3.155.
27. Visser EJ. Chronic post-surgical pain: epidemiology and clinical implications for acute pain management. Acute Pain. 2006;8(2):73–81. https://doi.org/10.1016/j.acpain.2006.05.002.
28. Richebé P, Capdevila X, Rivat C. Persistent postsurgical pain pathophysiology and preventative pharmacologic considerations. Anesthesiology: J Am Soc Anesthesiol. 2018;129(3):590–607. https://doi.org/10.1097/ALN.0000000000002238
29. Alfieri S, Rotondi F, Di Giorgio A, Fumagalli U, Salzano A, Di Miceli D, Ridolfini MP, Sgagari A, Doglietto G. Influence of preservation versus division of ilioinguinal, iliohypogastric, and genital nerves during open mesh herniorrhaphy. Ann Surg. 2006;243(4):553–8. https://doi.org/10.1097/01.sla.0000208435.40970.00.
30. Clarke H, Poon M, Weinrib A, Katznelson R, Wentlandt K, Katz J. Preventive analgesia and novel strategies for the prevention of chronic post-surgical pain. Drugs. 2015;75(4):339–51. https://doi.org/10.1007/s40265-015-0365-2.

31. Bailey M, Corcoran T, Schug S, Toner A. Perioperative lidocaine infusions for the prevention of chronic postsurgical pain. Pain 2018;n1. https://doi.org/10.1097/j.pain.0000000000001273
32. Ortiz MP, Godoy MCM, Schlosser RS, Ortiz RP, Godoy JPM, Santiago ES, Rigo FK, Beck V, Duarte T, Duarte MMF, Menezes MS. Effect of endovenous lidocaine on analgesia and serum cytokines: double-blinded and randomized trial. J Clinic Anesthesia. 2016;35:70–7. https://doi.org/10.1016/j.jclinane.2016.07.021
33. Hahnenkamp K, Durieux ME, Hahnenkamp A, Schauerte SK, Hoenemann CW, Vegh V, Theilmeier G, Hollmann MW. Local anaesthetics inhibit signalling of human NMDA receptors recombinantly expressed in Xenopus laevis oocytes: role of protein kinase C. Br J Anaesth. 2006;96(1):77–87. https://doi.org/10.1093/bja/aei271.
34. Wan X, Wang W, Liu J, Tong T. Estimating the sample mean and standard deviation from the sample size, median, range and/or interquartile range. BMC Med Res Methodol. 2014;14(1). https://doi.org/10.1186/1471-2288-14-135
35. Kranke P, Jokinen J, Pace NL, Schnabel A, Hollmann MW, Hahnenkamp K, Eberhart LH, Poepping DM, Weibel S. Continuous intravenous perioperative lidocaine infusion for postoperative pain and recovery. Cochrane Database Syst Rev. 2015. https://doi.org/10.1002/14651858.cd009642.pub2.
36. Katz J, Clarke H, Seltzer Z. Preventive analgesia. Anesth Analg. 2011;113(5):1242–53. https://doi.org/10.1213/ane.0b013e31822c9a59.
37. Grigoras A, Lee P, Sattar F, Shorten G. Perioperative intravenous lidocaine decreases the incidence of persistent pain after breast surgery. Clin J Pain. 2012;28(7):567–72. https://doi.org/10.1097/ajp.0b013e31823b9cc8.
38. Albi-Feldzer A, Mouret-Fourme EE, Hamouda S, Motamed C, Dubois PY, Jouanneau L, Jayr C. A double-blind randomized trial of wound and intercostal space infiltration with ropivacaine during breast cancer surgery. Anesthesiology. 2013;118(2):318–326. https://doi.org/10.1097/aln.0b013e31827d88d8
39. Onan B, Onan IS, Kilickan L, Sanisoglu I. Effects of epidural anesthesia on acute and chronic pain after coronary artery bypass grafting. J Card Surg. 2013;28(3):248–53. https://doi.org/10.1111/jocs.12086.
40. Gungor S, Fields K, Aiyer R, Valle AGD, Su EP. Incidence and risk factors for development of persistent postsurgical pain following total knee arthroplasty. Medicine. 2019;98(28): e16450. https://doi.org/10.1097/md.0000000000016450.
41. Ilfeld BM, Khatibi B, Maheshwari K, Madison SJ, Esa WAS, Mariano ER, Kent ML, Hanling S, Sessler DI, Eisenach JC, Cohen SP, Mascha EJ, Ma C, Padwal JA, Turan A. Ambulatory continuous peripheral nerve blocks to treat postamputation phantom limb pain: a multicenter, randomized, quadruple-masked, placebo-controlled clinical trial. Pain. 2020;162(3):938–55. https://doi.org/10.1097/j.pain.0000000000002087.
42. Weinstein EJ, Levene JL, Cohen MS, Andreae DA, Chao JY, Johnson M, Hall CB, Andreae MH. Local anaesthetics and regional anaesthesia versus conventional analgesia for preventing persistent postoperative pain in adults and children. Cochr Database Syst Rev. 2018. https://doi.org/10.1002/14651858.cd007105.pub3.
43. Park S-K, Yoon S, Kim BR, Choe SH, Bahk J-H, Seo J-H. Pre-emptive epidural analgesia for acute and chronic post-thoracotomy pain in adults: a systematic review and meta-analysis. Reg Anesth Pain Med. 2020;45(12):1006–16. https://doi.org/10.1136/rapm-2020-101708.
44. Albi-Feldzer A, Dureau S, Ghimouz A, Raft J, Soubirou J-L, Gayraud G, Jayr C. Preoperative paravertebral block and chronic pain after breast cancer surgery: a double-blind randomized trial. Anesthesiol. 2021;135(6):1091–103. https://doi.org/10.1097/ALN.0000000000003989.
45. Steyaert A, Lavand'homme P. Prevention and treatment of chronic postsurgical pain: a narrative review. Drugs. 2018;78(3):339–54. https://doi.org/10.1007/s40265-018-0866-x.
46. McNicol ED, Schumann R, Haroutounian S. A systematic review and meta-analysis of ketamine for the prevention of persistent post-surgical pain. Acta Anaesthesiol Scand. 2014;58(10):1199–213. https://doi.org/10.1111/aas.12377.
47. Nielsen RV, Fomsgaard JS, Siegel H, Martusevicius R, Nikolajsen L, Dahl JB, Mathiesen O. Intraoperative ketamine reduces immediate postoperative opioid consumption after spinal

fusion surgery in chronic pain patients with opioid dependency. Pain. 2017;158(3):463–70. https://doi.org/10.1097/j.pain.0000000000000782.
48. Kang C, Cho AR, Kim KH, Lee Eun-A, Lee HJ, Kwon JY, Kim H, Kim E, Baik JS, Kim C. Effects of intraoperative low-dose ketamine on persistent postsurgical pain after breast cancer surgery: a prospective, randomized, controlled, double-blind study. Pain Physic. 2020;23(1):37–47. https://pubmed.ncbi.nlm.nih.gov/32013277/
49. Ouellet M, Percival MD. Mechanism of acetaminophen inhibition of cyclooxygenase isoforms. Arch Biochem Biophys. 2001;387(2):273–80. https://doi.org/10.1006/abbi.2000.2232.
50. Lakdja F, Dixmérias F, Bussières E, Fonrouge JM, Lobéra A. [Preventive analgesic effect of intraoperative administration of ibuprofen-arginine on postmastectomy pain syndrome]. Bulletin Du Cancer. 1997;84(3):259–63. https://pubmed.ncbi.nlm.nih.gov/9207871/
51. Fransen M, Anderson C, Douglas J, MacMahon S, Neal B, Norton R, Woodward M, Cameron ID, Crawford R, Lo SK, Tregonning G, Windolf M. Safety and efficacy of routine postoperative ibuprofen for pain and disability related to ectopic bone formation after hip replacement surgery (HIPAID): randomised controlled trial. BMJ. 2006;333(7567):519. https://doi.org/10.1136/bmj.38925.471146.4f.
52. Amr YM, Yousef AAA-M. Evaluation of efficacy of the perioperative administration of venlafaxine or gabapentin on acute and chronic postmastectomy pain. Clin J Pain. 2010;26(5):381–5. https://doi.org/10.1097/ajp.0b013e3181cb406e.
53. Wong K, Phelan R, Kalso E, Galvin I, Goldstein D, Raja S, Gilron I. Antidepressant drugs for prevention of acute and chronic postsurgical pain. Anesthesiol. 2014;121(3):591–608. https://doi.org/10.1097/aln.0000000000000307.
54. Schmidt PC, Ruchelli G, Mackey SC, Carroll IR. Perioperative gabapentinoids. Anesthesiol. 2013;119(5):1215–21. https://doi.org/10.1097/aln.0b013e3182a9a896.
55. Pandey CK, Navkar DV, Giri PJ, Raza M, Behari S, Singh RB, Singh U, Singh PK. Evaluation of the optimal preemptive dose of gabapentin for postoperative pain relief after lumbar diskectomy. J Neurosurg Anesthesiol. 2005;17(2):65–8. https://doi.org/10.1097/01.ana.0000151407.62650.51.
56. Theisen K, Jacobs B, Macleod L, Davies B. The United States opioid epidemic: a review of the surgeon's contribution to it and health policy initiatives. BJU Int. 2018;122(5):754–9. https://doi.org/10.1111/bju.14446.
57. Keyes KM, Rutherford C, Hamilton A, Barocas JA, Gelberg KH, Mueller PP, Feaster DJ, El-Bassel N, Cerdá M. What is the prevalence of and trend in opioid use disorder in the United States from 2010 to 2019? Using multiplier approaches to estimate prevalence for an unknown population size. Drug Alcohol Depend Rep. 2022;3: 100052. https://doi.org/10.1016/j.dadr.2022.100052.
58. Diagnostic and Statistical Manual of Mental Disorders, Fifth Edition. Washington, DC: American Psychiatric Association; 2013. p. 541.
59. National Academies of Sciences E, and Medicine; Health and Medicine Division; Board on Health Sciences Policy; Committee on Medication-Assisted Treatment for Opioid Use Disorder. Barriers to broader use of medications to treat opioid use disorder. Washington (DC): National Academies Press, 2019.
60. Sharma B, Bruner A, Barnett G, Fishman M. Opioid use disorders. Child Adolesc Psychiatr Clin N Am. 2016;25(3):473–87. https://doi.org/10.1016/j.chc.2016.03.002.
61. Hayhurst CJ, Durieux ME. Differential opioid tolerance and opioid-induced hyperalgesia. Anesthesiol. 2016;124(2):483–8. https://doi.org/10.1097/aln.0000000000000963.
62. Chia Y-Y, Liu K, Wang J-J, Kuo M-C, Ho S-T. Intraoperative high dose fentanyl induces postoperative fentanyl tolerance. Canadian J Anesthesia/J Canadien D'anesthésie. 1999;46(9):872–7. https://doi.org/10.1007/bf03012978.
63. Collard V, Mistraletti G, Taqi A, Asenjo JF, Feldman LS, Fried GM, Carli F. Intraoperative esmolol infusion in the absence of opioids spares postoperative fentanyl in patients undergoing ambulatory laparoscopic cholecystectomy. Anesth Analg. 2007;105(5):1255–62. https://doi.org/10.1213/01.ane.0000282822.07437.02.

64. Shah A, Hayes CJ, Martin BC. Characteristics of initial prescription episodes and likelihood of long-term opioid use—United States, 2006–2015. MMWR. Morbid Mortal Weekly Rep. 2017;66(10):265–69. https://doi.org/10.15585/mmwr.mm6610a1
65. American Society of Anesthesiologists Task Force on Preanesthesia Evaluation; Pasternak LR, Arens JF, Caplan RA, Connis RT, Fleisher LA, Flowerdew R, Gold BS, Mayhew JF, Nickinovich DG, Rice LJ, Roizen MF, Twersky RS. Practice advisory for preanesthesia evaluation: an updated report by the American society of anesthesiologists task force on preanesthesia evaluation. Anesthesiology. 2012;116(3):522–38.
66. Barreveld A, Mendelson A, Deiling B, Armstrong C, Viscusi E, Kohan L. Caring for our patients with opioid use disorder in the perioperative period: a guide for the anesthesiologists [Review of Caring for Our Patients with Opioid Use Disorder in the Perioperative Period: A Guide for the Anesthesiologists] 2023.
67. Kohan L, Potru S, Barreveld AM, Sprintz M, Lane O, Aryal A, Emerick T, Dopp A, Chhay S, Viscusi E. Buprenorphine management in the perioperative period: educational review and recommendations from a multisociety expert panel. Reg Anesth Pain Med. 2021;46(10):840–59. https://doi.org/10.1136/rapm-2021-103007.
68. Zhao S, Chen F, Feng A, Han W, Zhang Y. Risk factors and prevention strategies for postoperative opioid abuse. Pain Res Manag. 2019;2019:1–12. https://doi.org/10.1155/2019/7490801.
69. Meyer LA, Lasala J, Iniesta MD, Nick AM, Munsell MF, Shi Q, Wang XS, Cain KE, Lu KH, Ramirez PT. Effect of an enhanced recovery after surgery program on opioid use and patient-reported outcomes. Obstet Gynecol. 2018;132(2):281–90. https://doi.org/10.1097/AOG.0000000000002735.
70. Fleischman AN, Tarabichi M, Foltz C, Makar G, Hozack WJ, Austin MS, Chen AF. Cluster-Randomized trial of opiate-sparing analgesia after discharge from elective hip surgery etable 1. Int Committ Med J Edit Data Shar State J Am Coll Surg 2019;229(4):335–345e5. https://doi.org/10.1016/j.jamcollsurg.2019.05.026
71. Sordo L, Barrio G, Bravo MJ, Indave BI, Degenhardt L, Wiessing L, Ferri M, Pastor-Barriuso R. Mortality risk during and after opioid substitution treatment: systematic review and meta-analysis of cohort studies. BMJ. 2017;357: j1550. https://doi.org/10.1136/bmj.j1550.
72. Mojtabai R, Mauro C, Wall MM, Barry CL, Olfson M. Medication treatment for opioid use disorders in substance use treatment facilities. Health Aff. 2019;38(1):14–23. https://doi.org/10.1377/hlthaff.2018.05162.
73. PL 117–328: Consolidated Appropriations Act, 2023 | Food and Nutrition Service. (n.d.). Retrieved 19 Mar 2023, https://www.fns.usda.gov/pl-117-328
74. Ward EN, Quaye AN-A, Wilens TE. Opioid use disorders. Anesth Analg. 2018;127(2):539–47. https://doi.org/10.1213/ane.0000000000003477.
75. Harrison TK, Kornfeld H, Aggarwal AK, Lembke A. Perioperative considerations for the patient with opioid use disorder on buprenorphine, methadone, or naltrexone maintenance therapy. Anesthesiol Clin. 2018;36(3):345–59. https://doi.org/10.1016/j.anclin.2018.04.002.

The Implications of the Opioid Epidemic for the Treatment of Perioperative Pain

Nan Xiang, Denise Courtney, Shivana Ramsingh, Rebecca Donald, and Sudheer Potru

Abstract The opioid epidemic in the United States and around the world has significant implications for the use of opioids in the management of acute and chronic pain. The perioperative period is often the initial exposure to opioids for many patients and may be an inflection point for particularly vulnerable patients. Adjusting expectations and consistent messaging from the surgical, anesthesiology, nursing, and other teams when appropriate is likely to result in the best outcomes for the patient.

Keywords Opioid crisis · Opioid epidemic · Fentanyl · Substance use disorder · Addiction · Overdose

1 Introduction

The opioid epidemic, declared a U.S. public health emergency in 2017, refers to a modern crisis involving substantially increased rates of misuse, abuse, and overdose deaths attributed to the opioid class of drugs. Since 1999, the United States has experienced an estimated one million deaths from drug overdoses, the majority of which involve opioids and, more recently, specifically fentanyl [1]. With over 10,0000

N. Xiang · S. Potru (✉)
Department of Anesthesiology, Emory University, Atlanta, GA, USA
e-mail: sudheer.potru@emory.edu; sudheer.potru@emory.edu

N. Xiang
e-mail: nan.xiang@emory.edu

D. Courtney
Atlanta VA Healthcare System, Decatur, GA, USA
e-mail: denise.courtney@va.gov

S. Ramsingh
University of West Indies, St. Augustine, Trinidad and Tobago

R. Donald
Department of Anesthesiology, Vanderbilt University, Nashville, TN, USA
e-mail: rebecca.donald@vumc.org

A. Abd-Elsayed and K. Schroeder (eds.), *Perioperative Pain Management*,
https://doi.org/10.1007/978-3-031-67648-2_4

deaths annually, drug overdose is now the number one cause of unintentional death in the U.S. and has contributed to an unprecedented decline in life expectancy [2–4]. In addition to the impact on mortality, consequences of the opioid epidemic include (1) rising rates of human immunodeficiency virus (HIV) and hepatitis C virus (HCV) infections; (2) escalating rates of perinatal morbidity and mortality; and (3) an estimated one trillion dollars in financial burden to the U.S. economy [5–9].

In this chapter, we seek to explain the origins of the opioid epidemic in the United States, review the evolution of the epidemic itself, discuss mitigation strategies, and describe perioperative evidence-based patient management in the current prescribing environment.

Background of the Opioid Epidemic

While the opioid epidemic clearly has numerous causes, the origin story for this crisis can largely be traced back to a series of events beginning in the 1990s. In 1996, Purdue Pharma utilized already-existing extended-release medication technology to bring to market a high-dose oxycodone product known as OxyContin. Although oxycodone was an old drug, the approval of this new formulation was based on the Food and Drug Administration's assessment that OxyContin's delayed absorption reduced the potential for eventual opioid abuse. Upon approval, Purdue began an aggressive marketing campaign that resulted in billions of dollars in revenue for the company and a flood of prescription opioids into communities [10]. Citing narrowly focused medical literature to increase drug sales, Purdue claimed that OxyContin was safe and effective for chronic pain, with little addiction potential [10]. Purdue's assertion that OxyContin was largely nonaddictive was based on a New England Journal of Medicine letter to the editor published in 1980 by physicians from Boston University Medical Center; this brief letter summarized findings of a non-peer-reviewed, retrospective study evaluating 1,1882 hospitalized patients that received at least one dose of an opioid medication while admitted [10, 11]. The review found that only four patients who received an opioid became addicted, leading the authors to conclude that 'the development of addiction is rare in medical patients with no history of addiction" [11]. Similarly, Purdue's significant push to expand opioid use for chronic nonmalignant pain was based on a retrospective review of just 38 patients that concluded opioid therapy to be a "safe, salutary, and more humane" option for treating chronic pain [12]. Purdue later pled guilty to felony misbranding and violating federal anti-kickback laws for making false claims related to OxyContin and paying physicians to write more and higher-dose OxyContin prescriptions [13].

Until the early 2000s, opioids were primarily being used to treat acute pain, but rates of opioid prescribing for chronic noncancer pain began to increase substantially; in 2012, the national opioid dispensing rate peaked at 255 million prescriptions [14, 15]. Aggressive pharmaceutical marketing and increased focus on the treatment of uncontrolled pain in the medical community (including the pain as the "fifth vital sign" initiative) resulted in widespread acceptance for the use of opioids for non-cancer pain [10, 16]. Lack of standardization of curriculum and training for physicians in the areas of pain management and substance use disorders (SUDs) may have contributed to expanded opioid prescribing.

However, the opioid epidemic is certainly a result of a multisystem failure. Many rural and socioeconomically disadvantaged communities experienced challenges with access to specialty pain management care, as well as poverty and mental health comorbidities, making them particularly vulnerable to opioid use. Prescription opioids often entered these communities at unprecedented rates through "pill mills" run by unscrupulous clinicians and entrepreneurs as well as true illicit drug dealers. Clinicians at these facilities across the country prescribed and dispensed hundreds of thousands of opioid tablets without standard workup or physical exam, and sometimes without even having seen the patient at all [17]. Although law enforcement became increasingly aware of the contributors to opioid abuse and diversion, physicians practicing medicine and writing prescriptions was considered outside of the purview of traditional law enforcement [18]. In recent years, the pharmaceutical distributors that shipped millions of opioid pills to pill mills have faced lawsuits for failure to monitor and report suspicious orders [19].

Characteristics of the United States health care system played a role in the rise of the opioid crisis as healthcare facilities commonly rely on volume-based care rather than value-based care for revenue. Furthermore, prescription opioids are often more financially accessible than other pain treatments like physical therapy, interventional procedures, or other non-medication-based treatment modalities [20]. Many prescription drug plans cover common opioids but either provide limited coverage or require prior authorization for less addictive pain medications, interventional procedures, or medications used to treat opioid use disorder [20, 21]. Also exacerbating the ongoing crisis was pharmaceutical industry influence on lawmakers, federal regulatory bodies, professional medical organizations, and patients through direct-to-consumer advertising, as well as American socioeconomic and cultural factors, including the so-called "pill for every ill" mentality [22]. Now, with over two million Americans currently diagnosed with opioid use disorder, the opioid epidemic is ongoing and continues to evolve [23].

Evolution of the Opioid Epidemic

The opioid epidemic has emerged in waves distinguished by the types of opioids contributing to overdose deaths. The first wave, which began around 1996, was dominated by prescription opioids. The abundance of prescription opioids facilitated their illegal distribution and non-medical use; between 1992 and 2003 the number of people misusing prescription drugs increased by 90% [24, 25]. Opioid-related deaths paralleled this increase in both medical and nonmedical use of prescribed opioids; in 2007, commonly prescribed opioids were involved in 78% of opioid overdose deaths [26]. As previously noted, the total number of opioid prescriptions dispensed peaked at more than 260 million in 2012, but from 2012 to 2021, the rates of opioid prescribing decreased in all 50 states with a national decrease of 46.4% during this time period [27]. Despite this decrease, prescription opioids still played a prominent role in opioid overdose deaths, but the percentage of deaths involving only prescription opioids gradually fell with increasing rates of heroin and fentanyl use [26].

The second wave of the opioid epidemic was marked by the transition to heroin, an illicitly produced semisynthetic opioid derived from the opium poppy, beginning roughly around 2010. As deaths attributable to opioids began to rise in the early 2000s, state and federal laws were passed with the intention of reducing supply, demand, and harm of prescribed opioids [25]. The National All Schedules Prescription Electronic Reporting (NASPER) Act was passed in 2005, which provided for the establishment of prescription drug monitoring programs (PDMPs) in each state [24]. PDMPs led to greater vigilance about possible opioid misuse, doctor shopping, or prescription opioid diversion and further curbed opioid prescribing. According to a study by Dowell et al., the combination of more restrictive prescribing laws and increasing use of PDMPs led to the reduction in opioid prescriptions by 8% and prescription overdose deaths by 12% from 2006 to 2013 [28].

In addition to the development of PDMPs and the passage of legislation creating greater restrictions and scrutiny related to opioid prescribing, other measures were taken to bring greater attention to the dangers of prescription opioids. In 2011, the Centers for Disease Control (CDC) declared deaths from prescription opioids an "epidemic." This was followed in 2012 with the development of a new "Policy Academy" by the American Medical Association to address the growing problem of prescription opioids [27]. Finally, in 2016, the initial CDC Guideline for Prescribing Opioids for Chronic Pain was published. The stated goal of these guidelines was to provide guidance about responsible opioid prescribing for primary care providers who may not have had formal training in pain management or addiction medicine. In the wake of this publication, however, many states passed additional laws to limit the supply of opioids. In addition, limitations on opioid prescriptions by pharmacies and insurers have created additional pressure on clinicians to stop or avoid prescribing opioids [20]. While there was likely a benefit realized from reducing the number of opioid pills in circulation, many patients treated with opioids for years and/or decades were (and have been) left searching for other clinicians to prescribe their medications.

Unfortunately, the ongoing demand for and reduced availability of prescription opioids coincided with the influx of heroin into the United States from international markets. Heroin also saw a dramatic decrease in price during this time, making it easier to access and cheaper to obtain than other illicit prescription opioids [25]. The increasing ease of access to a more potent yet cheaper opioid prompted many users of prescription opioids to transition to heroin as their drug of choice [20]. A study by Cerdá and colleagues found that those with a history of prescription opioid misuse were 13 times more likely to start using heroin than those who had no history of prescription opioid misuse [29]. As heroin began to dominate the illicit opioid market, deaths involving heroin also began to rise; from 2010 to 2017, deaths involving heroin increased **fivefold**. The percentage of opioid deaths involving heroin peaked at 41% in 2015, but even while the percentage of deaths involving heroin decreased, the overall number of deaths involving heroin continued to increase. It was only after 2017 that deaths involving heroin finally began to decline [26].

The United States entered the third and most deadly wave of the opioid epidemic around 2013, when synthetic opioids began to dominate the illicit drug market. As previously discussed, synthetic opioids, particularly fentanyl, began to gradually supplant heroin as the predominant illicit opioid for several reasons. First, fentanyl can be produced inexpensively in a lab from chemicals that are both easy to obtain and not tightly regulated abroad; Mexico remains the primary source of illicit fentanyl with many of the requisite chemicals being purchased from China. Second, since fentanyl is 50 to 100 times as potent as heroin, smaller quantities can be transported, so the drug is more easily smuggled and distributed [25]. In addition, there is a large online market for illicit drugs, facilitating the purchase of unregulated opioids [30] (Fig. 1).

The increased potency of fentanyl and its related compounds has undoubtedly contributed to the dramatic rise in opioid overdose deaths during the opioid epidemic. With the ever-changing landscape of the illicit opioid market, the content and potency of illicit drugs have become unpredictable, making it at times impossible for users to know what they are consuming. According to the 2021 DEA Fentanyl Profiling Programming Report, the purity of the 666 fentanyl powder samples (representing more than 778 kg of drug) analyzed ranged from 0.1 to 75.6% with an average purity of 14.4%. The fentanyl content of the pressed pills (commonly marketed by drug dealers as oxycodone, OxyContin, or Percocet) also varies significantly, with the average amount of fentanyl increasing from 1.3 mg/tablet in 2017 to 2.2 mg/tablet in 2022 [31]. Finally, opioid deaths are being increasingly attributed to synthetic fentanyl analogs whose chemical structure can easily be manipulated to evade detection by law enforcement. The potency of these compounds varies significantly. From

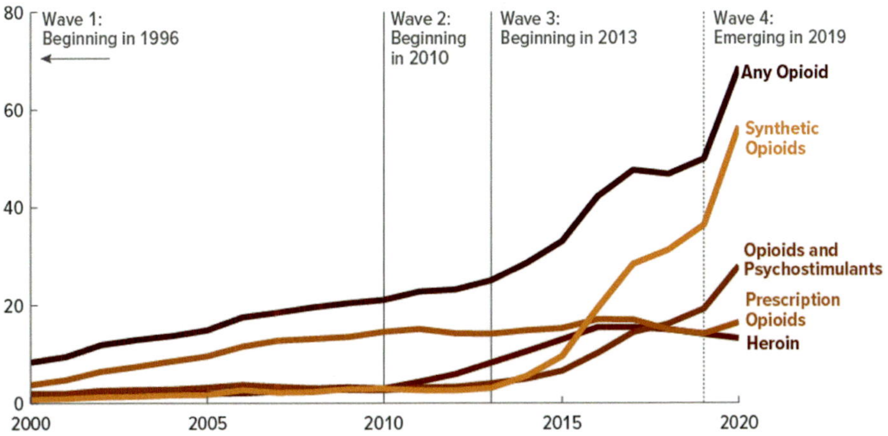

Fig. 1 The Waves of the Opioid Epidemic. https://www.cbo.gov/publication/58532

2019 to 2020, deaths involving synthetic opioids increased by over 56% and in 2020, synthetic opioids were involved in over 82% of opioid-involved deaths. This represents an 18-fold increase from the number of deaths involving synthetic opioids in 2013; users are caught unaware of fentanyl's potency and many have suffered unintentional overdoses [1].

A fourth wave of the opioid epidemic appears to be emerging at the time of this writing, as synthetic opioids are increasingly used in combination with psychostimulants such as methamphetamines or cocaine as well as other CNS depressants such as xylazine, an alpha-2-agonist utilized primarily as a tranquilizer in animals [32]. Some individuals intentionally combine opioids with stimulants to not only enhance the euphoria from the opioids but also to counteract what some perceive as the unpleasant effects of opioids [32]. Other users unwittingly consume combination drugs, as synthetic opioids and stimulants are increasingly combined by drug dealers or suppliers [25]. Not only do deaths due to psychostimulants in combination with synthetic opioids continue to rise, but deaths attributable to stimulants alone have also been steadily rising; overdose deaths due to psychostimulants alone increased 2.3-fold from 2015 to 2020 [33].

The Impact of COVID-19 on the Opioid Epidemic

The death rate during the third wave of the opioid epidemic saw an inflection point in the spring of 2020 coinciding with the start of the COVID-19 pandemic. From December 2019 to December 2020, more than 9,3000 Americans died of drug overdoses, which was an increase of 29.4% from the prior 12 months [34]. First, the increased stress and isolation from the pandemic led to an increase in substance use, both in quantity and frequency of use. According to the CDC, by June 2020, 13% of Americans reported starting or increasing substance use as a way to cope with the stress of the pandemic [35]. Escalating use in isolation due to social distancing, the increased potency of illicit opioids, and reduced access to harm reduction (including safe injection sites, medical practitioners, and medications for OUD) likely contributed to the escalation in opioid overdose deaths.

For patients with opioid use disorder (OUD) who were already in treatment, disruptions in care, particularly access to FDA-approved medications for OUD (methadone, buprenorphine, and naltrexone) and mental health services contributed to risk of relapse and overdose deaths for this vulnerable and marginalized patient population. Additionally, for this patient population that relies heavily on social support for recovery, the isolation from the pandemic proved particularly detrimental [36].

While the COVID-19 pandemic compounded the challenges of the opioid epidemic, it also led to implementation of several policies that positively impacted the trajectory of OUD care. This included easier access to care and initiation of MOUD treatment with buprenorphine via telehealth without the requirement of performing an in-person visit. Additionally, many Opioid Treatment Programs (OTPs, also known as methadone clinics), which usually require daily visits for methadone dispensing, allowed patients on a stable treatment regimen to obtain 14–28 days of medication at a time and several have continued this practice for stable patients. Finally, the increasing use of virtual meetings by groups such as Alcoholics Anonymous and Narcotics Anonymous provided social and emotional support for those who rely on community social support for recovery [36].

Measures to Mitigate the Opioid Crisis

On October 26th, 2017, the Department of Health and Human Services (HHS), noting the escalating numbers of overdose deaths, declared the opioid crisis a national public health emergency (NPHE) in the United States of America; this was later extended several times and is ongoing [37]. Legislation related to the opioid crisis includes the Comprehensive Addiction and Recovery Act (CARA, 2016), the 21st Century CURES Act (2016), the Substance Use-Disorder Prevention that Promotes Opioid Recovery and Treatment (SUPPORT) for Patients and Communities Act (2018), the Opioid Crisis Response Act (2018), the more recent State Opioid Response Grant Authorization Act (2022), and the Medication Access and Training Expansion Act (MATE, 2022).

While addressing the specifics of each law would make this chapter excessively long and is likely out of the scope of this text, these statutes effectively are attempting to do the following [38–41]:

1. Provide improved education to teenagers and parents regarding the dangers of opioids (and other drugs) by expanding prevention programs.
2. Improve social and educational programs to support reduction of stigma related to SUDs and SUD care as well as promote recovery programs and strategies.
3. Increase access to harm reduction strategies such as syringe exchange programs and safe injection sites.
4. Improve access to MOUD treatment, including requiring Medicaid coverage of methadone, buprenorphine, and naltrexone. The CARA and SUPPORT statutes also initially expanded of the scope of practice of multiple practitioners to prescribe buprenorphine; however, the MATE Act ultimately resulted in elimination of the so-called “X-waiver”, removing patient caps and limitations from buprenorphine to improve access as well.
5. Strengthen state prescription drug monitoring programs to include more substances as well as to link to other states’ PDMP programs to provide comprehensive prescribing information.

6. Expand access to naloxone, which is now over-the-counter as of early 2023(43).
7. Educate health care practitioners about the care of patients with SUDs.
8. Increase funding for trial and state opioid response efforts.
9. Increase funding to law enforcement agencies to provide more robust resources to stop the flow of illicit drugs across the U.S. borders.
10. Improve criminal justice reform, including expansion of drug courts, to reduce penalties and promote recovery for SUDs.

Perioperative Consequences of the Opioid Epidemic

It behooves the anesthesiologist and pain physician to understand the consequences of opioid use, including opioid-induced constipation, nausea and vomiting, depression, worsening of sleep apnea, decreased cognitive function, and development of tolerance and physical dependence [43]. Chronic use can also lead to the development of opioid use disorder (OUD), the desire to obtain and take opioids (either prescribed or illicit) without regard to personal, social, or professional consequences [44]. According to the CDC, an estimated quarter of all patients receiving long-term opioid therapy in a primary care setting suffer from OUD [45].

Chronic opioid use also impacts the post-operative period. Multiple studies have shown an association between preoperative chronic opioid use and increased postoperative complications, increased healthcare utilization such as length of hospital stay or discharge to a rehabilitation facility, and delayed recovery and wound healing; these associations occurred in various surgical specialties, including but not limited to elective abdominal surgery, foot and ankle surgery, total knee and hip arthroplasty, and posterior lumbar fusion for degenerative spine disease [46–49]. In fact, in a retrospective study by Santosa 2020, patients who had been classified with "medium" and "high" preoperative opioid use –which was based on oral morphine equivalents and duration of ongoing opioid therapy –were found to have increased postoperative mortality compared to the opioid naïve control group [50]. Nadarajah et al. found that patients undergoing shoulder surgery with preoperative opioid prescriptions appear to experience higher levels of postoperative pain, decreased function, and decreased satisfaction [51]. Waljee et al. found that chronic opioid use was associated with longer hospital length of stay, hospital readmission, and increased financial costs for care [46].

While preoperative opioid use appears to be associated with negative outcomes in the postoperative period, one must also consider how undergoing a surgical procedure can potentially contribute to chronic opioid use. The impetus to completely eliminate postoperative pain due to both social and marketing determinants may have resulted in the exposure of many opioid-naïve patients to high opioid regimens postoperatively. Compounding the situation is the lack of an established workflow for guiding patients from acute perioperative pain management to outpatient chronic pain management.

In a landmark study, Brummett et. al examined over 3,6000 opioid-naïve patients who had undergone "major" and "minor" surgeries between 2012 and 2015 and found that 6.5% of the major surgery patients and 5.9% of the minor surgery patients were still filling opioid prescriptions between 90 and 180 days postoperatively [52]. There was not a statistical difference between the major and minor surgery groups; patient risk factors for persistent postoperative opioid use included tobacco use, alcohol and other SUDs, anxiety, depression, and preoperative pain disorders such as back pain and centralized pain. Notably, the number of oral morphine equivalents prescribed, was also associated with an increased rate of persistent postoperative opioid use, though the authors note the overall effect size was small. This and other studies support the existence of modifiable patient factors that seem to predominantly contribute to the risk of persistent postoperative opioid use, while the predicted or actual magnitude of surgical pain does not appear to be a major differentiator [52, 53].

Other retrospective cohort studies have shown similar findings. Clarke et. al found that approximately 3.1% of a total of 3,9000 opioid-naïve patients in Canada from 2003 to 2010 were still receiving opioid medications more than 90 days following surgery [54]. Alam's 2012 retrospective cohort study in Canada demonstrated that opioid-naïve patients undergoing short-stay surgery were 44% more likely to become long-term opioid users within 1 year if they received an opioid prescription within 7 days after surgery [55]. Not surprisingly, preoperative opioid use is associated with longer duration of postoperative opioid use, with studies reporting 64–77% of chronic opioid users continuing to fill opioid prescriptions several months after surgery [53]. More than 20% of patients arriving for elective surgery are already taking opioids, a sizable portion of the surgical patient population [53].

In summary, opioid-naïve patients are at risk of developing persistent postoperative opioid use while individuals already on chronic opioids are also unable to consistently wean from their opioid regimens following surgery, even if these surgeries may be improving their underlying pain generators. This suggests that the surgical procedure is often an inflection point adding to the population of patients on chronic opioids. A combination of patient risk factors (some modifiable), perioperative management, and postoperative opioid prescribing practices may play a significant role in this process.

Preoperative

The first "intervention" point is at the time of surgical procedure scheduling, with identification of patients who may be at increased risk for persistent postoperative opioid use. As previously noted, there are multiple patient characteristics that increase such risk, and established questionnaires such as the Opioid Risk Tool (ORT) aim to use self-reported data to predict the risk of opioid misuse. However, recent studies suggest that revisions to the ORT may be needed to maintain their validity and its applicability to the postoperative period is unclear [56–58].

2 Opioid Risk Tool—OUD (ORT–OUD) [58]

This tool should be administered to patients upon an initial visit prior to beginning or continuing opioid therapy for pain management. A score of 2 or lower indicates low risk for future opioid use disorder; a score of >/= 3 indicates high risk for opioid use disorder.

Revised Opioid Risk Tool

Category	Yes	No
Personal history of illicit drug use [1]		
Personal history of alcohol misuse [1]		
Personal history of prescription drug misuse [1]		
Family history of illicit drug use [1]		
Family history of alcohol misuse [1]		
Family history of prescription drug misuse [1]		
Age between 16 and 45 years old [1]		
History of depression [1]		
History of ADHD, OCD, bipolar disorder, schizophrenia [1]		
Total		

Adapted from Cheatle et al. [58].

For patients at increased risk for persistent opioid use (and those for whom increased or chronic opioid use could potentially be harmful), it is important to provide appropriate expectations for severity of postoperative pain, as Waljee et al. have shown that appropriate analgesic expectations correlated with lower reported postoperative pain [59]. Additionally, a discussion about non-opioid therapies for analgesia as well as the expected course for postoperative recovery can be beneficial. Furthermore, in patients with a history of chronic pain and on chronic opioid therapy, care coordination with their prescribing physician is essential. A clear roadmap for timely follow-up with the surgeon to assess appropriate recovery as well as a return visit for the patient's prescribing physician can provide clarity and reassurance. For at-risk patients without a chronic pain practitioner, discussion of a possible postoperative consultation with a pain specialist may be appropriate. While addressed in other areas of this text, a similar approach can be taken with patients suffering from substance use disorders. For SUD patients, close collaboration between the surgical, anesthesia, and SUD treatment teams is likely to improve the rate of follow-up as well as outcomes [60].

In patients on chronic opioids, a discussion should be held regarding potential tapering of the regimen prior to surgery. While tapering strategies vary, one study recommends a reduction 10% per week over multiple weeks with collaboration between the surgical, anesthesia, and primary care or pain management services [61]. A small study evaluating the effects of preoperative reduction of opioids on patients undergoing total knee or hip arthroplasty found that a 50% reduction preoperatively resulted in improvements in multiple activity indices (compared to patients who did not taper); furthermore, this study showed similar outcomes between individuals who weaned opioids and the patients who were opioid naïve [62]. In a retrospective cohort study by Jain, where chronic opioid users (defined as having used > 5000 oral morphine equivalents over the previous year) were stratified based on timing of their most recent prescription, those with the longest abstinence from opioids prior to spine surgery showed significantly lower risk of long-term postoperative opioid use [63]. Notably, however, risks associated with weaning can include increased use of illicit substances, depression and suicidality, and risk of overdose [64]. Additionally, the importance of ensuring patient buy-in regarding the perioperative process, managing expectations, and ensuring perioperative pain control cannot be overstated.

Perioperative/Intraoperative

Intraoperatively, several care areas may influence post-operative opioid use. Several specialties have worked to develop enhanced recovery after surgery (ERAS) protocols, which focus on improving perioperative care, minimizing complications, and accelerating recovery [65]. Multimodal analgesia and the implementation of regional anesthesia can help to minimize the adverse effects of opioid medications in the recovery process.

The use of opioid-sparing pain regimens has become increasingly commonplace in the perioperative realm. Commonly used medications include acetaminophen, non-steroidal anti-inflammatory drugs (NSAIDs) such as ibuprofen and celecoxib, neuropathic medications such as gabapentin and pregabalin, intravenous alpha-2 adrenergic agonists such as dexmedetomidine and clonidine, as well as intravenous N-methyl-D-aspartate (NMDA) antagonists such as ketamine [66, 67]. Incidentally, there are no data to demonstrate that use of fentanyl near the start of a general anesthetic to either treat "pain" or blunt the response to sympathetic stimulation resulting from laryngoscopy has any bearing on postoperative opioid use.

The data behind opioid-free anesthetic plans is less clear. Opioid-free regimens often involve the use of dexmedetomidine, lidocaine, and/or ketamine infusions. In a Cochrane meta-analysis of 23 trials related to use of intravenous lidocaine infusion, there was not clear evidence of improved pain scores, early gastrointestinal recovery, postoperative nausea, or opioid consumption with the therapy [68]. The use of dexmedetomidine infusions is similarly unclear with some studies showing decreased pain scores and opioid use in the first 24 hour, along with decreased nausea/vomiting, though other studies showed no difference in opioid use while also observing bradycardia and hypotension [66, 69, 70]. Several meta-analyses were performed that attempted to elucidate the benefits of intravenous ketamine. Laskowski showed a reduction of total opioid consumption in patients who received intravenous ketamine boluses or infusions, particularly in thoracic, upper abdominal, and major orthopedic surgical groups, with a noted improvement in postoperative nausea and vomiting but an increased incidence of hallucinations and nightmares [71]. Jouguelet-Lacoste evaluated 5 meta-analyses and 39 clinical trials that showed use of low-dose ketamine infusions defined as less than 1.2 mg/kg/hr reduced postoperative opioid consumption by 40%, while no reports of major complications in the first 48 hour [72]. Lastly, Klatt's systematic review and meta-analysis found insufficient evidence to support a reduction in chronic pain with perioperative ketamine use [73].

Another common aspect of a multimodal anesthetic plan is the usage of regional anesthesia techniques, which has increased over the past decade. Regional anesthesia encompasses neuraxial blockade or peripheral nerve blockade. For many surgical specialties regional anesthesia remains a key component of the multi-modal analgesia plan, including orthopedic joint surgery, ERAS protocols for abdominal surgeries such as sleeve gastrectomy and the procedure-specific postoperative pain management (PROSPECT) guidelines for thoracic surgery and elective caesarean section [66, 67, 74, 75].

Regional anesthesia was associated with improved pain scores and decreased opioid use, primarily in hip replacement surgery, periarticular elbow surgery, and tibial plateau fracture surgery, although these small retrospective studies do not extend past three months postoperatively [76–78]. In contrast, there are numerous studies that do not show a significant effect of regional anesthesia on postoperative opioid use. Munsch et al. studied the effects of regional anesthesia for hip arthroscopy, which took the form of L1/L2 nerve root blocks or pericapsular nerve group (PENG) block targeting the articular branches of the femoral and obturator nerves for the hip joint [79]. The study found no significant differences in postoperative opioid prescription, opioid refill requests, or number of pain-related phone calls or office encounters. Trasolini et al. studied the effect of regional anesthesia for shoulder arthroscopic procedures, finding no significant difference in the patterns of filled postoperative opioid prescriptions between those who received a nerve block and those who did not. However, among preoperative opioid users, there was a statistically significant decrease of opioid prescription filling in the first two weeks postoperatively in the group who received a nerve block [80]. In another study by Cunningham, the use of regional anesthesia for surgical fixation of pelvic and acetabular fractures actually showed an association with an increase in inpatient and outpatient opioid use [81].

Regardless of specific interventions, a multimodal approach using both opioid and non-opioid medications is ideal for providing postoperative analgesia. Regional nerve blocks certainly have a role as well, although their impact on postoperative opioid use is equivocal. Involvement of a dedicated acute pain service, particularly for patients noted to be at increased risk for postoperative opioid use with history of OUD, is a good starting point in optimizing perioperative pain care.

With respect to patients with a history of OUD, care is needed to avoid overprescription of opioids that may place the patient at risk for relapse balanced with the need to achieve adequate pain control; uncontrolled pain itself can result in relapse. If the patient is already treated with medications for OUD, such as buprenorphine or methadone, the current expert opinion is to maintain these medications in the perioperative period. For buprenorphine, the recommendations from the Multi-Society

Working Group on opioid use disorder are generally to continue the preoperative dose through the perioperative period [60]. Additional strategies in the perioperative period include (1) splitting the doses into two or three doses per day for improved analgesic effect; (2) potentially increasing above preoperative doses in the setting of severe pain; and (3) adding short-acting full mu-opioid agonists, non-opioid medications, regional anesthesia techniques, as well as non-pharmacologic interventions such as ice packs, positioning, relaxation techniques, and psychosocial support [60]. Kohan et al. recommend continuing methadone at the patient's usual dose, while supplementing with additional mu-opioid agonists. Typically, methadone is delivered as a single daily dose in an opioid treatment program; however, the single dose can be divided into three times per day dosing for improved analgesia. Maintenance of OUD medications can help avoid cravings, decrease the risk of relapse, and help transition back to an appropriate outpatient regimen at discharge.

Postoperative

Surgeons, anesthesiologists, primary care physicians, and pain specialists all have responsibilities in the postoperative period, including monitoring the healing process, assessing for the adequacy of pain control, monitoring pain medication use with a mindset toward gradual tapering of opioids, and consideration of safer pain control options if needed.

One the initial inflection points in post-operative pain management is the selection of a regimen appropriate for the procedure. There has been evidence to suggest that the amount of opioids prescribed can be significantly decreased from historical practices without compromising pain scores or patient satisfaction [53]. Subsequent follow-up is needed with the patient to monitor pain symptoms and encourage gradual weaning and (hopefully) eventual cessation of opioids. A standardized weaning schedule may be challenging to apply for all patients, but it may be helpful as a starting point and as a means to guide discussion and expectations. In a randomized controlled trial, Hah et al. investigated the efficacy of motivational-interviewing (MI) along with guided opioid tapering for a group of patients undergoing total knee and hip arthroplasty [82]. The intervention for the MI-Opioid Taper consisted of a scheduled 25% opioid dose reduction every seven days coupled with weekly phone calls made by a pain physician that reviewed medication adherence, reviewed response to medication, advised on opioid weaning, provided support for the patient's efforts, provided education on pain management and drug misuse, and discussed over-utilization of opioids if applicable. The results of the MI-Opioid Taper study showed that patients who underwent the motivational interviewing taper as compared to those who did not receive weekly phone calls, had a 62% increase in the rate of return to baseline opioid use, the primary outcome, as well as 53% increase in the rate of complete postoperative opioid cessation (compared to those who did not) [82].

One important aspect of postoperative care for patients is an emphasis on collaboration across specialties. If continued opioid prescriptions past several months postoperatively are requested, this is often referred to a primary care physician or a chronic pain specialist. For patients without a history of chronic pain, establishing care at a new chronic pain clinic can be challenging logistically, whether due to wait times in the scheduling queue, insurance limitations, or local and regional opioid prescribing policies. Without care coordination and preemptive planning, it is possible patients may feel abandoned as they recover from surgery, which should be avoided.

The Perioperative Surgical Home (PSH) is one model that focuses on interdisciplinary collaboration and aims to guide a patient through a surgical process, beginning from the initial decision to undergo surgery and into the recovery and rehabilitation phase post-discharge [83]. Vetter's review of the PSH model notes the need to address inadequate treatment of postoperative pain, to minimize opioid-related side effects, and to improve upon opioid prescribing patterns so as to avoid negative outcomes. One concept of the PSH for the postoperative period is the establishment of a transitional pain service or clinic (TPS), which usually includes a team of pain specialists, internal medicine providers, addiction medicine specialists, mental health providers, licensed social workers, and advanced practice nurses [83]. The goal of the clinic or service is to optimize pain control, wean patients off high-dose opioids, decrease unnecessary readmissions, reduce healthcare costs, and minimize disability related to chronic post-surgical pain.

One of the earliest models for a TPS originated at Toronto General Hospital, which was established in 2014 [84]. The services that were provided included "multimodal medication optimization by anesthesiologists, postsurgical physical therapy and acupuncture, and a pain psychology intervention consisting of pain education, mindfulness training, brief hypnosis, and a form of cognitive–behavioral treatment called acceptance and commitment therapy (ACT)" [84]. There have been two cohort studies investigating the TPS at this institution, with additional randomized controlled trials ongoing. One team studied the effect of ACT on patients at increased risk for chronic postsurgical pain and persistent opioid use; the use of ACT in this cohort showed greater reductions in opioid use, pain interference, and depressed mood as compared to the non-ACT group, despite starting at a higher level for each category [85]. A separate study evaluating opioid consumption in the transitional pain clinic found that, at the conclusion of the six month study period, opioid-naïve patients had reduced consumption by 69%, with 46% having completely weaned off; in the opioid-experienced group, opioid use was reduced by 44% and 29% of patients had been completely weaned off [86]. Similar programs have been started at other institutions, which is often dependent upon incentivizing institutional support in the form of improved quality of care and decreased system costs, buy-in from surgeons, and collaboration of providers across multiple disciplines [87].

Key Takeaways

1. While the elements that created the opioid epidemic are multifactorial, its impacts on American society and healthcare as a whole have been profound and continue to reverberate.
2. While surgery remains a launching point for chronic opioid use and OUD in some, multidisciplinary teams can play a major role in significantly reducing the likelihood of a poor outcome.
3. Setting reasonable expectations for pain and opioid use in the perioperative period is critical to ensure medication stewardship and appropriate taper or discontinuation of opioids.

References

1. Synthetic Opioid Overdose Data | Drug Overdose | CDC Injury Center [Internet]. https://www.cdc.gov/drugoverdose/deaths/synthetic/index.html. Cited 25 Dec 2022
2. Products—Vital Statistics Rapid Release—Provisional Drug Overdose Data [Internet]. Available from: https://www.cdc.gov/nchs/nvss/vsrr/drug-overdose-data.htm. Cited 25 Dec 2022
3. Odds of Dying—Data Details—Injury Facts [Internet]. https://injuryfacts.nsc.org/all-injuries/preventable-death-overview/odds-of-dying/data-details/. Cited 14 Sep 2022
4. Dowell D, Arias E, Kochanek K, Anderson R, Guy GPJ, Losby JL, et al. Contribution of opioid-involved poisoning to the change in life expectancy in the United States, 2000–2015. JAMA. 2017;318(11):1065–7.
5. Hodder SL, Feinberg J, Strathdee SA, Shoptaw S, Altice FL, Ortenzio L, et al. The opioid crisis and HIV in the USA: deadly synergies. Lancet Lond Engl. 2021;397(10279):1139–50.
6. Suryaprasad AG, White JZ, Xu F, Eichler BA, Hamilton J, Patel A, et al. Emerging epidemic of hepatitis C virus infections among young nonurban persons who inject drugs in the United States, 2006–2012. Clin Infect Dis Off Publ Infect Dis Soc Am. 2014;59(10):1411–9.
7. Whiteman VE, Salemi JL, Mogos MF, Cain MA, Aliyu MH, Salihu HM. Maternal opioid drug use during pregnancy and its impact on perinatal morbidity, mortality, and the costs of medical care in the United States. J Preg. 2014;2014:1–8.
8. Azuine RE, Ji Y, Chang HY, Kim Y, Ji H, DiBari J, et al. Prenatal risk factors and perinatal and postnatal outcomes associated with maternal opioid exposure in an urban, low-income, multiethnic us population. JAMA Netw Open. 2019;2(6): e196405.
9. Florence C, Luo F, Rice K. The economic burden of opioid use disorder and fatal opioid overdose in the United States, 2017. Drug Alcohol Depend. 2021;218: 108350.
10. Van Zee A. The promotion and marketing of oxycontin: commercial triumph, public health tragedy. Am J Public Health. 2009;99(2):221–7.
11. Porter J, Jick H. Addiction rare in patients treated with narcotics. N Engl J Med. 1980;302(2):123.
12. Portenoy RK, Foley KM. Chronic use of opioid analgesics in non-malignant pain: report of 38 cases. Pain. 1986;25(2):171–86.
13. Marks JH. Lessons from corporate influence in the opioid epidemic: toward a norm of separation. J Bioethical Inq. 2020;17(2):173–89.
14. Gray BM, Vandergrift JL, Weng W, Lipner RS, Barnett ML. Clinical knowledge and trends in physicians' prescribing of opioids for new onset back pain, 2009–2017. JAMA Netw Open. 2021;4(7): e2115328.
15. U.S. Opioid Dispensing Rate Maps | Drug Overdose | CDC Injury Center [Internet]. Available from: https://www.cdc.gov/drugoverdose/rxrate-maps/index.html. Cited 14 Sep 2022

16. Morone NE, Weiner DK. Pain as the fifth vital sign: exposing the vital need for pain education. Clin Ther. 2013;35(11):1728–32.
17. Hirsch R. The opioid epidemic: it's time to place blame where it belongs. Mo Med. 2017;114(2):82–90.
18. McGreal C. American overdose: the opioid tragedy in three acts. London: Guardian Faber; 2019.
19. Haffajee RL, Mello MM. Drug companies' liability for the opioid epidemic. N Engl J Med. 2017;377(24):2301–5.
20. DeWeerdt S. Tracing the US opioid crisis to its roots. Nat. 2019;573(7773):S10–2.
21. Amid Opioid Crisis, Insurers Restrict Pricey, Less Addictive Painkillers—ProPublica [Internet]. Available from: https://www.propublica.org/article/insurers-limit-coverage-of-pricey-less-addictive-painkillers. Cited 14 Sep 2022
22. Dasgupta N, Beletsky L, Ciccarone D. Opioid crisis: no easy fix to its social and economic determinants. Am J Public Health. 2018;108(2):182–6.
23. Medications to Treat Opioid Use Disorder Research Report: Overview | NIDA [Internet]. Available from: https://nida.nih.gov/publications/research-reports/medications-to-treat-opioid-addiction/overview. Cited 14 Sep 2022
24. National All Schedules Prescription Electronic Reporting Act (NASPER) [Internet]. Available from: https://www.nasper.org/. Cited 5 Feb 2022
25. The Opioid Crisis and Recent Federal Policy Responses | Congressional Budget Office [Internet]. Available from: https://www.cbo.gov/publication/58221. Cited 22 Dec 2022
26. NIHCM [Internet]. Visualizing the impact of the opioid overdose crisis. Available from: https://nihcm.org/publications/visualizing-the-impact-of-the-opioid-overdose-crisis. Cited 22 Dec 2022
27. AMA Overdose Epidemic Report 2022.pdf [Internet]. Available from: https://www.ama-assn.org/system/files/ama-overdose-epidemic-report.pdf. Cited 22 Dec 2022
28. Dowell D, Zhang K, Noonan RK, Hockenberry JM. Mandatory provider review and pain clinic laws reduce the amounts of opioids prescribed and overdose death rates. Health Aff Proj Hope. 2016;35(10):1876–83.
29. NIHCM [Internet]. Visualizing the impact of the opioid overdose crisis. Available from: https://nihcm.org/publications/visualizing-the-impact-of-the-opioid-overdose-crisis (2022). Cited 22 Dec 2022
30. Jalali MS, Botticelli M, Hwang RC, Koh HK, McHugh RK. The opioid crisis: a contextual, social-ecological framework. Health Res Policy Syst. 2020;18(1):87.
31. CY 2021 Fentanyl Profiling Program (FPP) [Internet]. Available from: https://www.dea.gov/documents/2022/2022-08/2022-08-22/cy-2021-fentanyl-profiling-program-fpp. Cited 25 Dec 2022
32. Donald RR, Patel S, Smith M, Clayton S, Potru S. Common street drug names for the anesthesiologist and pain physician. Reg Anesth Pain Med. 2023;48(7):365–74.
33. Abuse NI on D. National Institute on Drug Abuse. Overdose death rates. Available from: https://nida.nih.gov/research-topics/trends-statistics/overdose-death-rates (2022). Cited 22 Dec 2022
34. A time of crisis for the opioid epidemic in the USA—The Lancet [Internet]. Available from: https://www.thelancet.com/journals/lancet/article/PIIS0140-6736(21)01653-6/fulltext. Cited 5 Feb 2022
35. https://www.apa.org [Internet]. Substance use during the pandemic. Available from: https://www.apa.org/monitor/2021/03/substance-use-pandemic. Cited 5 Feb 2022
36. Abuse NI on D. National Institute on Drug Abuse. COVID-19 & Substance Use. Available from: https://nida.nih.gov/research-topics/comorbidity/covid-19-substance-use (2022). Cited 5 Feb 2022
37. Ongoing emergencies | CMS [Internet]. Available from: https://www.cms.gov/about-cms/what-we-do/emergency-response/current-emergencies/ongoing-emergencies. Cited 15 Sep 2022
38. Three Things to Know About the SUPPORT Act Reauthorization—Opioid Principles [Internet]. Available from: https://opioidprinciples.jhsph.edu/three-things-to-know-about-the-support-act-reauthorization/. Cited 5 Sep 2023

39. The Medication Access and Training Expansion (MATE) Act | ACCME [Internet]. Available from: https://accme.org/mate-act. Cited 15 Sep 2022
40. Five Key Highlights from the Comprehensive Addiction And Recovery Act (CARA) [Internet]. Available from: https://abetterliferecovery.com/comprehensive-addiction-and-recovery-act-cara/. Cited 15 Sep 2023
41. H.R. 2466, State Opioid Response Grant Authorization Act—Congressman David Trone [Internet]. Available from: https://trone.house.gov/h-r-2466/. Cited 15 Sep 2022
42. FDA Approves First Over-the-Counter Naloxone Nasal Spray | FDA [Internet]. Available from: https://www.fda.gov/news-events/press-announcements/fda-approves-first-over-counter-naloxone-nasal-spray. Cited 15 Sep 2022
43. Wang D, Yee BJ, Grunstein RR, Chung F. Chronic opioid use and central sleep apnea, where are we now and where to go? a state of the art review. Anesth Analg. 2021;132(5):1244–53.
44. Strang J, Volkow ND, Degenhardt L, Hickman M, Johnson K, Koob GF, et al. Opioid use disorder. Nat Rev Dis Prim. 2020;6(1):3.
45. Prescription Opioids | Opioids | CDC [Internet]. Available from: https://www.cdc.gov/opioids/basics/prescribed.html. Cited 15 Sep 2022
46. Waljee JF, Cron DC, Steiger RM, Zhong L, Englesbe MJ, Brummett CM. Effect of preoperative opioid exposure on healthcare utilization and expenditures following elective abdominal surgery. Ann Surg. 2017;265(4):715–21.
47. Pagan DN, Hernandez VH, Reddy GB, D'Apuzzo MR. Chronic opioid use independently increases complications and resource utilization after primary total joint arthroplasty. J Arthroplasty. 2023;38(6):1004–9.
48. Ridenour R, Kowalski C, Ba D, Liu G, Bible J, Garner M, et al. Opioid use, perioperative risks, and associated postoperative complications in foot and ankle surgery. Foot Ankle Spec. 2022;15(6):528–35.
49. Jain N, Phillips FM, Weaver T, Khan SN. Preoperative chronic opioid therapy: a risk factor for complications, readmission, continued opioid use and increased costs after one- and two-level posterior lumbar fusion. Spine. 2018;43(19):1331–8.
50. Santosa KB, Lai YL, Oliver JD, Hu HM, Brummett CM, Englesbe MJ, et al. Preoperative opioid use and mortality after minor outpatient surgery. JAMA Surg. 2020;155(12):1169–71.
51. Nadarajah V, Meredith SJ, Jauregui JJ, Smuda MP, Medina S, Gilotra MN, et al. Preoperative opioid use in patients undergoing shoulder surgery. Shoulder Elb. 2021;13(3):248–59.
52. Brummett CM, Waljee JF, Goesling J, Moser S, Lin P, Englesbe MJ, et al. New persistent opioid use after minor and major surgical procedures in US adults. JAMA Surg. 2017;152(6): e170504.
53. Larach DB, Hah JM, Brummett CM. Perioperative opioids, the opioid crisis, and the anesthesiologist. Anesthesiology. 2022;136(4):594–608.
54. Clarke H, Soneji N, Ko DT, Yun L, Wijeysundera DN. Rates and risk factors for prolonged opioid use after major surgery: population based cohort study. BMJ. 2014;348: g1251.
55. Alam A, Gomes T, Zheng H, Mamdani MM, Juurlink DN, Bell CM. Long-term analgesic use after low-risk surgery: a retrospective cohort study. Arch Intern Med. 2012;172(5):425–30.
56. Clark MR, Hurley RW, Adams MCB. Re-assessing the validity of the opioid risk tool in a tertiary academic pain management center population. Pain Med Malden Mass. 2018;19(7):1382–95.
57. Khoury LH, Stephens J, Brown S, Chatha K, Girshfeld S, Lozano Leon JM, et al. Application of risk assessment tools to predict opioid usage after shoulder surgery. JSES Int. 2022;6(5):833–42.
58. Cheatle MD, Compton PA, Dhingra L, Wasser TE, O'Brien CP. Development of the revised opioid risk tool to predict opioid use disorder in patients with chronic nonmalignant pain. J Pain. 2019;20(7):842–51.
59. Waljee J, McGlinn EP, Sears ED, Chung KC. Patient expectations and patient-reported outcomes in surgery: a systematic review. Surgery. 2014;155(5):799–808.
60. Kohan L, Potru S, Barreveld AM, Sprintz M, Lane O, Aryal A, et al. Buprenorphine management in the perioperative period: educational review and recommendations from a multisociety expert panel. Reg Anesth Pain Med. 2021;46(10):840–59.

61. McAnally H. Rationale for and approach to preoperative opioid weaning: a preoperative optimization protocol. Perioper Med Lond Engl. 2017;6:19.
62. Nguyen LCL, Sing DC, Bozic KJ. Preoperative reduction of opioid use before total joint arthroplasty. J Arthroplasty. 2016;31(9 Suppl):282–7.
63. Jain N, Phillips FM, Malik AT, Khan SN. Preoperative opioid weaning before major spinal fusion: simulated data. Real-World Insights Spine. 2021;46(2):80–6.
64. Oliva EM, Bowe T, Manhapra A, Kertesz S, Hah JM, Henderson P, et al. Associations between stopping prescriptions for opioids, length of opioid treatment, and overdose or suicide deaths in US veterans: observational evaluation. BMJ. 2020;m283.
65. Ashok A, Niyogi D, Ranganathan P, Tandon S, Bhaskar M, Karimundackal G, et al. The enhanced recovery after surgery (ERAS) protocol to promote recovery following esophageal cancer resection. Surg Today. 2020;50(4):323–34.
66. Feray S, Lubach J, Joshi GP, Bonnet F, Van de Velde M. PROSPECT guidelines for video-assisted thoracoscopic surgery: a systematic review and procedure-specific postoperative pain management recommendations. Anaesthesia. 2022;77(3):311–25.
67. Li JW, Ma YS, Xiao LK. Postoperative pain management in total knee arthroplasty. Orthop Surg. 2019;11(5):755–61.
68. Weibel S, Jelting Y, Pace NL, Helf A, Eberhart LH, Hahnenkamp K, et al. Continuous intravenous perioperative lidocaine infusion for postoperative pain and recovery in adults. Cochrane Database Syst Rev. 2018;6(6):CD009642.
69. Olausson A, Svensson CJ, Andréll P, Jildenstål P, Thörn SE, Wolf A. Total opioid-free general anaesthesia can improve postoperative outcomes after surgery, without evidence of adverse effects on patient safety and pain management: a systematic review and meta-analysis. Acta Anaesthesiol Scand. 2022;66(2):170–85.
70. Salomé A, Harkouk H, Fletcher D, Martinez V. Opioid-free anesthesia benefit-risk balance: a systematic review and meta-analysis of randomized controlled trials. J Clin Med. 2021;10(10).
71. Laskowski K, Stirling A, McKay WP, Lim HJ. A systematic review of intravenous ketamine for postoperative analgesia. Can J Anaesth J Can Anesth. 2011;58(10):911–23.
72. Jouguelet-Lacoste J, La Colla L, Schilling D, Chelly JE. The use of intravenous infusion or single dose of low-dose ketamine for postoperative analgesia: a review of the current literature. Pain Med Malden Mass. 2015;16(2):383–403.
73. Klatt E, Zumbrunn T, Bandschapp O, Girard T, Ruppen W. Intra- and postoperative intravenous ketamine does not prevent chronic pain: a systematic review and meta-analysis. Scand J Pain. 2015;7(1):42–54.
74. Ibrahim M, Elnabtity AM, Hegab A, Alnujaidi OA, El Sanea O. Combined opioid free and loco-regional anaesthesia enhances the quality of recovery in sleeve gastrectomy done under ERAS protocol: a randomized controlled trial. BMC Anesthesiol. 2022;22(1):29.
75. Roofthooft E, Joshi GP, Rawal N, Van de Velde M. PROSPECT guideline for elective caesarean section: updated systematic review and procedure-specific postoperative pain management recommendations. Anaesthesia. 2021;76(5):665–80.
76. Pascarella G, Costa F, Del Buono R, Pulitanò R, Strumia A, Piliego C, et al. Impact of the pericapsular nerve group (PENG) block on postoperative analgesia and functional recovery following total hip arthroplasty: a randomised, observer-masked, controlled trial. Anaesthesia. 2021;76(11):1492–8.
77. Cunningham DJ, LaRose MA, Zhang GX, Au S, MacAlpine EM, Paniagua AR, et al. Regional anesthesia reduces inpatient and outpatient perioperative opioid demand in periarticular elbow surgery. J Shoulder Elbow Surg. 2022;31(2):e48-57.
78. Cunningham DJ, LaRose M, Zhang G, Patel P, Paniagua A, Gadsden J, et al. Regional anesthesia associated with decreased inpatient and outpatient opioid demand in Tibial plateau fracture surgery. Anesth Analg. 2022;134(5):1072–81.
79. Munsch MA, Via GG, Roebke AJ, Everhart JS, Ryan JM, Vasileff WK. Patient-specific factors, but neither regional anesthesia nor hip-specific cryotherapy, predict postoperative opioid requirements after hip arthroscopy for femoroacetabular impingement (FAI) syndrome. J Clin Orthop Trauma. 2022;28: 101848.

80. Trasolini NA, Bolia IK, Kang HP, Essilfie A, Mayer EN, Omid R, et al. National trends in use of regional anesthesia and postoperative patterns of opioid prescription filling in shoulder arthroscopy: a procedure-specific analysis in patients with or without recent opioid exposure. Orthop J Sports Med. 2020;8(6):2325967120929349.
81. Cunningham DJ, Robinette JP, Paniagua AR, LaRose MA, Blatter M, Gage MJ. Regional anesthesia does not decrease opioid demand in pelvis and acetabulum fracture surgery. Eur J Orthop Surg Traumatol Orthop Traumatol. 2022;32(7):1357–70.
82. Hah JM, Trafton JA, Narasimhan B, Krishnamurthy P, Hilmoe H, Sharifzadeh Y, et al. Efficacy of motivational-interviewing and guided opioid tapering support for patients undergoing orthopedic surgery (MI-Opioid Taper): a prospective, assessor-blind, randomized controlled pilot trial. EClinicalMedicine. 2020;28: 100596.
83. Vetter TR, Kain ZN. Role of the perioperative surgical home in optimizing the perioperative use of opioids. Anesth Analg. 2017;125(5):1653–7.
84. Katz J, Weinrib AZ, Clarke H. Chronic postsurgical pain: from risk factor identification to multidisciplinary management at the Toronto general hospital transitional pain service. Can J Pain Rev Can Douleur. 2019;3(2):49–58.
85. Abid Azam M, Weinrib AZ, Montbriand J, Burns LC, McMillan K, Clarke H, et al. Acceptance and Commitment Therapy to manage pain and opioid use after major surgery: preliminary outcomes from the Toronto general hospital transitional pain service. Can J Pain Rev Can Douleur. 2017;1(1):37–49.
86. Clarke H, Azargive S, Montbriand J, Nicholls J, Sutherland A, Valeeva L, et al. Opioid weaning and pain management in postsurgical patients at the Toronto general hospital transitional pain service. Can J Pain Rev Can Douleur. 2018;2(1):236–47.
87. Mikhaeil J, Ayoo K, Clarke H, Wąsowicz M, Huang A. Review of the transitional pain service as a method of postoperative opioid weaning and a service aimed at minimizing the risk of chronic post-surgical pain. Anaesthesiol Intensive Ther. 2020;52(2):148–53.

Genetics of Acute Pain

Danial Shams

Abstract Pain is one of the primary complaints following surgery and has major impacts on recovery, not to mention the costs (emotionally, physically, and financially) on the individual and society at large. In fact, survey studies show more than 70% of patients report moderate to extreme pain after surgery, with more than 70% also complaining of these same levels of pain after discharge [1]. This makes the treatment of acute post-operative pain an important mainstay of today's surgical and acute pain services. There is a growing body of literature describing the role that genetics may play in how and to what degree a person perceives pain. Further research into these topics may help guide future practitioners in identifying those patients at greatest risk for the development of significant post-operative and chronic pain. In addition, an individual's genetic makeup may contribute to the ability to develop individualized treatment plans that result in safer and more efficacious treatments.

Keywords Acute pain · Pain · Genetics · Chronic pain · COMT · GCH1 · SCN9A · CYP2D6 · OPRM1

1 Introduction

Pain is both universal and incredibly personal. It is experienced by all animals, including humans, at some point in their lives; it is an evolutionary advantage which allows organisms to protect themselves from injury. Yet, given the same type of injury or trauma, there still exists incredible interindividual variability in the perception of intensity and duration of pain. This variation is likely secondary to an intricate interconnection of environmental and genetic factors. As our knowledge of pain genetics has improved, certain genes and their products have been identified

D. Shams (✉)
Department of Anesthesiology, Vanderbilt University Medical Center, Nashville, TN, USA
e-mail: danial.shams@vumc.org

A. Abd-Elsayed and K. Schroeder (eds.), *Perioperative Pain Management*,
https://doi.org/10.1007/978-3-031-67648-2_5

which can possibly answer some of the questions surrounding this perception variability. This chapter briefly reviews pain pathways, discusses genetically inherited pain disorders, and postulates on future directions of research in regard to the genetics and treatment of acute pain.

2 Anatomy of Pain Pathways

Nociceptors

In the most basic way, pain is sensed peripherally and transmitted to the brain via the spinal cord. On a less superficial level, noxious stimuli are detected by a specific set of peripheral nerve fibers called nociceptors, leading to action potentials which carry the signal to the spinal cord. It is generally accepted that there are two major classes of nociceptors, Aδ fibers and C fibers. Aδ fibers are small- to medium-diameter, myelinated fibers which are important for well-localized, fast pain (or "first pain"). C fibers, on the other hand, are small-diameter, unmyelinated fibers responsible for poorly localized slow pain (or "second pain") [2]. However, if looked at more closely, even further divisions can be found for both types of fibers. Aδ fibers can be subdivided into Type I and II Aδ fibers, mediating mechanical/chemical and heat stimuli, respectively, while C fibers are believed to be incredibly heterogenous, as well as polymodal, being both heat and mechanically sensitive [3]. These nociceptors can also be differentiated based on which types of receptors and channels are expressed on their axons and cell bodies. These channels can grant the ability to sense noxious heat (TRPV1), cold sensation between 10 and 30 °C (TRPM8), acidic environments (ASICs), and various chemicals (TRPA1) [4].

Ascending Pathways

Noxious signals are transmitted from peripheral nociceptors to the dorsal root ganglia (DRG) and trigeminal ganglion in the body and face, respectively. From here, primary afferent nerve fibers synapse upon second-order neurons within the dorsal horn of the spinal cord, which is itself distinctly stratified into laminae. These second order neurons then ascend to the brain via the five main ascending pathways, the spinothalamic, spinoreticular, spinomesencephalic, cervicothalamic, and spinohypothalamic tracts [2].

The spinothalamic tract is the primary pain pathway, arising from lamina I and V-VII, and finally terminating in the thalamic nuclei; lesions within this tract cause significant to complete loss of nociception on the contralateral side of the body. The spinoreticular tract arises from laminae VII and VIII and terminates within the reticular formation and thalamus; it is thought to be involved in automatic responses to pain. The spinomesencephalic tract contains axons from laminae I and V which terminate in a multitude of places, including the mesencephalic reticular formation, periaqueductal gray, and parabrachial nucleus (which itself projects to the amygdala); this tract is thought to contribute to the emotional aspect of pain and be involved in descending modulatory pathways. The cervicothalamic tract has a function similar to the spinothalamic tract but contains axons from laminae III and IV. Finally, the spinohypothalamic tract contains axons from laminae I, V, and VIII which then synapse to the hypothalamic nuclei; this regulates the endocrine and cardiovascular responses to pain [2, 4]. The signal is then carried to the cortical structures, such as the prefrontal cortex, the somatosensory cortex, the anterior cingulate gyrus, and the insular cortex, none of which are in and of themselves essential to pain regulation, but all of which are critical components in the perception and response to painful stimuli.

3 Heritability of Pain

When discussing heritability within the human population, twin studies are one of the classic tools implemented to determine what role, if any, genetics play in a particular phenotype. Typically, pairs of monozygotic (MZ) and dizygotic (DZ) twins are compared, assuming that environmental influences will be similar across the population. If the concordance between MZ is greater than the DZ concordance, heritability can then be calculated. However, pain is such a broad phenotype with the possibility of multifactorial traits, that other forms of study may also be important. These include family analyses and genetic association studies to evaluate single nucleotide polymorphisms (SNPs) [5]. Additionally, a distinction needs to be made from genetic contributions to pain conditions and experimental pain responses. Below, we will break down the heritability of pain conditions themselves as well as the heritability of enhanced sensitivity to pain.

Twin Studies

Numerous pain phenotypes have been evaluated with twin studies to hunt for evidence of heritability. As noted above, given the differences present in pain phenotypes, this is not always an easy task; however, the genetic heritability has been indicated in several pain phenotypes.

Headaches

One of the most studied of these phenotypes is headaches, including migraines, tension, recurrent, and temporomandibular joint disorders (TMD). Twin studies looking at heritability in migraines have demonstrated a consistent, though wide, range, estimating the heritability to range anywhere from 33–77% [6]. The largest study, which included data from almost 30,000 pairs across eight countries, found the overall heritability to be 46%, or nearly half [7]; this value is corroborated by multiple additional studies. Tension-type headaches have also been found to demonstrate heritability of almost 50%, with the largest study reporting heritability of 48% for men and 44% for women [8].

Back and Neck Pain

In addition to headaches, back and neck pain, particularly low back pain, has been the subject of multiple twin studies. This has proved to be difficult given a large discrepancy in the definition of low back pain, but a meta-analysis of these studied found an overall heritability of just over one-third, or 34% [6]. The heritability of neck pain was found to be similar, although, once again, significant heterogeneity existed within the data sets, making a meta-analysis difficult.

Other Pain Modalities

In addition to headaches and back/neck pain, twin studies have been conducted for other pain phenotypes, with significant heritability found in some, but not in others (usually due to inadequate data). These include irritable bowel syndrome (IBS), found to have heritability of around 25%, rheumatoid arthritis, with heritability of nearly 50%, and chronic widespread pain (CWP), also with heritability around 50%. Studies evaluating osteoarthritis contained small sample data, making it difficult to reach any sort of conclusion regarding heritability; this remained true for carpal tunnel syndrome, ankylosing spondylitis, psoriatic arthritis, and gout [5, 6].

Experimental Pain Phenotypes

Experimental pain studies have attempted to unlock how pain is processed independent of the disease processes themselves. These pain sensitivity studies have sought to increase physiologic understanding through measuring responses to cold and heat pain. Just as with twin studies examining heritability for known pathologies, twin studies looking at experimental phenotypes also contained significant variability; they do, however, suggest there is heritability for experimental pain responses, likely more for cold-pressor pain (~50% heritability) than for heat pain measures (~25% heritability). Additional studies have also demonstrated correlations between pain tolerance and sex, ethnicity, and psychological traits (i.e. fear of pain, pain catastrophization). It has been established repeatedly that women have lower pain tolerance than men [9, 10], however, women are more likely to have their pain under-treated post-operatively and instead receive sedatives rather than analgesics compared to men [11]. Asians have also been shown to suffer from greater experimental pain perception compared to non-Hispanic Whitess [9, 12].

Psychological traits have also exhibited a correlation with experimental and experiential pain, just as they are risk factors for developing chronic pain post-operative pain. In a study by Patanwala et al., the Pain Catastrophizing Scale (PCS) and Fear of Pain Questionnaire-III (FPQ-III) were both revealed to correlate well with pain tolerance in cold water tests; those who were higher on the catastrophizer or fear of pain scales were much quicker to remove their hands from cold water baths than their counterparts who scored lower [9]. Unfortunately, there is lack of studies examining the relationship between experimental pain and clinical pain phenotypes. Further study into this could lead to a finetuning of experimental models looking at pain processes in the future [5, 13].

4 Candidate Genes

Multiple studies have explored the connection between genetics and pain, both for specific pain conditions as well as for experimental pain responses. Many of these are related to chronic pain conditions, such as temporomandibular disorders (TMD) or those mentioned above within the twin studies, but others have looked at the presence of SNPs in experimentally induced pain. See Table 1 for a brief overview.

Ion Channels

Ion channels vary in their molecular structure but are all membrane proteins which help to transport ions into or out of the cell. Broadly speaking, they are separated into voltage-gated and ligand-gated channels. Of the more than 400 channel genes encoded within the human genome and the ten known subtypes of voltage-gated sodium channels, $Na_V 1.7$, 1.8, and 1.9 are expressed almost exclusively within nociceptive neurons [14]. One of these, the $Na_V 1.7$, has been found to be associated with the ability to sense pain and is encoded by the *SCN9A* gene; a loss-of-function mutation within this gene causes familial insensitivity to pain. This, of course, may lead to significant complications, such as accidental trauma, burns, or skin ulcers. Studies also show that lesions within this gene may decrease post-operative pain sensitivity.

Table 1 Genes, their respective proteins, and their role in human pain

Encoding gene	Protein	Function	Phenotype
SCN9A	$Na_V1.7$ sodium channel	Voltage-gated sodium channel	Increased risk of sciatica, OA, post-lumbar discectomy, and phantom limb pain [24]
CACNA1A	$Ca_V2.1$ calcium channel	Voltage-gated calcium channel	Increased risk of neuropathic pain after mastectomy [25]
COMT	Catecholamine-*O*-methyltransferase	Catecholamine degradation	Higher enzyme activity leads to increased sensitivity to pain [17]
GCH1	GTP cyclohydrolase 1	BH_4 synthesis	Decreased sensitivity to experimental pain [18]
OPRM1	Mu-opioid receptor	Opioid signaling	Decreased analgesic response to morphine [19]
MC1R	Melanocortin-1 receptor	Controls type of melanin being produced	Red hair, fair skin, increased pain sensitivity and opioid requirements [21]
CYP2D6	Cytochrome P450, family 2, subfamily D, polypeptide 6	Drug metabolism	Gene duplication results in increased sensitivity to codeine [23]

On the contralateral side of this, a gain-of-function mutation within this same gene may lead to primary erythromelalgia, characterized by burning pain in the extremities, or paroxysmal extreme pain disorder (PEPD), characterized by mandibular, ocular, and rectal pain. Studies have shown a correlation between this gene and increased risk of sciatica, osteoarthritis (OA), pancreatitis, and post-lumbar discectomy pain [15].

Similar gain-of-function and loss-of-function mutations have been found in other ion channels, leading to variations of familial hemiplegic migraines (FHM). These mutations have been identified within $Ca_V2.1$ calcium channels, Na–K ATPase, and the $Na_V1.1$ sodium channel [4]. Even potassium channels have been recognized in pain pathologies. The voltage-gated potassium channel, $K_V9.1$, has a variant which leads to greater pain and decreased post-operative pain improvement in patients undergoing lumbar discectomy and amputees with phantom limb pain or neuropathic pain.

Catecholamine-O-Methyltransferase (COMT)

The COMT gene is one of the better studied SNPs in the field of pain genetics. The met158val SNP has been identified as a contributor in the observed differences in human responses to pain. The COMT gene encodes a protein that is involved in catecholamine degradation; the $val^{158}met$ SNP results in higher enzyme activity which then leads to an increased sensitivity to pain, leading to an increased morphine requirement in cancer patients [16]. A 3-year prospective trial identified 3 main haplotypes (low, average, and high pain sensitive) of the COMT gene based on responses to experimental pain. They then found that having even one low pain sensitive haplotype reduces the risk of developing TMD [17].

Guanosine Triphosphate (GTP) Cyclohydrolase 1 (GCH1)

GCH1 is the catalyst in the rate limiting step of the conversion of GTP to tetrahydrobiopterin (BH_4). BH_4 is involved the production of nitric oxide and citrulline, eventually leading to the production of serotonin and breakdown of phenylalanine to tyrosine [16]. It was initially found to be involved in neuropathic and inflammatory pain in animal research; further human research helped to identify variants which led to a decrease in the risk of developing chronic pain and a reduction in experimental pain sensitivity [18].

OPRM1 Gene

The opioid mu-receptor is encoded by the OPRM1 gene. This gene has multiple variants, though the 118 A > G is the most extensively studied and has been found to be associated with human responses to analgesia and pain. Patients with this SNP have been found to have a decreased response to morphine, both in pain relief and pupillary miosis. While the full reason for this effect is unknown, it is believed that this SNP leads to decreased effects of opioids in the areas of the brain most strongly associated with processing pain intensity [15, 19].

Melanocortin Receptor (MC1R)

It has been a long-standing saying that those with red-hair and fair skin require more anesthesia to remain sedated and greater analgesia to remain comfortable following surgery. While this was not initially accepted within the medical community itself, multiple SNPs in the MC1R gene have now been identified which demonstrate the phenotype of fair skin, red-hair, and increased pain sensitivity. It is postulated that MC1R is expressed in glial cells and the periaqueductal gray as well, thereby leading to this correlation [20, 21]. Thus, individuals with these SNPs require high doses of pain medication compared to those without. Interestingly, however, female carriers of these variants show greater analgesic effects to k-opioid analgesics where male carriers do not, demonstrating an additional sex-specific response within the k-opioid system [22, 23].

Cytochrome P450 2D6 (CYP2D6)

The P450 system is involved in the metabolism of many medications. The 2D6 polypeptide catalyzes codeine to morphine, a metabolic conversion necessary to illicit the clinical effects desired from analgesic administration. On its own, codeine has a 200 times lower affinity at the mu-opioid receptors than morphine; therefore, it depends strongly on this conversion for its clinical effects. Duplications of this gene thus lead to faster metabolism of codeine to morphine, thus increasing its effectiveness. The opposite is true for "poor metabolizers" lacking a functional CYP2D6 gene, whereby codeine will have minimal to no analgesic effect. These genetic variants are also relatively common; gene multiplications are found among nearly 3% of Caucasians and nonfunctional genes are found among 7% of Caucasians [23]. This means that nearly 10% of the Caucasian population gets no pain relief from codeine, as opposed to 0.5% of the African-American or Asian populations.

5 Future Directions

The future of genetics and its role in pain perception and management remains wide open for additional research and breakthroughs. As the rapid production of the COVID-19 vaccine has shown us, new techniques are constantly being developed which can be applied to the realm of pain and, more specifically, acute pain. This being said, additional studies are needed to account for the variability seen in the human population regarding pain phenotypes and pain reporting. As our understanding of how genetic constitution impacts perioperative analgesia improves, we will ideally begin to leverage this enhanced insight to create truly patient centered treatments, currently seen only in science fiction. Using genotypic information as a guide to analgesic therapy could be in the near future; for instance, nerve growth factor, NGF (a topic not covered in this chapter), has been identified as a target after a SNP from a single family demonstrated a hereditary insensitivity to pain. This led to the production of an NGF-inhibiting antibody called tanezumab, which can function as an analgesic for OA pain [26]. In this same vein, it is possible that a blockade of GCH1 may lead to the prevention of cancer pain or that selective $Na_V1.7$ inhibitors may reduce pain sensitivity [16]. Additionally, with the continued rise of artificial intelligence (AI), the research may advance at an even quicker clip.

Key Points

1. Pain perception is a delicate and complicated procedure and variations at any step of the signaling pathway, from the nociceptors to the cortical structures, may lead to increased or decreased pain sensitivities.
2. Identification of various genes via animal research can be combined with cohort analyses of humans to pinpoint bottlenecks and targets for future, genetically driven treatments.
3. Rapid advancement of research in this field will lead to further targets for analgesics and, hopefully, the analgesics themselves.

References

1. Gan TJ, Habib AS, Miller TE, White W, Apfelbaum JL. Incidence, patient satisfaction, and perceptions of post-surgical pain: results from a US national survey. Curr Med Res Opin. 2014;30:149–60.
2. Kandel ER, Schwartz JH, Jessell TM, Siegelbaum SA, Hudspeth AJ, eds. 24: Pain. In: Principles of neural science, Fifth Edition., 2000.
3. Basbaum AI, Bautista DM, Scherrer G, Julius D. Cellular and molecular mechanisms of pain. Cell. 2009;139:267–84.
4. Renthal W. Pain genetics. In: Rosenberg's molecular and genetic basis of neurological and psychiatric disease, 2015:1089–100.
5. Fillingim R, Wallace M, Herbstman D, Ribeiro-Dasilva M, Staud R. Genetic contributions to pain: a review of findings in humans. Oral Dis. 2008;14:673–82.
6. Nielsen C, Knudsen G, Steingrímsdóttir Ó. Twin studies of pain. Clin Genet. 2012;82:331–40.
7. Mulder EJ, van Baal C, Gaist D, Kallela M, Kaprio J, Svensson DA, Nyholt DR, Martin NG, MacGregor AJ, Cherkas LF, Boomsma DI, Palotie A. Genetic and environmental influences on migraine: a twin study across six countries. Twin Res. 2003;6:422–31.
8. Russell MB, Levi N, Kaprio J. Genetics of tension-type headache: A population based twin study. Am J Med Genet Part B Neuropsychiatric Genet. 2007;144B:982–6.
9. Patanwala AE, Norwood C, Steiner H, Morrison D, Li M, Walsh K, Martinez M, Baker SE, Snyder EM, Karnes JH. Psychological and genetic predictors of pain tolerance. Clin Transl Sci. 2019;12:189–95.
10. Pieretti S, Giannuario AD, Giovannandrea RD, Marzoli F, Piccaro G, Minosi P, Aloisi AM. Gender differences in pain and its relief. Ann dell'Ist Super di sanita. 2016;52:184–9.
11. Calderone KL. The influence of gender on the frequency of pain and sedative medication administered to postoperative patients. Sex Roles. 1990;23:713–25.
12. Cong X, Tan Z, Weidig T. Sex, Race, and Genomics of Pain. In: Dorsey SG, Starkweather AR, editors. Genomics of pain and co-morbid symptoms., 2020:181–91.
13. Angst MS, Phillips NG, Drover DR, Tingle M, Ray A, Swan GE, Lazzeroni LC, Clark JD. Pain sensitivity and opioid analgesia: a pharmacogenomic twin study. Pain. 2012;153:1397–409.
14. Venter JC, Adams MD, Myers EW, Li PW, Mural RJ, Sutton GG, Smith HO, Yandell M, Evans CA, Holt RA, Gocayne JD, Amanatides P, Ballew RM, Huson DH, Wortman JR, Zhang Q, Kodira CD, Zheng XH, Chen L, Skupski M, Subramanian G, Thomas PD, Zhang J, Miklos GLG, Nelson C, Broder S, Clark AG, Nadeau J, McKusick VA, Zinder N, et al. The Sequence of the human genome. Sci. 2001;291:1304–51.

15. James S. Human pain and genetics: some basics. Br J Pain. 2013;7:171–8.
16. Lötsch J. Genetic variability of pain perception and treatment—clinical pharmacological implications. Eur J Clin Pharmacol. 2011;67:541–51.
17. Diatchenko L, Slade GD, Nackley AG, Bhalang K, Sigurdsson A, Belfer I, Goldman D, Xu K, Shabalina SA, Shagin D, Max MB, Makarov SS, Maixner W. Genetic basis for individual variations in pain perception and the development of a chronic pain condition. Hum Mol Genet. 2005;14:135–43.
18. Tegeder I, Costigan M, Griffin RS, Abele A, Belfer I, Schmidt H, Ehnert C, Nejim J, Marian C, Scholz J, Wu T, Allchorne A, Diatchenko L, Binshtok AM, Goldman D, Adolph J, Sama S, Atlas SJ, Carlezon WA, Parsegian A, Lötsch J, Fillingim RB, Maixner W, Geisslinger G, Max MB, Woolf CJ. GTP cyclohydrolase and tetrahydrobiopterin regulate pain sensitivity and persistence. Nat Med. 2006;12:1269–77.
19. Reyes-Gibby CC, Shete S, Rakvåg T, Bhat SV, Skorpen F, Bruera E, Kaasa S, Klepstad P. Exploring joint effects of genes and the clinical efficacy of morphine for cancer pain: OPRM1 and COMT gene. Pain. 2007;130:25–30.
20. Kwon AH, Flood P. Genetics and gender in acute pain and perioperative opioid analgesia. Anesthesiol Clin. 2020;38:341–55.
21. Mogil JS, Wilson SG, Chesler EJ, Rankin AL, Nemmani KVS, Lariviere WR, Groce MK, Wallace MR, Kaplan L, Staud R, Ness TJ, Glover TL, Stankova M, Mayorov A, Hruby VJ, Grisel JE, Fillingim RB. The melanocortin-1 receptor gene mediates female-specific mechanisms of analgesia in mice and humans. Proc National Acad Sci. 2003;100:4867–72.
22. Edwards RR. Genetic predictors of acute and chronic pain. Curr Rheumatol Rep. 2006;8:411–7.
23. Lötsch J, Geisslinger G. Current evidence for a genetic modulation of the response to analgesics. Pain. 2006;121:1–5.
24. Reimann F, Cox JJ, Belfer I, Diatchenko L, Zaykin DV, McHale DP, Drenth JPH, Dai F, Wheeler J, Sanders F, Wood L, Wu T-X, Karppinen J, Nikolajsen L, Männikkö M, Max MB, Kiselycznyk C, Poddar M, te Morsche RHM, Smith S, Gibson D, Kelempisioti A, Maixner W, Gribble FM, Woods CG. Pain perception is altered by a nucleotide polymorphism in SCN9A. Proc National Acad Sci. 2010;107:5148–53.
25. Habib AS, Kertai MD, Cooter M, Greenup RA, Hwang S. Risk factors for severe acute pain and persistent pain after surgery for breast cancer: a prospective observational study. Reg Anesthesia Pain Med. 2019;44:192.
26. LN E, ST J, BC A, Masoud M, SD L, SM D, BM T. Tanezumab for the treatment of pain from osteoarthritis of the knee. New Engl J Med. 2010;363:1521–31.

Pain Management Consent Considerations

Elizabeth Wilson and Kristopher Schroeder

Abstract Healthcare professionals must consider patients as collaborators in the process of healthcare decision making. In matters of perioperative pain management, it is important to consider and include patients in decisions that may be impacted by their personal history of pain management/analgesic administration, value system/thought process regarding pain management, and the relative impact of potential complications related to analgesic procedures and opioid analgesics. To make these decisions, healthcare professionals must consider the ability of patients to make decisions in the setting of pain and polypharmacy and if the use of adjunct/surrogate decision makers may be appropriate/beneficial. In addition, it is important to consider how information is conveyed and the degree of detail that is required to ensure that patients are equipped to make a decision that best aligns with their belief system and values. Finally, patient decisions must be respected, and they must know that they possess the autonomy to be ultimately responsible for the decisions that will impact their healthcare delivery.

Keywords Consent · Capacity · Competency · Surrogate · Disclosure

1 Introduction

Healthcare professionals are required to obtain consent prior to performing procedures and administering medications. However, this practice has evolved greatly over time and continues to do so as patients desire more involvement in their healthcare decision making process. In many cases, healthcare professionals may struggle with the best course of action regarding what to disclose, what not to disclose, to

E. Wilson · K. Schroeder (✉)
Department of Anesthesiology, University of Wisconsin School of Medicine and Public Health, Madison, WI, USA
e-mail: Kmschro1@wisc.edu

E. Wilson
e-mail: Elizabeth.wilson@wisc.edu

A. Abd-Elsayed and K. Schroeder (eds.), *Perioperative Pain Management*,
https://doi.org/10.1007/978-3-031-67648-2_6

whom, and via what platform. Delivering too much information increases the potential risk that patients may fail to focus on important details or become unnecessarily concerned with incredibly rare outcomes. In contrast, a consent discussion that is too limited from the patient's perspective may foster a feeling in patients and their families that there is an effort to hide information or that healthcare professionals are limited in their interest in caring for patients. High-intensity/acuity situations (i.e. obstetrics and emergency departments), efforts to obtain consent in patients with limited capacity (i.e. in the setting of inebriation or polypharmacy), special patient populations (i.e. athletes, language barriers, and pediatrics), dealing with unknown consequences of a proposed intervention in the setting of pre-existing neurologic disease, and working with procedural learners/trainees can conspire to complicate the ability to achieve a satisfying consent discussion. However, there are a number of considerations and processes that, once utilized, can contribute to a more satisfying and appropriate consent process.

2 Historical Perspectives

There are, unfortunately, a series of historical landmark cases and studies that highlight inappropriate, inadequate, or omitted consent processes for research or clinical activities and it is shocking how recently one might peer back into our collective history to observe episodes of consent misconduct. An early leader in the fight for ethical research conduct was Henry K. Beecher, an anesthesiologist, who was instrumental in stopping a wide range of inappropriate clinical trials that included exposing unknowing participants to live viruses and injected cancer cells [1]. It wasn't until 1972 that the Tuskegee Syphilis Study was finally terminated after a whistle blower brought to light the abuse of these research subjects [2]. In similar ways, historical disclosure for clinical patients has also been equally disturbing and contemporaneously paternalistic. In 1914, litigation established that "Every human being of adult years and sound mind has a right to determine what shall be done with his own body." However, it took more than 40 additional years for the term "informed consent" to become recognized within the medicolegal domain [3]. Medical paternalism resulted in many patients being passive participants in their medical care and patients were frequently told, not asked, what medical therapies they might accept. As recently as the 1960's, it was common practice to withhold a cancer diagnosis from patients and, at that time, 90% of physicians preferred to not share this information with their patients [4]. Even in 2010, 55% of surveyed anesthesiologists and surgeons felt that the consent process was inappropriate since patients remember little of what is disclosed to them. In addition, nearly 30% of those surveyed believed that there was no need to disclose major risks with an incidence greater than 1/100 [5]. It is important to acknowledge the complicated history and continued evolution of informed consent to fully understand how the process of consent has ascended in its level of (perceived) importance and now represents a critical element of the patient-physician relationship.

The current state of consent for perioperative regional anesthesia procedures was best described by a 2007 survey study. In this study, 79 respondents answered a variety of questions related to their standard disclosure of information prior to the performance of regional anesthesia procedures. Of note, 26% of respondents reported that they only disclosed medical risk for medicolegal purposes instead of aiding patients in an informed decision-making process. In addition, the study found that disclosure of common and benign/low severity complications for peripheral regional and neuraxial procedures was completed by most respondents. As an example, 71% of respondents disclosed a risk of local pain following an interscalene block. However serious complications including paralysis (21%), seizures (39%), pneumothorax (37%), cardiac arrest (18%), and death (28%) were disclosed much less frequently. This same pattern held for spinal anesthesia where 73% of study participants disclosed a risk of local pain/discomfort but information for paralysis (43%), cardiac arrest (18%), and death (32%) was much less frequently divulged. The etiology for the poor risk disclosure for serious adverse events is likely multifactorial but could include not wanting to frighten patients prior to a procedure, not wanting to have patients decline a procedure, an unclear understanding of risk on the part of the providers, or a lack of provider comfort discussing issues of such magnitude. In addition, this study found that the incidences of severe complications disclosed for a number of potentially serious adverse events did not correlate well with what was available in the contemporary literature [6]. The results of this study indicate that, even for experts, there is additional work that needs to be done to ensure that our patients remain an active and informed participant in decisions relevant to medical management [7].

The reality is that a real or perceived lack of an adequate consent process and documentation may now be utilized as a legal strategy to paint a physician as uncaring and inattentive to detail. If for no other reason than the avoidance of medico-legal entanglements, it behooves our profession to embrace the tenets of contemporary consent discussions and documentation.

3 Consent

The consent process can be distilled into four distinct components that must be satisfied to ensure that the patients are appropriately positioned to participate in medical decision making.

Required Elements of Informed Consent:

1. Voluntariness
2. Disclosure
3. Understanding
4. Capacity

At first glance, voluntariness may seem the most obvious of the four consent elements. To satisfy this element of consent, patients must make a decision regarding their own health and the plan for care delivery without coercion and, ultimately, grant permission for treatment to proceed. In this process, it is critically important that patients are aware that they possess the ability to make the ultimate decision regarding delivery of medical and procedural care. In many cases, patients may not feel that they have the ability to impact the course of care delivery and efforts should be made to correct this perception. Ensuring voluntariness may be as simple as validating that the consent process contains the exact phrase "this is your decision to make and only you can grant permission for us to proceed." In some cases, voluntariness may be complicated by a variety of dynamics that might arise in the perioperative arena. For example, patients may present with a family member or other person (i.e., athletic trainer/agent/coach) who may seek to impose their ideas and values regarding treatment preferences on the patient. Patients need to know that no amount of procedural momentum removes their ability to terminate a procedure or change the direction of a treatment plan.

Disclosure is a key component of the consent process that is frequently misunderstood and poorly applied. For the purposes of medical intervention (whether medicinal or procedural), it is important to disclose the reported purpose of the proposed intervention. Patients should not present to the operating room or procedural area without a clear understanding of why they are there. Patients need to know the risks, benefits and potential complications of the proposed intervention and how their pre-existing medical conditions impact each of those. As mentioned previously, the results of the Brull et. Al. study highlight our profession's collective unease with disclosure of risks of substantial consequence [6]. An effort needs to be made to ensure that rare but serious risks are disclosed to patients. In the event that a healthcare professional finds discussing these sorts of rare events uncomfortable, there are a number of alternatives including pre-prepared printed and audiovisual modalities that can augment the conversation. This risk disclosure discussion should be tailored to the individual patient and the act of customizing this discussion helps to galvanize a strong relationship between the healthcare professional and the patient. For example, if the patient is a professional athlete there may be more time spent discussing the potential risks of long-term motor weakness or the potential for a delayed return to sport following a regional anesthesia procedure. In patients with pre-existing neurologic disease, it may be incredibly appropriate to disclose that there are unknown risks associated with the provision of regional anesthesia techniques and that there may be an unknown elevated risk associated with undergoing these procedures. In patients with a history of opioid abuse or misuse, it may be appropriate to discuss how the application of regional anesthesia techniques may be an important component of limiting the need for post-procedural opioid administration.

Beyond the risks of a proposed intervention, it is important to disclose clinical alternatives. For example, alternatives to regional anesthesia may include additional doses of opioid or other analgesics. In discussions of analgesic alternatives, it is important to acknowledge that there are risks associated with these procedures/therapeutics and efforts should be made to provide a reasonable risk/benefit discussion for these alternatives [8]. It is also important to disclose that there may be risks associated with delaying or foregoing a certain procedure [9]. For example, there is evidence to suggest that foregoing an epidural blood patch following an inadvertent dural puncture may increase the risk of chronic headache and low back pain [10].

With the proliferation of available regional anesthesia procedures and trainees of multiple disciplines, disclosure of personal procedure experience may also be an appropriate component of the consent discussion. It is also appropriate to disclose to patients if a medication is being used in an off-label fashion or if there is limited data yet available to support the use of a particular agent. While these discussions have the potential to be uncomfortable, they do help to strengthen relationships with patients and demonstrate empathy and caring.

Obviously, it would be impossible to disclose every possible risk potentially associated with a given intervention or medication. Therefore, it is important to consider those risks that possess a threshold incidence level or that might be of particular importance to a patient. In the United States, disclosure thresholds are subject to state-specific disclosure standards that vary from state to state and include the reasonable patient standard, the professional standard or a hybrid version. The reasonable patient standard requires physicians to disclose information to an extent that would be expected by a reasonable patient whereas the professional standard should encompass elements of disclosure expected by a reasonable medical practitioner under the same or similar conditions. Where this distinction becomes important is in a medicolegal setting. States with the reasonable patient disclosure standard encounter medical malpractice verdicts in favor of plaintiffs more frequently than states with a professional standard of disclosure [11]. These standards are highly variable and can change over time with changes in case law. It is therefore important to establish a good working relationship with your hospital's legal team to better understand the medicolegal environment that exists as a guide to local disclosure norms.

The next component of consent requires patients to understand their condition and appreciate the risks and benefits of a proposed procedure or treatment modality. Assessing understanding and capacity can be difficult but there are some pathways/techniques that may be helpful. One simple modality for assessing understanding and capacity is the "teach back" method. In this exercise, patients are simply asked to provide a description of the proposed intervention and, in so doing, demonstrate the ability to retain and process relevant and important information. Grisso and Applebaum further clarified questions that might be asked to further evaluate a patient's ability to understand their situation and the proposed intervention. These authors have proposed that understanding can be assessed by asking the patient the following questions [12].

Please tell me in your own words:

1. The problem with your health now.
2. The recommended treatment.
3. The possible risks and benefits of the treatment.
4. Alternatives to the proposed treatment.
5. The risks and benefits of avoiding the proposed treatment.

Finally, patients need to have adequate capacity to make decisions regarding their medical treatment. The terms consent and capacity are frequently and erroneously utilized in an interchangeable fashion. As has previously been made clear here, consent is a process that requires a number of elements to ensure that patient autonomy and self-determination is respected. Capacity is the ability of an individual to weigh available information and communicate a decision or preference. Capacity determinations are generally made by the clinician obtaining consent and these determinations can be occasionally challenging [13]. What makes capacity determinations unique is that they are intervention specific—meaning that patients may have the capacity to make some decisions but lack the capacity to make larger and more meaningful/impactful decisions [14]. For example, a patient exposed to significant opioid analgesics may have the capacity to make a decision regarding intravenous line placement or antibiotic therapeutics. However, this same patient may lack the capacity to make a determination regarding a surgical procedure or therapeutic agent associated with the potential for significant risk. While any clinician caring for a patient has the ability to make assessments of patient capacity, there are clinical tools that may have utility in aiding these assessments. For example, the MacArthur test and Mini-Mental State Examination (MMSE) may have a role in aiding in capacity assessments when there is a lack of clear capacity consensus [15, 16].

The ideal scenario for how information should be conveyed to patients has yet to be determined. Certainly, the classic approach of sitting with the patient and having a discussion of the risks and benefits of a proposed intervention has a certain appeal and familiarity. These discussions offer tremendous value as an opportunity to build rapport and establish a relationship between the patient and the healthcare professional. With an oral consent process, it becomes important for the healthcare professional to diligently document relevant aspects of the consent discussion. The important take-away with this approach is that if the consent discussion documentation is not completed, it would be difficult to later "prove" that it had taken place. There may be some benefits associated with the use of prepared video, multi-media or print material. When compiling this material, it is important to consider that the average American reads at the 8th grade reading level and that, in general, currently available medical information and consent materials are beyond the reading capabilities of many of our patients [17, 18]. The American Society of Anesthesiologists has created decision guides for neuraxial anesthesia that help explain these procedures and offer patients opportunities to reflect and generate questions prior to interacting with their anesthesiologist. These initiatives may offer the promise of ensuring that patients arrive for surgery already informed regarding the proposed procedure with ample opportunity to reflect and weigh potential risks and benefits [19].

Despite our collective best efforts to provide a thoughtful and complete consent discussion for our patients, it seems that, in many circumstances, we may be failing to effectively deliver information in a manner that induces significant procedural recall. A study of patients receiving consent information at a dedicated preoperative clinic two weeks prior to a planned surgical procedure revealed that on the day of surgery, 26% of patients could not recall any risks related to anesthesia, 37% could not recall any major risks, and 84% could not recall any minor risks [20]. When the ability to recall consent and risk discussions for regional anesthesia procedures has been evaluated, the data demonstrates that patient recall of risks is incredibly low. In one study of patients presenting for shoulder arthroplasty and interscalene nerve block, risk recall was significantly worse for the interscalene block than for the surgical procedure and 45% of patients were unable to recall a single risk related to the provision of interscalene analgesia [21]. In a study of 125 patients presenting for arthroscopic shoulder surgery and interscalene block, only 21% of patients were able to remember all four major risks (long-term nerve damage, seizure, life-threatening event, and damage to the covering of the lung) immediately following a scripted consent discussion [22].

Given the limitations related to consent discussions, there is an evolving body of literature suggesting that these discussions might be augmented via the utilization of a variety of presentation formats. In one study, a small, laminated information card was presented to women interested in labor analgesia. All women had the standard consent discussion with an anesthesiologist but those women who were also able to refer to this laminated information card had a significant improvement in recall of the process and potential risks [23]. In another study of laboring women, patients were asked to certify that they had read a form detailing the benefits and risks of epidural analgesia. This study demonstrated that the addition of a written consent form improved recall and improved the women's subjective ability to "remember and appreciate the different anesthetic options, risks, and procedures [24]."

4 Unique Consent Circumstances

There are a number of patient populations where the informed consent process may take on heightened importance or be subject to additional significant considerations. Athletes are one example where the stakes associated with a potential adverse event related to a regional anesthesia technique can be incredibly high. In one high profile case of litigation following a peripheral regional anesthesia procedure, a professional athlete sought $180 million in damages after they failed to return to their sport following knee surgery and an adductor canal block [25]. In athletes and other highly skilled individuals (dancers, musicians, etc.), it is important to consider and discuss the implications of any possible post-procedure decrement in motor or sensory function. For example, limited studies have indicated that femoral nerve blocks performed for anterior cruciate ligament repair have been associated with persistent strength deficits at six months, an increased time until athletes are able to return to sport, and an increased risk of re-injury [26, 27]. These patients may also suffer from significant financial pressure and lack of autonomy that may impose undue pressure while these athletes weigh their individual risk/benefit profile [28, 29].

The involvement of trainees represents an additional layer of complexity that should be discussed with patients and requests to limit trainee involvement should be honored. What is not yet well codified is how detailed these consent discussions need to be so that patients are aware of the experience level of who is caring for them but not unduly concerned about the lack of trainee experience [30, 31]. Beyond traditional modeling behavior, there is some evidence to suggest that simulation may have a role in preparing anesthesia trainees to better deliver consent information [32].

Obstetric patients represent another patient population where the acuity of the event, ongoing pain, and dynamic changes in patient condition can introduce challenges in the consent process. However, it is important to consider that, despite occasional time pressures, these patients generally wish to know all the risks associated with epidural analgesia prior to proceeding [33]. In addition, it is likely fair to conclude that other patients in pain are similarly interesting in being informed of relative risks and benefits associated with proposed analgesic interventions. Obstetric patients do represent a wonderful model for how patients in pain can be consented for interventional procedures. In one study of obstetric patients, those in pain had similar recall of epidural risks compared to those who were not in pain at the time of risk disclosure. In addition, those women who had a consent discussion while in pain were generally satisfied with the communication relevant to the procedure [34].

In a similar fashion, patients with language or other barriers to understanding consent discussions represent a patient population that requires additional consideration. There is substantial evidence describing a decreased rate of regional anesthesia and analgesia for an array of obstetric and surgical populations in patients with language barriers [35, 36]. The etiology of this difference may be multi-factorial but the convenience of the healthcare professional should not be a consideration for the avoidance of analgesic interventions and procedures. Substantial interpretive services and language lines are now ubiquitously available and there should therefore be no real reason to avoid standard consent discussions with these patients.

There are circumstances where regional anesthesia may be requested following a surgical procedure where either the anesthesia professional failed to discuss the proposed intervention, the surgical procedure unexpectedly converts to one that is substantially more extensive, or patients have more pronounced difficulties with analgesic management than anticipated. The consent process in postoperative patients can certainly be compromised secondary to polypharmacy and delirium. In fact, previous research has demonstrated that delirium in the recovery room is incredibly common (35%) and multiple cognitive domains are impacted. Even in patients who appear awake, significant deficits may remain [37]. In these circumstances, it may be helpful to consider if patients have the capacity to consent to a procedure that is more limited in potential risks (i.e., in the setting of pre-existing neurologic disease, is it possible that patients might possess the capacity to consent to fascial plane but not epidural analgesia). It may also be helpful in these scenarios to enlist the assistance of surrogate decision makers or people who know the patient and can reaffirm that the patient would normally consent to the proposed intervention or procedure. Finally, conversion to more extensive surgical procedures is not an uncommon event and therefore including and documenting a regional anesthesia consent discussion for all patients undergoing laparoscopic surgery may satisfactorily avoid most consent consternations.

There are circumstances where patients initially refuse regional anesthesia but later change their mind after encountering the pain associated with their surgical procedure. Practitioners of obstetric anesthesia will frequently encounter this situation when patients present with a pre-commitment directive or birth plan that outlines how they would like to avoid epidural analgesia but change course when they encounter significant pain in the process of delivery [38]. The management of these Ulysses contracts can be challenging because they pit the autonomous wishes of the patient against themselves [39]. Should the lucid wishes of a patient who has prepared their perioperative analgesic plan be honored or should the autonomy of the patient who may be altered via poly-pharmacy but who now has a more thorough understanding of the discomfort associated with a surgical/labor procedure/process be allowed to make a decision regarding their analgesic management? Sadly, there are no easy answers in these situations. Ideally, there would be an opportunity to discuss with patients their hesitancy to accept a therapeutic regimen or procedure. In this conversation, if might also be helpful to discuss with the patient what the management course will be if the patient does change their mind following their surgical procedure and thorough documentation of this conversation is absolutely essential.

5 Conclusion

In conclusion, informed consent is more than a discrete conversation, form, video, software platform, or interactive demonstration. Rather, informed consent is a process that requires time to engage with patients and determine/discuss information material to their values and current medical condition to adequately develop a patient centered care plan. Through active engagement in this process, significant benefits will be realized for both the provider and patient. Patient safety will be enhanced as patients are given the opportunity to disclose additional information during the consent discussions that could potentially impact the relative risk of certain adverse outcomes. Additionally, both patient and healthcare professional satisfaction will be improved by establishing rapport and strengthening relationships during the informed consent process.

Key Takeaways

1. Key elements of consent include voluntariness, disclosure, understanding, and capacity.
2. Informed consent is best accomplished as a process instead of a discrete event.
3. Individual patient characteristics and values need to be considered when presenting consent information.
4. Risks material to proposed interventions must be disclosed and efforts should be made to ensure the accuracy of risk disclosure information.

References

1. Schwenzer KJ. Best practice & research in anaesthesiology issue on new approaches in clinical research ethics in clinical research. Best Pract Res Clin Anaesthesiol. 2011;25:569–82.
2. Jones J. Bad blood: the tuskeegee syphilis experiments. 2nd ed. New York: Free Press; 1993.
3. Tierney S, Perlas A. Informed consent for regional anesthesia. Curr Opin Anesthesiol. 2018;31:614–21.
4. Open D. What to tell cancer patients: a study of medical attitudes. JAMA. 1961;175:1120–8.
5. Jamjoom AAB, White S, Walton SM, Hardman JG, Moppett IK. Anaesthetists' and surgeons' attitudes towards informed consent in the UK: an observational study. BMC Med Ethics. 2010;11:2. https://doi.org/10.1186/1472-6939-11-2.
6. Brull R, McCartney CJL, Chan VWS, Liguori GA, Hargett MJ, Xu D, Abbas S, El-Beheiry H. Disclosure of risks associated with regional anesthesia: a survey of American regional anesthesiologists. Reg Anesth Pain Med. 2007;32:7–11.
7. Domino KB. Informed consent for regional anesthesia: what is necessary? Reg Anesth Pain Med. 2007;32:1–2.
8. White SM, Baldwin TJ. Consent for anaesthesia. Anaesthesia. 2003;58:760–74.
9. Waisel DB, Truog RD. Informed consent. Anesthesiol. 1997;87:968–78.
10. Niraj G, Mushambi M, Gautham P, Patil A, Kelkar A, Hart E, Nurmikko T. Anaesthesia. 2021;76:1068–76.
11. Studdert DM, Mello MM, Levy MK, Gruen RL, Dunn EJ, Oral J, Brennan TA. J Empir Leg Stud. 2007;4:103–24.
12. Grisso T, Appelbaum PS. Assessing competence to consent to treatment: a guide for physicians and other health professionals. New York: Oxford University Press; 1998.
13. Orr T, Baruah R. Consent in anesthesia, critical care and pain medicine. BJA Educ. 2018;18:135–9.
14. McCombe K, Bogod D. Regional anesthesia: risk, consent and complications. Anaesthesia. 2021;76:18–26.
15. Appelbaum PS. Assessment of patients' competence to consent to treatment. N Engl J Med. 2007;357:1834–40.
16. Etchells E, Darzins P, Silberfeld M, et al. Assessment of patient capacity to consent to treatment. J Gen Intern Med. 1999;14:27–34.
17. Paasche-Orlow MK, Taylor HA, Brancati FL. Readability standards for informed-consent forms as compared with readability. N Engl J Med. 2003;348:721–6.
18. Tait AR, Teig MK, Voepel-Lewis T. Informed consent for anesthesia: a review of practice and strategies for optimizing the consent process. Can J Anesth. 2014;61:832–42.
19. https://www.asahq.org/standards-and-guidelines/resources-from-asa-committees. Accessed 28 Feb 2023.
20. Gillies A, Gillies R, Weinberg L. Patient recollections of perioperative anaesthesia risks. Anaesth Intensive Care. 2013;41:247–50.
21. Zarnegar R, Brown MRD, Henley M, Tidman V, Pathmanathan A. Patient perceptions and recall of consent for regional anaesthesia compared with consent for surgery. J R Soc Med. 2015;108:451–6.
22. Bai JW, Abdallah FW, Cohn M, Ladowski S, Madhusudan P, Brull R. Say what? Patients have poor immediate memory of major risks of interscalene block disclosed during the informed consent discussion. Reg Anesth Pain Med. 2019;44:981–5.
23. White LA, Gorton P, Wee MYK, Mandal N. Written information about epidural analgesia for women in labour: did it improve? Int J Obstet Anesth. 2003;12:93–7.
24. Gerancher JC, Grice SC, Dewan DM, Eisenach J. An evaluation of informed consent prior to epidural analgesia for labor and delivery. Int J Obstet Anesth. 2000;9:168–73.
25. https://www.si.com/nfl/2018/11/07/minnesota-vikings-sharrif-floyds-180-million-lawsuit-against-dr-james-andrews. Accessed 21 Feb 2023.

26. Luo TD, Ashraf A, Dahm DL, Stuart MJ, McIntosh AL. Femoral nerve block is associated with persistent strength deficits at 6 months after anterior cruciate ligament reconstruction in pediatric and adolescent patients. Am J Sports Med. 2015;43:331–6.
27. Everhart JS, Hughes L, Abouljoud MM, Swank K, Lewis C, Flanagan DC. Femoral nerve block at time of ACL reconstruction causes lasting quadriceps strength deficits and may increase short-term risk of re-injury. Knee Surg Sports Traumatol Arthrosc. 2020;28:1894–900.
28. Bunch WH, Dvonch VM. Informed consent in sports medicine. Clin Sports Med. 2004;23:183–93.
29. Meyer P, Schroeder K. Regional anesthesia in the elite athlete. Clin Sports Med. 2022;41:291–302.
30. Dierdorf SF. Anesthesia and informed consent. Current Opin Anesthesiol. 2002;15:349–50.
31. Waisel DB, Lamiani G, Sandrock NJ, Pascucci R, Trug RD, Meyer EC. Anesthesiology trainees face ethical, practical, and relational challenges in obtaining informed consent. Anesthesiol. 2009;110:480–6.
32. Bashir MA, Khan AA, Khan SA. Assessment of informed consent and the impact of simulation on anesthesia trainees: assessment of informed consent and the impact of simulation on anesthesia trainees. Cureus. 13(11): e19787. https://doi.org/10.7759/cureus.19787
33. Jackson A, Henry R, Avery N, VanDenKerkhof E, Milne B. Informed consent for labour epidurals: what labouring women want to know. Can J Anesth. 2000;47:1068–73.
34. Burkle CM, Olsen DA, Sviggum HP, Jacob AK. Parturient recall of neuraxial analgesia risks: impact of labor pain vs no labor pain. J Clin Anesth. 2017;36:158–63.
35. Bansal V. Anesthesiology and the non-english speaking patient. Anesthesiol. 2017;127:716–7.
36. Togioka BM, Seligman KM, Werntz MK, Yanez ND, Noles LM, Treggiari MM. Education program regarding labor epidurals increases utilization by Hispanic Medicaid beneficiaries: a randomized controlled trial. Anesthesiol. 2019;131:840–9.
37. Banerji A, Sleigh JW, Voss LJ, Garcia PS, Gaskell AL. Deconstructing delirium in the post anaesthesia care unit. Front Aging Neurosci. 2022;14: 930434. https://doi.org/10.3389/fnagi.2022.930434.
38. Burcher P. The Ulysses contract in obstetrics: a woman's choices before and during labour. J Med Ethics. 2013;39:27–30.
39. Willigenburg TV. Protecting autonomy as authenticity using Ulysses contracts. J Med Philos. 2005;30:395–409.

Perioperative Pain Management: Miscellaneous (Monitoring, Risk Assessment)

Edwin Amirianfar, Alexander Bautista, and Alaa Abd-Elsayed

Abstract Managing pain in the perioperative period is imperative, but careful consideration must be taken into account in order to properly, yet safely, administer medications to treat pain. Factors to consider for patients who are receiving both opioid and non-opioid pain medications, include age, chronic medical conditions, opioid naivety/tolerance Bethell et al. (Pharmacoepidemiol Drug Saf 29:504–9, 2020 [1]). Therefore, it is imperative to understand a patient's medical history in order to achieve adequate pain relief, while also creating a customized treatment plan to mitigate side effects.

Keywords Monitoring · Assessment · Risks · Pain management · Pain scale · Cannabis use · Opioid use disorder

High Risk Patients

1 Elderly

The elderly population, defined as patients over the age of 65, are at elevated risk for the development of a number of postoperative complications including an increased risk of postoperative delirium and functional decline [2, 3]. With advances in medical

E. Amirianfar (✉) · A. Bautista
Department of Anesthesiology and Perioperative Medicine, University of Louisville, Louisville, KY, USA
e-mail: Edwin.Amirianfar@louisville.edu

A. Bautista
e-mail: alexander.bautista@louisville.edu

A. Abd-Elsayed
University of Wisconsin-Madison, AnesthesiologyMadison, USA
e-mail: abdelsayed@wisc.edu

A. Abd-Elsayed and K. Schroeder (eds.), *Perioperative Pain Management*,
https://doi.org/10.1007/978-3-031-67648-2_7

management and surgical techniques, this patient population is now exposed to surgery more often than in the past with over 310 million surgeries performed per year [4].

With aging, functional changes occur in multiple organs that should be considered when prescribing medications to address pain. Functional changes occur that can affect the respiratory, cardiovascular, gastrointestinal, and renal systems [5]. Furthermore, metabolism and body mass composition are also affected in the aging population [5]. Aging impacts body mass composition through increases in total body water and reductions in lean body mass. This can affect the volume of distribution for medications as hydrophilic drugs will have a smaller apparent volume of distribution while lipophilic drugs will have an increased volume of distribution with a prolonged half-life [5, 6]. Drug absorption is also affected by aging, including a reduction in first-pass metabolism, which can lead to increased plasma concentrations of drugs (i.e. opioids) [5]. Furthermore, hepatic changes, either as a result of liver disease or normal aging, can also affect metabolism, including reductions in cytochrome P450 activity in the liver, which can alter first-pass metabolism and significantly increase bioavailability [5]. Aging also affects the respiratory system, where structural changes include a loss of lung elastic recoil, increased chest wall rigidity and a decrease in the force generation from respiratory muscles, which leads to a reduction in pulmonary function [7]. The changes in lung function play a role in the elderly population as they are more prone to the adverse effects of many of these pain medications.

Due to the age-related changes seen in the elderly, opioid monotherapy should be utilized with caution because the risk of adverse events associated with elevated opioid doses may be increased in these patients [8]. Multimodal analgesia utilizes various medication classes with different mechanisms of action to adequately control pain, while also limiting the adverse events associated with any particular analgesic class [9]. These multimodal analgesic medications include acetaminophen, NSAIDs, gabapentinoids, and ketamine. [9] Regional anesthesia, which includes both peripheral nerve blocks and neuraxial anesthesia, is another mode of analgesia that can assist with managing pain in the perioperative period in elderly patients. Peripheral nerve blocks consist of identifying a peripheral nerve and infiltrating it with an anesthetic agent with the goal of blocking transmission and inhibiting pain signaling [10]. Neuraxial anesthesia is the placement of local anesthetic in the proximity of the central nervous system and includes spinal, epidural, and caudal anesthesia [11]. Neuraxial anesthetics work by blocking nerve signal connections to the spinal cord to prevent the transmission of pain and also prevent spinal reflex inhibition of diaphragmatic and gastrointestinal function thereby hastening the return of bowel activity following surgery [8]. Peripheral and neuraxial anesthesia are considered safe in the elderly population and have shown that they are associated with decreased pain scores, a decreased need for postoperative analgesic medications, earlier ambulation, earlier return of bowel function, and improved mental status [2]. Common procedures where regional anesthesia can be used include thoracotomy, colectomy, and a variety of extremity procedures including joint arthroplasty or fracture repair [2]. Possible adverse events of regional anesthesia include nerve damage, hematoma, infection, and intravascular injection of local anesthetic [12]. In addition, the presence of local anesthetic systemic toxicity (LAST) from injection into vasculature presents with immediate seizures, which is more likely to occur in elderly patients likely due to decreased circulating plasma proteins and diminished hepatic function [12, 13].

2 Obstructive Sleep Apnea

Obstructive sleep apnea (OSA) is another medical diagnosis that should be considered in patients in the perioperative period. There are approximately 1 billion people affected globally by OSA making this an incredibly common diagnosis. Frequently, patients may present without a diagnosis of OSA and a thorough preoperative discussion may unveil a constellation of findings suggestive of the diagnosis [14]. The STOP-Bang questionnaire is an effective screening tool for OSA which includes asking patients about their snoring, tiredness, observed apnea, blood pressure, body mass index, age, neck size, and gender [15]. Providing adequate analgesia for patients with OSA may be difficult as opioids can be associated with a decrease in hypoxic and hypercapnic ventilatory drive that can further exacerbate nocturnal desaturation events [16]. In patients with OSA, the utilization of multimodal analgesia, including NSAIDs, acetaminophen, tramadol, ketamine, pregabalin, regional blocks or catheters may be helpful in decreasing the need for opioids [17]. Regional anesthesia approaches should consider the impact of diminished diaphragmatic function and potentially preferentially select approaches that avoid impacting the pulmonary system. Oral opioids should be the preferred route of administration following surgery, as patients with OSA are more likely to have oxygen desaturations with intravenous opioids [17]. Although there are no evidence-based guidelines, it would be appropriate to monitor these patients more closely in the postoperative period for any oxygen desaturations [18]. In certain patients (i.e. those with severe OSA or in whom large doses of postoperative opioid administration are anticipated), it may be prudent to error on the side of inpatient monitoring until patients can be more safely discharged.

3 Opioid Use Disorder

Opioid use disorder (OUD) is a chronic disease characterized by tolerance, craving, inability to control the use, and continued use despite adverse consequences [19]. Patients with OUD have a significant impairment and disability in daily activities at home and work [20]. This subset of patients can pose a challenge in terms of finding the right balance of adequate acute pain control without compromising the patient's road to recovery. Patients oftentimes encounter unfair treatment and are misjudged by providers because of the stigma associated with their condition. Inadequate pain relief, withdrawal symptoms and an increased relapse rate are common concerns in the perioperative setting [21].

It is imperative that a multidisciplinary team approach is utilized to successfully manage the analgesic needs of these patients. A referral to an acute pain service, substance use disorder team, psychologist and obtaining a thorough pain management history from the provider managing OUD is crucial. A urine toxicology screen testing for substances being used to treat OUD such as methadone, buprenorphine, opioids and illicit substances are helpful to gather objective information. The online prescription drug monitoring program databases should also be reviewed for confirmation of prescribed analgesics [22].

Patients who are at higher risk for opioid misuse and concomitant high anxiety levels and catastrophizing may benefit from further evaluation and categorization through use of the Pain Catastrophizing Scale. It has been shown that negative thinking can affect anxiety levels and may also trigger drug craving [23]. The utilization of the opioid risk tool can help guide postoperative pain management by screening patients with chronic pain who may be at high risk for relapse if opioid analgesics are prescribed.

Patients with OUD also have a higher tolerance to opioid medications and this must be taken into consideration when developing an appropriate pain regimen. For patients receiving opioid agonist therapy (OAT) with methadone or buprenorphine, their home dosage should be confirmed and continued in the perioperative period [17]. It is thought that patients on buprenorphine may require higher doses of opioids to displace buprenorphine from the mu opioid receptors in order to achieve adequate pain control [24]. Therefore, providers may need to administer higher starting doses of opioid medications in this population as compared to the opioid naïve population. Patients on OAT therapy should also receive oral and/or IV opioids with the use of patient-controlled anesthesia (PCA) [25]. However, patients with low doses of buprenorphine (considered 2 to 8 mg per day) may benefit from more frequent buprenorphine dosing (i.e. every 6 to 8 h) which will allow the drug to provide enhanced analgesic effects. The American Society of Regional Anesthesia recommends against the discontinuation of buprenorphine in the perioperative period for patients with OUD as this practice may be associated with an increased risk of relapse and overdose.

On the day of surgery, patients consuming chronic opioid analgesics should take their usual dose of oral opioid the morning of their surgery and should receive their daily maintenance dose preoperatively before the induction of general, spinal or regional anesthesia [26]. If a patient is unable to receive oral intake (i.e. preoperative fasting), the oral opioid dose should be converted to the IV dose of morphine [26]. Intraoperatively, further opioid administration should be guided by vital signs, specifically heart rate and blood pressure, and pupil dilation [26]. The Analgesia Nociception Index may also be used for guidance of opioid medication dosing, but the utility of this may be limited in patients who have severe arrhythmias, atrial fibrillation, implanted pacemakers, cardiopulmonary bypass, and those on antimuscarinic drugs [27].

A multimodal approach to pain management should be strongly considered in this patient population where the utility of escalating opioid doses is frequently limited. For example, the use of non-steroidal anti-inflammatory drugs (NSAIDs), acetaminophen, and regional anesthesia techniques should be strongly considered. The use of NSAIDs in the perioperative period may be associated with adverse effects that limit the applicability of these agents, including an increased risk of bleeding and kidney injury, which increases with higher dosage, concomitant anticoagulant use and higher COX-1 selectivity [28].

Post-operative pain management should always be individualized. The patient and the provider should be partners when determining which medication should be used while weighing a patient's history of analgesic management with the risks and benefits of proposed treatment options. Regardless of the type of surgical intervention, analgesic management plans should include pharmacologic non-opioid medications, regional anesthesia when appropriate and non-pharmacological interventions. In choosing which medication to use, i.e. methadone, buprenorphine and naltrexone, the providers should consider the patient's preference, drug interactions, and existing cardiac conduction problems such as prolonged QT interval. If the use of opioids is inevitable, patients should be made aware of the risk and benefits associated with opioid administration and the patients' addictionologist should be included as a decision-making collaborator.

It is necessary to educate patients and family members of opioid safe practices including safe medication use, storage and disposal, follow-up appointments, monitoring for signs and symptoms of cravings, withdrawals and anxiety. It is necessary for these patients to have close monitoring and encouragement for them to continue their OUD treatment and be provided with support as necessary [22].

4 Cannabis Use

"Cannabis" refers to products derived from the plant *Cannabis sativa* and includes marijuana, which contains significant amounts of tetrahydrocannabinol (THC) [29]. Marijuana is the most commonly used federally illegal drug in the United States and it is estimated that 30% of marijuana users have cannabis use disorder (CUD), which is defined as problematic cannabis use leading to impairment or distress that includes impaired control, continued use despite social/medical problems, craving, tolerance and withdrawal [30, 31]. The American Society of Regional Anesthesia and Pain Medicine have created guidelines as a response to the increased use of cannabis. One study showed that patients who were cannabis users experienced more postoperative pain and higher opioid consumption [32]. These guidelines recommend screening all patients for cannabis use, type of cannabis used, amount, frequency, and time and route of last consumption [33].

The various patient populations discussed may pose difficulties in managing pain. Specific tools to monitor and assess treatment should be implemented to assist providers in addressing pain. Although these are mostly subjective, they can give the provider an idea of whether or not the interventions are providing any benefit.

Monitoring

As analgesia with opioid medications is frequently required following surgery, healthcare professionals must be aware of the potential side effects that they can cause, the most serious of which remains sedation and respiratory depression [34]. Respiratory depression occurs through activation of μ-opioid receptors at specific sites in the central nervous system, including the respiratory rhythm generating area in the pons [35].

The PRediction of Opioid-induced respiratory Depression IN patients monitored by capnoGraphY (PRODIGY) trial created a risk prediction tool that accurately predicts respiratory depression in patients receiving parenteral opioids [36]. The PRODIGY Risk Prediction Tool consists of five different domains: age, sex, previous opioid use, presence of sleep disordered breathing, and presence of chronic heart failure (CHF). Each domain is designated a score and the sum of each domain is totaled. If the total score is less than 8 points, then the patient is considered low risk for respiratory depression. If the total score is 8 to 14, the patient is considered intermediate risk for respiratory depression. High risk of respiratory depression is considered 15 points or higher. See the table below that describes the PRODIGY Risk Prediction Tool (Table 1).

Table 1 PRODIGY risk score tool

Risk factors	Scoring criteria	Points	Score
Patient age (years)	Age < 60 Age 60–69 Age 70–79 Age ≥ 80	= 0 points = 8 points = 12 points = 16 points	
Sex	Male Female	= 8 points = 0 points	
Previous opioid use	Opioid naïve Previous opioid use	= 3 points = 0 points	
Sleep disordered breathing (SDB)	Known SDB or high STOP-BANG score	= 5 points = 0 points	
Chronic heart failure (CHF)	Coexisting CHF No known CHF	= 7 points = 0 points	
Total PRODIGY risk score			

5 Assessment

Pain assessment plays an important role for practitioners when they are prescribing pain medication. One study showed that poor pain assessment was the single most important barrier to adequate pain management [37]. Many different tools are used for pain assessment in patients perioperatively, including the Visual Analog Scale (VAS), Oswestry Disability Index, and the Functional assessment.

6 VAS

The VAS was the most frequently used scale in one study comparing different pain assessment tools (Fig. 1) [38]. The VAS is known to be a simple tool that is easy to understand for those that are cognitively intact and its ease of use is convenient in the clinical setting [39, 40]. The VAS is a line that is 100 mm in length that is labeled from 0 to 100 mm, corresponding to "no pain" and "worst possible pain," respectively, as seen in Fig. 2. As this is on a millimeter scale, patients are asked to mark where their pain intensity is on the VAS, with 101 possible levels of pain intensity [41]. Studies have shown that ranges on the VAS from 0 to 4 mm can be considered no pain, 5 to 44 mm as mild pain, 45 to 74 mm as moderate pain, and 75 mm to 100 mm as severe pain [42]. Assessing responses to analgesics should correlate with the mode of administration of the medication and expected time to maximal effect, where intravenous administration of opioids are typically assessed 15 to 30 min after administration and oral medications are reassessed at 45–60 min following administration [43]. The minimal clinically important difference is a change of 10 mm on the VAS, with acceptable pain control after surgery being less than 33 mm [44].

Fig. 1 Visual analog scale

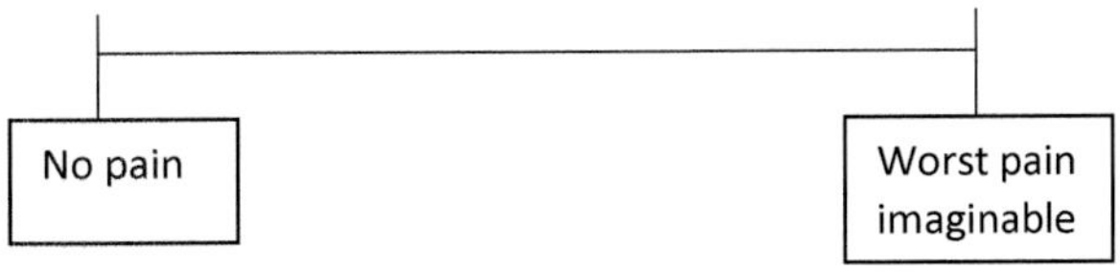

Fig. 2 Numeric rating scale

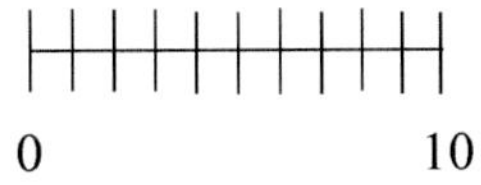

7 Numerical Rating Scale (NRS)

The Numerical Rating Scale (NRS) evaluates patients' pain from a scale, usually 0 to 10, See Fig. 2 [45]. Compared to the VAS, this scale has a certain amount of options (i.e. in a 0 to 10 point scale there are 11 possible options) whereas the VAS can have unlimited answers options. The NRS has been validated as a pain assessment measuring tool that has similar validity to other pain scales and strongly correlated with VAS [46].

8 Oswestry Disability Index

Introduced in 1980, the Oswestry Disability Index (ODI) is the most commonly used outcome-measure questionnaire for low back pain in the hospital setting and consists of ten sections, scored from 0 to 5 for each answer for a total possible score of 50 [47, 48]. The statements are scored on a scale from 0 to 5 with 0 representing no disability and 5 representing most severe disability. This score is then multiplied by 2 and is then converted into a percentage. An ODI of 0–20% represents minimal disability, 21–40% represents moderate disability, 41–60% represents severe disability, 61–80% represents severely crippled, 81–100% represents patients are bed bound [49]. Studies have shown that patients with LBP but no disability have an average ODI of 11.88, while those who have LBP with disability have an average ODI of 22.07 [50]. Studies have shown that the ODI is reliable and easy to use in clinical practice for patients with low back pain [51]. In the year 2000, modifications were made to the ODI with changes in wording of statements in multiple sections, now called version 2.0, and is now preferred over the original version [52].

9 Functional Pain Scale

Another way to assess pain is in terms of its relation to a patient's functional status and their ability to attend to their daily duties/activities. The Functional Pain Scale (FPS) evaluates a patient's pain and its effect on their daily activities on a scale of 0 (indicating no pain) to 10 (indicating immobilizing pain) [53]. Table 2 describes the different levels of pain with their appropriate descriptors. Pain is considered "mild" if from 1 to 3, "moderate" if from 4 to 6, and "severe" if 7 or higher [53]. These numbers will correlate to different activities of daily living, sleep habits and communicability with others and has the potential to give the clinician a more objective assessmentof a patient's pain and their response to medications. The FPS does have its limitations though, including its use in those with lower education, as the FPS has some words that require a level of reading comprehension/understanding that may exceed the ability of some patients [53].

Table 2 Functional pain scale description and definition

Description	Definition
No pain (0)	No pain
Minimal (1)	Hardly noticeable/no impact on ADL's/ sleep not affected and able to use passive distraction for comfort
Mild (2)	Noticeable when not distracted/no impact on ADL's/sleep only slightly affected and able to use both passive and active distraction for comfort
Uncomfortable (3)	Pain is present but can complete all ADL's/ sleep is slightly affected and passive distraction only give marginal relief
Moderate (4)	Constantly aware of pain but can complete ADLs with modification/sleep marginally affected at times/ passive distraction is of no use, but active distraction gives some relief
Distracting (5)	Aware of pain/ able to complete some ADL's but limited by pain/sleep is affected and active distraction are only slightly useful
Distressing (6)	Pain is present/unable to complete most ADLs limited by pain/ sleep is difficult and active distraction is only marginal
Unmanageable (7)	Pain interfere with normal ADL's/nothing seems to help/ sleep is very difficult/active distractions are very difficult to concentrate on
Intense (8)	Cannot complete any ADLs without much assistance/ cannot concentrate/ conversation is difficult/ unable to sleep and unable to use distraction
Severe (9)	Cannot do any ADL's even with assistance can barely talk/ unable to sleep and unable to use distraction
Immobilizing (10)	Unable to move or talk due to intensity of pain/unable to sleep and unable to use distraction

10 Conclusion

Pain management in the perioperative period may pose a challenge to many practitioners and a detailed history is imperative in customizing a pain regimen to create an individualized plan for each patient. One must consider whether or not a patient is high risk and should take this into account when creating a treatment plan. Assessing pain response to different interventions may also be difficult as most of the tools used are subjective and include the VAS, NRS, and ODI. The FPS can help provide the practitioner more of an objective view of how the patient's current pain status is and help further guide treatment.

11 Key Takeaway Points

1. Each patient must have their pain regimens customized including those who are considered high risk.
2. Utilizing the various pain scales can help providers assess patients' response to pain.
3. Using a multimodal approach to analgesia can help patients achieve pain relief, while also mitigating side effects.

References

1. Bethell J, Neuman MD, Bateman BT, et al. Age and postoperative opioid prescriptions: a population-based cohort study of opioid-naïve adults. Pharmacoepidemiol Drug Saf. 2020;29(4):504–9. https://doi.org/10.1002/pds.4964.
2. Shellito AD, Dworsky JQ, Kirkland PJ, et al. Perioperative pain management issues unique to older adults undergoing surgery: a narrative review. Ann Surg Open. 2021;2(3): e072. https://doi.org/10.1097/AS9.0000000000000072.
3. Hill MV, McMahon ML, Stucke RS, Barth RJ Jr. Wide variation and excessive dosage of opioid prescriptions for common general surgical procedures. Ann Surg. 2017;265(4):709–14. https://doi.org/10.1097/SLA.0000000000001993.
4. Dobson GP. Trauma of major surgery: a global problem that is not going away. Int J Surg. 2020;81:47–54. https://doi.org/10.1016/j.ijsu.2020.07.017.
5. Drenth-van Maanen AC, Wilting I, Jansen PAF. Prescribing medicines to older people-how to consider the impact of ageing on human organ and body functions. Br J Clin Pharmacol. 2020;86(10):1921–30. https://doi.org/10.1111/bcp.14094.
6. Shi S, Klotz U. Age-related changes in pharmacokinetics. Curr Drug Metab. 2011;12(7):601–10. https://doi.org/10.2174/138920011796504527.
7. Scott-Warren V, Maguire S. Physiology of ageing, Anaesthesia and Intens Care Med. 2017;18(1):52–54. ISSN 1472-0299,https://doi.org/10.1016/j.mpaic.2016.10.015
8. Nordquist D, Halaszynski TM. Perioperative multimodal anesthesia using regional techniques in the aging surgical patient. Pain Res Treat. 2014;2014: 902174. https://doi.org/10.1155/2014/902174.
9. Schwenk ES, Mariano ER. Designing the ideal perioperative pain management plan starts with multimodal analgesia. Korean J Anesthesiol. 2018;71(5):345–52. https://doi.org/10.4097/kja.d.18.00217.
10. Folino TB, Mahboobi SK. Regional anesthetic blocks. In: StatPearls. Treasure Island (FL): StatPearls Publishing; 29 Jan 2023.
11. Olawin AM, Das M J. Spinal anesthesia. In: StatPearls. Treasure Island (FL): StatPearls Publishing; 27 June 2022.
12. Kent CD, Bollag L. Neurological adverse events following regional anesthesia administration. Local Reg Anesth. 2010;3:115–23. https://doi.org/10.2147/LRA.S8177.
13. Fukuda T, Kakiuchi Y, Miyabe M, Kihara S, Kohda Y, Toyooka H. Free lidocaine concentrations during continuous epidural anesthesia in geriatric patients. Reg Anesth Pain Med. 2003;28(3):215–20. https://doi.org/10.1053/rapm.2003.50131.
14. Malhotra A, Ayappa I, Ayas N, et al. Metrics of sleep apnea severity: beyond the apnea-hypopnea index. Sleep. 2021;44(7):zsab030. https://doi.org/10.1093/sleep/zsab030

15. Pivetta B, Chen L, Nagappa M, et al. Use and performance of the STOP-bang questionnaire for obstructive sleep apnea screening across geographic regions: a systematic review and meta-analysis. JAMA Netw Open. 2021;4(3):e211009. Published 1 Mar 2021. https://doi.org/10.1001/jamanetworkopen.2021.1009
16. Weil JV, McCullough RE, Kline JS, Sodal IE. Diminished ventilatory response to hypoxia and hypercapnia after morphine in normal man. N Engl J Med. 1975;292(21):1103–6. https://doi.org/10.1056/NEJM197505222922106.
17. Bolden N, Smith CE, Auckley D, Makarski J, Avula R. Perioperative complications during use of an obstructive sleep apnea protocol following surgery and anesthesia. Anesth Analg. 2007;105(6):1869–70. https://doi.org/10.1213/01.ane.0000295223.31946.b5.
18. Kaw R, Gali B, Collop NA. Perioperative care of patients with obstructive sleep apnea. Curr Treat Options Neurol. 2011;13(5):496–507. https://doi.org/10.1007/s11940-011-0138-5.
19. Taylor JL, Samet JH. Opioid use disorder. Ann Intern Med. 2022;175(1):ITC1-ITC16. https://doi.org/10.7326/AITC202201180
20. Centers for Disease Control and Prevention. Opioid Basics | CDC's Response to the Opioid Overdose Epidemic | CDC. www.cdc.gov. Published 17 June 2021. https://www.cdc.gov/opioids/basics/index.html
21. Herscher M, Fine M, Navalurkar R, Hirt L, Wang L. Diagnosis and management of opioid use disorder in hospitalized patients. Med Clin North Am. 2020;104(4):695–708. https://doi.org/10.1016/j.mcna.2020.03.003.
22. Ward EN, Quaye AN, Wilens TE. Opioid use disorders: perioperative management of a special population. Anesth Analg. 2018;127(2):539–47. https://doi.org/10.1213/ANE.0000000000003477.
23. Koob GF, Volkow ND. Neurobiology of addiction: a neurocircuitry analysis. Lancet Psychiatry. 2016;3(8):760–73. https://doi.org/10.1016/S2215-0366(16)00104-8.
24. Kohan L, Potru S, Barreveld AM, et al. Buprenorphine management in the perioperative period: educational review and recommendations from a multisociety expert panel. Reg Anesth Pain Med. 2021;46(10):840–59. https://doi.org/10.1136/rapm-2021-103007.
25. Sritapan Y, Clifford S, Bautista A. Perioperative management of patients on buprenorphine and methadone: a narrative review. Balkan Med J. 2020;37(5):247–52. https://doi.org/10.4274/balkanmedj.galenos.2020.2020.5.2.
26. Coluzzi F, Bifulco F, Cuomo A, et al. The challenge of perioperative pain management in opioid-tolerant patients. Ther Clin Risk Manag. 2017;13:1163–1173. Published 5 Sep 2017. https://doi.org/10.2147/TCRM.S141332
27. Daccache G, Jeanne M, Fletcher D. The analgesia nociception index: tailoring opioid administration. Anesth Analg. 2017;125(1):15–7. https://doi.org/10.1213/ANE.0000000000002145.
28. Sheth KR, Bernthal NM, Ho HS, et al. Perioperative bleeding and non-steroidal anti-inflammatory drugs: an evidence-based literature review, and current clinical appraisal. Medicine (Baltimore). 2020;99(31): e20042. https://doi.org/10.1097/MD.0000000000020042.
29. National Center for Complementary and Integrative Health. Cannabis (Marijuana) and Cannabinoids: What You Need to Know. NCCIH. Published November 2019. https://www.nccih.nih.gov/health/cannabis-marijuana-and-cannabinoids-what-you-need-to-know
30. Centers for Disease Control and Prevention. Addiction | Health Effects | Marijuana | CDC. www.cdc.gov. Published 9 Sept 2021. https://www.cdc.gov/marijuana/health-effects/addiction.html
31. Kerridge BT, Pickering R, Chou P, Saha TD, Hasin DS. DSM-5 cannabis use disorder in the national epidemiologic survey on alcohol and related conditions-III: gender-specific profiles. Addict Behav. 2018;76:52–60. https://doi.org/10.1016/j.addbeh.2017.07.012.
32. Cannabis use increases pain after surgery, study shows. www.asahq.org. https://www.asahq.org/about-asa/newsroom/news-releases/2022/10/cannabis-use-increases-pain-after-surgery-study-shows
33. All Patients Should be Screened for Cannabis Use Before Surgery, First U.S. Guidelines Recommend. The American Society of Regional Anesthesia and Pain Medicine (ASRA). https://www.asra.com/news-publications/asra-update-item/asra-updates/2023/01/03/all-patients-should-be-screened-for-cannabis-use-before-surgery-first-u.s.-guidelines-recommend

34. Jarzyna D, Jungquist CR, Pasero C, et al. American society for pain management nursing guidelines on monitoring for opioid-induced sedation and respiratory depression. Pain Manag Nurs. 2011;12(3):118-145.e10. https://doi.org/10.1016/j.pmn.2011.06.008.
35. Boom M, Niesters M, Sarton E, Aarts L, Smith TW, Dahan A. Non-analgesic effects of opioids: opioid-induced respiratory depression. Curr Pharm Des. 2012;18(37):5994–6004. https://doi.org/10.2174/138161212803582469.
36. Khanna AK, Bergese SD, Jungquist CR, et al. Prediction of opioid-induced respiratory depression on inpatient wards using continuous capnography and oximetry: an international prospective, observational trial. Anesth Analg. 2020;131(4):1012–24. https://doi.org/10.1213/ANE.0000000000004788.
37. Von Roenn JH, Cleeland CS, Gonin R, Hatfield AK, Pandya KJ. Physician attitudes and practice in cancer pain management. A survey from the Eastern cooperative oncology group. Ann Intern Med. 1993;119(2):121–126. https://doi.org/10.7326/0003-4819-119-2-199307150-00005
38. Hjermstad MJ, Fayers PM, Haugen DF, et al. Studies comparing numerical rating scales, verbal rating scales, and visual analogue scales for assessment of pain intensity in adults: a systematic literature review. J Pain Symptom Manage. 2011;41(6):1073–93. https://doi.org/10.1016/j.jpainsymman.2010.08.016.
39. Reed MD, Van Nostran W. Assessing pain intensity with the visual analog scale: a plea for uniformity. J Clin Pharmacol. 2014;54(3):241–4. https://doi.org/10.1002/jcph.250.
40. Younger J, McCue R, Mackey S. Pain outcomes: a brief review of instruments and techniques. Curr Pain Headache Rep. 2009;13(1):39–43. https://doi.org/10.1007/s11916-009-0009-x.
41. Williamson A, Hoggart B. Pain: a review of three commonly used pain rating scales. J Clin Nurs. 2005;14(7):798–804. https://doi.org/10.1111/j.1365-2702.2005.01121.x.
42. Jensen MP, Chen C, Brugger AM. Interpretation of visual analog scale ratings and change scores: a reanalysis of two clinical trials of postoperative pain. J Pain. 2003;4(7):407–14. https://doi.org/10.1016/s1526-5900(03)00716-8.
43. Wells N, Pasero C, McCaffery M. Improving the quality of care through pain assessment and management. In: Hughes RG editors. Patient safety and quality: an evidence-based handbook for nurses. Rockville (MD): Agency for Healthcare Research and Quality (US); April 2008.
44. Myles PS, Myles DB, Galagher W, et al. Measuring acute postoperative pain using the visual analog scale: the minimal clinically important difference and patient acceptable symptom state. Br J Anaesth. 2017;118(3):424–9. https://doi.org/10.1093/bja/aew466.
45. Haefeli M, Elfering A. Pain assessment. Eur Spine J. 2006;15Suppl 1(Suppl 1):S17–S24. https://doi.org/10.1007/s00586-005-1044-x
46. Adeboye A, Hart R, Senapathi SH, Ali N, Holman L, Thomas HW. Assessment of functional pain score by comparing to traditional pain scores. Cureus. 2021;13(8):e16847. Published 3 Aug 2021. https://doi.org/10.7759/cureus.16847
47. Fairbank JC, Couper J, Davies JB, O'Brien JP. The Oswestry low back pain disability questionnaire. Physiotherapy. 1980;66(8):271–3.
48. Mehra A, Baker D, Disney S, Pynsent PB. Oswestry disability index scoring made easy. Ann R Coll Surg Engl. 2008;90(6):497–9. https://doi.org/10.1308/003588408X300984.
49. Yeh J. Vertebroplasty and kyphoplasty. Orthopaedic bone cements. Published online 2008:74–91. https://doi.org/10.1533/9781845695170.1.74
50. Tonosu J, Takeshita K, Hara N, et al. The normative score and the cut-off value of the Oswestry Disability Index (ODI). Eur Spine J. 2012;21(8):1596–602. https://doi.org/10.1007/s00586-012-2173-7.
51. Vianin M. Psychometric properties and clinical usefulness of the Oswestry Disability Index. J Chiropr Med. 2008;7(4):161–3. https://doi.org/10.1016/j.jcm.2008.07.001.
52. Fairbank JC, Pynsent PB. The Oswestry disability index. Spine (Phila Pa 1976). 2000;25(22):2940–2952. https://doi.org/10.1097/00007632-200011150-00017
53. Adeboye A, Hart R, Senapathi SH, Ali N, Holman L, Thomas HW. Assessment of functional pain score by comparing to traditional pain scores. Cureus. 2021;13(8):e16847. Published 3 Aug 2021. https://doi.org/10.7759/cureus.16847

Review of Eras Pain Management Protocols

George Yacoub, Clara Nemr, and Alaa Abd-Elsayed

Abstract This chapter focuses on summarizing and reviewing recent literature evaluating common pain management strategies employed by Enhanced Recovery After Surgery (ERAS) protocols. ERAS protocols that promote effective pain management focus on the use of multimodal analgesia methods and the implementation of nerve blocks to reduce pain and opioid consumption in the postoperative setting. Recent literature review shows particularly strong support for the incorporation of perioperative administration of Cox-inhibitors in combination with NSAIDs, glucocorticoids, and central a-2 agonists, as well as the incorporation of an appropriate nerve block. Multimodal analgesia, in addition to administration of a neural block, are well established methods that serve the goal of reducing postoperative pain, opioid consumption, and postoperative nausea and vomiting.

Keywords ERAS · Enhanced recovery after surgery · Pain management · Multimodal Analgesia · Neural block

1 Introduction

Enhanced Recovery After Surgery (ERAS) is a patient-focused program that aims to create specialized surgical protocols with the goal of reducing a patient's stress response to surgery, enhancing physiological performance, and expediting the recovery process. In addition, this multidisciplinary approach works to reduce

G. Yacoub (✉)
University of Michigan Medical School, Ann Arbor, MI, USA
e-mail: geyacoub@med.umich.edu

C. Nemr
Chicago College of Osteopathic Medicine, Midwestern University, Downers Grove, IL, USA
e-mail: clara.nemr@midwestern.edu

A. Abd-Elsayed
Department of Anesthesia, University of Wisconsin School of Medicine and Public Health, Madison, WI, USA
e-mail: abdelsayed@wisc.edu

A. Abd-Elsayed and K. Schroeder (eds.), *Perioperative Pain Management*,
https://doi.org/10.1007/978-3-031-67648-2_8

expenses, shorten hospital stays, and mitigate postoperative complications and readmissions [1]. The ERAS term was coined in 2001 by a group of surgeons led by Professor Ken Fearon and Professor Olle Ljungqvist to create an evidence-based multimodal perioperative care pathway for patients undergoing major surgery. At that time, physicians were practicing in a manner that failed to reflect published evidence-based guidance and best practice. Further enhancements occurred following the implementation of a common patient database and efforts to sustain compliance and collaboration among medical centers, ultimately improving patient care. In 2010, the ERAS Society for Perioperative Care was founded and quickly added membership institutions with multidisciplinary interest in improvements in perioperative patient care [2]. Basic ERAS protocols include preoperative patient guidance/education, baseline nutrition assessment and supplementation, elimination/limited fasting in the perioperative period, avoidance of nasogastric tubes, introduction of carbohydrate intake up to two hours before surgery, implementation of standardized anesthetic and pain management procedures (such as epidurals and non-opioid pain relief) and initiating early patient mobilization [3].

2 Preoperative ERAS Guidelines

ERAS preoperative protocols require patients to receive counseling prior to surgery. Patient education can be in the form of an in-person class, multimedia content, virtual reality, or telephone interview. Counseling information is generally provided for the patient and their support infrastructure and generally includes recovery expectations and planning, fasting guideline review and timing of carbohydrate drink consumption, prescription fulfillment, provision of contact information for questions that may arise as surgery approaches, and meeting with an ERAS coordinator, anesthesiologist, and surgeon. In addition, targeted history and physical examinations are performed to ensure optimization and preemptively address any medical titration or diagnostic requirements. Surgical optimization may include both medical and psychological interventions that aid in facilitating the recovery profile of patients. These interventions might include preoperative training relevant to deep breathing exercises, guided-imagery, and alcohol smoking abstinence for 4 weeks prior to surgery, anemia therapy, endocrinology consult for diabetics, O-NET screening for chronic pain patients, and showering with chlorhexidine-based scrub before surgery [4].

3 ERAS Guidelines: Multimodal Analgesia for Perioperative Care

Pain management is a crucial component of ERAS protocols. Specifically, multimodal analgesia involves the simultaneous utilization of diverse techniques and medications to deliver effective pain relief while minimizing reliance on opioids and reducing opioid-related side effects [4]. Preemptive analgesic approaches have demonstrated an ability to reduce pain, opioid requirements, inflammation, nausea, and vomiting [5, 6]. Regional anesthetic techniques linked to perioperative multimodal analgesia include intrathecal morphine, thoracic epidural, transversus abdominis plane (TAP) block, and erector spinae plane block (ESPB). Systemic medications encompass lidocaine, acetaminophen, nonsteroidal anti-inflammatory drugs (NSAIDs), gabapentinoids, dexamethasone, NMDA receptor antagonists, and central α-2 agonists [7].

4 Intrathecal Morphine

Intrathecal morphine (ITM) therapy promotes postoperative analgesia through preoperative injection of 3–20 mcg/kg of morphine into the cerebrospinal fluid, activating Mu-opioid receptors in the dorsal horn of the spinal cord [8]. Morphine exhibits hydrophilic characteristics in comparison to other opioids, resulting in an extended stay in the cerebrospinal fluid and a prolonged duration of action. Intravenous (IV) morphine and intrathecal morphine share similar side effects, however smaller doses of morphine are administered intrathecally [9]. A meta-analysis performed by Musa et al. evaluates the effects of intrathecal morphine in the pediatric spine surgery setting, shows that ITM administration reduces total postoperative opioid consumption at 24 and 48 h and increases the time until analgesic rescue. Furthermore, this study showed no significant increase in incidence of respiratory depression, nausea and vomiting, or pruritus with ITM use [10]. A similar meta-analysis study was performed by Wang et al. but focuses on adult spinal surgery and shows that ITM administration significantly reduces postoperative pain up to 24 h and reduces analgesic consumption. ITM was shown to be associated with increased incidence of pruritus in this study, but not any other opioid related side effects including respiratory depression or nausea and vomiting [11]. A meta-analysis study performed by Ryu et al. and focuses on the Cesarean setting shows that ITM administration significantly reduces postoperative pain and morphine consumption, and is especially more effective when combined with a ilioinguinal nerve and anterior transversus abdominis plane block [12]. A randomized control trial by Cheah et al. shows ITM administration in the setting of primary total joint arthroplasty reduces postoperative pain, nausea and vomiting, and improves patient ambulation, but has no significant effect on total opioid consumption [13].

5 Thoracic Epidural Analgesia

Thoracic epidural analgesia provides excellent pain relief in patients undergoing upper abdominal, colorectal, thoracic, and gynecological surgeries. Thoracic epidural analgesia blocks pain fibers from the thoracic sympathetic chain ganglia and is administered through a catheter placed in the epidural space around the spinal cord [14]. The thoracic epidural space consists of valveless veins connecting to the azygos vein and the basivertebral plexus. Infusions of local anesthetics or opioids within the epidural space travel towards the nerve roots and through the intervertebral foramina [15]. Epidural analgesia minimizes opioid requirements, enhances the ability of patients to breathe and cough, improves respiratory function, facilitates mobility, and reduces ileus. Common side effects of epidural infusions include hypotension, pruritus, and urinary retention [7]. Serious side effects including local anesthetic systemic toxicity, epidural hematoma, and sustained nerve injury are rare. A systematic review and meta-analysis were conducted by Daghmouri et al. to evaluate a variety of analgesic techniques and their impact on postoperative pain in the laparoscopic colonic surgery setting. Their study shows that postoperative administration of thoracic epidural analgesia is associated with significant postoperative pain reduction at 24 h and faster bowel function recovery, but a longer length of stay [16]. A similar study by Lin et al. analyzing the effects of regional pain management techniques in the video-assisted thoracic surgery setting showed postoperative thoracic epidural analgesia administration to be associated with lower resting pain compared to other strategies [17]. A similar meta- analysis study by Luo et al. that evaluates analgesic techniques in breast and thoracic surgery setting showed that thoracic epidural analgesia is significantly less effective at reducing pain compared to other thoracic analgesic techniques [18]. A systematic review by Hughes et al. evaluating the effectiveness of thoracic epidural analgesia in the open abdominal surgery setting shows thoracic epidural analgesia to be associated with significantly reduced postoperative pain when compared to patient-controlled systemic opioids postoperatively [19].

6 Transversus Abdominis Plane Block

The transversus abdominis plane (TAP) block is a mode of analgesia that functions via the administration of local anesthetics between the transversus abdominis and internal oblique muscles. The block anesthetizes thoracolumbar nerves innervating the anterior abdominal wall and is used in the setting of a variety of abdominal surgeries [20]. When used for postoperative analgesia following abdominal surgery, TAP blocks have been shown to reduce pain and opioid consumption [21]. Risks associated with ultrasound-guided abdominal TAP blocks include visceral organ injury, bleeding/hematoma formation, local anesthetic systemic toxicity (including ventricular arrhythmia and seizures), and transient femoral nerve palsy [22]. Daghmouri et al.'s meta-analysis of analgesic techniques in the laparoscopic colonic surgery setting showed TAP blocks were associated with lower postoperative pain scores at 24 h, reduced opioid consumption, shorter length of stay, and faster bowel function recovery [16]. Systematic review and meta-analysis by Brogi et al. evaluating the effects of TAP block on postoperative pain showed that TAP block is associated with significant postoperative pain reduction at 6, 12, and 24 h and reduced opioid consumption in the gynecological, appendectomy, inguinal, bariatric, and urological surgery setting [21]. However, a similar meta-analysis by Shin et al. focusing on effects of TAP blocks in the laparoscopic hysterectomy setting showed no significant effect of using a TAP block on postoperative pain or opioid consumption [23]. Ding et al.'s meta-analysis study on laparoscopic gynecologic surgeries shows, with high confidence, that TAP block in combination with adjuvant analgesia significantly reduces postoperative pain and opioid consumption at 24 h, especially when combined with paracetamol and NSAIDs [24]. While classic approaches to TAP blocks are effective for anesthetizing the lower abdomen, subcostal technique modifications may extend analgesia and prove effective for upper abdominal procedures as well.

7 Erector Spinae Plane Block

Erector spinae plane block (ESPB) is an additional analgesic modality that has been reported to provide effective analgesia following a large number of spine, abdominal, breast, and thoracic surgical procedures. The mechanism of analgesia following ESPB is, as of yet, a matter of contention but proposed mechanisms include the blockade of ventral rami of spinal nerves, sympathetic nerve fibers, and intercostal nerves [25]. The ESPB is performed by injecting a local anesthetic between the anterior fascia of the erector spinae muscle group and the tip of the transverse process of either thoracic or lumbar vertebra. ESPB is conceptually both safer and easier to perform than a paravertebral block and procedural ease is enhanced through an ability to realize extended dermatomal analgesia following a single injection [26]. A meta-analysis was performed by Ma et al. to explore the analgesic effect of ESPB in spine surgery where they found that preoperative ESPB significantly reduces postoperative pain, opioid consumption, and post operative nausea and vomiting (PONV) [27]. A similar study by Koo et al. focused on thoracic surgeries also demonstrated that ESPB use is associated with lower postoperative pain scores [28]. Viderman et al. in a meta-analysis study focusing on abdominal surgery showed that ESPB use is associated with lower postoperative opioid consumption and an extended duration until rescue analgesia is required [29]. A meta-analysis by Cui et al. that included studies in the breast, orthopedic, thoracoscopic, cholecystectomy, nephrolithotomy, and cardiac surgery settings demonstrated that ESPB reduced postoperative opioid consumption at 24 h, PONV, and prolonged the time until rescue analgesia was required [30].

8 Lidocaine

Lidocaine, a local anesthetic, provides multimodal pain control by inhibiting propagation of nerve impulses through blocking voltage-gated sodium channels in neurons, preventing depolarization [7]. Perioperative lidocaine infusions decrease pain, opioid usage, ileus duration, nausea, and length of stay. In addition, lidocaine infusions mitigate the proinflammatory effects caused by surgery by blocking polymorphonuclear neutrophil priming [31]. The mechanism by which lidocaine inhibits intracellular G-protein signaling molecules explains the low concentrations of active lidocaine needed and its prolonged duration of effect at those low concentrations [32]. A systematic review was performed by Chu et al. in 2020 that evaluated the role of IV lidocaine in the management of acute and chronic postoperative pain. Chu et al.'s study demonstrated that dosing guidelines for IV lidocaine are inconsistent. Different studies performed a starting intraoperative IV lidocaine bolus ranging from 1.5–2 mg/kg. Maintenance doses ranged from 1.5 mg/kg/hr to 3 mg/kg/hr. The studies also differed on the use of post-operative continuous IV infusions, with some studies discontinuing IV lidocaine postoperatively and others performing a continuous infusion that ranged in duration between 4–24 h postoperatively. Furthermore, the efficacy of IV lidocaine in reducing pain and reducing opioid use and side effects has not been shown to be consistent across the studies. Some studies demonstrate lidocaine's efficacy in reducing pain while no significant pain reduction is found in other studies across a variety of different surgical specialties including laparoscopic abdominal, open abdominal, breast, and ENT surgeries [33]. A systematic review by Boswell et al. that focuses on cardiac surgery shows that perioperative IV lidocaine administration has not been shown to significantly reduce pain or improve surgical outcomes [34]. Stone et al. published ERAS guidelines for minimally invasive gynecologic surgery that recommends not including IV lidocaine broadly due to lack of literature evidence supporting its benefits [35]. A randomized clinical trial by Casas-Arroyave et al. demonstrated intravenous lidocaine demonstrates comparable efficacy to thoracic epidural analgesia in controlling acute postoperative pain following major abdominal surgery at the 24-h postoperative mark [36].

9 Acetaminophen and NSAIDS

Acetaminophen is a fundamental component of many supplementary analgesic treatment regimens where it has demonstrated an ability to decrease postoperative pain and opioid requirements. Acetaminophen reduces the release of proinflammatory and pain-amplifying mediators, leading to antinociceptive effects at peripheral sites [37]. Oral and IV acetaminophen are both available for administration, however IV acetaminophen may be more feasible in anesthetized patients or with contraindications to oral intake and peaks faster in cerebrospinal fluid [38]. NSAIDs mechanism of action is the inhibition of cyclooxygenase (COX) enzymes. COX converts arachidonic acid into prostaglandins, prostacyclins, and thromboxanes, with the therapeutic effects arising from the lack of these eicosanoids. Thromboxanes contribute to platelet adhesion, while prostaglandins induce vasodilation, elevate the hypothalamic temperature set-point, and participate in anti-nociception [39]. The combination of NSAIDs and acetaminophen results in a much more significant reduction of postoperative pain and opioid consumption than acetaminophen alone [37]. Meta-analysis of a variety of studies in different fields including thoracic, orthopedic, gynecological, obstetric, and general surgery demonstrated that postoperative co-administration of paracetamol, NSAIDs, and COX-2 inhibitors with patient-controlled analgesia morphine resulted in a significant reduction of morphine administration in the first 24 h post-surgery. Co-administration of NSAIDs significantly reduced morphine administration and significantly reduced the risk of PONV [38]. A meta-analysis by Heybati et al. evaluating the effects of non-opioid analgesic administration perioperatively in the adult cardiac surgery setting demonstrated, with moderate to high confidence, that acetaminophen use significantly reduces postoperative pain at 24 h [40]. A meta-analysis study by Ding et al. evaluated nonopioid analgesics and regional techniques for perioperative pain management in laparoscopic gynecological surgery. With a high confidence level, they found that NSAID administration, with and without acetaminophen, significantly reduces total opioid consumption at 24 h, and co-administration with acetaminophen and a topical analgesic or a peripheral nerve block reduces pain at 24 h [24]. Use of prophylactic acetaminophen combined with NSAIDs is shown to reduce morphine intake, reduce post-operative pain, and significantly improve patient ambulation in total knee arthroplasties more effectively than using acetaminophen or NSAIDs alone [41]. Implementation of ERAS pathways prior to elective cesarean section was shown to drive an eightfold increase in IV acetaminophen use and a twofold decrease in morphine use controlling for age, race, ethnicity, pre-pregnancy body mass index, and patient reported pain score. Furthermore, there was a significant increase in the proportion of patients reporting acceptable pain scores, decrease in outpatient opioid prescription on discharge, decrease in hours to postsurgical ambulation, and decrease in hours to postsurgical solid intake [42].

10 Gabapentinoids

Gabapentinoids are structural analogs of the inhibitory neurotransmitter γ-aminobutyric acid (GABA) and are antiepileptic, anticonvulsant drugs used to treat neuropathic pain. When administered preoperatively, gabapentinoids block hyperalgesia surrounding wounds in postoperative patients [43]. In addition, gabapentinoids are effective for reducing perioperative pain, development of chronic pain, and surgically related nausea and vomiting [7]. However, current literature does not provide sufficient evidence supporting the routine perioperative administration of gabapentinoids to provide significant pain reduction. Furthermore, dosing guidelines are unclear with different studies administering gabapentin ranging from 600–1200 mg and pregabalin ranging from 100–300 mg. Timing of administration also varied between studies with administration being either preoperative, postoperative, or both [44–47]. Verret et al. performed a meta-analysis in 2020 evaluating the role of gabapentinoids in the management of acute and chronic postoperative pain. The meta-analysis included data from a variety of surgical specialties like orthopedic, spinal, non-endoscopic abdominal, endoscopic abdominal, ophthalmologic, maxillofacial, ENT, plastic, breast, thoracic and cardiac surgeries. The results show a mild analgesic effect of gabapentinoids at 6, 12, 24, and 48 h, but not at 72 h. However, this effect on pain control was determined to not be clinically significant since it did not exceed the minimal clinically important difference for any of the time points measured. The results show that administration of gabapentinoids reduced opioid administration with a mean difference of 8 mg IV morphine equivalents. However, the difference observed in opioid administration is not supported by a high degree of evidence in this analysis. Furthermore, the group observed a statistically significant increased incidence of adverse side effects from gabapentinoid administration including dizziness and visual disturbance [46]. Stone et al. similarly advise against the use of gabapentinoids in their ERAS guidelines for minimally invasive gynecologic surgeries due to the FDA reported side effects of respiratory depression when using gabapentinoids in combination with opioids [35]. A similar meta-analysis performed by Fiore et al. in 2023 that specifically focuses on craniotomies showed with a low degree of confidence that gabapentin administration slightly reduced postoperative pain at 24 h without evidence of pain reduction at any other time points [47]. Overall, literature evidence to support the broad use of gabapentinoids in ERAS protocols is inconsistent and controversial as of now.

11 Glucocorticoids and Dexamethasone

Dexamethasone, a glucocorticoid drug, is commonly used to reduce perioperative pain and PONV. Glucocorticoids bind to the glucocorticoid receptors (GR) expressed throughout the body, inducing or repressing transcription of genes through binding directly to DNA [48]. This mechanism of action is used to treat inflammation, allergies, asthma, arthritis, skin, and kidney conditions [49]. Important side effects related to dexamethasone administration include impaired wound healing, muscle atrophy, and hypertension [48]. A meta-analysis by Weibel et al. that evaluated the effectiveness of different prophylactic pharmacologic interventions demonstrated that > 4 mg IV dexamethasone administration prior to surgery or at anesthesia induction is effective at reducing PONV [50]. A systematic review by Korwin-Kochanowska on hallux valgus RCT studies found evidence that preoperative administration of dexamethasone reduces postoperative pain [51]. A systematic review study by Macfater et al.

shows that prophylactic administration of dexamethasone and ondansetron on anesthesia induction and haloperidol administration at the end of surgery reduces postoperative pain intensity and opioid use in Laparoscopic sleeve gastrectomies [52, 53]. Anger et al. conducted a systematic review study with the intention of developing guidelines for the management of postoperative pain after primary elective total hip arthroplasty. This group found a significant value for the incorporation of dexamethasone in perioperative multimodal analgesia- causing reduced pain, earlier patient ambulation, reduced morphine consumption, and reduced PONV. 10 mg of perioperative dexamethasone had a significant effect on reducing postoperative pain, opioid consumption in the first 24 h, and correlates with early ambulation and a shorter length of hospital stay. Furthermore, 10 mg dexamethasone administration 24 h postoperatively reduced morphine consumption on day two and was associated with a shorter length of stay when compared with a single dose [54]. In addition, a systematic review by Singh et al. showed that both intravenous and perineural administration of dexamethasone decrease the occurrence of rebound pain following a peripheral nerve block administered for postoperative pain management [55].

12 NMDA Receptor Antagonists and Ketamine

Ketamine is an NMDA receptor antagonist commonly administered as a general anesthetic induction agent and multimodal perioperative pain management adjunct. Typically used in conjunction with opioids, ketamine enhances opioid effects and contributes to the alleviation of chronic pain [56]. In higher dosages, the use of ketamine is suboptimal owing to undesirable effects, including hallucinations, nightmares, nausea, dizziness, and blurred vision. Additionally, evidence regarding the efficacy of lower doses in managing acute postoperative pain has been inconclusive [57]. Current literature does not provide sufficient evidence to support the routine use of ketamine perioperatively to reduce postoperative pain. Furthermore, the dosing of ketamine across different studies varied greatly with studies providing an induction bolus ranging from 0.1 mg/kg to 1 mg/g and continuous IV infusions postoperatively for 24 h ranging from 2 mcg/kg/hr to 250 mcg/kg/hr [58–60]. Meyer-Friebem et al. conducted a systematic review and meta-analysis to evaluate the effects of perioperative ketamine on postoperative pain management and found, with low confidence, that ketamine had mild and insignificant pain reducing effects. However, they found, with moderate confidence, a significant effect on reducing morphine consumption post-operatively. They did not include a meta-analysis of the ketamine-related adverse effects due to the low quality of evidence. Their study mainly included randomized controlled trials in spine surgery and lower limb orthopedic surgery settings [58]. A meta-analysis by Wang et al. looking at the effects of ketamine on pain management in Cesarean sections showed that Ketamine administration reduces pain and reduces opioid consumption postoperatively. This study also did not include an analysis of ketamine-related side effects due to the low amount of evidence [59]. A randomized, prospective, double-blinded, and placebo-controlled study by Loftus et al. indicates that administering intraoperative ketamine can result in decreased opiate usage during the 48 h following surgery in patients with chronic pain and opiate dependency. Furthermore, ketamine may contribute to lower opioid consumption and reduced pain intensity throughout the entire postoperative period [61]. A meta-analysis by Mariscal et al. showed that ketamine administration had no significant effect on postoperative pain but significantly reduced postoperative opioid administration in adolescent idiopathic scoliosis patients undergoing spinal fusion [60]. Overall, the literature studying the benefits of including ketamine in multimodal analgesia is inconsistent and inconclusive. Furthermore, there is a lack of sufficient data analyzing the significance and prevalence of ketamine-related adverse effects including hallucinations, confusion, and prolonged intubation.

13 Central α-2 Agonists

Central α-2 agonists inhibit norepinephrine release from presynaptic neurons and centrally induce analgesia via the locus coeruleus [62]. These effects block withdrawal symptoms in opioid users but also reduce a patient's need for additional anesthetics or sedatives [63]. Despite being shown to reduce postoperative pain and opioid consumption, alpha-2 agonists, like dexmedetomidine and clonidine, are associated with adverse events including bradycardia, hypotension, and sedation. A meta-analysis was conducted by Yu et al. evaluating randomized control trials in a variety of operative settings including thoracic, breast, gynecological, urological, and abdominal surgeries to evaluate the effect of dexmedetomidine on postoperative pain and opioid consumption. These studies evaluated in this analysis used dexmedetomidine for inducing or maintaining anesthesia, or both. The studies all used a narrow dosing range of 0.1–1 mcg/kg for bolus administrations and 0.1-1mcg/kg/hr for anesthesia maintenance. This study shows that the use of dexmedetomidine significantly reduces postoperative pain at the 2 and 4 h mark and significantly reduces the need for postoperative rescue analgesia. Furthermore, the use of dexmedetomidine reduces PONV occurrence and opioid consumption. However, side effects reported include significant increase in risk of bradycardia and significantly prolonged time until extubation for patients in the dexmedetomidine group [64]. Heybati et al. performed a similar analysis with the goal of determining the effects of different analgesics specifically in the adult cardiac surgery setting. Their analysis shows, with moderate to high confidence, that use of clonidine or dexmedetomidine significantly reduces postoperative pain at the 24-h mark [40]. Ding et al.'s meta-analysis study on laparoscopic gynecologic surgeries shows, with high confidence, that dexmedetomidine administration reduces postoperative pain and opioid consumption at 24 h [24]. A meta-analysis by Wang et al. analyzing the effects of perioperative dexmedetomidine (0.5-2mcg/kg) on postoperative pain in the primary total hip or knee arthroplasty setting shows that dexmedetomidine significantly reduced pain at 24 h and risk of PONV but was associated with significantly increased risk of bradycardia [65].

14 Conclusion

ERAS protocols are an imperative component of contemporary perioperative anesthetic and analgesic care. Effective implementation of these protocols promises an opportunity to optimize patient outcomes and speed recovery. A key component of ERAS pathways includes multimodal analgesia, a strategy that combines various analgesic techniques to effectively manage pain while minimizing the reliance on opioids. This approach reduces postoperative pain and opioid-related side effects. Integrating multimodal analgesia into ERAS protocols has improved patient comfort, facilitated early mobilization, and contributed to a faster overall recovery. The combined impact of ERAS and multimodal analgesia emphasizes a comprehensive and patient-focused strategy in surgical care, promoting improved results and a more streamlined healthcare experience.

References

1. El Tahan MR, Pahade A, Gómez-Ríos MÁ. Enhanced recovery after surgery: comes out to the Sun. BMC Anesthesiol. 2023;23(1):274.
2. Melnyk M, Casey RG, Black P, Koupparis AJ. Enhanced recovery after surgery (ERAS) protocols: time to change practice? Can Urol Assoc J. 2011;5(5):342–8.
3. Caughey AB, Wood SL, Macones GA, Wrench IJ, Huang J, Norman M, et al. Guidelines for intraoperative care in cesarean delivery: enhanced recovery after surgery society recommendations (Part 2). Am J Obstet Gynecol. 2018;219(6):533–44.
4. Lassen K. Consensus review of optimal perioperative care in colorectal surgery: enhanced recovery after surgery (ERAS) group recommendations. Arch Surg [Internet]. 2009 Oct 1 [cited 2023 Dec 2];144(10):961. Available from: http://archsurg.jamanetwork.com/article.aspx?doi=10.1001/archsurg.2009.170
5. Apfel CC, Turan A, Souza K, Pergolizzi J, Hornuss C. Intravenous acetaminophen reduces postoperative nausea and vomiting: a systematic review and meta-analysis. Pain [Internet]. 2013 May [cited 2023 Dec 2];154(5):677–89. Available from: https://journals.lww.com/00006396-201305000-00010
6. Tan M, Law LSC, Gan TJ. Optimizing pain management to facilitate enhanced recovery after surgery pathways. Can J Anesth/J Can Anesth [Internet]. 2015 Feb [cited 2023 Dec 2];62(2):203–18. Available from: http://link.springer.com/10.1007/s12630-014-0275-x
7. Simpson JC, Bao X, Agarwala A. Pain management in enhanced recovery after surgery (ERAS) protocols. Clin Colon Rectal Surg [Internet]. 2019 Mar [cited 2023 Oct 8];32(2):121–8. Available from: https://www.ncbi.nlm.nih.gov/pmc/articles/PMC6395101/
8. Pitre L, Garbee D, Tipton J, Schiavo J, Pitt A. Effects of preoperative intrathecal morphine on postoperative intravenous morphine dosage: a systematic review protocol. JBI Database of Systematic Rev Implementation Reports [Internet]. 2018 Apr [cited 2023 Dec 2];16(4):867–70. Available from: https://journals.lww.com/01938924-201804000-00011
9. Meylan N, Elia N, Lysakowski C, Tramèr MR. Benefit and risk of intrathecal morphine without local anaesthetic in patients undergoing major surgery: meta-analysis of randomized trials. British J Anaesthesia [Internet]. 2009 Feb [cited 2023 Dec 2];102(2):156–67. Available from: https://linkinghub.elsevier.com/retrieve/pii/S0007091217345269

10. Musa A, Acosta FL, Tuchman A, Movahedi R, Pendi K, Nassif L, et al. Addition of intrathecal morphine for postoperative pain management in pediatric spine surgery: a meta-analysis. Clinical Spine Surgery: A Spine Publication [Internet]. 2019 Apr [cited 2023 Nov 21];32(3):104–10. Available from: https://journals.lww.com/01933606-201904000-00004
11. Wang J, Sun H, Sun WT, Sun HP, Tian T, Sun J. Efficacy and safety of intrathecal morphine for pain control after spinal surgery: a systematic review and meta-analysis. European Rev Med Pharmacol Sci [Internet]. 2021 Mar [cited 2023 Nov 21];25(6):2674–84. Available from: https://doi.org/10.26355/eurrev_202103_25431
12. Ryu C, Choi GJ, Jung YH, Baek CW, Cho CK, Kang H. Postoperative analgesic effectiveness of peripheral nerve blocks in cesarean delivery: a systematic review and network meta-analysis. JPM [Internet]. 2022 Apr 14 [cited 2023 Dec 3];12(4):634. Available from: https://www.mdpi.com/2075-4426/12/4/634
13. Cheah JW, Sing DC, Hansen EN, Aleshi P, Vail TP. Does intrathecal morphine in spinal anesthesia have a role in modern multimodal analgesia for primary total joint arthroplasty? The J Arthroplasty [Internet]. 2018 Jun [cited 2023 Dec 3];33(6):1693–8. Available from: https://linkinghub.elsevier.com/retrieve/pii/S0883540318300342
14. McLeod G, Cumming C. Thoracic epidural anaesthesia and analgesia. Continuing Education in Anaesthesia Critical Care and Pain [Internet]. 2004 Feb [cited 2023 Dec 2];4(1):16–9. Available from: https://linkinghub.elsevier.com/retrieve/pii/S1472261517300055
15. Sudheshna KD, Gopinath R, Ayya SS, Kar P, Kumar RV. High vs mid thoracic epidural analgesia—a comparative study on the ease of insertion and effects on pain, hemodynamics, and oxygenation in patients undergoing thoracotomies. Ann Card Anaesth. 2019;22(4):383–7.
16. Daghmouri MA, Chaouch MA, Oueslati M, Rebai L, Oweira H. Regional techniques for pain management following laparoscopic elective colonic resection: a systematic review. Annals of Medicine and Surgery [Internet]. 2021 Dec [cited 2023 Nov 21];72:103124. Available from: https://linkinghub.elsevier.com/retrieve/pii/S2049080121010748
17. Lin J, Liao Y, Gong C, Yu L, Gao F, Yu J, et al. Regional analgesia in video-assisted thoracic surgery: a bayesian network meta-analysis. Front Med (Lausanne). 2022;9: 842332.
18. Luo G, Tao J, Zhu J, Xie K, Ni C. Comparison of analgesic effects of different regional blocks in video-assisted thoracic and breast surgeries: a network meta-analysis and systematic review. Pain Phys. 2022;25(5):339–54.
19. Hughes MJ, Ventham NT, McNally S, Harrison E, Wigmore S. Analgesia after open abdominal surgery in the setting of enhanced recovery surgery: a systematic review and meta-analysis. JAMA Surg [Internet]. 2014 Dec 1 [cited 2023 Nov 21];149(12):1224. Available from: http://archsurg.jamanetwork.com/article.aspx?doi=10.1001/jamasurg.2014.210
20. Charlton S, Cyna AM, Middleton P, Griffiths JD. Perioperative transversus abdominis plane (TAP) blocks for analgesia after abdominal surgery. Cochrane Pain, Palliative and Supportive Care Group, editor. Cochrane Database of Systematic Reviews [Internet]. 2010 Dec 8 [cited 2023 Dec 2]; Available from: https://doi.wiley.com/10.1002/14651858.CD007705.pub2
21. Brogi E, Kazan R, Cyr S, Giunta F, Hemmerling TM. Transversus abdominal plane block for postoperative analgesia: a systematic review and meta-analysis of randomized-controlled trials. Can J Anesth/J Can Anesth [Internet]. 2016 Oct [cited 2023 Nov 21];63(10):1184–96. Available from: http://link.springer.com/10.1007/s12630-016-0679-x
22. Tsai HC, Yoshida T, Chuang TY, Yang SF, Chang CC, Yao HY, et al. Transversus abdominis plane block: an updated review of anatomy and techniques. BioMed Research International [Internet]. 2017 [cited 2023 Dec 2];2017:1–12. Available from: https://www.hindawi.com/journals/bmri/2017/8284363/
23. Shin JH, Balk EM, Gritsenko K, Wang A, Plewniak K, Shaparin N. Transversus abdominis plane block for laparoscopic hysterectomy pain: a meta-analysis. JSLS [Internet]. 2020 [cited 2023 Nov 21];24(2):e2020.00018. Available from: https://www.ncbi.nlm.nih.gov/pmc/articles/PMC7234801/
24. Ding X, Ma Y, Ma Y, Chen C, Zhang X, Duan Q, et al. Efficacy of non-opioid analgesics and regional techniques for perioperative pain management in laparoscopic gynecological surgery: a systematic review and network meta-analysis. Int J Surg. 2023;109(11):3527–40.

25. Yang X, Zhang Y, Chen Y, Xu M, Lei X, Fu Q. Analgesic effect of erector spinae plane block in adults undergoing laparoscopic cholecystectomy: a systematic review and meta-analysis of randomized controlled trials. BMC Anesthesiol [Internet]. 2023 Jan 6 [cited 2023 Dec 2];23(1):7. Available from: https://bmcanesthesiol.biomedcentral.com/articles/10.1186/s12871-023-01969-6
26. Forero M, Adhikary SD, Lopez H, Tsui C, Chin KJ. The erector spinae plane block: a novel analgesic technique in thoracic neuropathic pain. Regional Anesthesia and Pain Medicine [Internet]. 2016 [cited 2023 Dec 2];41(5):621–7. Available from: https://rapm.bmj.com/lookup/doi/10.1097/AAP.0000000000000451
27. Ma J, Bi Y, Zhang Y, Zhu Y, Wu Y, Ye Y, et al. Erector spinae plane block for postoperative analgesia in spine surgery: a systematic review and meta-analysis. Eur Spine J [Internet]. 2021 Nov [cited 2023 Nov 22];30(11):3137–49. Available from: https://link.springer.com/10.1007/s00586-021-06853-w
28. Koo CH, Lee HT, Na HS, Ryu JH, Shin HJ. Efficacy of erector spinae plane block for analgesia in thoracic surgery: a systematic review and meta-analysis. J Cardiothoracic and Vascular Anesthesia [Internet]. 2022 May [cited 2023 Nov 23];36(5):1387–95. Available from: https://linkinghub.elsevier.com/retrieve/pii/S105307702100536X
29. Viderman D, Aubakirova M, Abdildin YG. Erector spinae plane block in abdominal surgery: a meta-analysis. Front Med [Internet]. 2022 Feb 23 [cited 2023 Nov 23];9:812531. Available from: https://www.frontiersin.org/articles/10.3389/fmed.2022.812531/full
30. Cui Y, Wang Y, Yang J, Ran L, Zhang Q, Huang Q, et al. The effect of single-shot erector spinae plane block (ESPB) on opioid consumption for various surgeries: a meta-analysis of randomized controlled trials. J Pain Res. 2022;15:683–99.
31. Dunn LK, Durieux ME. Perioperative use of intravenous lidocaine. Anesthesiology [Internet]. 2017 Apr 1 [cited 2023 Dec 2];126(4):729–37. Available from: https://pubs.asahq.org/anesthesiology/article/126/4/729/19830/Perioperative-Use-of-Intravenous-Lidocaine
32. Hollmann MW, McIntire WE, Garrison JC, Durieux ME. Inhibition of mammalian Gq protein function by local anesthetics. Anesthesiology [Internet]. 2002 Dec 1 [cited 2023 Dec 2];97(6):1451–7. Available from: https://pubs.asahq.org/anesthesiology/article/97/6/1451/40283/Inhibition-of-Mammalian-Gq-Protein-Function-by
33. Chu R, Umukoro N, Greer T, Roberts J, Adekoya P, Odonkor CA, et al. Intravenous lidocaine infusion for the management of early postoperative pain: a comprehensive review of controlled trials. Psychopharmacol Bull. 2020;50(4 Suppl 1):216–59.
34. Boswell MR, Moman RN, Burtoft M, Gerdes H, Martinez J, Gerberi DJ, et al. Lidocaine for postoperative pain after cardiac surgery: a systematic review. J Cardiothorac Surg. 2021;16(1):157.
35. Stone R, Carey E, Fader AN, Fitzgerald J, Hammons L, Nensi A, et al. Enhanced recovery and surgical optimization protocol for minimally invasive gynecologic surgery: an AAGL white paper. J Minimally Invasive Gynecol [Internet]. 2021 Feb [cited 2023 Nov 4];28(2):179–203. Available from: https://linkinghub.elsevier.com/retrieve/pii/S155346502030385X
36. Casas-Arroyave FD, Osorno-Upegui SC, Zamudio-Burbano MA. Therapeutic efficacy of intravenous lidocaine infusion compared with thoracic epidural analgesia in major abdominal surgery: a noninferiority randomised clinical trial. British J Anaesthesia [Internet]. 2023 Nov [cited 2023 Dec 3];131(5):947–54. Available from: https://linkinghub.elsevier.com/retrieve/pii/S0007091223004865
37. Ong CKS, Seymour RA, Lirk P, Merry AF. Combining paracetamol (Acetaminophen) with nonsteroidal antiinflammatory drugs: a qualitative systematic review of analgesic efficacy for acute postoperative pain. Anesthesia and Analgesia [Internet]. 2010 Apr [cited 2023 Dec 3];110(4):1170–9. Available from: https://journals.lww.com/00000539-201004000-00030
38. Maund E, McDaid C, Rice S, Wright K, Jenkins B, Woolacott N. Paracetamol and selective and non-selective non-steroidal anti-inflammatory drugs for the reduction in morphine-related side-effects after major surgery: a systematic review. British J Anaesthesia [Internet]. 2011 Mar [cited 2023 Nov 8];106(3):292–7. Available from: https://linkinghub.elsevier.com/retrieve/pii/S0007091217329902

39. Ghlichloo I, Gerriets V. Nonsteroidal anti-inflammatory drugs (NSAIDs). In: StatPearls [Internet]. Treasure Island (FL): StatPearls Publishing; 2023 [cited 2023 Dec 3]. Available from: http://www.ncbi.nlm.nih.gov/books/NBK547742/
40. Heybati K, Zhou F, Lynn MJ, Deng J, Ali S, Hou W, et al. Comparative efficacy of adjuvant nonopioid analgesia in adult cardiac surgical patients: a network meta-analysis. J Cardiothoracic and Vascular Anesthesia [Internet]. 2023 Jul [cited 2023 Nov 21];37(7):1169–78. Available from: https://linkinghub.elsevier.com/retrieve/pii/S105307702300188X
41. Lubis AM, Maruanaya S, Tantri AR, Pontoh LAP, Ifran NNPPS. The use of combination paracetamol and ibuprofen in postoperative pain after total knee arthroplasty, a randomized controlled trial. Pain Physician. 2021;24(8):E1199–204.
42. Hedderson M, Lee D, Hunt E, Lee K, Xu F, Mustille A, et al. Enhanced recovery after surgery to change process measures and reduce opioid use after cesarean delivery: a quality improvement initiative. Obstet Gynecol. 2019;134(3):511–9.
43. Turan A, Karamanlioglu B, Memis D, Usar P, Pamukçu Z, Türe M. The analgesic effects of gabapentin after total abdominal hysterectomy: anesthesia and analgesia [Internet]. 2004 May [cited 2023 Dec 3];1370–3. Available from: http://journals.lww.com/00000539-200405000-00033
44. Patel AS, Abrecht CR, Urman RD. Gabapentinoid use in perioperative care and current controversies. Curr Pain Headache Rep [Internet]. 2022 Feb [cited 2023 Nov 8];26(2):139–44. Available from: https://link.springer.com/10.1007/s11916-022-01012-2
45. Wick EC, Grant MC, Wu CL. Postoperative multimodal analgesia pain management with nonopioid analgesics and techniques: a review. JAMA Surg [Internet]. 2017 Jul 1 [cited 2023 Nov 8];152(7):691. Available from: http://archsurg.jamanetwork.com/article.aspx?doi=10.1001/jamasurg.2017.0898
46. Verret M, Lauzier F, Zarychanski R, Perron C, Savard X, Pinard AM, et al. Perioperative use of gabapentinoids for the management of postoperative acute pain. Anesthesiology [Internet]. 2020 Aug 1 [cited 2023 Nov 8];133(2):265–79. Available from: https://pubs.asahq.org/anesthesiology/article/133/2/265/109137/Perioperative-Use-of-Gabapentinoids-for-the
47. Fiore G, Porto E, Pluderi M, Ampollini AM, Borsa S, Legnani FG, et al. Prevention of postoperative pain after elective brain surgery: a meta-analysis of randomized controlled trials. Medicina (Kaunas). 2023;59(5):831.
48. Ramamoorthy S, Cidlowski JA. Corticosteroids: mechanisms of action in health and disease. Rheum Dis Clin North Am. 2016;42(1):15–31, vii.
49. De Oliveira GS, Almeida MD, Benzon HT, McCarthy RJ. Perioperative single dose systemic dexamethasone for postoperative pain. Anesthesiology [Internet]. 2011 Sep 1 [cited 2023 Dec 3];115(3):575–88. Available from: https://pubs.asahq.org/anesthesiology/article/115/3/575/11126/Perioperative-Single-Dose-Systemic-Dexamethasone
50. Weibel S, Rücker G, Eberhart LH, Pace NL, Hartl HM, Jordan OL, et al. Drugs for preventing postoperative nausea and vomiting in adults after general anaesthesia: a network meta-analysis. Cochrane Database Syst Rev. 2020;10(10):CD012859.
51. Korwin-Kochanowska K, Potié A, El-Boghdadly K, Rawal N, Joshi G, Albrecht E, et al. PROSPECT guideline for hallux valgus repair surgery: a systematic review and procedure-specific postoperative pain management recommendations. Reg Anesth Pain Med. 2020;45(9):702–8.
52. on behalf of the PROSPECT collaborators, Macfater H, Xia W, Srinivasa S, Hill AG, Van De Velde M, et al. Evidence-based management of postoperative pain in adults undergoing laparoscopic sleeve gastrectomy. World J Surg [Internet]. 2019 Jun [cited 2023 Nov 17];43(6):1571–80. Available from: http://link.springer.com/10.1007/s00268-019-04934-y
53. Benevides ML, Oliveira SSDS, De Aguilar-Nascimento JE. The combination of haloperidol, dexamethasone, and ondansetron for prevention of postoperative nausea and vomiting in laparoscopic sleeve gastrectomy: a randomized double-blind trial. OBES SURG [Internet]. 2013 Sep [cited 2023 Nov 17];23(9):1389–96. Available from: http://link.springer.com/10.1007/s11695-013-0923-1

54. Anger M, Valovska T, Beloeil H, Lirk P, Joshi GP, Van De Velde M, et al. PROSPECT guideline for total hip arthroplasty: a systematic review and procedure-specific postoperative pain management recommendations. Anaesthesia [Internet]. 2021 Aug [cited 2023 Nov 20];76(8):1082–97. Available from: https://associationofanaesthetists-publications.onlinelibrary.wiley.com/doi/10.1111/anae.15498
55. Singh NP, Makkar JK, Chawla JK, Sondekoppam RV, Singh PM. Prophylactic dexamethasone for rebound pain after peripheral nerve block in adult surgical patients: systematic review, meta-analysis, and trial sequential analysis of randomised controlled trials. British J Anaesthesia [Internet]. 2023 Oct [cited 2023 Dec 3];S0007091223005184. Available from: https://linkinghub.elsevier.com/retrieve/pii/S0007091223005184
56. Laskowski K, Stirling A, McKay WP, Lim HJ. A systematic review of intravenous ketamine for postoperative analgesia. Can J Anesth/J Can Anesth [Internet]. 2011 Oct [cited 2023 Dec 3];58(10):911–23. Available from: http://link.springer.com/10.1007/s12630-011-9560-0
57. Himmelseher S, Durieux ME, Weiskopf RB. Ketamine for perioperative pain management. Anesthesiology [Internet]. 2005 Jan 1 [cited 2023 Dec 3];102(1):211–20. Available from: https://pubs.asahq.org/anesthesiology/article/102/1/211/7320/Ketamine-for-Perioperative-Pain-Management
58. Meyer-Frießem CH, Lipke E, Weibel S, Kranke P, Reichl S, Pogatzki-Zahn EM, et al. Perioperative ketamine for postoperative pain management in patients with preoperative opioid intake: a systematic review and meta-analysis. J Clinical Anesthesia [Internet]. 2022 Jun [cited 2023 Dec 3];78:110652. Available from: https://linkinghub.elsevier.com/retrieve/pii/S0952818022000083
59. Wang J, Xu Z, Feng Z, Ma R, Zhang X. Impact of ketamine on pain management in cesarean section: a systematic review and meta-analysis. Pain Phys. 2020;23(2):135–48.
60. Mariscal G, Morales J, Pérez S, Rubio-Belmar PA, Bovea-Marco M, Bas JL, et al. Meta-analysis of the efficacy of ketamine in postoperative pain control in adolescent idiopathic scoliosis patients undergoing spinal fusion. Eur Spine J [Internet]. 2022 Dec [cited 2023 Nov 20];31(12):3492–9. Available from: https://link.springer.com/10.1007/s00586-022-07422-5
61. Loftus RW, Yeager MP, Clark JA, Brown JR, Abdu WA, Sengupta DK, et al. Intraoperative ketamine reduces perioperative opiate consumption in opiate-dependent patients with chronic back pain undergoing back surgery. Anesthesiology. 2010;113(3):639–46.
62. Giovannitti JA, Thoms SM, Crawford JJ. Alpha-2 Adrenergic receptor agonists: a review of current clinical applications. Anesthesia Progress [Internet]. 2015 Mar 1 [cited 2023 Dec 3];62(1):31–8. Available from: https://meridian.allenpress.com/anesthesia-progress/article/62/1/31/24911/Alpha2-Adrenergic-Receptor-Agonists-A-Review-of
63. Mukhtar AM, Obayah EM, Hassona AM. The use of dexmedetomidine in pediatric cardiac surgery. Anesthesia and Analgesia [Internet]. 2006 Jul [cited 2023 Dec 3];103(1):52–6. Available from: https://journals.lww.com/00000539-200607000-00010
64. Yu DH, Shen X, Lai L, Chen YJ, Liu K, Shen QH. Application of dexmedetomidine as an opioid substitute in opioid-free anesthesia: a systematic review and meta-analysis. Pain Phys. 2023;26(6):E635–49.
65. Yang Q, Ren Y, Feng B, Weng X. Pain relieving effect of dexmedetomidine in patients undergoing total knee or hip arthroplasty: a meta-analysis. Medicine [Internet]. 2020 Jan [cited 2023 Nov 21];99(1):e18538. Available from: https://journals.lww.com/10.1097/MD.0000000000018538

Preoperative Preparation for Regional Anesthesia

Melanie Donnelly and Peter W. Coleman

Abstract Patients present for surgery with a myriad of concerns that may impact perioperative pain management and functional recovery. In addition, these patients may present with complicated analgesic regimens, be exposed to unprescribed analgesics, or have a history of abuse and discussions with patients regarding these factors can simultaneously build rapport and improve adherence with collaboratively constructed analgesic plans. Regional anesthesia is a unique analgesic component which may either be the sole anesthetic for a surgery, or a critical part of postoperative pain management. It may also be an additional source of stress and anxiety for patients and their friends and family on the day of surgery. As a component of a comprehensive perioperative analgesic discussion, adequate preoperative preparation for regional anesthesia may not only improve patient satisfaction and reduce anxiety, but also improve patient outcomes.

Keywords Regional Anesthesia · Preoperative education · Postoperative pain · Patient centered · Decision aids

1 Introduction

Preoperative patient education improves multiple endpoints of patient care. The anesthesiologist often faces barriers to timely involvement in preoperative preparation. Regional anesthesia is a unique and beneficial modality which, while an important part of many perioperative plans, is often poorly introduced to patients prior to the day of surgery. Several approaches to preoperative preparation, including web based

M. Donnelly (✉) · P. W. Coleman
Anesthesiology, Medical College of Wisconsin, Wauwatosa, WI, USA
e-mail: mdonnelly@mcw.edu

P. W. Coleman
e-mail: peter.coleman@cuanschutz.edu

P. W. Coleman
Anesthesiology, University of Colorado, Aurora, USA

A. Abd-Elsayed and K. Schroeder (eds.), *Perioperative Pain Management*,
https://doi.org/10.1007/978-3-031-67648-2_9

and written modalities, have demonstrated not only improved patient satisfaction and decreased patient anxiety but also improved patient outcomes. These may be applied to preoperative preparation for regional anesthesia.

2 Discussion

In 2001, the Institute of Medicine established a framework for the assessment of health care quality. A component of this framework included the domain of "patient-centered" care which is "Providing care that is respectful of and responsive to individual patient preference, needs and values and ensuring that patient values guide all clinical decisions" [1]. Supporting this principle, the American Pain Society published guidelines in 2016 which recommend "...patient and family centered individually tailored education to the patient, including information on treatment options for the management of postoperative pain...." The guidelines also promote the use of a shared decision-making process to create an individually tailed pain management plan. It has been shown that patient engagement and collaborative decision-making processes between providers and patients in healthcare, result in improved health outcomes [2, 3]. The demonstrated benefits of preoperative education include decreased length of stay, increased patient and family satisfaction, reduced opioid use, and reduced patient anxiety [4, 5].

In the course of providing anesthesia care and perioperative pain management, unique challenges to providing patient centered care and comprehensive preoperative education may emerge [6]. One of the major barriers is related to the typical timing of a preoperative visit between a patient and their anesthesiologist. In many medical centers, anesthesiologists only become involved with patient care on the day of surgery in the preoperative holding area. By this time, patients have made the decision to proceed with surgery and it is more likely that this preoperative conversation focuses on medical history and planned anesthetic pathways rather than on the patients' overall goals of health and values exploration. As Clapp so aptly pointed out, when the anesthesiologist meets patients on the day of surgery, the anesthesia and consent process may be seen by the patient as part of a "package of care that has already been decided upon in the surgeon's office" [7]. Clapp also points out that the anesthesia concerns in this setting may be subordinate to concerns specifically related to the surgical plan. Additionally, there is frequently intense time pressure in the preoperative day of surgery environment, with anesthesiologists often being allotted only 5–10 min with a patient prior to surgery. In this short time period, it would be challenging to have the necessary conversations to accomplish collaborative decision making about patient care. Further, patients may be anxious or overwhelmed by the unfamiliarity of the environment, the prospect of post-operative pain, the idea of total loss of control when "going under" or any number of other legitimate psychological stressors.

There are a number of reasons to implement pre-operative education programs or pathways that focus on anesthesia and surgery prior to the day of surgery. The most common stressors for patients having surgery are “lack of knowledge and fear of the unknown” which can lead to anxiety about and around the experience [8]. Both of these can be, at least partially, alleviated with preoperative contact and effective preoperative education [8]. Given the constraints around time and contact with patients on the day of surgery, there may be some benefit to creating workflows and materials that would provide preoperative education to patients regarding anesthesia. These could incorporate decision aids to further prepare patients to have more informed conversations with their anesthesiologists on the day of surgery.

Perioperative surgical home literature has demonstrated that early patient engagement can be beneficial to both the patient and healthcare system by supporting patients in their decision making, establishing expectations around surgery and anesthesia, and opening the lines of communication [3]. In joint arthroplasty patients and those having colonic surgery, it has been demonstrated that preoperative education and counseling can be part of a care pathway which may lead to lessened complication rates and lower readmission rates [3, 9, 10].

3 Patient Outcomes

In order to optimize postoperative recovery, patients must understand what support they will benefit from and what to expect during the recovery process. Barriers to patients’ experiencing optimal recovery include preoperative anxiety, which has been shown to be a predictor of higher pain scores for a wide range of surgeries [11]. Even in what might be considered minor surgery, preoperative mental state can have a large impact on postoperative recovery [11].

Fear and anxiety surrounding anesthesia and surgery may be the result of fear of the unknown and knowledge deficits about the process. Patients indicate that some concerns about anesthesia include fear of dying during anesthesia (8–55%), being awake during anesthesia (5–54%), postoperative pain (5–65%) and post-operative nausea (5–48%) [12] Though many studies have discovered the positive impact on anxiety related to preoperative education[14–17], there are some that demonstrate no improvement in anxiety [12, 18].

Preoperative education for patients regarding anesthesia has been predominantly shown to reduce anxiety surrounding the surgical experience and improve satisfaction. One group examined the impact of preoperative education on anxiety levels before surgery in patients scheduled for total joint arthroplasty [13]. The preoperative education provided included pamphlets and a video prepared by the American Society of Regional Anesthesia and Pain Medicine (now ASRA Pain Medicine). In this study, sharing preoperative education materials was shown to significantly minimize the increase in anxiety on the day of surgery. Interestingly, despite this positive finding, about 70% of both the intervention group and control group reported that anesthesia options for surgery had not been discussed prior to meeting with their anesthesia professionals on the day of surgery. These findings did indicate that those patients in the intervention group were more likely to prefer regional anesthesia and

90% of the intervention group recommended that others having surgery watch the videos and read the pamphlets they received [13].

Recent work in this area has demonstrated that the addition of a short 12-min video at the preoperative visit, in addition to usual care of a preoperative clinic visit and short briefing with the anesthesiologist on day of surgery, reduced preoperative anxiety and resulted in vital sign maintenance closer to baseline in the preoperative period [14]. This study targeted patients who would be offered a spinal anesthetic, and the video specifically discussed spinal anesthesia, the surgical procedure, and addressed "common myths" about surgery and anesthesia. Another group had similar findings with a preoperative video on spinal anesthesia demonstrating an ability to reduce anxiety and hemodynamic parameter deviation from preoperative baseline [15]. A different group also examined the impact of an instructional video on anxiety in patients being offered regional anesthesia [16]. The authors examined the impact of a short [7, 9] for patients who were scheduled to receive either a brachial plexus block or a spinal anesthetic. This video was viewed 2 weeks prior to surgery during the patient's preoperative assessment. Anxiety levels immediately prior to and following surgery were found to be lower in the group who viewed the video.

Another benefit of preoperative education is related to patient expectations about pain control and the postoperative process. Halawi et al. found that the most important predictor of admission to an extended care facility, following admission for total joint arthroplasty, was related to patient expectations [19]. Patient expectations are a modifiable factor which can be influenced by preoperative processes and educational efforts [19]. Postoperative opioid consumption has also been shown to be influenced by preoperative patient education and a reframing of analgesic benchmarks that might be expected to require opioid analgesics. Yajnik et al. examined the impact of using a simple educational tool created by the regional anesthesia group for patient education [20]. This patient education card introduced the patient to the analgesic options available to them following surgery. This card was reviewed prior to block placement in preoperative holding, at the time of admission to the floor, and on daily pain management team rounds visits. Utilization of this education framework was associated with a significant reduction in postoperative analgesic administration [20]. Other studies have demonstrated that the impact of preoperative education may extend well beyond what is typically considered a part of the postoperative phase of care. In one study, preoperative education regarding opioid use was shown to reduce opioid dependence following rotator cuff repair two years following surgery. The intervention used included preoperative opioid education delivered verbally, via video, and paper materials [5]. Khorfan examined a comprehensive intervention that aimed to reduce postoperative opioid use in general surgery patients [21]. In this study, changes to education were comprehensively expanded to include provider education, standardized patient materials, setting pain management goals and expectation, and installing an opioid waste disposal site. In this study 71% of patients reported receiving preoperative education, 87% reported receiving postoperative education, and 65% reported receiving both [21]. Those who received preoperative education reported feeling more prepared to manage their pain following surgery. Postoperative education alone was not associated with feeling prepared to manage pain, and receiving both pre and postoperative education provided the most patient preparedness for pain management. Preoperative education and a feeling a preparedness to manage pain were associated with a diminished postoperative opioid requirement. These findings support the effectiveness of preoperative education programs that seek to improve patient preparedness to manage pain following surgery and reduced opioid use in the postoperative period [21] Patient education on opioid use and abuse was studied as part of a much broader intervention implemented to improve the use multimodal postoperative pain management strategies and lessen opioid prescribing in a general surgery population. In those patients presented with enhanced education offerings, dramatically fewer opioids were prescribed, increased levels of non-opioid medications were utilized to address pain complaints, and patients overwhelmingly (81%) reported good or excellent pain control [22].

Patient satisfaction can also be impacted by the provision of preoperative education efforts that focus on the process and plan for delivery of anesthesia. A patient education handout used in a multilingual patient population demonstrated significant improvements in patient satisfaction. The patients enrolled in this study indicated that they better understood the role of anesthesiologists, options related to anesthesia and options for pain control after being exposed to the educational pamphlet prior to their surgical procedure [12]. When examining patient satisfaction in surgical populations, it has been consistently demonstrated that the addition of a video or multimedia interface to a patient's preoperative education platform improves satisfaction over brochures or in person verbal interactions [17, 23, 24].

4 Regional Anesthesia

In studies examining patient concerns about anesthesia, it has been noted that approximately 27% of patients considering regional anesthesia were concerned about permanent paralysis, back injury, and seeing the procedure [25]. It has been demonstrated that a preoperative appointment with an anesthesiologist can improve the acceptance rate of regional anesthesia and reduce anxiety about the process. Patients undergoing total joint arthroplasty had a preoperative appointment with an anesthesiologist prior to surgery where an assessment was performed and a discussion about the relative merits and risks of general vs spinal anesthesia was conducted. Patients were surveyed before and after these visits and the impact of this visit resulted in patient preference for spinal anesthesia increasing from 39 to 76%. Forty-seven percent of those patients who changed their mind from initially desiring general anesthesia to ultimately requesting spinal anesthesia indicated that it was because they felt more knowledgeable about the anesthesia choices available to them. The implementation of preoperative anesthesia discussions was also associated with a significant decrease in anxiety related to the upcoming surgery [26].

Decision aids represent effective tools that can be implemented at various points in a patient's health care journey to assist in determining "preference sensitive" decisions. Preference sensitive decisions are frequently those where there is little clinical benefit associated with one path versus the other but where there may be value- or experience-based reasons why one therapeutic path is selected above another. In the context of preference sensitive decisions, the use of decision aids has been shown to result in decreased indecision, improved patient engagement, and improved satisfaction with the decision making process [27]. In addition, the use of decision aids has been shown to help establish clearer expectations around care, lessen anxiety in decision making and foster a better overall understanding of the healthcare options [27]. In this context, decision aids are tools used to facilitate discussions between healthcare professionals and patients. They are not meant to be a substitute for physician consultation. Ideally, decision aids can be incorporated into the process of shared decision making during anesthesia care discussions. The shared decision-making process is similarly employed when there is no medically best choice and patient preferences play a role in determining next steps in the patient's healthcare journey. Figure 1 depicts the shared decision making process and the critical steps in the process [28]. Decision aids are ideally utilized during these types of patient encounters and can facilitate collaborative decision making around patient care [27].

Regional anesthesia and pain management strategies frequently fall into this category of preference sensitive decision making. As such, decision aids can provide substantial assistance in the process of shared analgesic decision making between the patient and the anesthesia professional [27, 29]. The ASA has developed decision aids for both peripheral nerve blocks and neuraxial nerve blocks. The use of

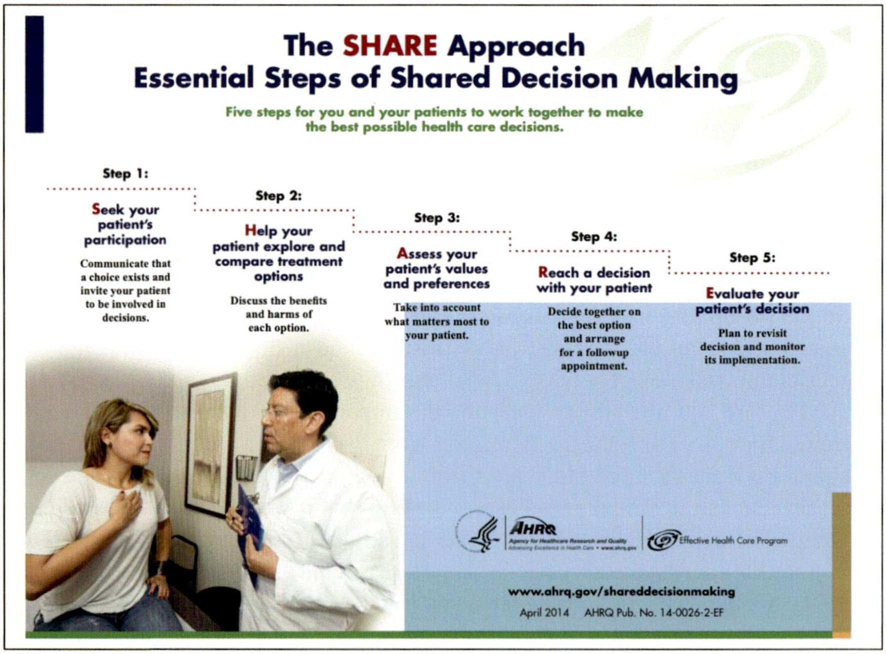

Fig. 1 The SHARE approach [28]

these aids has been associated with an increased degree of patient engagement in the preoperative regional anesthesia discussion and an improved understanding of regional anesthesia [30]. Further research seeks to evaluate the impact of similar decision aids in the setting of planned Monitored Anesthesia Care [27].

5 Modality of Education

Multiple preoperative education modalities have been examined without one yet emerging as the clearly superior method. Studies evaluating patient preference for delivery of education have demonstrated that they would prefer to obtain education via a pamphlet or in a preoperative visit. Video education dissemination and group information session were less preferred modalities for preoperative education [25]. There has been an extensive use of web-based tools for surgical education that have demonstrated improvements in patient satisfaction and engagement across multiple surgical specialties [31]. Video based information concerning anesthesia has been demonstrated as beneficial in a number of studies [13, 16]. Ensuring that language included in education offerings is targeted at an appropriate reading level will ensure that delivery is accessible to patients. Timing of educational endeavors should aim to begin in the preoperative phase and ideally in the surgeon's office after the decision has been made to proceed with surgery [4]. Preoperative education should then continue through any presurgical encounter up to and including the day of surgery.

The perioperative surgical home (PSH) has been defined as "a micro-healthcare system centered on the patient from the time of the decision for surgery to the physical and social recovery as an outpatient up to 30 days after discharge from the hospital with a triple aim of improving (i) clinical outcomes and the (ii) patient experience, as well as (iii) reducing healthcare costs" [32]. This model of care is patient-centric and requires that caregivers and family members are engaged as partners in care. This model of care will often include patient education, patient centered optimization and evaluation prior to surgery [32]. Patient counseling and education fit easily into the PSH model of care to improve outcomes for patients and organizations. Shared decision making and values-based decision making are critical strategies in this construct [33]. A recent literature review demonstrated that the implementation of the PSH often resulted in decreased length of stay, decreased use of postoperative opioids and increased likelihood of discharge to home [34]. Of the eleven manuscripts included in this review, all but one identified preoperative education and counseling as a critical part of the PSH.

6 Conclusion

Preoperative education is a critical part of patient care and can aid in the process of setting patient expectations surrounding the surgical experience, reducing anxiety, improving patient satisfaction, reducing long and short term opioid use, and encouraging patient engagement in decision making about their surgical and anesthetic care. Multiple education modalities have been developed and evaluated but more research is needed to determine the optimal content, timing and delivery method in regards to regional anesthesia preoperative education. There are potential benefits of this work which may extend beyond the preoperative and immediate postoperative period and this is another area that should be targeted for further exploration. Decision aids are known as useful adjuncts in the shared decision making process and have demonstrated efficacy in reducing decisional conflict and anxiety and facilitating values-based decision making for individual patients. More research is needed in this area to further define how these tools impact patient experiences and utilization of health care resources.

The preponderance of work in this area supports efforts to provide preoperative anesthesia education for patients prior to the day of surgery. A wide variety of approaches have achieved success in improving perioperative outcomes by providing preoperative education on anesthesia and regional anesthesia. The decision aids created by the ASA are evidence-based and readily available tools which should be more widely utilized. These aids represent a valuable adjunct in achieving a more patient centered approach to conversations about regional anesthesia with patients.

7 Key Takeaways

1. Preoperative education about anesthesia, whether in-person, video or static, decreases patient anxiety and may improve outcomes.
2. Preoperative education about regional anesthesia improves acceptance of regional anesthesia and decreases patient anxiety.
3. Decision aids can help facilitate improved patient participation and decision making.
4. The perioperative surgical home may provide a framework for the incorporation of preoperative education for regional anesthesia.

References

1. Crossing the Quality Chasm: A New Health System for the 21st Century. (2001). https://doi.org/10.17226/10027
2. Chou R, Gordon DB, de Leon-Casasola OA, Rosenberg JM, Bickler S, Brennan T, Carter T, Cassidy CL, Chittenden EH, Degenhardt E, Griffith S, Manworren R, McCarberg B, Montgomery R, Murphy J, Perkal MF, Suresh S, Sluka K, Strassels S, Wu CL. Management of postoperative pain: a clinical practice guideline from the American pain society, the American society of regional anesthesia and pain medicine, and the American society of anesthesiologists' committee on regional anesthesia, executive committee, and administrative council. J Pain. 2016;17(2):131–57. https://doi.org/10.1016/J.JPAIN.2015.12.008.
3. Kash BA, Zhang Y, Cline KM, Menser T, Miller TR. The perioperative surgical home (PSH): a comprehensive review of US and Non-US studies shows predominantly positive quality and cost outcomes. Milbank Q. 2014;92(4):796–821. https://doi.org/10.1111/1468-0009.12093.
4. Kruzik N. Benefits of preoperative education for adult elective surgery patients. AORN J 2009;90(3). https://doi.org/10.1016/J.AORN.2009.06.022
5. Cheesman Q, DeFrance M, Stenson J, Weekes D, Feldman J, Abboud J, Austin L. The effect of preoperative education on opioid consumption in patients undergoing arthroscopic rotator cuff repair: a prospective, randomized clinical trial-2-year follow-up. J Shoulder Elbow Surg. 2020;29(9):1743–50. https://doi.org/10.1016/J.JSE.2020.04.036.
6. Tylee MJ, Rubenfeld GD, Wijeysundera D, Sklar MC, Hussain S, Adhikari NKJ. Anesthesiologist to patient communication: a systematic review. JAMA Network Open 2020;3(11). https://doi.org/10.1001/JAMANETWORKOPEN.2020.23503
7. Clapp JT, Fleisher LA, Lane-Fall MB. Decision aids are a solution, but to which problem? Anesth Analg. 2019;128(5):837–8. https://doi.org/10.1213/ANE.0000000000003974.
8. Helms LJ. Video education to improve preoperative anxiety in the Bariatric surgical patient: a quality improvement project. J Perianesthesia Nursing : Official J Amer Soc PeriAnesthesia Nurses. 2020;35(5):467–71. https://doi.org/10.1016/J.JOPAN.2020.01.012.
9. Carli F, Charlebois P, Baldini G, Cachero O, Stein B. An integrated multidisciplinary approach to implementation of a fast-track program for laparoscopic colorectal surgery. Canadian J Anaesthesia = J Canadien d'anesthesie 2009;56(11):837–842. https://doi.org/10.1007/S12630-009-9159-X
10. Jones S, Alnaib M, Kokkinakis M, Wilkinson M, st Clair Gibson A, Kader D. Pre-operative patient education reduces length of stay after knee joint arthroplasty. Annals of the Royal College of Surgeons of England. 2011;93(1):71–75. https://doi.org/10.1308/003588410X12771863936765
11. Nilsson U, Dahlberg K, Jaensson M. Low preoperative mental and physical health is associated with poorer postoperative recovery in patients undergoing day surgery: a secondary analysis from a randomized controlled study. World J Surg. 2019;43(8):1949–56. https://doi.org/10.1007/S00268-019-04995-Z.
12. Ortiz J, Wang S, Elayda MA, Tolpin DA. Preoperative patient education: can we improve satisfaction and reduce anxiety? Rev Bras Anestesiol. 2015;65(1):7–13. https://doi.org/10.1016/J.BJAN.2013.07.009.
13. Bondy LR, Sims N, Schroeder DR, Offord KP, Narr BJ. The effect of anesthetic patient education on preoperative patient anxiety. Reg Anesthesia and Pain Med. 1999;24(2):158–164. https://doi.org/10.1016/S1098-7339(99)90078-0
14. Rajput S, Tiwari T, Chaudhary A. Effect of preoperative multimedia based video information on perioperative anxiety and hemodynamic stability in patients undergoing surgery under spinal anesthesia. J Family Med Primary Care. 2021;10(1):237. https://doi.org/10.4103/JFMPC.JFMPC_1544_20.
15. Dias R, Baliarsing L, Barnwal NK, Mogal S, Gujjar P. Role of pre-operative multimedia video information in allaying anxiety related to spinal anaesthesia: a randomised controlled trial. Indian J Anaesth. 2016;60(11):843–7. https://doi.org/10.4103/0019-5049.193681.

16. Jlala HA, French JL, Foxall GL, Hardman JG, Bedforth NM. Effect of preoperative multimedia information on perioperative anxiety in patients undergoing procedures under regional anaesthesia. Br J Anaesth. 2010;104(3):369–74. https://doi.org/10.1093/BJA/AEQ002.
17. Yeşilyurt DS, Findik ÜY. Effect of preoperative video information on anxiety and satisfaction in patients undergoing abdominal surgery. Comput Inform Nursing: CIN. 2019;37(8):430–6. https://doi.org/10.1097/CIN.0000000000000505.
18. Salzwedel C, Petersen C, Blanc I, Koch U, Goetz AE, Schuster M. The effect of detailed, video-assisted anesthesia risk education on patient anxiety and the duration of the preanesthetic interview: a randomized controlled trial. Anesth Analg. 2008;106(1):202–9. https://doi.org/10.1213/01.ANE.0000287665.96156.72.
19. Halawi MJ, Vovos TJ, Green CL, Wellman SS, Attarian DE, Bolognesi MP. Patient expectation is the most important predictor of discharge destination after primary total joint arthroplasty. J Arthroplasty. 2015;30(4):539–42. https://doi.org/10.1016/J.ARTH.2014.10.031.
20. Yajnik M, Hill JN, Hunter OO, Howard SK, Kim TE, Harrison TK, Mariano ER. Patient education and engagement in postoperative pain management decreases opioid use following knee replacement surgery. Patient Educ Couns. 2019;102(2):383–7. https://doi.org/10.1016/J.PEC.2018.09.001.
21. Khorfan R, Shallcross ML, Yu B, Sanchez N, Parilla S, Coughlin JM, Johnson JK, Bilimoria KY, Stulberg JJ. Preoperative patient education and patient preparedness are associated with less postoperative use of opioids. Surgery. 2020;167(5):852–8. https://doi.org/10.1016/J.SURG.2020.01.002.
22. Sheldon RR, Weiss JB, Do WS, Forte DM, Carter PL, Eckert MJ, Sohn VY. Stemming the tide of opioid addiction-dramatic reductions in postoperative opioid requirements through preoperative education and a standardized analgesic regimen. Mil Med. 2020;185(3–4):436–43. https://doi.org/10.1093/MILMED/USZ279.
23. Huber J, Ihrig A, Yass M, Bruckner T, Peters T, Huber CG, Konyango B, Lozankovski N, Stredele RJF, Moll P, Schneider M, Pahernik S, Hohenfellner M. Multimedia support for improving preoperative patient education: a randomized controlled trial using the example of radical prostatectomy. Ann Surg Oncol. 2013;20(1):15–23. https://doi.org/10.1245/S10434-012-2536-7.
24. Pager CK. Randomised controlled trial of preoperative information to improve satisfaction with cataract surgery. Br J Ophthalmol. 2005;89(1):10–3. https://doi.org/10.1136/BJO.2004.048637.
25. Lee A, Gin T. Educating patients about anaesthesia: effect of various modes on patients' knowledge, anxiety and satisfaction. Curr Opin Anaesthesiol. 2005;18(2):205–8. https://doi.org/10.1097/01.ACO.0000162842.09710.D5.
26. Raghavan G, Shyam V, Murdoch JAC. A survey of anesthetic preference and preoperative anxiety in hip and knee arthroplasty patients: the utility of the outpatient preoperative anesthesia appointment. J Anesth. 2019;33(2):250–6. https://doi.org/10.1007/S00540-018-02608-Y.
27. Southerland WA, Beight LJ, Shapiro FE, Urman RD. Decision aids in anesthesia: do they help? Curr Opin Anaesthesiol. 2020;33(2):185–91. https://doi.org/10.1097/ACO.0000000000000832.
28. The SHARE Approach Essential Steps of Shared Decision Making. Content last reviewed September 2020. Agency for Healthcare Research and Quality;Rockville, MD:2020. https://www.ahrq.gov/health-literacy/professional-training/shared-decision/tools/share-poster.html
29. Domino K, Posner K, Sween L, Shapiro F. Improving patient-centered care delivery in 2017: introducing pre-anesthesia decision aids. ASA Monitor 2017;81:10–13.
30. Posner K, Mincer S, Harvey A, Xue A, Van Norman G, Domino K. Regional Anesthesia decision aids in the pre-anesthesia clinic improve patient engagement and knowledge. ASA Abstracts. 25 Oct 2015. <ASA/content/asaabstracts/2015/REGIONAL ANESTHESIA AND ACUTE PAIN/abs_a2846.htm>
31. Seeman K. The importance of quality perioperative patient education. (2019);23(1):94–101. https://doi.org/10.1080/15398285.2019.1574525

32. Desebbe O, Lanz T, Kain Z, Cannesson M. The perioperative surgical home: an innovative, patient-centred and cost-effective perioperative care model. Anaesthesia, Critical Care and Pain Med. 2016;35(1):59–66. https://doi.org/10.1016/J.ACCPM.2015.08.001.
33. Elhassan A, Elhassan I, Elhassan A, Sekar K, Cornett E, Urman R, Kaye A. Perioperative surgical home models and enhanced recovery after surgery. J Anaesthesiol Clin Pharmacol. 2019;35(Suppl 1):46–50. https://doi.org/10.4103/JOACP.JOACP_47_18.
34. Cline KM, Clement V, Rock-Klotz J, Kash BA, Steel C, Miller TR. Improving the cost, quality, and safety of perioperative care: a systematic review of the literature on implementation of the perioperative surgical home. J Clinical Anesthesia. 2020;63. https://doi.org/10.1016/J.JCLINANE.2020.109760

The Role of Inpatient/Acute Pain Services for Perioperative Pain Management

Hari Kalagara, Asaf Gans, Lauren Gatewood, and Sindhuja Nimma

Abstract Pain management is a significant concern for patients undergoing surgery. This chapter delves into the many roles an Inpatient Pain Service (IPS) or Acute Pain Service (APS) team can play in perioperative pain management. The APS team is a dedicated group of anesthesiologists, anesthesia fellows and residents, nurses, and technicians who work together to aid in safe and effective perioperative pain management. Its goals are to help reduce opioid consumption, reduce delays in hospital discharge, improve patient satisfaction, maximize patient safety, and answer patient questions. The IPS team helps place and manage peripheral and neuraxial nerve blocks/catheters, manage intravenous (IV) lidocaine and ketamine infusions, manage patient-controlled analgesia (PCA) pumps, or implement a combination of these techniques. There are tremendous benefits to implementing these strategies, including reducing the side effects of opioids, facilitating participation in rehabilitation, and improving pain control. Members of the APS team should be experts in choosing the best pain relief intervention, managing, and troubleshooting perioperative pain, identifying contraindications to different interventions, recognizing regional anesthesia and medication-induced emergencies and side effects. This chapter may serve as a guide for a successful acute pain service and the scope of practice within its different roles.

Keywords Acute pain service · Regional anesthesiology · Inpatient pain service · Perioperative care · Pain management · Peripheral nerve block · Peripheral nerve catheters · Epidural catheters · Ketamine infusion · Lidocaine infusion · Acute pain consultation · Chronic pain · Multidisciplinary team

H. Kalagara (✉) · A. Gans · L. Gatewood · S. Nimma
Department of Anesthesiology and Perioperative Medicine, Mayo Clinic, Jacksonville, FL 32224, USA
e-mail: Kalagara.Hari@mayo.edu

L. Gatewood
e-mail: Gatewood.Lauren@mayo.edu

S. Nimma
e-mail: Nimma.Sindhuja@mayo.edu

A. Abd-Elsayed and K. Schroeder (eds.), *Perioperative Pain Management*,
https://doi.org/10.1007/978-3-031-67648-2_10

1 Introduction

The acute pain service (APS) or inpatient pain service (IPS) is a dedicated, multidisciplinary team specializing in perioperative pain management of inpatient surgical patients. Pain management is a significant concern for patients undergoing surgery, and inadequate pain management is often the cause of hospital discharge delays [1–3]. The APS team as an organized unit was first described in the late 1980s. Soon after, hospitals worldwide adopted this concept and developed it into an organized establishment addressing many patient concerns by incorporating education, research, and clinical care [4].

In most established academic and private practice hospitals, the APS team is led by physician anesthesiologists with fellowship-level training or expertise in regional anesthesiology and acute pain medicine [5]. However, the inpatient APS functions best as an integrated team that includes physicians, nurses, technicians, residents, fellows, nurse practitioners, and other medical professionals. Since pain is universal to all post-surgical patients, it is essential to understand the APS team's role in addressing individual patient pain management strategies through assessment and implementation of data-driven management protocols. This team assumes a variety of roles in their efforts to address pain control, improve continuity of care, enhance patient education, drive research endeavors, and, most importantly, promote patient safety. In the following sections, we address the numerous roles of the inpatient APS team in managing perioperative pain.

2 Peripheral Nerve Catheters

Before the utilization of peripheral nerve blocks for upper and lower extremity surgeries, surgeons and anesthesiologists depended heavily on opioids to manage acute postoperative pain. While multimodal analgesia is strongly encouraged, opioids remain a potent problem. Given the recent opioid crisis, non-pharmacological interventions have gained increasing attention in addressing intraoperative and postoperative pain [5]. Peripheral nerve catheters (PNC) are typically placed before surgery in a dedicated preoperative area, immediately post-operatively in the postanesthesia care unit (PACU), and at times in the operating room (OR). The APS team examines the patient's preoperative history and scheduled surgery and identifies indications and contraindications to offering a nerve block to ultimately establish post-operative pain expectations.

From performing a peripheral nerve block to following up with the patient postoperatively, the inpatient APS team plays an incredibly important role. The APS team decides the local anesthetic of choice and technique (i.e., single shot block versus peripheral nerve catheter) after a discussion with the surgical team and the patient. Peripheral nerve catheters are more challenging to place than single-shot injections; however, they offer longer-lasting pain control compared to a single-shot approach. While the anesthesiologist, resident, or fellow will ultimately perform the block and administer sedation, the integrated team of nurses and technicians help with the time-out process prior to needle insertion; help position the patient, set up the block tray supplies, and ensure proper documentation either on a paper chart or electronic medical record.

After performing a peripheral nerve catheter, a member of the APS team will evaluate the patient by performing a sensory and motor exam to ensure a successful block. Once the scheduled surgery is completed, patients with nerve catheters can either be sent home with a home catheter device or be admitted overnight for observation. The APS team is responsible for following up with patients in either discourse. If the patient is sent home with a catheter, the patient and a family member are educated on how to use the pain pump device and troubleshoot common catheter or pump-related issues. They are also provided with a phone number to call anytime with concerns. A member of the APS team, either a resident, fellow, or nurse, will follow up with the patient daily until the catheter is removed. For patients staying overnight in the hospital, the on-call APS team members will assess the patient overnight and during morning rounds to ensure adequate pain control. They will help troubleshoot any patient or catheter-related issues. The team will also evaluate the catheter dressing site to ensure the insertion site is clean and dry with no obvious signs of infection and that the catheter is not displaced or dislodged. The concentration of local anesthetic, rate of infusion, total volume, and maximum dose per hour is determined and titrated by the APS team. Based on physical exam findings and subjective patient experience, the settings of basal and bolus LA infusions can be adjusted to ensure more significant pain relief and patient satisfaction. The team will additionally assess the nurse-reported pain scores, opioid utilization, diet progression, and primary team services' communication to determine expected patient disposition. Depending on the hospital system, nurses, physical therapists, surgeons, internal medicine physicians, sub-specialty physicians, and social workers may work together with the patient. In the end, however, all teams must work cohesively to ensure an expedited and smooth recovery process for the patient. It is important to note that effective communication of the expectation of pain with a nerve block is integral to improving patient satisfaction and reducing patient anxiety. Recently with growing use of interfascial plane blocks, continuous catheters can be placed for these blocks also to enable prolonged postoperative analgesia, for example erector spinae plane (ESP) block catheters or serratus anterior plane (SAP) block catheters for patients with rib fractures.

Apart from ensuring adequate postoperative pain control, assessing patients for any side effects or complications of a peripheral nerve catheter is imperative. Specifically, every patient should be evaluated for local anesthetic systemic toxicity (LAST), which can initially present with mild symptoms, such as tinnitus, perioral numbness, and metallic taste. If not immediately recognized and treated, LAST can progress to agitation, confusion, seizures, arrhythmia, cardiac arrest, and even death [6]. It is imperative that all members of the inpatient pain team are educated on how to recognize and treat LAST. In summary, an inpatient APS team should be able to work as an integrative team to evaluate and troubleshoot peripheral nerve catheters, offer a multimodal pain plan, eloquently and concisely manage patient expectations, and systematically approach any deviations from the expected course or unexpected complications. Unfortunately, not all healthcare systems have the resources, financial ability, or trained personnel to offer nerve catheters or establish an organized inpatient pain team for catheter follow-up. These groups often resort to single-shot blocks and either a nurse or physician may or may not follow up with the patients postoperatively.

3 Home Catheters

There are many benefits associated with peripheral nerve catheters, including postoperative analgesia, decreased opioid consumption, improved participation in rehabilitation, and increased patient satisfaction. When performed appropriately, there are minimal side effects [27–29]. However, persistent safety concerns may limit enthusiasm for discharging patients with a peripheral nerve catheter. Physicians remain concerned over the potential for catheter migration in an unmonitored setting, the potential for local anesthetic systemic toxicity, and injuries associated with an anesthetized extremity. One way to address these concerns is through the utilization of dilute concentrations of local anesthetics, which, if delivered intravascularly, should only produce minimal symptoms [30]. This, in conjunction with a direct phone line to an available physician or nurse, allows an APS team to monitor their patients closely, troubleshoot malfunctioning catheters, and answer questions. Thirty percent of patients utilized this phone resource even though they were discharged with verbal and written instructions [31]. While not every hospital system has the resources or infrastructure to support the ability to discharge patients with peripheral nerve catheters, the patient benefits of peripheral nerve catheters should strongly argue for integrating them into a multimodal analgesic paradigm. Having an APS team will help to manage these home catheters more effectively on a regular basis in a systematic manner.

4 Single Shot Blocks

When a nerve catheter is not indicated, or a specific surgery does not necessitate long-term pain control, a single shot nerve block, paravertebral block (PVB) or interfascial plane (IFP) blocks can be offered for postoperative pain control. The duration of a single shot block depends not only on the anatomical location of the block and the patient's age but also on the local anesthetic of choice and what adjuvants are added (i.e., adrenaline, dexamethasone, dexmedetomidine, clonidine, buprenorphine) with the local anesthetic. On average, a single shot block with ropivacaine or bupivacaine can last between 12–24 h. Single shot blocks, for example, are typically offered for outpatient procedures such as upper and lower extremity surgeries, breast lumpectomy or mastectomy, arterio-venous fistula creation, etc. Most patients are discharged from the hospital, and follow-up on post-operative day one depends on the expectations of the current inpatient APS practice. Some centers do offer single shot intrathecal (spinal) opioid injections for certain surgeries preoperatively especially for ERAS programs. If the patient is admitted overnight, a member of the APS team, depending on the institution, may evaluate the patient to assess pain scores and overall patient satisfaction. Some APS teams may not have an organized way of following up single shot blocks, and patients will only have follow-up with the APS team as necessary if concerns arise. However, the ability to routinely assess patients following regional anesthesia procedures offers an opportunity for enhanced quality improvement initiatives and rapid intervention in circumstances where block resolution is delayed or results in significant patient discomfort.

5 Neuraxial Catheters

For major surgeries such as open abdominal or pelvic surgery, extensive lower extremity surgery, or thoracic surgery, a thoracic or lumbar epidural catheter can be offered for intraoperative and postoperative analgesia [7]. Contraindications to neuraxial catheters include patient refusal, history of spine surgery, spine hardware, coagulopathy, bacteremia, signs of infection at the anticipated needle insertion site, or hemodynamic instability. A neuraxial catheter can be considered if the benefits outweigh the risks after a collaborative discussion occurs between the patient, surgical team, and anesthesiologist. The entire APS team is involved in patient care during the procedure. For example, the APS technician will help position the patient appropriately while the nursing team performs a pre-procedure safety check (time-out) to ensure the correct patient is undergoing the correct surgery and the correct block is being performed. The physician will place the epidural catheter and direct sedation administration while the nursing staff can help document procedure details, including the spinal level of insertion, depth of needle and catheter, type of catheter used, and any complications noted during the placement or during the test dose administration [7]. After the successful placement of the epidural, the APS team will dictate the local anesthetic of choice, rate of infusion, as well as the number of bolus doses allowed every hour.

Similar to the management of peripheral nerve catheters, there is a systematic approach to evaluating epidural catheters, such as evaluating the sensory and motor blockade of a neuraxial catheter, assessing pain scores, opioid usage, oral intake, and ambulation. A discussion with the surgical service should also occur, outlining their plans for removing surgical tubes and drains, expected disposition, and methods for diagnostic or therapeutic studies. This information can help guide the optimal duration of therapy and limit epidural catheter duration dependent complications including infection [8]. Some centers prefer paravertebral (PVB) catheters for thoracic and other major abdominal surgeries instead of epidurals to enable postoperative analgesia and to overcome the risks and limitations of these central neuraxial blocks.

Based on the ASRA anticoagulation guidelines, the APS team ensures proper discontinuation of anticoagulants before neuraxial blockade. They also dictate which anticoagulants can be administered while a neuraxial catheter is in place and at what doses and frequencies, how extended anticoagulation should be held before neuraxial catheter manipulation or removal, and when anticoagulants can be reinitiated once a neuraxial catheter is removed [9]. Before the placement of any neuraxial block, it is imperative that the entire APS team is familiar with appropriate anticoagulation recommendations.

It is well known that epidurals can cause hemodynamic perturbations via sympathectomy and its associated vasodilation. It is also well known that the perioperative period is associated with significant fluid shifts and potential blood loss. The combination of inadequate resuscitation and iatrogenic sympathectomy can cause hypotension and associated sequela. Therefore, an inpatient APS team needs to be cognizant of a patient's fluid status, needs for vasopressor support, and changes in labs consistent with hemoconcentration or hemodilution [10]. Another critical aspect of evaluating a patient with a neuraxial catheter is to assess their gastrointestinal function by assessing their ability to tolerate PO medication and have bowel movements or pass flatus. Along the same lines, it is also important to evaluate for nausea and vomiting. A patient that can tolerate a PO diet without nausea while also demonstrating a return of gastrointestinal motility through passing flatus is likely making strides toward utilizing PO medication for pain control and discontinuing the neuraxial catheter. This comes into play often with abdominal surgeries and the potential for ileus and small bowel obstruction. If the patient cannot tolerate PO/NG medications, then pain control options include neuraxial or IV medication, which are incompatible with progression to discharge and may worsen nausea and potential ileus. A neuraxial catheter, in and of itself, should decrease the incidence of postoperative ileus by decreasing opioid consumption and via blockade of the sympathetic fibers that slow gastrointestinal transit [11–12].

Sometimes, even when a neuraxial catheter is placed convincingly and without problems, maintaining an effective and safe block is challenging. It is important to know how to troubleshoot common problems and know when there is a concerning finding. Common issues the inpatient APS team encounters include no sensory or one-sided sensory blocks, epidural catheter migration, inadequate local anesthetic dosing, hypotension, infection, or erythema at the insertion site, etc [13]. To effectively care for patients with any neuraxial block, the inpatient APS team must be a well-educated team of individuals trained to assess the indications and contraindications of offering the procedure and manage neuraxial-related side effects and complications.

6 Lidocaine Infusion

A peripheral or neuraxial nerve block procedure involves bathing targeted nerves in local anesthetic to disrupt the pain signaling pathway from the periphery to the central nervous system. However, if the APS team determines there is a contraindication to performing such a procedure, administering intravenous lidocaine can benefit selected patients. Numerous articles have illustrated systemic lidocaine's anti-inflammatory and cytokine reduction properties [14]. While the mechanism of action for lidocaine on peripheral nerves is via sodium channel blockade, the mechanism of action for intravenous lidocaine infusion at therapeutic doses is believed to be via blockade of the muscarinic and NMDA receptors [14–15].

IV lidocaine has been used as part of a multimodal analgesic regimen for many types of surgery. For a specific subset of surgeries, there seems to be a decrease in opioid consumption, length of hospital stay, pain scores, occurrences of postoperative ileus, and postoperative nausea and vomiting. While a reduction is noted in most studies, it may not be statistically or clinically significant [15–16]. The subset of surgeries with the most evidence-based support for IV lidocaine is abdominal surgery and genitourinary surgery, specifically laparoscopic abdominal surgery and radical retropubic prostatectomy [17]. Some patients may show particular benefit when opioid medications have been deemed ineffective or if they have been shown to have acute hyperalgesia [15]. In contrast, the administration of intravenous lidocaine for obstetric and breast surgery did not show improvement in their incidence of pain, postoperative nausea, and vomiting, opioid consumption, or length of stay [16].

Due to lidocaine's potential to block cardiac sodium channels, significant cardiac disease can be considered a relative contraindication. Additionally, IV lidocaine infusions should be used cautiously in patients with significant renal or hepatic dysfunction due to altered metabolism. Seizure disorders, neurologic disorders, and breastfeeding patients may also represent relative contraindications to intravenous lidocaine infusions [16]. Therefore, if the APS department at a particular institution oversees patients on IV lidocaine infusions, the team must be well educated on the signs and symptoms of LAST. Typically, to initiate a lidocaine infusion, a loading dose of 1.5 mg/kg ideal body weight is given over 10 min, followed by an infusion of 1.5 mg/kg/hr ideal body weight. Infusions may be considered for 24 h following surgery but may be discontinued sooner if side effects are noted [16]. An APS team's role in IV lidocaine infusion management should include appropriate patient selection and initiation of the infusion, dosing, and titration, answering questions regarding side effects or concerns while also ensuring that patients don't receive additional nerve blocks or fascial plane blocks with local anesthetics while the IV lidocaine is running. Because of the potential for neurologic and cardiovascular abnormalities associated with IV Lidocaine infusions, having a dedicated APS team to oversee patient care is critical. Variations in clinical practices are seen where these patients are being managed postoperatively in the intensive care unit (ICU) or on general floors.

7 Patient Controlled Analgesia (PCA)

The benefits of opioid Intravenous Patient Controlled Analgesia (IV PCA) are well documented and include improved patient satisfaction and pain control when compared to nurse-administered opioid boluses, decreased anxiety due to enhanced patient feelings of control over their pain medication, and increased mobility and thus a reduced risk of deep vein thrombosis [18]. While there are documented benefits of IV PCA, there are multiple side effects, including nausea, drowsiness, constipation, and respiratory depression. Programming an IV PCA requires consideration of the initial loading dose, intermittent demand dose, lockout interval, and hourly limit. Numerous opioid medications are amenable to IV PCA, and common choices include morphine, hydromorphone, fentanyl, and sufentanil. The choice of opioid is patient dependent and outside the scope of this discussion.

While the primary medicine or surgical team manages the initiation, titration, and discontinuation of IV PCA at some institutions, this role is tasked to the inpatient APS team at other institutions. To evaluate a patient with an IV PCA, the APS team will do a thorough chart review and examine the patient to review pain scores, IV PCA settings, IV PCA bolus attempts, IV PCA boluses received, non-opioid analgesic orders, and reported side effects (respiratory depression, sedation, constipation, nausea, vomiting). If the patient reports unsatisfactory pain control without side effects (and appropriate IV PCA utilization, i.e. 2–3 demands per hour), increasing the intermittent bolus dose amount or frequency of the intermittent bolus dose is a consideration that could be discussed with the patient and primary team [19–20]. If, however, the patient reports opioid-related side effects and their pain is still unsatisfactory, a conversation with the patient that focuses on risks and benefits associated with IV PCA utilization and consideration of other non-opioid analgesic techniques may be beneficial. The optimal goal of any team managing the IV PCA is to transition the patient as quickly and safely as possible from IV PCA to an oral multimodal pain regimen in preparation for discharge. Respiratory rate monitoring with a priority on patient safety is critical to preventing opioid-related adverse events while using IV PCA.

8 Ketamine

Ketamine is a phencyclidine analog that is a dissociative anesthetic agent that reverses central sensitization and enhances descending pain-modulating pathways [21]. As an infusion, it has been used for many decades to treat acute and chronic pain and severe depression [22]. Recently, there has been a surge of use in the perioperative period in patients with refractory pain and post-surgical patients with chronic pain who are opioid-tolerant [22]. Because there is such wide variability in patient selection, indications, and monitoring, several associations, such as the American Society of Anesthesiologists (ASA) and the American Society of Regional Anesthesia and Pain

Medicine (ASRA), created consensus guidelines for the use of intravenous (IV) ketamine infusions.

Ketamine is increasingly being administered under an APS team's guidance in inpatient settings. Ketamine infusions are often started in patients undergoing surgery where the expected post-operative pain is severe such as might be encountered following open abdominal surgery, thoracic surgery, and spine surgery, or in opioid-dependent patients expected to have an acute exacerbation of a baseline chronic pain condition. In select patients with severe sleep apnea, ketamine is often used as an adjunct to limit opioid administration. While the decision to start a ketamine infusion is primarily made by the intraoperative anesthesiologist or primary surgical or critical care team, the APS team is often consulted to direct further management.

If the ketamine infusion is started in the operating room, a bolus dose of ketamine, typically 0.3–0.5 mg/kg, is given before an infusion of 0.1–0.2 mg/kg/hr is initiated [23]. At this infusion rate, the subanesthetic dose of serum ketamine concentration of 100–200 ng/ml is known to produce analgesia [24–25]. Perioperative ketamine infusions are typically continued through two postoperative days. The APS team is responsible for evaluating patients every day and titrating the ketamine infusion rate to improve patient comfort and minimize the occurrence and severity of side effects. It is generally recommended that the ketamine infusion rate not exceed 1mcg/kg/hr [26]. Ketamine should be avoided in patients with severe cardiovascular disease, active psychosis, pregnancy, severe hepatic dysfunction, and elevated intraocular or intracranial pressure. Ketamine infusions should also be titrated down or even stopped if the patient is experiencing side effects, including confusion, disorientation, changes in sensory perceptions such as auditory or visual hallucinations, or loss of motor coordination. In institutions with a dedicated inpatient APS team, the responsibility falls on this team of trained individuals to perform daily pain evaluations during morning rounds, assess the need to continue or discontinue the infusion, illicit the patient for side effects, and coordinate with the primary team to formulate a plan for a smooth transition off IV ketamine to multimodal oral pain medications. While not all institutions have a dedicated inpatient pain team, it is a significant advantage and a safety net to have a team trained to recognize indications, contraindications, dosing titration, and side effects of ketamine. These patients can be managed on regular floors with nursing team care coordination with APS support.

9 Consults

At any institution with an established APS team, a variety of perioperative responsibilities are shared among the team. One such responsibility is accepting and addressing consultations for the APS team to evaluate patients. Consultation requests for the APS team come in a variety of forms. For example, the primary team may request the APS team to perform an epidural blood patch (EBP) for a patient suffering from a post-dural puncture headache. At most institutions, the anesthesiologist will assist in placing an EBP. However, some requests may go directly to the chronic pain service or the neurosurgery team. If a patient has major aortic surgery and needs a spinal drain placed for protection from spinal cord ischemia, the APS team might be consulted to place and follow up on a spinal drain. Post-lung transplant, if a patient is difficult to wean from the ventilator due to pain, the APS team can be consulted to place either an epidural catheter or paravertebral blocks to help expedite extubation, improve respiratory mechanics, and enhance pain control. In any hospitalized patient with poorly controlled pain, the APS team might be asked to evaluate the patient for recommendations about opioid regimen changes, multimodal analgesia, potential regional anesthesia, IV ketamine or IV lidocaine initiation, or consultation for evaluation by chronic pain specialists. Patients with severe vascular disease with ischemic extremity pain may benefit from increased perfusion to the affected limb. The APS team can help perform extremity blocks that lead to a more localized sympathectomy and temporarily dilate extremity vasculature to improve blood flow. If patients have a history of opioid use disorder or are already taking medications like methadone and Suboxone, the APS team is often approached before surgery to evaluate the patient and make further recommendations for acute surgical pain management. Similarly, if a patient has a history of high baseline opioid consumption, the APS or chronic pain teams can consult to discuss perioperative medication plans and help set expectations.

10 Pros and Cons of APS Team

There are many considerations when addressing in-hospital pain. It has been shown that implementing an Acute Pain Service (APS) with dedicated physicians and nurses effectively improves post-operative analgesia, decreases adverse effects, and improves patient perception of care [30, 32]. These dedicated physicians and nurses are trained to be cognizant of the effects of peripheral and neuraxial catheters, different analgesic options, associated side effects with different medications and procedures, and troubleshooting inappropriately functioning analgesic therapies. While it is essential to recognize the benefits of an acute pain service, there is a cost associated with an acute pain service. It has been shown that there are inappropriate referrals to the acute pain service resulting in increased costs to the patient and occurrences where the patient received no benefit from the service [33]. Implementation of an APS can lead to improved patient outcomes. Keys to a successful APS include leadership by anesthesiologists, interdisciplinary coordination, education of patients and health care providers, standardization of regional anesthesia procedures, and systematic billing practices. Given the current focus on perioperative opioid use, an APS team can provide individualized inpatient pain management plans, institute multimodal analgesia options, and collaborate with other providers involved with perioperative pain management. In addition to taking care of patients, the APS team invests tremendous time and energy to train young nurses and physicians through education, research, and patient care. A dedicated, multidisciplinary team knowledgeable and trained to handle perioperative pain management is vital to successful patient care.

11 Key Points

- An inpatient/acute pain service is a multidisciplinary team specializing in perioperative pain management of mostly surgical and limited non-surgical patients.
- The acute pain service examines a patients' preoperative history and identifies indications and contraindications to regional anesthesia while establishing post-operative pain management strategies that seek to minimize opioid administration.
- The acute pain service team troubleshoots peripheral nerve and neuraxial blocks, offers multimodal pain plans, eloquently and concisely manages patient expectations, and systematically approaches deviations from the expected course to unexpected complications.
- Managing a successful acute pain service requires effective leadership, interdisciplinary coordination, education of patients and health care providers, standardization of regional anesthesia procedures, and systematic billing practices.

References

1. Jenkins K, Grady D, Wong J, et al. Post-operative recovery: day surgery patients' preferences. Br J Anaesth. 2001;86:272–4.
2. Warfield CA, Kahn CH. Acute pain management. Programs in U.S. hospitals and experiences and attitudes among U.S. adults. Anesthesiology 1995;83:1090–1094.
3. Pavlin DJ, Chen C, Penaloza DA, et al. Pain as a factor complicating recovery and discharge after ambulatory surgery. Anesth Analg. 2002;95:627–34.
4. Ready LB, Oden R, Chadwick HS, et al. Development of an anesthesiology-based postoperative pain management service. Anesthesiology 1988;68:100–106.
5. Tighe P, Buckenmaier CC, Boezaart AP, et al. Acute pain medicine in the United States: a status report. Pain Med 2015;16:1806–1826.
6. Dickerson DM, Apfelbaum JL. Local anesthetic systemic toxicity. Aesthet Surg J. 2014;34(7):1111–9. https://doi.org/10.1177/1090820X14543102.
7. Manion SC, Brennan TJ, Riou B. Thoracic epidural analgesia and acute pain management. Anesthesiology 2011;115:181–188. https://doi.org/10.1097/ALN.0b013e318220847c
8. Bomberg H, Bayer I, Wagenpfeil S, Kessler P, Wulf H, Standl T, Gottschalk A, Döffert J, Hering W, Birnbaum J, Spies C, Kutter B, Winckelmann J, Liebl-Biereige S, Meissner W, Vicent O, Koch T, Sessler DI, Volk T, Raddatz A. Prolonged catheter use and infection in regional anesthesia: a retrospective registry analysis. Anesthesiology 2018;128:764–773. https://doi.org/10.1097/ALN.0000000000002105
9. Horlocker T, Vandermeulen, E, Kopp S, et al. Regional anesthesia in the patient receiving antithrombotic or thrombolytic therapy. American society of regional Anesthesia and pain

medicine evidence-based guideliens (fourth edition). Reg Anesth Pain Med. 2018;43:263–309. https://doi.org/10.1097/AAP.0000000000000763

10. Holte K, Foss NB, Svensén C, Lund C, Madsen JL, Kehlet H. Epidural anesthesia, hypotension, and changes in intravascular volume. Anesthesiology 2004;100:281–286. https://doi.org/10.1097/00000542-200402000-00016
11. Zoumprouli A, Chatzimichali A, Papadimitriou S, Papaioannou A, Xynos E, Askitopoulou H. Gastrointestinal motility following thoracic surgery: the effect of thoracic epidural analgesia. A randomized controlled trial. BMC Anesthesiol. 2017;17(1):139. https://doi.org/10.1186/s12871-017-0427-y. PMID: 29037157; PMCID: PMC5644078.
12. McLeod GA, Cumming C. Thoracic epidural anaesthesia and analgesia, Continuing Educat Anaesthesia Critical Care and Pain. 2004;4(1): 16–19. https://doi.org/10.1093/bjaceaccp/mkh006
13. Hermanides J, Hollmann MW, Stevens MF, Lirk P. Failed epidural: causes and management. BJA: British J Anaesthesia 2012;109(2):144–154. https://doi.org/10.1093/bja/aes214
14. Kandil E, Melikman E, Adinoff B. Lidocaine infusion: a promising therapeutic approach for chronic pain. J Anesthesia Clinical Res. 8(1). https://doi.org/10.4172/2155-6148:1000697
15. Eipe N, Gupta S, Penning J. Intravenous lidocaine for acute pain: an evidence-based clinical update. BJA Education. 2016;16(9):292–298. https://doi.org/10.1093/bjaed/mkw008
16. The use of Intravenous Lidocaine for Postoperative Pain and Recovery: International consensus statement on efficacy and safety. Foo I, Anaesthesia 2021;76:238–250.
17. Dunn L, Durieux M. Perioperative use of intravenous lidocaine. Anesthesiology. 2017;126:729–37.
18. Choiniere M, Rittenhouse BE, Perreault S, et al. Efficacy and costs of patient-controlled analgesia versus regularly administered intramuscular opioid therapy. Anesthesiology. 1998;89:1377–88.
19. Badner NH, Doyle JA, Smith MH, Herrick IA. Effect of varying intravenous patient-controlled analgesia dose and lockout interval while maintaining a constant hourly maximum dose. J Clin Anesth. 1996;8:382–5.
20. Grass JA. Patient-controlled analgesia. Anesth Analg. 2005;101(5 Suppl):S44–61. https://doi.org/10.1213/01.ANE.0000177102.11682.20. PMID: 16334492.
21. Urban MK, Ya Deau JT, Wukovits B, Lipnitsky JY. Ketamine as an adjunct to postoperative pain management in opioid tolerant patients after spinal fusions: a prospective randomized trial. HSS J. 4(1):62–5. https://doi.org/10.1007/s11420-007-9069-9. Epub 2007 Dec 19. PMID: 18751864; PMCID: PMC2504281.
22. Schwenk ES, Viscusi ER, Buvanendran A, Hurley RW, Wasan AD, Narouze S, Bhatia A, Davis FN, Hooten WM, Cohen SP. Consensus guidelines on the use of intravenous ketamine infusions for acute pain management from the American society of regional anesthesia and pain medicine, the American academy of pain medicine, and the American society of anesthesiologists. Reg Anesth Pain Med. 2018;43(5):456–466. https://doi.org/10.1097/AAP.0000000000000806. PMID: 29870457; PMCID: PMC6023582.
23. Vadivelu N, Schermer E, Kodumudi V, Belani K, Urman RD, Kaye AD. Role of ketamine for analgesia in adults and children. J Anaesthesiol Clin Pharmacol. 32(3):298–306. https://doi.org/10.4103/0970-9185.168149. PMID: 27625475; PMCID: PMC5009833.
24. Domino EF, Zsigmond EK, Domino LE, Domino KE, Kothary SP, Domino SE. Plasma levels of ketamine and two of its metabolites in surgical patients using a gas chromatographic mass fragmentographic assay. Anesth Analg. 1982;61(2):87–92 PMID: 7198883.
25. Clements JA, Nimmo WS, Grant IS. Bioavailability, pharmacokinetics, and analgesic activity of ketamine in humans. J Pharm Sci. 1982;71(5):539–42. https://doi.org/10.1002/jps.2600710516. PMID: 7097501.
26. Schmid RL, Sandler AN, Katz J. Use and efficacy of low-dose ketamine in the management of acute postoperative pain: a review of current techniques and outcomes. Pain. 1999;82(2):111–25. https://doi.org/10.1016/S0304-3959(99)00044-5. PMID: 10467917.
27. Selander D. Catheter technique in axillary plexus block. Acta Anaesth Scand. 1977;21:324–9.

28. Dahl J, Christiansen C, Daugaard J, Schultz P, Carlsson P. Continuous blockade of the lumbar plexus after knee surgery-postoperative analgesia and bupivacaine plasma concentrations. A controlled clinical trial. Anaesthesia. 1988;43:1015–8.
29. Capdevila X, Barthelet Y, Biboulet P, Ryckwaert Y, Rubenovitch J, d'Athis F. Effects of perioperative analgesic technique on the surgical outcome and duration of rehabilitation after major knee surgery. Anesthesiology. 1999;91:8–15.
30. Narinder, R. Chapter 78. Acute pain service: organization, function, and implementation. NYSORA Textbook of Regional Anesthesia and Acute Pain Management. Admir Hadzic. McGraw Hill;2007. https://accessanesthesiology.mhmedical.com/content.aspx?bookid=413&sectionid=39828240
31. Ilfeld B, Morey T, Enneking F. Continuous infraclavicular brachial plexus block for postoperative pain control at home: a randomized, double-blinded, placebo-controlled study. Anesthesiology. 2002;96:1297–304.
32. Mitra S, Jain K, Singh J, Jindal S, Saxena P, Singh M, Saroa R, Ahuja V, Kang J, Garg S. Does an acute pain service improve the perception of postoperative pain management in patients undergoing lower limb surgery? A prospective controlled non-randomized study. J Anaesthesiol Clin Pharmacol. 2020;36(2):187–194. https://doi.org/10.4103/joacp.JOACP_104_19. Epub 2020 Jun 15. PMID: 33013033; PMCID: PMC7480304.
33. Sussman M, Goodier E, Fabri I, Borrowman J, Thomas S, Guest C, Bantel C. Clinical benefits, referral practice and cost implications of an in-hospital pain service: results of a service evaluation in a London teaching hospital. Br J Pain. 11(1):36–45. https://doi.org/10.1177/2049463716673667. Epub 2016 Oct 11. PMID: 28386403; PMCID: PMC5370625.
34. Webb CAJ, Kim TE. Establishing an acute pain service in private practice and updates on regional Anesthesia billing. Anesthesiol Clin. 36(3):333–344. https://doi.org/10.1016/j.anclin.2018.04.005. PMID: 30092932.
35. Cohen SP, Vase L, Hooten WM. Chronic pain: an update on burden, best practices, and new advances. Lancet. 397(10289):2082–2097. https://doi.org/10.1016/S0140-6736(21)00393-7. PMID: 34062143
36. Manion SC, Brennan TJ, Riou B. Thoracic epidural analgesia and acute pain management. Anesthesiology. 2011;115:181–188. https://doi.org/10.1097/ALN.0b013e318220847c
37. Brown, D.L. Spinal, epidural, and caudal anesthesia. Miller RD editors. Miller's Anesthesia, 6th ed. Philadelphia:Elsevier Churchill Livingstone.
38. Kay, J. Epidural troubleshooting—anaesthesia (2018). Available at: https://www.anaesthesia.org.au/pain/pdf/pain.pdf. Accessed 2 Jan 2023
39. Kay, J. Epidural troubleshooting—anaesthesia (2018). Available at: https://anaesthesia.org.au/pain/pdf/hypotension.pdf. Accessed 2 Jan 2023
40. Ameer MA, Knorr TL, Munakomi S, et al. Spinal epidural abscess. [Updated 2022 Nov 17]. StatPearls [Internet]. Treasure Island (FL):StatPearls Publishing;2022. Available from: https://www.ncbi.nlm.nih.gov/books/NBK441890/
41. Khairat A, Waseem M. Epidural Hematoma. [Updated 2022 Aug 7]. StatPearls [Internet]. Treasure Island (FL):StatPearls Publishing;2022. Available from: https://www.ncbi.nlm.nih.gov/books/NBK518982/
42. Kumar K, Singh SI. Neuraxial opioid-induced pruritus: an update. J Anaesthesiol Clin Pharmacol. 2013;29(3):303–7. https://doi.org/10.4103/0970-9185.117045. PMID: 24106351; PMCID: PMC3788225.
43. Owen H, Plummer JL, Armstrong I, et al. Variables of patient-controlled analgesia: I Bolus size. Anaesthesia. 1989;44:7–10.
44. Klein SM. Beyond the hospital: continuous peripheral nerve blocks at home Anesthesiology. 2002;96:1283–5.

Pain and the Transition from Acute to Chronic

Adeeb Oweidat, Rofayda Gad, Yair Rubin, Alain Harb, Nour El Hage Chehade, and Amro Khalili

Abstract Chronic post-surgical pain reduces quality of life, challenging to treat, and has economic impact. Factors that predispose patients to development of chronic post-surgical pain may be potential targets for identification and prevention of transition from acute to chronic pain. This involves a multidisciplinary perioperative plan that begins at the preoperative clinic and continues beyond healing phase of surgery.

Keywords Types of pain · Neuroplasticity · Epigenetics

A. Oweidat (✉)
Associate Program Director for Regional Anesthesia and Acute Pain, University of Iowa Hospital and Clinic, Iowa City, USA
e-mail: adeeb.oweidat@gmail.com

R. Gad
Instructor of Anesthesiology NYU Hospital, Iowa City, USA
e-mail: Rofayda.Y.Gad@gmail.com

Y. Rubin
Clinical Associate Professor of Anesthesia, Medical Director, Non OR Anesthesia Services, University of Iowa Hospital and Clinic, Iowa City, USA
e-mail: yair-rubin@uiowa.edu

A. Harb
Assistant Professor of Anesthesiology, University of Miami, Miller School of Medicine, Miami, Florida, USA
e-mail: alain.ch.harb@gmail.com

N. El Hage Chehade
Assistant Professor of Anesthesiology, Cleveland Clinic, Cleveland, USA
e-mail: ELHAGEN2@ccf.org

A. Khalili
Instructor of Clinical Anesthesiology, Division of Cardiovascular Anesthesia, American University of Beirut Medical Center, Beirut, Lebanon
e-mail: amero.kh@hotmail.com

A. Abd-Elsayed and K. Schroeder (eds.), *Perioperative Pain Management*,
https://doi.org/10.1007/978-3-031-67648-2_11

1 Introduction

The International Association for the Study of Pain (IASP) defines pain as the unpleasant sensory and emotional experience associated with actual or potential tissue damage. Though it is most often related to tissue damage, perception of the damage varies due to many factors: attitudes, beliefs, personality, social factors, non-modifying factors like gender and ethnicity, and underlying conditions such as comorbidities, mental stress, and substance abuse. Moreover, genetic associations affect a person's pain perception by orchestrating the entire mechanism [1].

2 Theories of Pain

- Gate Control theory (1965): This is the first theory of pain, which presented pain as a mind–body experience. The theory states that a stimulus must synapse at three different locations within the spinal cord: the fibers of the dorsal column and in the dorsal horn, the Substantia Gelatinosa, and the transmission cell. The Substantia Gelatinosa regulates the signals from the periphery; It will either block pain signals or allow them to enter the spinal cord's "neurological gate." The gate will open if the pain in the periphery is more intense than the non-painful positive stimuli. The signal is then transmitted in the spinal cord, ascends to the thalamus, where it is integrated, and then registered within the primary somatosensory cortex of the parietal lobe. A real-life example is demonstrated within pediatric medical care. Suppose a positive, non-painful stimulus (game or play) of high enough intensity and distraction is administered to the child simultaneously as a painful procedure. In that case, it closes the pain gate in the spinal cord, preventing the ascending propagation of the pain nerve signal from the procedure [2].
- Neuro-matrix Model: The neuro-matrix model was developed 30 years after the gate control theory following observations of amputees suffering from phantom limb pain. This model suggests that painful sensations originate in the central nervous system (CNS) rather than the periphery. The neuro-matrix consists of various areas within the CNS that contribute to pain perception signaling. Locations include the spinal cord, brainstem, thalamus, somatosensory cortex, motor cortex, prefrontal cortex, insular cortex, and limbic system. This model acknowledges that pain can be affected by cognitive and emotional factors [2].
- Biopsychosocial: This model hypothesizes that pain results from intricate biological, psychological, and sociological interactions. It supports the notion that the human body cannot be categorized when considering management options for pain. John D. Loeser, an anesthesiologist, was the first to implement this model. He proposed that four parts need to be taken into consideration in the treatment of pain: nociception (perceptive component), pain (sensory-discriminatory component), suffering (motivo-affective component), and pain behaviors (cognitive behavioral component). The biopsychosocial model of pain is also the closest

to incorporating genetic factors. The way we approach pain management today is based mainly on Loeser's four elements of pain, and failure to consider these elements can be viewed as an inadequate assessment of care [2].

Pain is a protective mechanism that serves an important role. However, if it persists long after resolving the triggering event, it loses its intended function. Typically, after cessation of nociceptive stimuli and tissue recovery, the body returns to its normal state, and pain is no longer experienced. If the pain does not diminish and instead continues beyond the expected healing timeline, the patient now has developed chronic pain [26]. Factors differentiating between acute and chronic pain include the cause, the duration, and the treatment approach (Table 1). The term transitional pain service has gained attention in recent years. Transitional pain services focus on trying to help surgical patients who are felt to be at risk of their acute pain evolving into chronic pain. This will be the main focus of the next section of this chapter [6, 7].

In 2016, The International Association for the Study of Pain further classified pain into three broad descriptive categories: nociceptive, neuropathic, and nociplastic. These categories are intended to provide information about the mechanisms underlying the pain, which can serve as targets for drug or non-drug treatments and facilitate communication between stakeholders (e.g., clinicians, patients, and researchers) [8].

- Nociceptive pain: Adaptive transient pain in response to a noxious stimulus (like an alarm that announces the presence of a potentially damaging stimulus). Nociceptive pain is caused by neural activity responding to potentially damaging stimuli such as postoperative tissue damage, post-exercise injuries, mechanical low back pain, and sickle cell crisis. Nociceptive pain is further divided into visceral and somatic pain [6].
- Neuropathic pain: Is initiated or caused by a primary lesion or damage of the somatosensory nervous system, including the peripheral and central neural structures, causing spontaneous pain and hyperalgesia (like an alarm that is constantly on even though there is no emergency or gives repeated false alarms). Proposed mechanisms associated with the initiation of neuropathic pain may include trauma, stroke, autoimmune diseases, and responses to toxic element exposure. Typical neuropathic pain includes postherpetic neuralgia, trigeminal neuralgia, complex

Table 1 Description of pain

Characteristic of pain	Cause	Duration of pain	Treatment strategy
Acute pain	Known	Short, Resolves after healing < 3 months	Self-limiting. Resolves after removing the underlying cause
Chronic pain	Mostly unknown—Related to Neuroplasticity of the CNS	Persists past healing for > 3 months	Attempt to accomplish pain control rather than cure

regional pain syndrome type II, central pain syndromes, and distal polyneuropathy due to various causes such as diabetes, HIV, and alcohol [6, 7].

- Nociplastic pain: the underlying mechanism is considered augmented CNS pain, sensory processing, and altered pain modulation [28]. It represents hypersensitivity to pain resulting from abnormal central processing of normal input (e.g., fibromyalgia, irritable bowel syndrome, tension-type headache, noncardiac chest pain) [6, 7]. This type of pain can occur in isolation, as often occurs in conditions such as fibromyalgia or tension-type headache, or as part of a mixed-pain state in combination with ongoing nociceptive or neuropathic pain, as might occur in chronic low back pain [9].

Furthermore, Pain can also be categorized into two broad categories: adaptive and maladaptive. Adaptive pain protects the organism from injury or promotes healing when damage has occurred. Maladaptive pain, in contrast, is a pathologic operation of the nervous system; it is a disease where pain is uncoupled from a noxious stimulus or healing tissue. Such pain may occur due to damage to the nervous system (neuropathic pain) or abnormal nervous system operation (functional pain). It is usually persistent or recurrent [6, 7].

3 Mechanism of Pain

Noxious stimuli are transduced to the dorsal horn of the spinal cord, where amino acid and peptide transmitters activate second-order neurons. Spinal neurons then transmit signals to the brain. The resultant actions by the individual involve sensory-discriminative, motivational-affective, and modulatory processes in an attempt to limit or stop the painful process. As we said, this is in normal conditions; however, Persistent, intense pain activates secondary mechanisms at the periphery and within the central nervous system that cause **allodynia, hyperalgesia, and hyperpathia,** which can diminish normal functioning [6].

Multiple mechanisms that can produce pain have been identified; they include nociception, peripheral sensitization, phenotypic switches, central sensitization, ectopic excitability, structural reorganization, and decreased inhibition.

Nociception: Represents the sole mechanism responsible for nociceptive pain and comprises the processes of transduction, conduction, transmission, and perception. Nociceptors have unmyelinated (C-fiber) or thinly myelinated (A- fiber) axons. The pathways and mechanisms involved in mediating nociceptive pain signals include four stages.

Transduction: It is the process by which painful mechanical, thermal, or chemical stimuli are encoded to generate electrical signals—the generator potentials. Pain or noxious stimuli are converted into electrical activity following activation of receptors sensitive to heat, cold, mechanical, or chemical stimuli in the unmyelinated C-fiber, thinly myelinated A-delta fiber, and myelinated A-beta fiber of the peripheral nociceptors. Depending on the neuron type, each group of neurons responds with slow, intermediate, or rapid velocity to different stimuli and pain thresholds. Once a generator potential reaches a threshold, an action potential is fired.

Conduction: The process by which an action potential is conducted along a nerve fibers membrane to reach the presynaptic membrane of synapsis between neurons in the spinal cord or brain. Pain or noxious stimuli are converted into electrical activity following activation of receptors sensitive to heat, cold, mechanical, or chemical stimuli in the unmyelinated C- fiber, thinly myelinated A-delta -fiber, and myelinated A-beta fiber of the peripheral nociceptors. Depending on the neuron type, each group of neurons responds with slow, intermediate, or rapid velocity to different stimuli and pain thresholds.

Transmission is when the action potential is passed from one nerve cell to another through a chemical or electrical synaptic connection. In the pain processing pathway, synaptic transmission from the first order to the second-order neurons occurs at the spinal cord's dorsal horn or the brainstem's sensory nucleus. The transmission from second to third-order neurons occurs in the brainstem's thalamus or the parabrachial nucleus.

Perception: Perception of pain is formed at the cortical level and usually serves as a warning. Normally, the threshold for pain should be sensitive enough to prevent damage but not hypersensitive to the extent of interfering with normal activities. Responses to pain include reflex withdrawal through a reflex pathway in the spinal cord or brainstem, purposeful pain avoidance and emotional reaction, cortical processing, and learning and memory that involve the hippocampus and other neural structures [6, 7].

It is worth noting that the transmission of pain signaling from the periphery to the central nervous system and cortex is plastic and can change over time in response to repeated stimuli. For example, the neuroplasticity of peripheral nociceptors can result in peripheral sensitization to stimuli, and this transition will be addressed in the next section [10, 11].

- Aβ fibers: are considered rapidly conducting and respond to mechanical stimuli with a low threshold.
- Aδ fibers: respond to heat, cold, and high-intensity mechanical stimuli and conduct with intermediate velocity.
- C fibers: conduct slowly and can respond to heat, mechanical or chemical stimuli.
- The interface between primary afferents and the spinal cord occurs in the laminae.
- Aβ fibers make synaptic connections with PKC + neurons in Laminae III-IV and ϒ wide dynamic range neurons (WDR) in lamina V.
- Aδ fibers make synaptic connections with spinothalamic projection neurons in outer lamina II and wide dynamic range (WDR) neurons in Lamina V. The WDR neurons are important as they have been implicated in "wind up" or sensitization of the spinal cord because the intensity of their response increases as the frequency of the incoming stimulus increases [6–9].
- C fibers make synaptic contacts with spinothalamic projection neurons in lamina I and Inner lamina II.

Visceral organs may also create pain symptomology. Visceral pain is mediated by visceral nerves that include sympathetic nerves (cervical, thoracic, and lumbar) and parasympathetic nerves (cranial nerve X and spinal nerves S2-4), with their cell bodies residing in the dorsal root ganglion (DRG) or visceral nerve ganglion (Nodose ganglion). The second-order neurons are localized in laminae I and II of the spinal cord or in the brainstem (Nucleus solitarius).

Electrical signals (action potentials) are transmitted to the dorsal horn of the spinal cord and then relayed via two primary ascending pathways, the spinothalamic (pain and temperature) and spinoparabrachial (likely mediates affective pain) tracts. The spinothalamic pathway projects into the thalamus and somatosensory cortex, while the spinoparabrachial pathway connects to the hippocampus's ventral medial nucleus and the amygdala's central nucleus [6, 7, 10, 11].

4 Nociceptors: Anatomy, Physiology, and Peripheral Sensitization

In some pathological circumstances, action potentials can be generated in locations other than the peripheral nerve endings. This phenomenon is called ectopic activity/discharge. Ectopically generated spikes can be conducted to the spinal cord and the peripheral nerve ending, where Substance P is released and has been related to neurogenic inflammation.

The sensory neuron cell body is a site critical for integrating neural activity. Proteins and signaling molecules are delivered to the soma via axonal transport mechanisms, possibly contributing to aberrant or ectopic activity under pathological conditions. Many of the proteins responsible for these processes have been identified under normal and pathological conditions [6, 7, 10, 11].

There are several different types of peripheral nociceptors involved in pain processing.

- *Thermal nociceptors* detect extreme temperatures, and mechanical nociceptors detect intensive pressure. These nociceptors comprise small diameter Aδ (Adelta) fibers that are thinly myelinated and conduct signals at a velocity of 5–30 m/s.
- *C fibers* are the primary neuronal type of polymodal nociceptors. These fibers are unmyelinated neurons with a slower conduction velocity of approximately one m/sec or less. These nociceptors are activated by high-intensity mechanical, chemical, and thermal stimuli.
- A third type of neuron involved in pain processing is the *Aβ neuron*. These neurons are large-diameter sensory fibers that contribute to the normal perception of stimulus quality, even though they do not respond directly to noxious stimuli. Activity in large-diameter fiber systems can modify pain perception and is believed to mediate allodynia in various pathological circumstances.

Both C and Aδ fibers can release glutamate and substance P (a neuropeptide). Substance P is thought to enhance and prolong the actions of glutamate. Substance P may activate more post-synaptic neurons as there is no reuptake mechanism.

5 Specific verus Diverse Nociceptors

Diverse nociceptors in the body respond to specific stimulation through the expression and activation of specific receptors/channels. For example.

- Mechano-transduction is mediated by TRPV4, ASIC-3, and the low threshold voltage-gated calcium channel (VGCC) CaV3.2.
- Thermo-transduction is mediated by TRPM8 (melastatin type 8) for cool, TRPV4 for warm, and TRPV1 (vanilloid type 1) for hot sensations.
- Chemoreceptors, through specific receptors/channels, can sense tissue acidosis (TRPV1 and ASIC-3), noxious organic compounds (e.g., aldehydes at TRPA1) and endogenous chemicals (e.g., ATP at P2X3).

In addition to specific nociceptors, some nociceptors express diverse channels/receptors that can respond to different stimulations, i.e. mechanical, thermal and chemical. These nociceptors are called polymodal nociceptors [6, 7, 10, 11].

Enhancing our collective understanding of how pain is signaled has become a target of much research in the first part of this century. This enhanced research activity has frequently focused on subtypes of the capsaicin receptor, which are cationic channels that form the "pain" receptors. The Transient Receptor Potential (TRP) is a family of receptor subtypes. Some respond to mechanical stimuli (mechanotransducer), whereas others are thermo-transducers (e.g., TRPV1 and TRPA1 subtype). TRPV1 agonists, agonists, and target destruction of TRPV1-expressing neurons are under investigation. Also note that the G Protein-coupled receptors (GPCR), tropomyosin-receptor-kinase (TRK), and Cytokine receptors are essential for modulating the sensitivity of nociceptors. Further understanding of these channels may lead to new targeted therapies [12, 13].

6 Transduction of the Painful Stimulus

Following the process of converting a stimulus to an electrical stimulus, the process of transduction propagates the signal from the periphery to the central nervous system. Any understanding of this process is crucial because it represents an additional area that may be impacted by either plasticity/remodeling and therapeutics [12, 13].

Generator Potential:

In the normal or naïve state, the stimulus activates multiple potential receptors. These mechanical, thermal, and/or chemical stimuli are transduced by specific receptors/channels into a membrane potential depolarization, called the "generator potential" in the nerve endings [6, 12].

Spike initiation:

Spike initiation is the next step in the pathway after the stimulus has interacted with a pain receptor to trigger a generator potential. Numerous ion channels play a role in the spike initiation and upstroke of the spike. The Na1.7, Nav1.8, and Nav1.9 are the most important sodium channels for spike initiation. It is important to understand that the anatomical distribution of the ion channels is critical to producing action potential generation and propagation. Several voltage-gated channels regulate the action potential threshold. All of these ion channels are potential therapeutic targets [6, 12, 13].

Spike propagation:

The ion channels underlying action potential propagation, such as Nav1.6, are distinct from those underlying spike initiation. Following an insult, similar to the pain receptors and spike initiation, the pattern of channel expression can change, including redistribution of NaV1.7 and/or NaV1.8 to the cell membrane. Therapies directed at sodium channel-blocking compounds, such as local anesthetics, TCAs, and some COX inhibitors, have been used to treat pain [6, 12, 13].

Cell body:

The cell body (soma) serves as the supply depot for the rest of the neuron, synthesizing and packaging the proteins, transmitters, and lipids. In nociceptive afferents, the VGSC NaV1.8 is the primary sodium channel in the cell for action potential generation [6, 12, 13].

7 Pro- and Anti-inflammatory Mediators and Receptors

- GPCRs (G-protein coupled receptors) are responsive to E-type prostaglandins (EP), bradykinin (B) types 1 and 2, and serotonin (5HT) types 1A, 2, and 7.
- Tyrosine receptor kinases (TRK) are responsive to trophic factors such as nerve growth factor (NGF) and artemin
- There are receptors for inflammatory cytokines such as TNF-α, interleukin 1-β, and IL-6.
- These inflammatory mediators and their receptors are up-regulated or phosphorylated, leading to increased excitability of nociceptive neurons [6, 12, 13].

8 How Acute Pain Turns into Chronic

According to the CDC, chronic pain is the leading cause of disability in the United States. In most circumstances, terminating acute nociception and full tissue recovery restores normal homeostasis and ends the pain process. However, repetitive nociceptive stimulation may result in a prolonged inflammatory process by activating lymphocytes and releasing TNF-a and interleukins. Chronic inflammation leads to a series of changes in the periphery, such as reduction of pain threshold in the primary afferent neurons, phosphorylation of protein kinases A and C, up-regulation of voltage-gated sodium channels and TRPV1 receptors in DRG, and increased production of substance P and CGRP in both the periphery and the spinal cord. This process is known as peripheral sensitization and involves complex maladaptive neuroplastic mechanisms at all levels of pain processing, from the periphery to the brain, that ultimately culminate in a chronic pain state [14].

Chronic pain After Surgery: [15]

Patient-specific

- Genotype
- Medical history, preoperative chronic pain, opioid use
- Psychological factors
- Past experiences

Medical/Surgical

- Type of surgery, reoperation, and related therapies
- Anesthesia and analgesia
- Severity/duration of acute post-operative pain

Predictors for Poor Postoperative Pain [15]:

- Age
- Depression
- Catastrophizing
- Preexisting pain
- Preoperative use of opioids
- Prior surgery at same site
- Type of surgery
- Preexisting chronic pain

9 Peripheral Sensitization

In the periphery, sensitivity and maladaptive processes can spread beyond the site of the initial injury and result in secondary hyperalgesia. In addition, spinal cord neuronal excitability can produce an exaggerated response to non-painful stimuli (allodynia). Hyperalgesia and allodynia may have a biological protective role in that they cause the organism to protect and reduce movement of the affected area, thus limiting further tissue injury and allowing for healing. However, when sensitization extends far beyond the initial physical or temporal boundaries of the acute event, maladaptive chronic pain conditions can result in significant negative impacts on a patient's ability to function and manage their pain symptomology [14, 18].

10 Central Sensitization

As a result of a peripheral lesion that consistently generates pain impulses to the spinal cord, inhibitory interneurons involved in modulating painful nerve transmission impulses may die. Furthermore, glial cells may remodel neuronal synapses to intensify nociceptive transmission. The loss of inhibitory neuron function and enhancement of aberrant signaling pathways ultimately results in elevated responses to stimulation and the development within the CNS of additional second-order neuronal connections [12].

The spinal cord, DRG and dorsal horn neurons can be stimulated to express several genes and proteins implicated in enhancing the propagation of continuous nociceptive signals. The most notable change is increased mRNA coding for various receptors and ion channels such as Na and TRPV1. This change in receptor kinetics leads to the hyperexcitable state of chronic pain [14].

Another vital receptor type in the spinal cord is the NMDA. A tightly bound Mg plug normally keeps this receptor inactive during acute noxious stimulation. However, with continuous nociceptive stimulation a prolonged slow depolarization of the neurons in the dorsal horn causes a massive influx of calcium which displaces the Mg plug from the NMDA receptors. This then allows glutamate to bind to NMDA receptors which results in activation of NMDA receptors and the subsequent 'wind-up' phenomenon, which manifests as allodynia.

The wind-up process results in neuroplasticity.

Neuroplasticity is the physical remodeling of neuronal cytoarchitecture that from persistent acute pain leading to the transition from acute to chronic pain.

Another factor in central sensitization is loss of inhibitory neurons in the spinal cord and changes in the cortex and gray matter that further reduce the inhibitory signals coming from the brain [15–17].

11 Peripheral Nerve Injury and Its Effects on Spinal Dorsal Horn Interneuron Neuroplasticity in Chronic Pain

The dorsal horn of the spinal cord is composed broadly of excitatory and inhibitory neurons and is organized into six laminae. Sensory information from the peripheral tissues is transmitted through the afferent sensory neurons to the dorsal horn. The superficial laminae I and II receives nociceptive signals, while the deep laminae III to VI have non-nociceptive information transmitted to them. Integrated sensory information is then transferred to several brain regions, including the thalamus [16, 17].

Due to the relatively close anatomic location of the structures of each lamina, structural and functional neuroplasticity of the dorsal horn can induce pain perception alterations. When the somatosensory processing system is altered by peripheral injury, the information can be incorrectly sensed, often leading to normally non-noxious stimuli evoking pain sensation. This pain caused by non-noxious stimuli is called allodynia, and is a characteristic of neuropathic and nociplastic pain [16, 17].

An example of this neuroplastic change associated with allodynia can be seen with neuropeptide Y promoter (Npy) inhibitory interneurons. Outer lamina II Npy inhibitory interneurons send inhibitory gamma-aminobutyric acid (GABA) signals to projection neurons in lamina I. Additionally, the axons of Npy neurons also project to lamina III/IV cells, where the subtypes of interneurons are closely associated with noxious stimuli. After a peripheral nerve injury stimulus, there is a decreased Npy neuronal excitability resulting in pain like behavior with touch; This touch evoked pain is improved when the Npy interneuron excitability is increased.The synaptic modifications of the circuits in the spinal cord dorsal horn cause balanced changes in the neuronal projections to the brain in lamina 1 with regards to excitation and inhibition. This at least partially accounts for chronic pain development and maintenance [14, 17].

In the brain:

A pain matrix has been identified by radiological evidence. Functional magnetic resonance imaging and positron emission tomography scans have identified several essential pain centers and various changes in the pain matrix when sensitization occurs: the thalamus where the spinothalamic tract terminates (somatosensory discrimination), mid/anterior insula, anterior cingulated cortex and prefrontal cortex (affective and motivational components of pain), periaqueductal gray (PAG) and rostral ventromedial medulla (RVM) (fight-or-flight responses and stress-induced analgesia), reticular formation (regulating descending pathways), spinoparabrachial pathway to the hypothalamus and the amygdala (autonomic and sensory coordination). There is a strong correlation between chronic pain and mental status reflected in pathophysiologic changes in the pain matrix [14].

12 Endogenous Pain Inhibitory System

Top-down modulation of pain signals has long been observed. Physicians in WWII often noted soldiers with significant battlefield injuries who reported minimal pain. The endogenous pain inhibitory system is now widely accepted. It involves descending inputs from the hypothalamus, amygdala, and cingulate cortex that communicate with the thalamus and midbrain (periaqueductal gray) and then to the medulla—neurons within the medulla project to the spinal cord dorsal horn.

The inhibitory modulating pathways are sensitive to opioids and other agents, including cannabinoids serotonin and norepinephrine. The precise mechanism by which drugs interact with the inhibitory system is still incompletely understood, but activation of the inhibitory pathways is the end result. Activation of these pathways may be an important mechanism to decrease the development of chronic pain [17].

Epigenetics

Epigenetics refers to modifications in gene expression that do not require a change in genetic sequence; rather, changes in the environment alter gene expression. Despite in-depth evaluations examining the impact of pain modulation genetics and epigenetics, a paucity of valid, evidence-based information limits the clinical applicability of these pathways [2].

In contrast to the genetic determinism inherent in genomic studies, the field of epigenetics strives to understand environmental control over gene expression [3]. Epigenetic mechanisms of genetic pain associations reveal specific biological mechanisms that, with the presence or lack of specific gene(s), contribute to a delivered pain response and explain the difference in pain physiology. Epigenetic alterations, including DNA methylation, histone acetylation, and RNAi, are necessary for normal tissue specialization and neurologic development. However, these same modifications play a significant role in the induction of the chronic pain phenotype following neurologic injury [4].

Significant evidence highlights epigenetics's ability to modify general pain types, including inflammatory, neuropathic, visceral, and cancer-related pain. Each of these pain types may benefit from future therapeutics that utilize epigenetic targeting to maximize potential analgesic benefits, decrease chronic pain development, and limit side effects [5].

Preventing Acute Pain from Becoming Chronic

Unlearning' by the nervous system could be an important concept for unraveling the development of chronic pain in the future; however, currently, treating acute pain aggressively is an important strategy in pain management to prevent chronic pain. It is reasonable to assume that severe and persistent preoperative pain can lead to chronic pain development, so it is crucial to focus on aggressive pain management in the perioperative period. However, to date, the effectiveness of this approach has been equivocal [6].

It is not a surprise that chronic pain frequently develops after surgery. All of the aforementioned factors leading to peripheral and central sensitization are present during many surgical procedures, including an intense noxious input and secondary inflammation. There are limited studies that investigate how psychological factors influence chronic post-surgical pain, and the results are often contradictory. Some experts suggest that being in a hypervigilant state can cause chronic post-surgical pain. Fear of surgery and anxiety could also be contributing factors. It is known that certain regions of the brain, known as limbic regions, can influence the RVM. This area has descending projections that modulate the activity of the dorsal horn, which is involved in maintaining nerve injury-induced pain, mainly through a 5-HT3 mechanism. Therefore, emotional factors related to pain may have a neuroanatomic basis in humans [6].

A structured approach to blunting the development of chronic pain might include:

1. Predicting which patients might be at risk for elevated postoperative pain: Early recognition of patients with a high risk of developing chronic pain is imperative. Preoperative quantitative sensory testing (QST) has shown potential as a clinical tool to predict postoperative pain. It can be used to identify patient populations at high risk of developing acute postoperative pain and guide the use of pre-emptive, intraoperative, and postoperative analgesia [6].

The degree of acute pain is predictive of the development of chronic pain, and surgical types associated with significant postoperative pain are consistently found to simultaneously suffer more frequently from the development of chronic pain. In a study by Visser et al., amputation, sternotomy, and thoracotomy were the surgical procedures most likely to be associated with the development of chronic pain.

2. Implement appropriate preventative analgesia that aims to target receptors at various levels of the pain pathway to reduce overall neuronal excitability and improve analgesia. The principle of utilizing a multimodal analgesic approach is to provide synergistic pain control and minimize the therapeutic risks of any individual modality.

In the periphery:

Consider how the extent of tissue damage helps determine the severity of nociceptive stimulation, the length of the tissue healing process, the magnitude of inflammation, and how these factors can impact the risk of chronic pain development. This notion that links peripheral injury to chronic pain development reinforces the need to handle tissues carefully, avoid injuring nerves, and further the development of minimally invasive surgical techniques as a pathway to reducing the risk of chronic pain development.

Within the spinal cord:

The activation of NMDA receptors and wind-up phenomenon are important changes in the spinal cord that foster the transition from acute to chronic. The perioperative administration of NMDA receptor antagonists, including ketamine, nitrous oxide, magnesium, and methadone, should simultaneously reduce perioperative pain intensity, wind-up, and chronic pain [25].

These agents may also be beneficial in treating intractable pain and as adjuncts to multimodal pharmacological treatment plans. Unfortunately, treatment is frequently limited to short courses due to the development of side effects and addictive potential.

Adjuvants such as a-2-delta ligands binding to voltage-dependent calcium channels (gabapentin and pregabalin) are anti-neuropathic agents with probable preventative effects.

Local and regional anesthesia block the afferent transmission of pain signals, reducing pain sensitivity. In theory, reducing acute pain should reduce central neuroplasticity and, therefore, minimize the risk of the development of chronic pain [12].

In the brain matrix:

There is a strong link between individual preoperative expectations, psychological status, and postoperative pain intensity. Functional MRI studies have demonstrated changes in the centers of the brain matrix of patients with chronic pain. These centers are mainly responsible for mood, affect, and behavior. Predicting which patients with significant psychosocial stressors are more prone to chronic pain development appears reasonable [19–22].· Therefore, a biopsychosocial approach should be utilized in treating patients with a high risk of developing chronic pain.

13 Preventing Neuroplastic Changes

There are some exciting possibilities for preventing changes in the dorsal horn's neuroplasticity. One such possibility is the use of drugs that block 5-hydroxytryptamine-3 (5-HT3) receptors. Studies have shown that this method can have anti-nociceptive effects in humans by blocking the descending serotonergic facilitatory drive to the dorsal horn laminae. Additionally, while gabapentin interacts with the auxiliary $\alpha 2\delta$ subunit of voltage-gated Ca2 + channels, there is evidence that its actions also depend on the 5-HT3 receptor [6].

14 Prevention of Microglial Activation

There are drugs available that can modify or inhibit microglia, such as fluoracitrate, acetyl-l-carnitine, monocycline, and propentofylline. These drugs have been found to alleviate pain sensitivity. In diabetic peripheral neuropathy, microglial cells appear to play a significant role, as evidenced by an increased density of these cells in the dorsal spinal cord and thalamic nuclei of diabetic mice.

Cannabidiol has been found to have anti-nociceptive effects in mice. Specifically, when given at the same time as the onset of diabetic neuropathy, it was associated with reduced microglial density in the dorsal spinal cord and blunted elevation in phosphorylated p38 MAPK. Reducing microglial accumulation and activation in the spinal cord can limit neuropathic pain development, even after cannabidiol withdrawal. CB1 and CB2 agonists show anti-nociceptive effects until discontinued in established neuropathic pain. Early treatment to inhibit microglia in the CNS can prevent neuropathic pain in diabetic patients who commonly experience it. Microglial activation can be regulated through receptor modulation. P2X7 and P2X4 receptors are upregulated during nerve injury, and their deletion can attenuate neuropathic pain. CCR2 gene deletion blocks glial cell recruitment. An NF-κB inhibitor can prevent neuropathic pain development. ERK activation is also involved in neuroplasticity and maintains microglial expression of the pain phenotype [6].

In order to prevent chronic pain, it may be necessary to institute a program of preventive analgesia that encompasses the entire perioperative period from before the incision until final wound healing. Unfortunately, it is not known to what extent and for how long the blockade of pain signals would be required to prevent the establishment of chronic pain [23]. In addition, we cannot forget the effects of local and systemic inflammatory mediators in developing chronic pain. Again, it remains unclear if blocking pain signaling pathways without addressing inflammation provides meaningful reductions in chronic pain intensity or duration.

Approximately 7% of all major surgical interventions result in a pain disability problem one year later. This substantial pain burden requires a consideration of how the chronicity of this pain and the ongoing need for opioids might impact the recovery narrative for surgical patients. Building transitional pain services that employ a multi-faceted approach to monitoring opioid use after discharge from surgery and aiming to safely wean patients from opioids while maintaining effective pain management may ultimately be the solution that provides an encompassing approach for those patients who experience chronic pain.

The services offered by the TPS are broken down into three categories:

A) Introduction and optimization of multimodal analgesia to both improve pain management and facilitate weaning from opioids [24].
B) Leveraging non-pharmacologic interventions including physiotherapy and acupuncture.
C) Deploying psychological interventions by a trained pain psychology team around an acceptance and commitment therapy (ACT) model.

The TPS treats two types of patients: opioid-naïve patients without a preexisting pain condition and patients presenting with a preexisting pain condition or on preoperative opioid medications. The care of these patients is managed and coordinated by an interdisciplinary team composed of anesthesiologists, acute pain nurse practitioners, clinical psychologists, palliative care specialists, exercise physiologists, and patient-care coordinators.

Multiple pharmacologic interventions have been proposed to interfere with the development of chronic pain by modulating pain pathways at multiple locations. Continued research will be necessary to determine the effectiveness of these components and multi-modal approaches in reducing the development and severity of chronic pain.

Key Points:

- Nociceptors have free nerve endings in the skin and other tissues, mediating the transduction of external or internal chemical or physical stimuli into generator potentials. They transform generator potentials into action potentials that propagate toward the central nervous system and cause the release of neurotransmitters and neuromodulators into the superficial dorsal horn of the spinal cord or brainstem.
- Ectopic signaling (antegrade and retrograde) can be seen in pathology and contributes to neurogenic inflammation.

- Tissue insult leads to increased sensitivity of nociceptive terminals through increased density of several transducers and posttranslational modifications (phosphorylation).
- This is mediated by inflammatory mediators such as ATP, PGE2, NGF, and TNF-α from epithelial cells, resident (mast) cells, and recruited (macrophages) immune cells.
- Neuronal changes (neuroplasticity) in threshold and excitability increase nociceptors' sensitivity and ectopic activity (peripheral sensitization).
- Tissue insult can also affect potential action thresholds and spike initiation/propagation through modifications in membrane ion channels. All of these sites represent current and potential therapeutic targets.
- •Transitional pain service models employ a multi-faceted approach to monitoring opioid use after discharge from surgery and aim to wean patients from opioids while maintaining effective pain management safely.

References

1. Nirvanie-Persaud L, Millis RM. Epigenetics and pain: new insights to an old problem. Cureus. 2022;14(9):e29353. https://doi.org/10.7759/cureus.29353
2. Trachsel LA, Munakomi S, Cascella M. Pain theory. StatPearls Publishing, Treasure Island (FL); 2022.
3. Crow M, Denk F, McMahon SB. Genes and epigenetic processes as prospective pain targets. Genome Med. 2013;5:12. https://doi.org/10.1186/gm416.
4. Descalzi G, Ikegami D, Ushijima T, Nestler EJ, Zachariou V, Narita M. Epigenetic mechanisms of chronic pain. Trends Neurosci. 2015;38:237–46. https://doi.org/10.1016/j.tins.2015.02.001.
5. McGreevy K, Bottros MM, Raja SN. Preventing chronic pain following acute pain: risk factors, preventive strategies, and their efficacy. Eur J Pain Suppl. 2011;5(2):365–72. https://doi.org/10.1016/j.eujps.2011.08.013.PMID:22102847;PMCID:PMC3217302.
6. Voscopoulos C, Lema M. When does acute pain become chronic? BJA: British J Anaesthesia. 2010;105(1):i69–i85. https://doi.org/10.1093/bja/aeq323
7. Hiraga S-I, Itokazu T, Nishibe M, Yamashita T. Neuroplasticity related to chronic pain and its modulation by microglia. Inflammat Regenerat. 2022;42:15. https://doi.org/10.1186/s41232-022-00199-6.
8. Murphy AE, Minhas D, Clauw DJ, Lee YC. Identifying and managing nociplastic pain in individuals with rheumatic diseases: a narrative review. Arthritis Care Res (Hoboken). 2023;75(10):2215–22. https://doi.org/10.1002/acr.25104. Epub 2023 Mar 16 PMID: 36785994.
9. Fitzcharles MA, Cohen SP, Clauw DJ, Littlejohn G, Usui C, Häuser W. Nociplastic pain: towards an understanding of prevalent pain conditions. Lancet. 2021;397(10289):2098–110. https://doi.org/10.1016/S0140-6736(21)00392-5. PMID: 34062144.
10. Feizerfan A, Sheh G. Transition from acute to chronic pain, Continuing Educat Anaesthesia Critical Care and Pain. 2015;15(2):98–102. https://doi.org/10.1093/bjaceaccp/mku044
11. Buchheit T, Van de Ven T, Shaw A. Epigenetics and the transition from acute to chronic pain. Pain Med. 2012;13(11):1474–90. https://doi.org/10.1111/j.1526-4637.2012.01488.x. Epub 2012 Sep 14. PMID: 22978429; PMCID: PMC3501579.
12. Basbaum AI, Jessell TM. The perceppon of pain. In: Kandel ER, Schwartz JH, Jessell TM, editors. Principles of neural science. 4th ed. St. Louis, MO: McGraw-Hill; 2000. p. 479.

13. Vadivelu N, Sinatra R. Recent advances in elucidating pain mechanisms. Curr Opin Anaesthesiol. 2005;18:540–7.
14. Ossipov MH, Lai J, Malan TP Jr, Porreca F. Spinal and supraspinal mechanisms of neuropathic pain. Ann NY Acad Sci. 2000;909:12–24.
15. Kehlet H, Jensen T, Woolf C. Persistent postsurgical pain: risk factors and prevention. The Lancet. 2006;367:1618–25.
16. Wieseler-Frank J, Maier SF, Watkins LR. Central proinflammatory cytokines and pain enhancement. Neurosignals. 14;166–174.
17. Guilbaud G, Benoist JM, Levante A, et al. Primary somatosensory cortex in rats with pain-related behaviors due to a peripheral mononeuropathy auer moderate Res. 1992;92:227–245.
18. Baliki MN, et al. Nociception, pain, negative moods and behavior selection. Neuron. 2015;87:474–91.
19. Dolin S et al. Effectiveness of acute postoperative pain management: I. evidence from published data. Br J Anaesth. 2002;89(3):409–23.
20. Casey KL, Tran TD. Cortical mechanisms mediating acute and chronic pain in humans. In: Cervero F, Jensen TS, editors. Handbook of clin neurology. Boston: Elsevier; 2006. p. 159–77.
21. Woolf C. Pain: moving from symptom control toward mechanism-specific pharmacologic management. Ann Intern Med. 2004;140:441–51.
22. Chong MS, Bajwa ZH. Diagnosis and treatment of neuropathic pain. J Pain Symptom Manage. 2003;25:S4–11.
23. Scholz J, Woolf CJ. Can we conquer pain? Nat Neurosci. 2002;5:1062–7.
24. Katz J, Clarke H, Seltzer Z. Preventive analgesia: quo vadimus? Anesth Analg. 2011;113:1242–53.
25. Katz J, Weinrib A, Fashler SR, et al. The Toronto general hospital transitional pain service: development and implementation of a multidisciplinary program to prevent chronic postsurgical pain. J Pain Res. 2015;8:695–702. https://doi.org/10.2147/JPR.S91924.
26. Veehof MM, Oskam MJ, Schreurs KM, Bohlmeijer ET. Acceptance-based interventions for the treatment of chronic pain: a systematic review and meta-analysis. Pain. 2011;152:533–42. https://doi.org/10.1016/j.pain.2010.11.002.
27. Feizerfan A, Sheh G. Transition from acute to chronic pain. Continuing Educat Anaesthesia Critical Care and Pain. 2015;15(2):98–102. https://doi.org/10.1093/bjaceaccp/mku044.

Transitional Pain Clinic

Marianne Tanios, Maher Kodsy, Emma Fu, Vipul Dhumak, Brendan Astley, and Hesham Elsharkawy

Abstract Transition pain clinic are growing in importance in several parts of the world due to the need for an organized approach for treating pain. Those clinics can help transition patient from chronic pain to care in the acute setting and vice versa. This allows for continuity of care without interruption of pain treatment at any phase of management.

Keywords Chronic post-surgical pain · Transitional pain clinic · Multimodal pre-emptive analgesia · Acute pain management · Chronic pain management · Closing the gap

M. Tanios (✉) · E. Fu · V. Dhumak · B. Astley · H. Elsharkawy
Department of Anesthesiology, Case Western Reserve University—MetroHealth Medical Center, 2500 MetroHealth Drive, Cleveland, Ohio 44109, USA
e-mail: mtanios@metrohealth.org

E. Fu
e-mail: efu@metrohealth.org

V. Dhumak
e-mail: vdhumak1@metrohealth.org

B. Astley
e-mail: bastely@metrohealth.org

H. Elsharkawy
e-mail: helsharkawy@metrohealth.org

M. Kodsy
Department of Anesthesiology, Perioperative Services, Elyria Anesthesia Services, Inc., University Hospitals Elyria Medical Center, 630 East River Street, Elyria, OH 44035, USA
e-mail: maher.kodsy@UHospitals.org

A. Abd-Elsayed and K. Schroeder (eds.), *Perioperative Pain Management*,
https://doi.org/10.1007/978-3-031-67648-2_12

1 Introduction

The development of Chronic Postsurgical Pain (CPSP) is currently a major concern after surgery. Patients with CPSP utilize a disproportionate amount of healthcare resources, driving up costs and potentially leading to poor quality of life. Patients suffering from CPSP have limited treatment options and often are overly reliant on opioids.

Many patients are not overly burdened by pain in the early perioperative period when they are closely attended to by hospital clinicians or have undergone a procedure intended to alleviate pain. However, many patients experience a worsening of pain symptomatology when they are discharged from the hospital and have fewer options and resources available to address the pain that they are experiencing. Poorly controlled chronic postoperative pain is a concerning situation for those patients with preexisting pain, anxiety, depression, opioid tolerance, addiction, alcohol abuse and pain catastrophizing [1–4].

Pain is defined by the World Health Organization (WHO) as an unpleasant sensory and emotional experience associated with actual or potential tissue damage or described in terms of such damage. Multiple factors affect the pain experience of a given patient and this makes tackling the trajectory of pain challenging. Team collaboration between surgeons and anesthesia caregivers is of paramount importance to target postoperative pain from different perspectives and improve outcomes. In high-risk patients, a referral plan to a transitional pain clinic may be required to mitigate acute pain before it proceeds to chronic pain [5].

In most cases, recovery from surgery and the pain associated with the procedure progresses quickly as patients return to their baseline level of function. Despite the typically limited duration of recovery period, subjecting patients to poorly controlled pain is no longer acceptable and there is a need to implement proactive comprehensive approaches for pain management rather than utilizing reactive acute care only [6].

The main goal of the "Transitional Pain Clinic" is to focus on implementing predictive models to enhance care effectiveness in practice settings, decrease postoperative opioid use, and decrease healthcare costs.

2 Definition of CPSP

Our understanding of CPSP is growing and the complications that can arise from it can be life changing, often negatively affecting the patient's daily living activities. CPSP appears to be far more common in recent years than in the past. Recently, the WHO along with the International Association of the Study of Pain (IASP) thought to include chronic pain in the new International Classification of Diseases Eleventh Revision (ICD-11), and defined CPSP as pain that occurs after surgery/traumatic tissue injury and stays with the individual for a long time (at least 3 months) [7, 8].

The inclusion of CPSP in the new classification of ICD-11 highlights how this condition is now considered a disease rather than a symptom and that identification and diagnosis of pain needs to be addressed with a more specific long-term treatment plan [9].

3 Incidence of CPSP

According to the Center for Disease and Control (CDC), Chronic pain is the leading cause of disability in the USA [10]. The incidence of CPSP varies widely between 3 and up to 85% according to the type of surgery [8]. The exponential increase in surgical procedures worldwide and a conservative median incidence of CPSP around 20–30% at 6–12 months is anticipated to substantially increase new cases of CPSP [11].

A literature review that considered many study designs and variable assessments of perioperative pain outlined the incidence of CPSP according to the type of surgery. This review found that CPSP is very common after amputation (30–85%), craniotomy (7–65%), inguinal hernia (5–63%), cholecystectomy (3–56%), caesarean section (6–55%), total knee arthroplasty (TKA) (13–44%), thoracotomy (5–71%), mastectomy (11–57%), sternotomy (7–50%), vasectomy (0–37%), and less common among hip replacement (7–23%), and abdominal surgery (17–21%) [11].

4 Mechanisms of CPSP

The pathophysiological theory behind CPSP is thought to be related to peripheral (injury site) and central (spinal and supraspinal) sensitization after tissue/nerve injury. This sensitization stimulates inflammatory and immune mediators which in turn activates the peripheral and dormant nociceptive receptors leading to activation of the central pathway via pain signaling at N-methyl-D-aspartate (NMDA) receptors and glial cells [12].

The sustained release of this inflammatory cascade leads to pain symptoms such as hyperalgesia (increased pain sensitivity to noxious stimuli), allodynia (painful stimulation caused by non-painful stimuli), dysesthesia (unpleasant touch perception and tingling) and pain chronicity. Therefore, CPSP is a combination of somatic, inflammatory and neuropathic pain [13, 14].

5 Risk Factors

Evidence shows that CPSP could be related to perioperative pain levels and stimulation of nociceptive pathways [1]. Early identification of risk factors for CPSP can improve postsurgical outcomes and pain trajectories. CPSP is complex and can be attributed to many factors that include, but are not limited to:

- **Demographic risk factors**: Age (young), sex (female), high body mass index (BMI), pain sensitivity, lower educational level and socioeconomic status [15].
- **Preoperative chronic pain:** Patients with preexisting pain, poorly controlled acute pain, comorbidities, chronic pain diagnoses (e.g., fibromyalgia, migraine, low back pain), any coexisting psychological disorders are liable to experience CPSP [16].

  Preoperative pain is a strong predictor of CPSP [17].
- **Intraoperative related pain**: Surgical trauma, types of surgical procedures, (major, laparoscopic), surgical duration, incision site, nerve injury, ischemia, complications, anesthetic techniques (halogenated anesthesia, remifentanil) may result in opioid-induced hyperalgesia [18–20].
- **Postoperative acute pain:** Exacerbated from any complication related to electrocautery, re-operation, infection, bleeding, hematoma, organ rupture, compartment syndrome, radiation and chemotherapy [13].

Approximately 70% of patients suffer from hyperalgesia (neuropathic pain) during the transition period between acute and chronic pain and consequently develop an increased opioid requirement, tolerance and decreased pain control [21, 22].

- **Psychological factors**: Stress-related to surgery and accompanying fear, anxiety, diminished ability to cope with pain, lack of social support, depression and preexisting psychological disorders.

A prospective study predicted that CPSP after colorectal surgery is related to age, anxiety, depression, pain with movement 24 h after surgery, as well as the length of surgery. These are all factors that must be addressed in a post care plan that aims to mitigate CPSP development [2]. In the pediatric population, perioperative pain is related to anxiety, coping, and parental catastrophizing [23].

- **Genetic factors:** Identifying patients with polymorphisms that can lead to variable pain sensitivity and opioid use. Examples would be Catechol-O-Methyl Transferase (COMT) and melanocortin-1-gene expressed in women with red hair are associated with higher opioid use [20].

Montes et al. completed a study on 500 patients with CPSP and concluded that a gene-related encoding protein that mediates peripheral and central inflammatory response to tissue or nerve injury was unlikely but can't be completely excluded and more research is needed in the future [24].

The biopsychological model of pain related to social, behavioral and biological factors can modify pain experience [25].

6 Pediatric CPSP

Chronic Post-Surgical Pain (CPSP) in the pediatric population has been poorly described in the literature, related to its lower prevalence [26].

CPSP in pediatrics is defined as pain affecting the surgical area for more than 3 months postoperatively. Recent studies evaluating CPSP account for pain severity, frequency, social, physical, and functional limitations. The literature omits important data points like school days missed, social isolation and pain related anxiety (Fig. 1) [27].

A recent study reported that the prevalence of CPSP was 10.9% in children aged 6–18 years, after observing 258 patients [28]. In other studies, the prevalence of CPSP was found to be 22% with mixed surgical procedures and 13.5% with inguinal hernia repairs [29, 30].

Major orthopedic procedures, thoracotomies, and inguinal hernia repairs have a propensity for CPSP development in pediatric patients. As per Dugan et al. of those who reported pain, 28% missed some school days due to pain, 30% had trouble sleeping, and 42% reported that they sometimes missed time spent with friends due to pain [31].

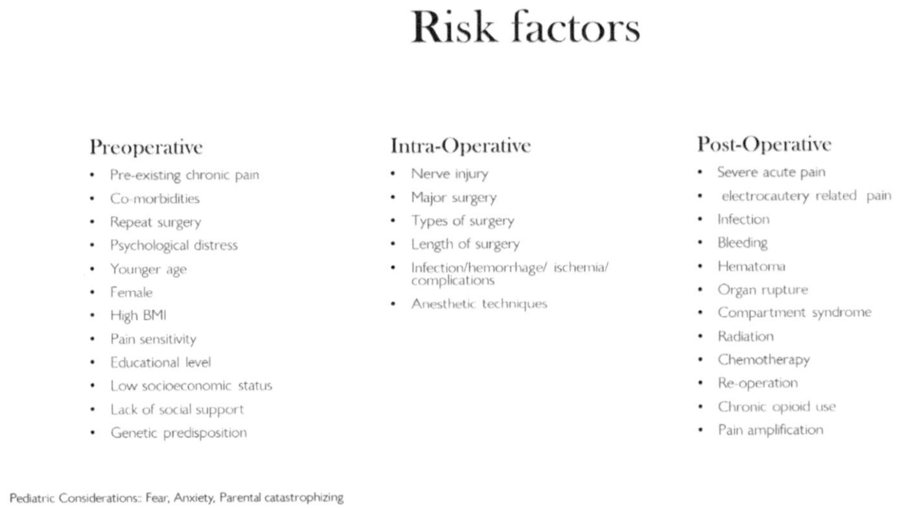

Fig. 1 Risk factors. Adapted from Rosenberger et al.[11] and Robins et al. [23]

7 Preoperative Pain Assessment

Presurgical risk modeling includes a consideration of risk factors including mental health and preoperative pain[32]. Schreiber et al. reported that a personalized pain plan was more effective than protocolization for controlling pain and preventing CPSP [33].

To aid in pain plan personalization efforts, utilization of the Patient Heath Questionnaire (PHQ-9) and General Anxiety Disorder Questionnaire (GAD-7) could assist in identifying patients at elevated for CPSP related to their preexisting anxiety and depression symptomology [20]. A systematic review on Quantitative Sensory Testing (QST) found a correlation of 4–54% between preoperative pain and CPSP development depending on experimental stimulation methods (heat, cold, pressure algometry, electrical, punctate mechanical stimulation, and induction of inflammatory injury). Although this approach reported positive results in a research setting, it is impractical in clinical settings [34, 35].

8 Prevention of CPSP and the Need for Post Discharge Pain Care

CPSP is a complex biopsychological phenomenon that, once initiated, is difficult to treat. The gap between acute and chronic pain is defined as the subacute pain period. This analgesic period, the "gray zone", generally extends between 10 days to 3 months into the postoperative period and is often following hospital discharge. This period is considered critical for identifying patients at increased risk and implementing strategies aimed at preventing CPSP. Strategic models focus on this time frame and may be referred to as "Transitional Pain Clinic" (TPC) and/or post discharge personalized pain care. In this timeframe, multimodal preemptive analgesics, nerve block, and cognitive behavior therapy represent a sampling of the multidisciplinary approaches that may be needed [21, 36, 37].

9 Persistent Perioperative Pain Clinic (PPPC) and Transitional Pain Clinic (TPC)

Many long-term physical, psychological, social, and economic effects can be seen due to chronic pain. They become more complex over time and may even become irreversible and refractory to treatment [38]. Evidence demonstrates that the development of chronic pain can be limited by proactively preventing peripheral and central sensitization to noxious stimulation by using multimodal analgesia[39]. Utilization of comprehensive multi- or interdisciplinary biopsychosocial approaches are needed to improve functioning after surgery and for prevention and treatment of CPSP [40].

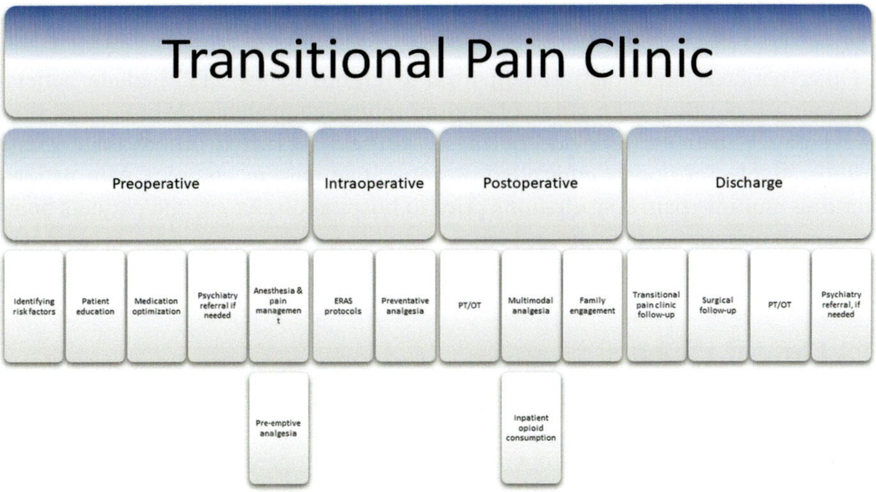

Fig. 2 Classification model of transitional pain clinic ERAS: Enhanced recovery after surgery PT/OT: Physical therapy/occupational therapy

Therefore, TPC, which can include psychological assessment and behavioral interventions, should be utilized to identify patients at risk for CPSP. The goals of the TPC are to adequately manage and monitor long-term pain with multimodal interventions, maintain function and activities of daily living, and reduce opioid consumption. TPC provides multidisciplinary pain management during inpatient stays and up to six months after hospital discharge [41–43].

The interdisciplinary team consists of nurse practitioners, physicians, psychologists and other allied health professionals, such as physiotherapists. Anesthesiologists and addictionologists tailor a patient's care plan to utilize multimodal analgesia and reduce opioid use when possible. Psychologists provide behavior interventions for pain and addiction. An important aspect to the success of the TPC is the patient's participation in understanding and showing commitment towards weaning from opioid-based pain management. Intensive follow-up with patients immediately post-discharge, bimonthly visits for two months after discharge and then monthly visits for three to six months have demonstrated a positive impact on pain outcomes and reducing opioid consumption (Fig. 2) [43].

10 Referral Criteria to TPC

The process should start with identifying risk factors for new persistent opioid use after surgery including tobacco use, alcohol and substance use disorders, mood disorders, anxiety and pain diagnosis prior to surgery. For example, the odds of chronic opioid therapy after lumbar fusion are increased in patients with clinically diagnosed depression, with 77% of those patients receiving chronic opioids versus 50% without a diagnosis of depression[42].

Other patients that would benefit from a referral to the TPC include patients consuming more than 90 mg/day of oral morphine equivalents (MEQ) on postoperative day 1, patients followed by the acute pain service for more than 3 days postoperatively for poorly controlled postoperative pain or complex pain patients requiring multiple pain consultations prior to hospital discharge, and patients being discharged on long-acting opioids [43].

11 Flow of Patients

The anesthesia team develops a pain management plan for the preoperative, intraoperative and immediately postoperative periods. Postoperatively, while the patient is in the hospital, physical and occupational therapy referrals should be attempted. Patients and family engagement are paramount. Necessary home healthcare referrals should be arranged. In-hospital opioid consumption should be monitored and weaned, if possible, with the aid of nonopioid medications and nonpharmacologic strategies.

On discharge, appointments should be made for the patient with the TPC to continue the opioid weaning process. Physical therapy/ occupational therapy (PT/ OT), social workers, home health care, and psychiatry referrals may also be required if not already involved.

Life-style modification including massage, acupuncture, music therapy, relaxation techniques, social support and other integrative medicine practices are useful tools in managing pain. These modalities offer temporary pain relief, likely by distracting the patient from thinking about their own pain symptoms [44].

Hypnosis is another alternative technique for stress reduction [45]. A large meta-analysis on pediatric and adult populations undergoing diverse surgical procedures found that hypnosis has a positive impact on emotional feelings related to stress. Shnur et al. documented that 15 min of hypnosis improved the patient's emotional state, mood, and anxiety compared to placebo [46].

Finally, the patient's primary care provider should be a critical component of the postoperative pain management transition team and should ultimately be comfortable managing the prescribed analgesic regimen.

12 Pre-emptive and Preventative Analgesic Regimen

Pre-emptive analgesia techniques are interventions that seek to block peripheral and central pain transmission before a noxious stimulus occurs. This would include local anesthesia given into the skin before an incision is made, ongoing IV (opioid, anesthesia) or regional/neuraxial local anesthesia during the noxious insult (surgery) and after the injury/throughout the recovery period. The goal of preventative analgesia is to enable early mobilization and to decrease the stress response perioperatively while minimizing side effects from any one analgesic technique. Preventative analgesia includes a combination of interventional techniques (nerve or fascial plane blocks) and pharmacologic therapies. A multimodal approach can allow for a reduction in opioid use, lower pain scores and decrease the length of hospital stay [47].

The use of perioperative regional anesthesia may or may not prevent CPSP. It has not been proven that regional anesthesia prevents CPSP after thoracotomy. Nor does perioperative regional anesthesia or preoperative genicular nerve neuroablation prevent CPSP in knee arthroplasty. However, after breast cancer surgery, in highly catastrophizing patients, paravertebral blocks may prevent CPSP intensity and diminish the surgical impact on daily life for up to a year [48].

13 Pharmacological Interventions of CPSP

The application of Enhanced Recovery after Surgery (ERAS) protocols using multimodal approaches to pain management could assist in mitigating postoperative pain and the development of CPSP. Medications used to treat pain include ketamine, gabapentinoids, anti-inflammatory, corticosteroids, intravenous lidocaine, alpha-2 agonists (clonidine, dexmedetomidine), and topical treatments (low-concentration capsaicin, 5% lidocaine patch, nitroglycerin transdermal patch, 5% amitriptyline cream, 0.5% ketamine, 2% amitriptyline/1% ketamine combination cream).

Although these medications are frequently used to treat acute postoperative pain, a recent meta-analysis pointed out that many pharmacological medications proved to be inefficient in reducing CPSP [49].

Ketamine

Current studies found that ketamine's effect on CPSP development is not promising. Although it was previously thought that ketamine use preoperatively can decrease postoperative opioid use, this may not be true. When taking a closer look at the available evidence, factors such as small sample size studied, ketamine dosage, timing and duration of use with different types of surgery, gave results that are inconclusive [49].

Gabapentinoids

Gabapentinoids are used preoperatively to reduce neuropathic pain especially when nerve damage is suspected during surgery. Unfortunately, a recent comprehensive study found that gabapentin is not useful for the prevention of CPSP. Although, it was effective for 3 months after total knee arthroplasty and cardiac surgery, more studies with larger sample sizes are needed to prove its effect on CPSP [49].

Non-steroid anti-inflammatory drugs (NSAIDs)

NSAIDs are beneficial in reducing secondary hyperalgesia and central sensitization but have no effect on CPSP. NSAID use may be limited in patients with impaired kidney functions, bleeding tendencies, and allergic reactions [50].

Acetaminophen

Acetaminophen is frequently used in perioperative management for its analgesic effect, but no study found an effect on CPSP [50].

Corticosteroids

A Cochrane review on 3 studies found that corticosteroids contributed to decreasing central sensitization to pain and had a positive effect on decreasing CPSP. In contrast, De Oliveira et al. reported that dexamethasone use did not decrease the incidence of CPSP in mastectomy patients [51].

IV Lidocaine

Based on the limited duration of IV lidocaine administration, it is not terribly surprising that reports of sustained pain control remain inconclusive. For example, the prevalence of pain at 6 months when the IV lidocaine infusion was given for 24 h or less showed statistically significant reductions in pain after breast surgery in 2 trials. However, no pain benefit was found at 3 months for the same procedure and the same infusion duration in other trials. Two recent reviews supported the use of IV lidocaine in treating CPSP in different types of surgery, but a larger multicenter clinical trial will be more beneficial in confirming the use of IV lidocaine [49, 52, 53].

14 Opioid Weaning and Pain Management

Opioid-induced hyperalgesia, a paradoxical increase in the patient's pain severity and decrease in pain tolerance may develop after short-term administration of opioids in the peri-operative period. While hyperalgesia is a clinically relevant issue, especially for patients with chronic pain, it can be overcome in the acute postoperative setting by a concurrent infusion of low-dose ketamine, for example. While intra-operative opioids should be used judicially, the difference in the operating room is unlikely to make a significant difference in patients' lives [54].

This elucidates a need for an institutional effort lead by a variety of services to wean patients from opioids. To do so, this should include educating providers who prescribe discharge analgesics about alternative options for pain management that include multimodal analgesic regimens.

For patients who cannot be immediately weaned off opioids, follow-up in a chronic pain or TPC should be arranged [54].

A patient-specific approach starting from preoperative risk assessment (risk factors are discussed earlier in this chapter), education, and setting realistic and achievable goals and expectations for postoperative pain could help decrease opioid use. Determining the need for discharge opioid prescriptions should also be based on inpatient opioid consumption.

It may be beneficial to give patients written prescriptions for over the counter (OTC) medications, as patients may perceive the medication as having greater efficacy than when dispensed OTC [55].

Treatment of acute pain with opioids for greater than 8 days can lead approximately 1 in 7 patients to continue to use opioids for up to 1 year. The rate for long-term opioid use increases to 30% for patients who use opioids for 31 days or more. [56].

As attention to opioid prescribing has increased, legislative bodies in certain states have started to limit the duration of initial opioid prescriptions for acute pain and professional guidelines are also recommending opioid tapers by 6 weeks after most major surgeries. However, the recommendations for opioid weaning are largely based on anecdotal experience [42].

15 The Role of Peripheral Nerve Stimulation

A variety of beneficial interventional CPSP treatment modalities have been described and implemented in clinical practice. Neuromodulation with peripheral nerve stimulation (PNS) for up to 60 days is commonly used with better outcomes on pain control. Over the last decade, there has been a growing interest in evaluating the efficacy and duration of pain relief with PNS for difficult to treat pain cases like CPSP and post amputation phantom limb pain. PNS placement can be achieved with ultrasound guidance and/or fluoroscopy. PNS is a proven technique that is safe, effective, and minimally invasive while still treating chronic, intractable post-surgical pain targeting different nerve locations [57].

Wilson et al. reported a significant reduction of pain scores with the use of PNS in a randomized-controlled trial (RCT) evaluating the impact of this technique on shoulder pain management[58]. Deer et al. reviewed 14 RCTs on patients with chronic refractory pain that included chronic migraine sufferers (occipital nerve), cluster headache (sphenopalatine ganglion), headache with fibromyalgia (C2 nerve), hemiplegic shoulder pain, failed back pain syndrome, extremity, trunk, and pelvic pain (tibial nerve). These patients were successfully treated with PNS and demonstrated the efficacy of percutaneously implanted stimulators in pain intensity reduction over multiple nerve locations [59]. Bouche et al. presented a case series describing the use of ultrasound-guided percutaneous PNS of the brachial plexus as well as supra-scapular nerve and reported pain reduction of more than 50% after one year in patients with CPSP and peripheral nerve injury [60].

Spinal cord stimulation (SCS) has been successfully used for phantom limb pain, chronic post thoracotomy pain, neuropathic pain of upper and lower limbs, cervical and spinal surgeries and complex regional pain syndrome [13, 61, 62].

16 Cryoanalgesia

Cryoneurolysis involves cooling targeted nerves to reversibly decrease their function and provides sustained pain relief that can last for weeks to months [44, 63].

24 RCTs examined the efficacy of cryoanalgesia for thoracotomy, herniotomy, nephrectomy and tonsillectomy and found positive outcomes in decreasing CPSP, post-operative opioid use and consequently nausea and constipation when compared to opioid analgesia only. This opioid-sparing technique can last beyond a patient's hospital discharge, and persistent pain control will hopefully translate into reductions in health care costs via a decreased incidence of readmission and emergency room visits. Furthermore, cryoanalgesia is inexpensive and is associated with less maintenance requirements compared to nerve blocks where there is a risk of local anesthetic toxicity and the burden to carry an infusion pump [64].

17 Radiofrequency Ablation

As a minimally invasive technique, Radio Frequency Ablation (RFA) has been widely accepted for treating chronic refractory post-surgical pain. Radiofrequency on targeted nerves alters pain pathways with thermal coagulation.

Two case reports documenting chronic chest pain after surgery noticed long-term pain relief with RFA [65]. Another case series focusing on intercostal neuralgia reported promising results in pain reduction with RFA [66]. Case series for hip pain with avascular necrosis used cooled RFA under fluoroscopic guidance and found a significant decrease in opioid use and pain scores [67].

18 Business Models of Transitional Pain Clinic

Toronto General hospital developed an innovative multidisciplinary approach for CPSP. It consists of a combination of opioid weaning with non-opioid medications, when possible, along with psychological assessment with Acceptance and Commitment Therapy (ACT).

The concept of ACT is based on behavioral interventions and stress reduction that can lead to reductions in pain-related complications. Implementation of this ACT behavioral management program was associated with a significant decrease in pain characteristics, opioid use, and depression compared to groups with no ACT intervention [68].

The Salt Lake City Veteran Affairs hospital established a multidisciplinary Transitional Pain Services (TPS) for patients undergoing orthopedic surgery, which resulted in reductions in opioid use. These pain services were financially supported by their hospitals [69, 70].

Both hospitals describe the effect of the model in terms of dollars where the savings from TPS outweighed its costs.

Unfortunately, most of the currently offered analgesic therapies are not routinely continued into the discharge period. However, to prevent pain sensitization and chronicity, a long-term therapeutic plan must be implemented and personalized for a given patient. Even with excellent in-hospital pain management, patients may be abruptly switched from an individual regimen to a standard oral regimen, then discharged with a non-personalized care plan. Thereafter, subsequent pain management is often inadequate. The result of this suboptimal care results in more pain, stress, and a decrease in the patient's quality of life. Patients who are discharged prematurely and without an adequate plan will only drain more costs from the healthcare system in the future if CPSP develops.

Duke Health succeeded in tackling patients at elevated risk for CPSP development through a clinical care model designed to decrease perioperative opioids and support the patient beyond the immediate perioperative period. This model consists of 3 different categories related to -1-psychological (cognitive behavioral, relaxation, and patient's favorite soft music therapy), -2- Medical (opioid weaning, multimodal approach) and -3-physical optimization (rehabilitation, anti-inflammatory, plant-based diet), and pain clinic (morphine and opioid weaning).

At Duke, the staff managing the TPS is also in charge of inpatient care services, thereby optimizing the continuum of care [71].

Vanderbilt has noticed that TPS can benefit patients through reinforcing ERAS pathways in the perioperative period. Strict adherence to these protocols has improved pain satisfaction on stratified high-risk patients (high-dose opioid (>60 MEDD) and opioid-use disorder), decreased health care expenses, and improved outcomes (pain control, opioid- dose adjustment, treatment of chronic conditions, and patient education). [72] [45].

Closing the Gap Between Acute and Chronic Pain: Practical Solutions

Preventing CPSP is better for healthcare systems and patients and should be the goal of perioperative analgesia. There are multiple pathways to CPSP prevention that might be considered, and a tailored and combined approach is more likely to be successful. Practical solutions could be achieved through the following:

Primary prevention of pain is defined as preventing acute pain with modeled approaches for the general population and high-risk groups.

Secondary prevention is defined as prevention of the transition from acute to chronic pain. Hence the many names of this period; subacute pain, persistent pain, and transitional pain.

Tertiary prevention is aimed at reducing the frequency, severity and disability related to chronic pain [10].

Macrae et al**.** suggested that preventing pain is like any other disease states that have a progression. As an example, controlling diabetes and smoking will prevent limb amputation and the development of phantom pain [73].

Chronic pain after surgery is costly and may be substantially contributing to the opioid epidemic. There are direct medical costs related to specialty evaluations, radiographic diagnosis, surgeries, procedures, medications (opioids, neuromodulators, antidepressants), and indirect costs related to job loss and disability. CPSP and persistent opioid use following surgery are some of the main reasons that clinicians and patients are voicing a need for "Transitional Pain Clinic" (TPC) [74].

The inclusion of healthcare experts from different specialties and business specialists is required to make the TPC sustainable. Education, fellowships, and the value of dual fellowships in Acute Pain Management (APM) and Chronic Pain Management (CPM) or dual staff coverage (acute and chronic) together should be encouraged. Involving stakeholders like academic chairs to contribute to funding fellowships for interested staff, special training, and electives may also reinforce participation. Attending society, meetings and courses related to pain medicine and continued practice expansion through the incorporation of ultrasound, nerve and interfascial blocks, X-ray, advanced procedures, neuromodulation, cryoanalgesia, and RFA will enhance practitioners' skills and improve confidence in applying new techniques.

Vital to the success of TPC is multidisciplinary collaboration and the creation of personalized plans for each individual patient. These plans should include a psychiatric evaluation that focuses on changing a patient's mentality on how to adapt to adverse situations and manage pain. Communication among the members may be enhanced through the establishment of regular meetings. Inclusion of substance use disorder and perioperative medicine education can be an important component of continued learning and practice expansion.

Expansion of funding for acute and chronic pain programs may help to shift the treatment paradigm from identifying risk factors associated with pain into ways to prevent the transition from acute to chronic pain earlier. These interventions may result in saving health care costs and making the TPC financially feasible as well.

19 Cost-Effectiveness Enhancement of Transitional Pain Clinic

At this point, optimizing the cost-effectiveness of the TPC dictates that utilization should be prioritized for high-risk patients and matched to the anticipated volume of major surgical procedures. Nesting the TPC within the perioperative surgical home should improve the ability to implement pre-emptive pain management strategies and plan postoperative TPC referral. Involving additional services related to preoperative preparation like psychiatry and addiction clinics will have a positive impact on the patient's behavior.

Machine learning algorithms can be useful tools for predicting patients at elevated risk for CPSP. Telehealth communication is an easy and accessible way of communication between patients and their caregivers. Future composite biomarkers to detect the underlying cause behind the transition of acute to chronic pain after surgery are under investigation through ongoing multicenter control trials. Clarke et al. suggested that analyzing a patient's DNA sequencing, blood and salivary pain biomarkers and their analgesic responses to medications will be a crucial step toward a personalized pain medicine [75]. The concept of "Traditional Pain Management" needs to change into "Transitional Pain Clinic" for treating acute pain before proceeding to chronic pain.

20 Practice and Research Gaps

Unfortunately, there remain many gaps between patient care in the perioperative period and the postoperative care needed to achieve long-term recovery. First and for most, acceptance of the clinician team and restrictive/myopic business models remain barriers to further TPC success. Second, discharging patients with interdisciplinary team support can overwhelm patients. Third, the greatest obstacle is to wean patients from opioids especially if they are dependents and reached the tolerance level. The goal of decreasing dependance on opioids is a noble target worthy of pursuit. Fourth, behavior and psychological support has a direct impact on the quality of recovery for these patients. Communication, early planning, and focusing on closing the gap while identifying patients with highly predisposing risk factors for CPSP are additional assets that should be considered to ensure the success of TPC.

Finally, obtaining approval from institutional leadership and securing financial investments required from hospitals and healthcare system represent critical steps in crafting a business plan that will ensure program sustainability and enhance recovery outcomes. CPSP mandates a comprehensive pain management strategy, hence the necessity for TPC [17, 76].

21 Future Directions

The future role of TPC is focusing on identifying analgesic gaps, leveraging expertise, and coordinating care to close gaps in pain care will help to ensure a place for this patient care modality.

Alternative approaches that can be easily implemented in most healthcare systems include the utilization of APM and CPM teams with enhanced collaboration and earlier patient stratification, consultations, referral to multidisciplinary teams and coordination with addiction, rehabilitation medicine, and psychiatry. Using existing resources represents an intriguing opportunity to enhance patient care without needing to identify novel revenue streams. Ideally, any intervention will result in decreasing length of stay, opioid weaning, reducing emotional distress, improving quality of life, less surgical follow-up, and increasing postoperative satisfaction. In a concurrent fashion, implementation of these workflows can be expected to reduce the incidence and severity of persistent postsurgical pain to where it can be more easily controlled.

22 Conclusion

Postoperative analgesic management continues to suffer from gaps in care that can be improved through the incorporation of advances in pain science and the inclusion of collaborative and multidisciplinary healthcare professionals.

While APM and CPM services play an essential role in perioperative pain management, they generally lack the ability to follow patients at timepoints largely removed from their surgical procedures. The inherent value of TPC is that they can continue to follow patients as they recover and work to diminish or eliminate the need for opioid analgesics. The value of this clinic may be difficult to measure, but decreased opioid consumption, hospital admissions, improved patient satisfaction, and a diminished community-based opioid burden are all immeasurable attributes of the services provided by TPC. As the field continue to evolve, future research should focus on types of surgeries and patient characteristics that are most likely to benefit from TPC and novel methodologies to improve the care provided to these patients.

23 Key Points

- Chronic postsurgical pain (CPSP) is the one of the most common causes of disability. Perioperative pain management should be proactive and utilize comprehensive approaches rather than reactive or mono-focal care.
- The Transitional Pain Clinic is designed to close the gap between acute and chronic pain. It encompasses perioperative pain management and a post discharge pain care plan.
- The Transitional Pain Clinic represents an important modality for treating acute pain before proceeding to chronic pain.
- Transitional Pain Clinics leverage multimodal approaches to analgesic management that strive to decrease opioid use, lower pain scores, improve quality of life, and reduce health care costs.

List of Abbreviations

TPC	Transitional Pain Clinic
CPSP	Chronic Post-Surgical Pain
ERAS	Enhanced recovery After Surgery
ICD-11	International Classification of Diseases Eleventh Revision
IASP	International Association for the study of Pain
CDC	Centers for Disease Control and Prevention
TKR	Total Knee Replacement
BMI	Body Mass Index
PPPC	Persistent Perioperative Pain Clinic
MEQ	Morphine Equivalents
MEDD	Morphine Equivalent Daily Dose
IV	Intra-Venous
NMDA	N-Methyl-D-Aspartate
COMT	Catechol-O-Methyl Transferase
RCT	Randomized-Control Trial
C2 nerve	Cervical 2 nerve
OTC	Over The Counter
PNS	Peripheral Nerve Stimulation
RFA	Radio Frequency Ablation
SCS	Spinal Cord Stimulation
TPS	Transitional Pain Services
APM	Acute Pain Management
CPM	Chronic Pain Management

References

1. Lewis GN, Rice DA, McNair PJ, Kluger M. Predictors of persistent pain after total knee arthroplasty: a systematic review and meta-analysis. Br J Anaesth. 2015;114(4):551–61. https://doi.org/10.1093/bja/aeu441. Epub 2014 Dec 26 PMID: 25542191.
2. Jin J, Chen Q, Min S, Du X, Zhang D, Qin P. Prevalence and predictors of chronic postsurgical pain after colorectal surgery: a prospective study. Colorectal Dis. 2021;23(7):1878–89. https://doi.org/10.1111/codi.15640. Epub 2021 Apr 5 PMID: 33738887.
3. Costelloe C, Burns S, Yong RJ, Kaye AD, Urman RD. An analysis of predictors of persistent postoperative pain in spine surgery. Curr Pain Headache Rep. 2020;24(4):11. https://doi.org/10.1007/s11916-020-0842-5. PMID: 32072357.
4. Hah JM, Cramer E, Hilmoe H, Schmidt P, McCue R, Trafton J, Clay D, Sharifzadeh Y, Ruchelli G, Goodman S, Huddleston J, Maloney WJ, Dirbas FM, Shrager J, Costouros JG, Curtin C, Mackey SC, Carroll I. Factors associated with acute pain estimation, postoperative pain resolution, opioid cessation, and recovery: secondary analysis of a randomized clinical trial. JAMA Netw Open. 2019;2(3): e190168. https://doi.org/10.1001/jamanetworkopen.2019.0168. Erratum in: JAMA Netw Open. 2022 Apr 1;5(4): e229747. PMID: 30821824; PMCID: PMC6484627.

5. Elsharkawy H, Clarke H, Schwenk E. Transitional pain services: closing the gap between acute and chronic pain. ASRA Pain Medicine News 2022;47. https://doi.org/10.52211/asra020123.011
6. Hesham E et al. Transitional pain services: closing the gap between acute and chronic pain. ASRA News 2023;48(1). https://doi.org/10.52211/asra020123.11
7. Treede RD, Rief W, Barke A, Aziz Q, Bennett MI, Benoliel R, Cohen M, Evers S, Finnerup NB, First MB, Giamberardino MA, Kaasa S, Kosek E, Lavand'homme P, Nicholas M, Perrot S, Scholz J, Schug S, Smith BH, Svensson P, Vlaeyen JWS, Wang SJ. A classification of chronic pain for ICD-11. Pain. 2015;156(6):1003–7. https://doi.org/10.1097/j.pain.0000000000000160.PMID:25844555;PMCID:PMC4450869.
8. Zhang Y, Zhou R, Hou B, Tang S, Hao J, Gu X, Ma Z, Zhang J. Incidence and risk factors for chronic postsurgical pain following video-assisted thoracoscopic surgery: a retrospective study. BMC Surg. 2022;22(1):76. https://doi.org/10.1186/s12893-022-01522-1.PMID:35236334;PMCID:PMC8892711.
9. Schug SA, Lavand'homme P, Barke A, Korwisi B, Rief W, Treede RD. IASP taskforce for the classification of chronic pain. The IASP classification of chronic pain for ICD-11: chronic postsurgical or posttraumatic pain. Pain. 2019;160(1):45–52. https://doi.org/10.1097/j.pain.0000000000001413. PMID: 30586070.
10. McGreevy K, Bottros MM, Raja SN. Preventing chronic pain following acute pain: risk factors, preventive strategies, and their efficacy. Eur J Pain Suppl. 2011;5(2):365–72. https://doi.org/10.1016/j.eujps.2011.08.013.PMID:22102847;PMCID:PMC3217302.
11. Rosenberger DC, Pogatzki-Zahn EM. Chronic post-surgical pain—update on incidence, risk factors and preventive treatment options. BJA Educ. 2022;22(5):190–196. https://doi.org/10.1016/j.bjae.2021.11.008. Epub 2022 Feb 24. PMID: 35496645; PMCID: PMC9039436.
12. Kodivalasa M. 14 ChapterChronicpost-surgicalpain (CPSP). Chronic pain management, 2021; 81.
13. Shipton EA. The transition from acute to chronic post surgical pain. Anaesth Intensive Care. 2011;39(5):824–36. https://doi.org/10.1177/0310057X1103900506. PMID: 21970126.
14. Pogatzki-Zahn EM, Segelcke D, Schug SA. Postoperative pain-from mechanisms to treatment. Pain Rep. 2017;2(2): e588. https://doi.org/10.1097/PR9.0000000000000588.PMID:29392204;PMCID:PMC5770176.
15. Schnabel A, Yahiaoui-Doktor M, Meissner W, Zahn PK, Pogatzki-Zahn EM. Predicting poor postoperative acute pain outcome in adults: an international, multicentre database analysis of risk factors in 50,005 patients. Pain Rep. 2020;5(4): e831. https://doi.org/10.1097/PR9.0000000000000831.PMID:32766467;PMCID:PMC7390596.
16. Glare P, Aubrey KR, Myles PS. Transition from acute to chronic pain after surgery. Lancet. 2019;393(10180):1537–46. https://doi.org/10.1016/S0140-6736(19)30352-6. PMID: 30983589.
17. Katz J, Seltzer Z. Transition from acute to chronic postsurgical pain: risk factors and protective factors. Expert Rev Neurother. 2009;9(5):723–44. https://doi.org/10.1586/ern.09.20. PMID: 19402781.
18. Salengros JC, Huybrechts I, Ducart A, Faraoni D, Marsala C, Barvais L, Cappello M, Engelman E. Different anesthetic techniques associated with different incidences of chronic post-thoracotomy pain: low-dose remifentanil plus presurgical epidural analgesia is preferable to high-dose remifentanil with postsurgical epidural analgesia. J Cardiothorac Vasc Anesth. 2010;24(4):608–16. https://doi.org/10.1053/j.jvca.2009.10.006. Epub 2009 Dec 16 PMID: 20005744.
19. Schug SA, Bruce J. Risk stratification for the development of chronic postsurgical pain. Pain Rep. 2017;2(6): e627. https://doi.org/10.1097/PR9.0000000000000627.PMID:29392241;PMCID:PMC5741327.
20. Richebé P, Capdevila X, Rivat C. Persistent postsurgical pain: pathophysiology and preventative pharmacologic considerations. Anesthesiology. 2018;129(3):590–607. https://doi.org/10.1097/ALN.0000000000002238. PMID: 29738328.

21. Lavand'homme P. Transition from acute to chronic pain after surgery. Pain. 2017;158(Suppl 1):S50–4. https://doi.org/10.1097/j.pain.0000000000000809. PMID: 28134653.
22. Jensen TS, Stubhaug A, Breivik H. Important development: extended acute pain service for patients at high risk of chronic pain after surgery. Scand J Pain. 2016;12(1):58–9.
23. Robins H, Perron V, Heathcote LC, Simons LE. Pain neuroscience education: state of the art and application in pediatrics. Children. 2016;3(4):43.
24. Montes A, Roca G, Sabate S, Lao JI, Navarro A, Cantillo J, Canet J. GENDOLCAT study group. Genetic and clinical factors associated with chronic postsurgical pain after hernia repair, hysterectomy, and thoracotomy: a two-year multicenter cohort study. Anesthesiology. 2015;122(5):1123–41. https://doi.org/10.1097/ALN.0000000000000611.. PMID: 25985024.
25. Nicholas MK. The biopsychosocial model of pain 40 years on: time for a reappraisal? Pain. 2022;13:10–97.
26. Nikolajsen L, Brix LD. Chronic pain after surgery in children. Curr Opin Anaesthesiol. 2014;27(5):507–12. https://doi.org/10.1097/ACO.0000000000000110. PMID: 25051264.
27. Torfreda Wells L, Bray J. Pediatric Regional Anesthesia and Chronic Postoperative Pain Jul 19, 2018, 12:18 PM
28. Batoz H, Semjen F, Bordes-Demolis M, Bénard A, Nouette-Gaulain K. Chronic postsurgical pain in children: prevalence and risk factors. A prospective observational study. Br J Anaesth. 2016;117(4):489–496. https://doi.org/10.1093/bja/aew260. Epub 2016 Oct 17. PMID: 28077537.
29. Pagé MG, Stinson J, Campbell F, Isaac L, Katz J. Identification of pain-related psychological risk factors for the development and maintenance of pediatric chronic postsurgical pain. J Pain Res. 2013;6:167–80. https://doi.org/10.2147/JPR.S40846. Epub 2013 Mar 5. PMID: 23503375; PMCID: PMC3594915.
30. Aasvang EK, Kehlet H. Chronic pain after childhood groin hernia repair. J Pediatr Surg. 2007;42(8):1403–8. https://doi.org/10.1016/j.jpedsurg.2007.03.042. PMID: 17706504.
31. Dugan MQ, Delgado JR, De Souza E, Anderson TA. Pediatric chronic post-surgical pain prevalence, pain scores, and quality-of-life: results of an exploratory patient survey at a single-center tertiary care children's hospital. J Anesth. 2022;36(5):606–611. https://doi.org/10.1007/s00540-022-03089-w. Epub 2022 Jul 13. Erratum in: J Anesth. 2022 Oct 12; PMID: 35829912.
32. Bande D, Moltó L, Pereira JA, Montes A. Chronic pain after groin hernia repair: pain characteristics and impact on quality of life. BMC Surg. 2020;20(1):147. https://doi.org/10.1186/s12893-020-00805-9.PMID:32631293;PMCID:PMC7336434.
33. Schreiber KL, Muehlschlegel JD. Personalization over protocolization. Anesthesiology. 2021;134(3):363–5. https://doi.org/10.1097/ALN.0000000000003695.PMID:33465232; PMCID:PMC8057682.
34. Werner MU, Mjöbo HN, Nielsen PR, Rudin A. Prediction of postoperative pain: a systematic review of predictive experimental pain studies. Anesthesiology. 2010;112(6):1494–502. https://doi.org/10.1097/ALN.0b013e3181dcd5a0. PMID: 20460988.
35. Persistent Perioperative Pain Podcast: Transitional Pain Service El-Sharkawy H, Gulur P. discuss the need for, implementation of, and results of creating a transitional pain service to help patients with persistent post surgical pain. Recorded 07/21/2019.
36. Glare P, Overton S, Aubrey K. Transition from acute to chronic pain: where cells, systems and society meet. Pain Managem. 2020;10(6):421–36. https://doi.org/10.2217/pmt-2019-0039. Epub 2020 Oct 28 PMID: 33111634.
37. Tiippana E, Hamunen K, Heiskanen T, Nieminen T, Kalso E, Kontinen VK. New approach for treatment of prolonged postoperative pain: APS out-patient clinic. Scand J Pain. 2016;12(1):19–24.
38. Fine PG. Long-term consequences of chronic pain: mounting evidence for pain as a neurological disease and parallels with other chronic disease states. Pain Med. 2011;12(7):996–1004. https://doi.org/10.1111/j.1526-4637.2011.01187.x. PMID: 21752179.
39. Andreae MH, Andreae DA. Regional anaesthesia to prevent chronic pain after surgery: a Cochrane systematic review and meta-analysis. Br J Anaesth. 2013;111(5):711–20. https://doi.org/10.1093/bja/aet213.

40. Thapa P, Euasobhon P. Chronic postsurgical pain: current evidence for prevention and management. Korean J Pain. 2018;31(3):155–173. https://doi.org/10.3344/kjp.2018.31.3.155. Epub 2018 Jul 2. PMID: 30013730; PMCID: PMC6037807.
41. Admiraal M, Hermanns H, Hermanides J, Wensing CG, Meinsma SL, Wartenberg HC, Hollmann MW. Study protocol for the TRUSt trial: a pragmatic randomised controlled trial comparing the standard of care with a transitional pain service for patients at risk of chronic postsurgical pain undergoing surgery. BMJ Open. 2021;11(8): e049676.
42. Wu CL, King AB, Geiger TM, Grant MC, Grocott MPW, Gupta R, Hah JM, Miller TE, Shaw AD, Gan TJ, Thacker JKM, Mythen MG, McEvoy MD. Fourth Perioperative quality initiative workgroup. American society for enhanced recovery and perioperative quality initiative joint consensus statement on perioperative opioid minimization in opioid-naïve patients. Anesth Analg. 2019;129(2):567–577. https://doi.org/10.1213/ANE.0000000000004194. PMID: 31082966; PMCID: PMC7261519.
43. Clarke H, Azargive S, Montbriand J, Nicholls J, Sutherland A, Valeeva L, Boulis S, McMillan K, Ladak SSJ, Ladha K, Katznelson R, McRae K, Tamir D, Lyn S, Huang A, Weinrib A, Katz J. Opioid weaning and pain management in postsurgical patients at the toronto general hospital transitional pain service. Can J Pain. 2018;2(1):236–47. https://doi.org/10.1080/24740527.2018.1501669.PMID:35005382;PMCID:PMC8730554.
44. Ye Y, Gabriel RA, Mariano ER. The expanding role of chronic pain interventions in multimodal perioperative pain management: a narrative review. Postgrad Med. 2022;134(5):449–57. https://doi.org/10.1080/00325481.2021.1935281. Epub 2021 Jun 8 PMID: 34033737.
45. Edwards DA, Hedrick TL, Jayaram J, Argoff C, Gulur P, Holubar SD, Gan TJ, Mythen MG, Miller TE, Shaw AD, Thacker JKM, McEvoy MD. POQI-4 working group. American society for enhanced recovery and perioperative quality initiative joint consensus statement on perioperative management of patients on preoperative opioid therapy. Anesth Analg. 2019;129(2):553–566. https://doi.org/10.1213/ANE.0000000000004018. PMID: 30768461.
46. Schnur JB, Kafer I, Marcus C, Montgomery GH. Hypnosis to manage distress related to medical procedures: a meta-analysis. Contemp Hypn. 2008;25(3–4):114–28. https://doi.org/10.1002/ch.364.PMID:19746190;PMCID:PMC2739386.
47. Vadivelu N, Mitra S, Schermer E, Kodumudi V, Kaye AD, Urman RD. Preventive analgesia for postoperative pain control: a broader concept. Local Reg Anesth. 2014;29(7):17–22. https://doi.org/10.2147/LRA.S62160.PMID:24872720;PMCID:PMC4012350.
48. Geradon P, Lavand'homme P. Use of regional analgesia to prevent the conversion from acute to chronic pain. Curr Opin Anaesthesiol. 2022;35(5):641–6. https://doi.org/10.1097/ACO.0000000000001175. Epub 2022 Aug 4 PMID: 35942702.
49. Carley ME, Chaparro LE, Choinière M, Kehlet H, Moore RA, Van Den Kerkhof E, Gilron I. Pharmacotherapy for the prevention of chronic pain after surgery in adults: an updated systematic review and meta-analysis. Anesthesiology. 2021;135(2):304–25. https://doi.org/10.1097/ALN.0000000000003837. PMID: 34237128.
50. Zhao-Fleming H, Hand A, Zhang K, Polak R, Northcut A, Jacob D, Dissanaike S, Rumbaugh KP. Effect of non-steroidal anti-inflammatory drugs on post-surgical complications against the backdrop of the opioid crisis. Burns and Trauma. 2018;1:6.
51. de Oliveira GS Jr, Bialek JM, Turan A, McCarthy RJ, Sessler DI. Perioperative dexamethasone and the development of chronic postmastectomy pain: a single-center observational cohort study. Reg Anesth Pain Med. 2015;40(5):539–44. https://doi.org/10.1097/AAP.0000000000000301. PMID: 26263077.
52. Chang YC, Liu CL, Liu TP, Yang PS, Chen MJ, Cheng SP. Effect of perioperative intravenous lidocaine infusion on acute and chronic pain after breast surgery: a meta-analysis of randomized controlled trials. Pain Pract. 2017;17(3):336–43.
53. Bailey M, Corcoran T, Schug S, Toner A. Perioperative lidocaine infusions for the prevention of chronic postsurgical pain: a systematic review and meta-analysis of efficacy and safety. Pain. 2018;159(9):1696–704.
54. Lirk P, Rathmell JP. Opioid-free anaesthesia: Con: it is too early to adopt opioid-free anaesthesia today. Europ J Anaesthesioll EJA. 2019;36(4):250–254.

55. Gridley C, Robles J, Calvert J, Kavoussi N, Winkler T, Jayaram J, ... Miller NL. (2020).
56. Brandal D, Keller MS, Lee C, Grogan T, Fujimoto Y, Gricourt Y, ... Cannesson M. (2017).
57. Helm S, Shirsat N, Calodney A, Abd-Elsayed A, Kloth D, Soin A, Shah S, Trescot A. Peripheral nerve stimulation for chronic pain: a systematic review of effectiveness and safety. Pain Ther. 2021;10:985–1002.
58. Wilson RD, Gunzler DD, Bennett ME, Chae J. Peripheral nerve stimulation compared to usual care for pain relief of hemiplegic shoulder pain: a randomized controlled trial. Amer J Phys Med Rehabilit/Assoc Acad Physiatrists. 2014;93(1):17.
59. Deer TR, Esposito MF, McRoberts WP, Grider JS, Sayed D, Verrills P, Lamer TJ, Hunter CW, Slavin KV, Shah JM, Hagedorn JM. A systematic literature review of peripheral nerve stimulation therapies for the treatment of pain. Pain Med. 2020;21(8):1590–603.
60. Bouche B, Manfiotto M, Rigoard P, Lemarie J, Dix-Neuf V, Lanteri-Minet M, Fontaine D. Peripheral nerve stimulation of brachial plexus nerve roots and supra-scapular nerve for chronic refractory neuropathic pain of the upper limb. Neuromodulation: Technol Neural Interface. 2017;20(7):684–9.
61. Subedi B, Grossberg GT. Phantom limb pain: mechanisms and treatment approaches. Pain Res Treat. 2011;14:2011.
62. Graybill J, Conermann T, Kabazie AJ, Chandy S. Spinal cord stimulation for treatment of pain in a patient with post thoracotomy pain syndrome. Pain Phys. 2011;14(5):441.
63. Trescot AM. Cryoanalgesia in interventional pain management. Pain Phys. 2003;6(3):345.
64. Park R, Coomber M, Gilron I, Shanthanna H. Cryoanalgesia for postsurgical pain relief in adults: a systematic review and meta-analysis. Annals of Med Surgery. 2021;1(69): 102689.
65. Abd-Elsayed A, Lee S, Jackson M. Radiofrequency ablation for treating resistant intercostal neuralgia. Ochsner J. 2018;18(1):91–93. PMID: 29559878; PMCID: PMC5855433.
66. Fiala KJ, Martens JM, Keith MK, Ghouse A, Abd-Elsayed A. Cooled radiofrequency ablation for intercostal neuralgia. Ochsner J. (2023).
67. Naber J, Lee N, Kapural L. Clinical efficacy assessment of cooled radiofrequency ablation of the hip in patients with avascular necrosis. Pain Managem. 2019;9(4):355–9.
68. Hughes LS, Clark J, Colclough JA, Dale E, McMillan D. Acceptance and commitment therapy (ACT) for chronic pain. Clin J Pain. 2017;33(6):552–68.
69. How We Do It: Salt Lake City Veterans Affairs Medical Center Transitional Pain Service Feb 1, 2021.
70. Buys MJ, Bayless K, Romesser J, Anderson Z, Patel S, Zhang C, Presson AP, Brooke BS. Opioid use among veterans undergoing major joint surgery managed by a multidisciplinary transitional pain service. Reg Anesth Pain Med. 2020;45(11):847–52.
71. How I Do It: Transition Pain Clinic, Duke Health Feb 1, 2021.
72. Building a Transitional Pain Service: Vanderbilt Experience. Feb 1, 2021, 00:45 AM by David A Edwards, MD, PhD.
73. Macrae WA. Chronic post-surgical pain: 10 years on. Br J Anaesth. 2008;101(1):77–86.
74. Sun EC, Mariano ER, Narouze S, Gabriel RA, Elsharkawy H, Gulur P, Merrick SK, Harrison TK, Clark JD. Making a business plan for starting a transitional pain service within the US healthcare system. Reg Anesth Pain Med. 2021;46(8):727–31.
75. Clarke H, Katz J, Flor H, Rietschel M, Diehl SR, Seltzer Z. Genetics of chronic post-surgical pain: a crucial step toward personal pain medicine. Can J Anaesth. 2015;62(3):294–303. https://doi.org/10.1007/s12630-014-0287-6. Epub 2014 Dec 4 PMID: 25471684.
76. Episode 36: Transitional Pain Service Jan 31, 2019.

Clinical Scenarios

Pain Management in the Setting of Language Barriers and Global Health

Michelle Kuei, Danielle Savino, and Matthew Swisher

Abstract There are multiple barriers to pain management in the United States and globally. Language, cultural and ethnic differences are significant factors with the increasing heterogeneity of the population globally. There are social, systemic, and biological elements to consider when examining pain disparities and creating appropriate pain management strategies in minority groups. Globally, in low- or middle-income countries (LMICs), pain disparities exist largely due to limited resources. Pain and surgical disease account for more than 30% of disease burden worldwide, with the majority of the burden in LMICs where there are significant barriers to pain and anesthesia care (Size et al. in Anaesthesia. 62:38–43, 2007; Lipnick MS, Dubowitz G, Wabule A. Regional anesthesia in resource-constrained environments. In: Atlas of ultrasound-guided regional anesthesia. Elsevier, Inc.; 2019. p. 405–1;). Patients often have poor or nonexistent analgesic options due to lack of staff available to administer analgesic medications, lack of opioids, education, and perceived safety of opioids. Patients then expect undertreatment of perioperative and acute pain to be the norm (Size et al. in Anaesthesia. 62:38–43, 2007). Regional techniques can be helpful in these situations, however, there needs to be adequate resources and trained professionals.

Keywords Language barriers · Global health · Resource-limited · Limited English proficiency · Language discordance · Ethnic discordance · Cultural competency · Low-.or middle-income countries

---

M. Kuei · D. Savino
Department of Anesthesiology, University of Wisconsin-Madison, Madison, WI, USA
e-mail: mkuei@wisc.edu

D. Savino
e-mail: dsavino@uwhealth.org

M. Swisher (✉)
Department of Anesthesiology, University of California San Diego, San Diego, CA, USA
e-mail: mwswisher@health.ucsd.edu

A. Abd-Elsayed and K. Schroeder (eds.), *Perioperative Pain Management*,
https://doi.org/10.1007/978-3-031-67648-2_13

1 Introduction

Language, cultural, and ethnic differences are barriers to pain management. Limited English proficiency is associated with worse health care outcomes and disparities in care, even when socioeconomic and insurance status are accounted for, suggesting that language and culture play an important role. With increasing linguistic and cultural diversity, both in the United States and globally, this becomes a significant factor in healthcare [3, 4]. While there are limited studies addressing language and cultural barriers to perioperative analgesia, pain management plans should be adjusted accordingly to effectively treat patients of diverse backgrounds.

This chapter also delves into barriers to and strategies for pain control in resource-limited settings. Anesthesia services have become a critical necessity in LMICs where there is a huge burden of untreated surgical conditions. These conditions are often easily treatable but have a high fatality rate due to limited access to surgical and anesthesia care [5]. With the increase in surgical volume, perioperative pain management becomes concurrently more important. Though pain is one of the top causes of disability-adjusted life years globally and pain management is considered a basic human right, unreliable pain control strategies are frequently present in resource-limited settings. Analgesia is viewed of lower priority than treatment of other disease processes [1, 2]. Pharmacologic, non-pharmacologic, and regional anesthesia techniques for pain control are, unfortunately, of varying availability in LMICs.

2 Language, Cultural, and Ethnic Differences

Pain assessments are often performed via self-report, so language is important in communicating pain. Since pain is complex, it is difficult to describe and assess with simple ratings. Language allows patients to convey the location, quality, and severity of their pain, in addition to associated symptoms of their pain and side effects of pain medications. This promotes a more comprehensive pain assessment. In predominantly English-speaking healthcare settings, studies have shown that patients with limited English proficiency have higher pain scores and fewer pain assessments performed. Thus, pain scales in multiple languages or pain scales that utilize images can be beneficial to facilitate adequate treatment of pain [3]. For example, one study found that Spanish-speaking children undergoing chemotherapy experienced pain that was unrecognized and therefore was not treated appropriately. The authors of this study hypothesized that the Spanish version of the pain tool should be used to better communicate these children's pain and avoid analgesic undertreatment [6].

Healthcare professionals caring for a patient with limited English proficiency should assess the clinical situation, degree of language gap, available resources, and patient preference [6]. Patients with limited English proficiency may not be able to effectively communicate their pain needs with healthcare professionals, leading to ineffective pain control, especially when interpreters are not readily available [3]. Language barriers can also lead to fewer interactions with healthcare professionals. If the language gap is substantial and/or there is a patient preference for interpretation services, a medical interpreter should be used [7]. Interpreters do not completely eradicate language barriers. However, they do improve communication between healthcare professionals and patients. However, healthcare professionals often underutilize dedicated interpreter services, instead, substituting their own limited language knowledge for clinical encounters. It can be viewed as more time consuming to treat patients with language discordance and use interpreter services [4]. In a study of hospitalized Spanish-speaking obstetrics/gynecology patients, it was found that use of interpreters was associated with better pain control, timely response to pain needs, ease of receiving pain medications, and perceived helpfulness of healthcare professionals as stewards of analgesic therapeutics [8].

The presence of a language-concordant healthcare professional or dedicated interpreter is associated with improved quality and outcomes, including decreased pain and improved physical and psychological well-being [4]. In a study of pain management in breast cancer patients, it was reported that Spanish speakers reported greater pain severity, distress, and barriers to pain management than English speakers. They also endorsed greater misconceptions about the doctor-patient relationship and pain management, likely due to poor communication with healthcare professionals [9]. Good communication allows healthcare professionals to set pain expectations and discuss different alternatives for pain management/treatment [8].

Another study investigated the association between parental English proficiency and pain management in pediatric surgical patients. It was found that children of limited English proficiency parents had fewer pain assessments and higher levels of pain recorded prior to receiving opioid analgesics compared with children of English proficient parents. However, children of limited English proficiency parents with ≥ 2 interpreter encounters each day had lower pain scores after medication administration and were more likely to receive opioids at pain levels similar to children with English proficient parents. These findings suggest that more frequent use of professional interpreters when assessing pain could reduce the disparity in pain management. This study also found that children with limited English proficiency parents used the nonverbal face pain scale more and the numeric pain rating scale (NRS) less than children with English proficient parents. Again, certain pain scales may be more appropriate for limited English proficiency patients, which should be taken into consideration for more effective pain assessment[10].

Studies have shown that pain ratings are only comparable between nurses and patients when the nurse is language concordant with the patient [11]. In a study exploring nurses' perspectives on caring for patients with limited English proficiency, language barriers were identified as the biggest obstacles in providing adequate, appropriate, and timely care. Communication was identified as the most important component of a nurse's role in the care of hospitalized patients. Certain situations were identified where the use of interpreters is not feasible, including when patients are under the influence of anesthesia or severe pain and anxiety. Often in the perioperative setting, especially with emergency surgery, interpreter services can be difficult to access. In these situations, there is the potential for novel technologies to assist in the management of language barriers [12].

In addition to recognizing increasing language diversity, there is growing heterogeneity of cultures and ethnicities. It is therefore important to understand how this diversity impacts pain management as well. There are persistent ethnic disparities in the prevalence, treatment, progression, and outcomes of pain-related conditions despite advances in pain management. These inequities have been demonstrated across a broad array of treatment settings. Ethnic minorities frequently receive inadequate or substandard healthcare. These patients may be less likely to receive pain medications, receive lower doses of pain medications, and have longer wait times in the emergency department. Their pain is also often underestimated by healthcare professionals. They are also less likely to be included as an active participant in decisions relevant to their medical treatment [11, 13, 14]. Understanding the institutionalized structure and mechanisms driving these differences in medical management is an important factor that might result in reductions in the disparities relevant to adequate pain treatment of ethnic minorities. There are sociocultural, healthcare system structural, and physiological factors that convalesce to complicate pain management. Because pain is a subjective experience, it can be easily influenced by any of these factors [11, 15].

Healthcare professionals are more likely to be responsive to pain communication with people from a concordant culture and are less likely to understand pain communication communicated by people from other cultures. Culture can determine how pain is perceived, experienced, and communicated. Different cultures have different expectations and may accept pain as a normal part of life/their medical condition and not a clinical problem that requires treatment. Other cultures may also display diverse pain coping strategies that can influence the pain experience. Each cultural and ethnic group has its own norms for the communication of pain and distress, both verbal and non-verbal. Some cultures and ethnic groups may display more emotion in the presence of pain, while others may be more stoic and downplay the pain. Patients may not ask for pain medications because they think it will be brought to them if they need it, or that non-verbal indicators would be sufficient to convey their pain. Patients may think that it is disrespectful or viewed as complaining to ask for pain medications, or that their pain should be more severe before conveying it to the healthcare professionals. Some cultures prefer alternative and complementary pain treatments to pain medications. Other sociocultural factors include family traditions, religious beliefs, and previous experiences. People who are more acculturated report similar levels of pain to people of the country to which they have emigrated [11, 15, 16].

Structurally, predominantly minority neighborhoods are less likely to stock opioids in their pharmacies. However, even when access is equal, different ethnic groups still use different amounts of pain medications. Certain ethnic groups will underreport pain and have a fear of medication dependency, tolerance, and side effects. Gaps in communication of pain occur from sociocultural beliefs, misperceptions, and language barriers [11, 15].

In a study of oncology patients at various treatment sites, it was found that 65% of minority patients (Hispanic and nonwhite backgrounds) received inadequate pain treatment compared with 50% of nonminority patients. Minority patients also received better pain management at community-based treatment settings. Various factors likely contribute to these findings, including concern for potential drug abuse, inability to pay for pain medications, barriers in accessing healthcare and filling prescriptions, and difficulty in healthcare professionals assessing pain due to differences in language and culture. Certain minority groups may also fear aggressive medical treatment and side effects of analgesics or lack assertiveness in seeking healthcare, thus making them less likely to report pain and reluctant to pursue pain management with stronger analgesics. Awareness of the risk for inadequate pain management in minority groups can be beneficial in improving pain assessment and treatment in these groups. There is also a need for patient education relevant to pain management in minority groups and public health education as it relates to pain [17, 18].

Biologically, ethnic differences in pain tolerance have been documented in a variety of pain-related conditions. This has been shown both clinically and in experimental pain studies across different ethnicities around the world. In general, those of ethnic minority backgrounds relative to the country in which they live demonstrate increased pain sensitivity in comparison to those of ethnic majorities. They have lower pain thresholds to various types of nociceptive stimulation, including thermal, ischemic, and pressure/mechanical pain. It has been suggested that endogenous pain-regulatory systems may account for ethnic differences in pain perception [11, 18, 19]. Furthermore, there are also biological ethnic differences in drug metabolism, dosing requirements, therapeutic responses, and side effects of analgesics. However, more studies need to be performed to elucidate the associated genetic factors [11, 15, 19].

Some studies have shown that western approaches to multi-disciplinary pain treatments are designed and delivered in a way that are more likely to benefit certain ethnic and cultural groups. Pain treatments and assessment tools should be culturally tailored to patients' backgrounds to improve outcomes. Healthcare professionals need to recognize the wide variation in pain expression and communication across cultures and ethnic groups. Cultural competence training amongst healthcare professionals is important. Healthcare professionals should develop knowledge and appreciation on culturally specific beliefs and attitudes held by their patients, even if they are not scientifically grounded. These medical professionals can then use this knowledge to adjust their patients' pain management plan. Further research should explore beliefs and expectations of pain management in different cultural groups to allow for integration with evidence-based pain management [11, 15, 16, 18, 20]. In addition, culturally appropriate treatment strategies that integrate cultural practices, philosophies, products, or environments should be considered as pathways to facilitate behavior change and provide a framework for patient-focused interventions. This can be achieved through social networks of community workers and recruiting individuals from the community with knowledge and training in pain management [15]. Studies have also shown that patients are more likely to actively participate in their treatment with healthcare professionals of the same background [19].

Medical professionals should be flexible in the way they approach pain management and treat pain in a culturally appropriate manner without biases and stereotyping. It has been shown that education focused on disparities in pain management led to increased physician confidence in their ability to identify potential barriers when treating minorities and increased confidence in their ability to implement strategies to minimize biases. Training healthcare professionals in communication skills, use of interpreters, and cultural competence are important interventions [11, 15, 16, 18, 20].

The mechanisms underlying ethnic and cultural differences in pain experiences are multifactorial and complex, thus more studies need to be performed to clarify the intricate variables and how to best address them. It is unknown which factors, if intervened upon, would have the greatest impact. Equalizing pain treatment across all patient groups will assume a place of increasing prominence as society grows more ethnically and culturally diverse. The increasing prevalence of pain can have debilitating socioeconomic and health ramifications for the individual and society. More pain research needs to be conducted and translated into practices and policies with a focus of reducing disparities in pain management [11, 15, 18, 20].

3 Pain Management in Global Health

Historically, pain management in resource-limited areas has been overlooked by the global medical community as more emphasis and resources are funneled toward issues deemed more pressing including communicable diseases [21]. Unfortunately this has led to a large gap in both knowledge/clinical training and resources for pain management, leaving many LMICs to either find alternative strategies for pain control or forgo the expectation of controlling pain altogether [21, 22]. With the lack of emphasis on pain management in LMICs, many barriers to appropriate pain management have developed, including lack of resources, education discrepancies, government policies, fear of opioid adverse effects, and more [23].

While pain management has in the past been neglected as an essential part of global health, there is hope for the future. As the global surgical burden increases, there will ultimately be an increased need for adequate perioperative pain management. Luckily, in recent years there has been a shift in global agendas to include both acute and chronic pain management as a fundamental human right [21, 24]. Organizations such as the World Health Organization (WHO) have emphasized the need to prioritize pain management and palliative care as part of universal health coverage [23, 25, 26].

The array of perioperative pain management strategies in LMICs around the world is difficult to encompass succinctly. This wide disparity is largely secondary to the fact that most LMICs are limited to what is available at the local patient, provider, and system levels [24, 27]. It is important to grasp the magnitude of discrepancy that exists from a resource allocation standpoint to understand pain management in LMICs. For example, morphine is a relatively inexpensive medication that has been declared essential by the WHO [23]. Despite this statement, its availability remains skewed.

It has been noted that the richest 10% of countries in the world continue to hold approximately 90% of distributed morphine equivalent opioids [21, 24]. Tramadol is a commonly utilized analgesic with more access to this weak opioid in LMICs due to its less direct effects [28]. Due to the lack of availability of opioids for many patients worldwide, other non-opioid strategies are often used. Additionally, even when opioids are available, many healthcare professionals in LMICs feel uncomfortable administering/prescribing them due to lack of understanding and experience utilizing them [23].

Non-opioid analgesics have long been a mainstay of perioperative pain management in countries of all resource levels. In fact, they are the first step noted in the WHO analgesic ladder for both acute and chronic pain management [29]. While it is difficult to ascertain exact data on the overall use of non-opioid analgesics throughout LMICs, paracetamol and diclofenac are often mentioned as part of the non-opioid analgesic ladder [22, 30]. Their use in treatment regimens is contingent on each community's access to non-opioid analgesics and may vary greatly.

Ketamine has long been relied on in LMICs as a means for both anesthesia and pain management. The organization, Médecins Sans Frontières/Doctors Without Borders, estimates that more than 50 countries globally depend on ketamine as part of multimodal analgesic plans, usually given concomitantly with tramadol and diclofenac for maximal effect [31]. In addition to ketamine's use as a perioperative analgesic in LMICs, it is crucial to note that ketamine remains vital as the primary anesthetic for many resource-limited countries [31, 32].

Many LMICs have developed resourceful, individualized adjuncts to medications as components of multimodal perioperative pain management pathways. For example, acupuncture has long been a staple of Eastern medicine and is used in countries of all resource levels [33]. Its ability to decrease both postoperative opioid requirements and postoperative nausea/vomiting makes it an ideal complementary medicine when considering multimodal pain management. Other studies have shown that approaches, such as talking with friends can be a successful option for nonpharmacologic pain management. One study from Ethiopia in 2019 found this to be the most common method of non-pharmacologic postoperative pain control with 88.3% of patients using it within 6 hours after surgery [34]. While these different methods of nonpharmacologic pain management are certainly important adjuvants in LMICs, they are not appropriate substitutes to pharmacologic pain management.

LMICs face significant barriers when it comes to providing adequate pain management, in both the acute and chronic setting. The first barrier that should be addressed is the historical lack of initiative in pain management with the past several decades focusing mainly on communicable diseases. With the expected exponential increase in surgical and anesthetic services worldwide, pain management has started to receive more recognition [22]. Along the same lines, the lack of resources, specifically opioid availability, in LMICs often severely limits the available approaches to pain management [21, 22]. In addition to lack of resources, limited training in pain management and lack of pain protocols have also been cited as a significant barrier to adequate pain control in LMICs. Several studies based in Rwanda have demonstrated that a fear of medication side effects and concern for incorrect decision making has negatively impacted evidence-based practice. One study found that only 46% of medical personnel interviewed had training in acute pain management [21]. Other barriers to pharmacologic pain management in LMICs include cultural beliefs about pain, fear of addiction, and government regulations of opioid administration.

4 Regional Techniques in Global Health

Unfortunately, there is minimal available data that addresses acute pain in LMICs and therefore identifying specific areas or surgical procedures requiring improvement is challenging. Studies are typically performed at healthcare centers with better resources and may poorly represent the acute pain situation in more rural settings where conditions are likely worse [1]. A survey conducted in Nigeria on postoperative pain demonstrated that 68.7% of patients reported moderate to unbearable pain 24 hours after surgery [35]. In addition to post-surgical pain, pain related to traumatic events accounts for a significant portion of the disease burden in LMICs and often requires pain management techniques similar to what might be required in the perioperative environment. Regional techniques are helpful in these situations [1].

Perioperative anesthesia-related morbidity and mortality is higher in LMICs due to lack of anesthesia infrastructure, trained professionals, equipment, basic monitors, safety protocols, and medications. There is often a lack of access to functioning anesthetic machines, basic airway equipment, capnography, monitors of neuromuscular blockade, and even oxygen. Previous research has demonstrated that there is a lower mortality rate with regional anesthesia compared to general anesthesia when used in these limited resource settings. For example, a study performed at Doctors Without Borders facilities, demonstrated that spinal anesthesia and regional anesthesia were associated with lower odds of perioperative death compared with general anesthesia with intubation [36]. Regional anesthesia helps avoid life-threatening perioperative airway and respiratory complications, especially in obstetrics. It can also improve pain control, shorten recovery room length of stay, and increase operating room efficiency, which all contributed to decreased healthcare costs. Regional anesthesia can decrease the need for opioids, which are in short supply in LMICs. It can also provide a less resource-intensive option than general anesthesia. Regional anesthesia is most beneficial for obstetric, trauma, and orthopedic patients, which represent the most common surgical cases in low- and middle-income countries [37–39]. Furthermore, during the COVID-19 pandemic, regional anesthesia has been recommended over general anesthesia to avoid aerosolization from airway management procedures. Minimizing aerosolizing can improve system health through decreasing infection in healthcare professionals who are already in short supply [37].

Neuraxial anesthesia is relatively easy to teach and perform, cost-effective, safe, and efficacious. It can be used for surgeries at and below the umbilicus. The equipment needed is minimal and less expensive than what is required for general anesthesia.

However, there is limited access to spinal needles that reduce the risk of post-dural puncture headaches. When there is a shortage of spinal needles, introducer needles from IV cannulas can be utilized [37, 40]. The shift to neuraxial anesthesia from general anesthesia for cesarean sections was slower in LMICs. In west Africa, anesthesia professionals were not providing spinal anesthesia due to personal preference and level of expertise. However, a retrospective study from Nigeria, demonstrated that there is a trend toward increasing spinal anesthesia utilization for cesarean sections [41]. A retrospective analysis on anesthetic procedures performed at healthcare facilities with medical professionals from Doctors Without Borders over a 6-year period was conducted. The study found that the most common type of anesthetic technique was spinal anesthesia (45.56%) and the most common procedure performed was cesarean section (35.54%) [36].

Anesthesia contributes disproportionately to maternal mortality in LMICs, mainly due to airway complications. A systematic review of obstetric morbidity and mortality in low- and middle-income countries showed that general anesthesia tripled the odds of maternal death as compared with neuraxial anesthesia. General anesthesia also doubled the odds of perinatal death and was associated with an increased risk of postpartum hemorrhage and low Apgar scores compared with neuraxial anesthesia [42]. Neuraxial anesthesia in obstetrics can provide safe anesthesia by avoiding airway manipulation, which decreases the risk of aspiration and desaturation. However, there needs to be education on physiological changes with neuraxial anesthesia to avoid high spinals and intraoperative hypotension [43].

Neuraxial techniques also provide analgesia after the cesarean section. There is poor labor analgesia in resource-limited environments. In a study of laboring women in Nigeria, 85.1% of women stated would want labor analgesia. However, only 38.9% of women received labor analgesia [44]. Therefore, more education and training programs can be beneficial. In Ghana, a program was implemented to teach local anesthesia professionals how to perform spinal anesthesia for cesarian sections. This training paradigm consisted of didactic and practical training, focusing on preanesthetic evaluation, management of an inadequate block, sterile technique, local anesthetic dosage, treatment of side effects, complication management, and hemodynamic monitoring. After the training, the use of spinal anesthesia for cesarian sections increased from 6% to 89% over 3 years, then to 97% in 5 years. This research suggests that spinal anesthesia can be efficiently provided in resource-limited settings with the development of appropriate protocols, staff education, and the availability of basic equipment and medications. The study authors also developed and implemented a single-shot spinal labor analgesia protocol. However, this protocol was not sustainable due to a shortage of anesthesia professionals [45]. Unfortunately, epidurals are rarely used in LMICs due to a paucity of epidural kits, infusion pumps, and trained staff to monitor and manage the epidural infusion and monitor for complications. Epidural catheter insertion is also more complicated to perform, more costly, and associated with more potential complications than spinals [45]. Epidural boluses can be performed manually if infusion pumps are the limiting factor. Single shot spinal analgesia can be utilized instead of epidurals, although single shot spinal analgesia is associated with a limited duration. Intrathecal opioids can be a reasonable alternative to epidurals as well, however the availability of preservative-free opioids may limit more widespread implementation [46, 47].

Despite frequent use of spinal blocks, peripheral nerve blocks are not routinely performed in LMICs. In a survey of Nigerian anesthesiologists, spinal anesthesia was regularly utilized. Whereas the majority of anesthesiologists reported either never or rarely performing an epidural or peripheral nerve block. When peripheral nerve blocks were performed, a nerve stimulator was typically used to appropriately target nerve structures [48].

In LMICs, there is widespread interest in performing peripheral nerve blocks, but insufficient training and lack of appropriately trained medical professionals. These medical professionals need to be educated on how to utilize ultrasound imaging, indications and contraindications to various regional techniques, and how to manage potential complications. There needs to be enough staff to follow-up with patients after their regional anesthetic, particularly if there are epidurals or nerve catheters involved. Anesthesia professionals are often poorly supported and difficult to recruit and retain in LMICs. There is a need for more in-depth training and regional anesthesia fellowships in LMICs to learn peripheral nerve and fascial plane blocks and for ultrasound training [37]. In a multicenter study in the Democratic Republic of the Congo and Ethiopia, 41 medical professionals were taught femoral, popliteal and forearm nerve blocks. Following this training program, this group demonstrated an ability to consistently provide regional anesthesia and were able to perform almost 1000 analgesic blocks with high success rates and no complications. The success of this program demonstrates that it is feasible to perform regional techniques in resource-limited areas successfully and safely [2]. Another study performed at a Nigerian healthcare center demonstrated that peripheral nerve blocks have been used successfully for orthopedic surgeries, particularly upper extremity surgeries. In this case, brachial plexus blocks were frequently utilized as the primary anesthetic thereby avoiding the need for general anesthesia and airway instrumentation [49].

Various techniques may be successfully utilized to provide regional anesthesia in LMICs including ultrasound-guided, landmark-based, or nerve stimulation. The preferred technique is locally dependent upon the equipment and trained medical professional availability. The safety profile associated with various nerve blocks and localization techniques may vary significantly. Generally, distal blocks and the use of ultrasound are associated with the highest safety profile. Lack of equipment may remain a barrier to the routine performance of peripheral nerve blocks. Sterile ultrasound gel and probe covers are usually unavailable in resource-limited settings. Thus, when performing ultrasound-guided nerve blocks, the provider should insert the block needle through a sterile-prepped area of skin away from the ultrasound probe as to not contaminate the needle. Probe covers can also be substituted with sterile gloves and adhesive dressings. Ultrasound gel in general can be difficult to obtain, so there may need to be substitutions with other lubricants/gels [2]. Some equipment, like block/spinal needles, are utilized after their expiration date. Specific peripheral nerve block needles that are blunted, insulated, and echogenic can be difficult to obtain, so instead, spinal needles or hypodermic needles can be utilized. It is assumed that sharper needles, like spinal needles, may be more likely to injure nerve structures, but there is not clear evidence on needle type with relation to nerve injury. However, needle tips can be blunted sterilely if the provider prefers. Needle echogenicity/visibility on ultrasound can be increased by roughening the outer needle layer with a surgical blade, using a guidewire, or performing the block with saline hydrodissection [2]. Ultrasound imaging equipment remains limited and costly in LMICs. This imaging modality has become more affordable with handheld devices that can be connected to cell phones or laptops. Recent ultrasound technology has also become more durable, portable, and equipped with longer battery lives, which is helpful in resource-limited settings where electricity can be unreliable. Some machines are also more streamlined with fewer and more user-friendly controls to help with the learning curve. Ultrasound maintenance can also be expensive and this is a required consideration if equipment donation is contemplated [37]. Lastly, basic monitors still need to be available for regional anesthesia as well [50].

In addition to equipment shortages, medications in LMICs are frequently in shortage as well. Local anesthetics are not always readily available and can have quality control issues resulting from inadequate storage conditions, inconsistent sourcing, or utilization beyond printed expiration dates. The actual concentration of the prepared local anesthetic may be different from the concentration reported on the label. There may not be standard concentrations of local anesthetics available either, so diluting the medication and paying close attention to the drug label is important. Single-use vials may need to be used across multiple patients and reused over several days, putting patients at elevated risk for infection. Furthermore, the amount of local anesthetic needed to perform a single peripheral block can be used for multiple spinals, which then contributes to the shortage of local anesthetics. The local anesthetic is arguably more beneficial if saved for neuraxial anesthesia [2, 50]. In a study of anesthesia resources in Uganda, 30% of anesthesia professionals stated that they never had local anesthetic for neuraxial anesthesia and 28% stated that they only sometimes had local anesthetic available [51]. Lipid emulsion and vasopressors are also frequently unavailable, which affects the safety of performing regional and neuraxial anesthesia. Vasopressors are often needed during neuraxial anesthesia. Using smaller volumes, short-acting, and lower concentration of local anesthetics may be the safer option when lipid emulsion is not readily available [2, 50].

There are additional logistical and safety considerations associated with implementing regional anesthesia programs in resource-limited areas. Although regional anesthesia has the potential to increase efficiency, it can also have the opposite effect if appropriate workflow and protocols are not in place. This needs to be tailored to individual healthcare settings by local healthcare professionals. There is a huge learning curve and logistical barriers, which can decrease efficiency with initial implementation of regional techniques. Discussions also need to be held on if the benefits of regional anesthesia outweigh the risks and how to ensure adequate supply and quality of equipment and medications. Medical professionals need to learn both how to perform the regional techniques and how to manage complications, such as Local Anesthetic Systemic Toxicity (LAST) or loss of an airway. Although regional anesthesia, particularly under ultrasound-guidance, is generally considered to be low risk, the data on the safety of regional anesthesia is mainly in well-resourced settings with trained medical professionals. More studies need to be conducted on the safety of regional anesthesia in resource-limited settings. The degree of safety that is acceptable and "bare minimum" requirements to administer regional anesthesia needs to be established. There needs to be guidelines on who can provide regional anesthesia, how much training is needed, and if lipid emulsion and vasopressors need to be present [2].

Other factors include institutional practices and healthcare professional preferences. For example, a study in Ghana demonstrated that local surgeons were performing inguinal hernia repairs under local anesthetic infiltration half as frequently as visiting surgeons from abroad [52]. Healthcare professionals are more comfortable with techniques they are familiar with. For example, anesthesia professionals prefer to use ketamine, even if neuraxial anesthesia or local anesthetic infiltration would be appropriate [50].

Regional anesthesia in LMICs has the potential to reduce morbidity and mortality, while increasing efficiency. However, there needs to be adequate resources, trained medical professionals, and workflow and safety protocols. More studies need to be performed on safety and access to supplies in resource-limited settings.

5 Training Opportunities in Global Health

As anesthesiology residency programs have become more common and well developed in many LMICs, the desire for subspecialty anesthesia training has expectedly grown. There are two main options for residents and attendings in LMICs to obtain this subspecialty training: 1) out-of-country fellowship training, and 2) in-country/local fellowship training. Both training options have advantages and disadvantages for anesthesia personnel of LMICs. Since many LMICs do not have the availability of in-country subspecialty training yet, the only available option is pursuing an out-of-country fellowship. Out-of-country fellowship training requires an anesthesiologist to leave one's country to join an established fellowship program usually in a higher-income country for a period of time in order to become an expert in that subspecialty before returning. The advantage of this particular avenue is that the trainee can learn at an established program with subspecialty experts usually without a substantial lack of local resources and/or teaching impairing their fellowship training [53]. The World Federation of Societies of Anaesthesiologists (WFSA) has established a number of subspecialty training programs (critical care, pediatric anesthesia, regional anesthesia, cardiac anesthesia, pain management, thoracic anesthesia, and obstetric anesthesia) of varying durations for anesthesiologists from LMICs with the goal of providing subspecialty training for applicants in local geographic regions [54].

The major disadvantages of out-of-country fellowship training include: 1) lack of funding, 2) lack of opportunities, 3) medical migration, 4) learning outside of one's home context, and 5) inability to translate the learning upon returning [55]. While WFSA has greatly increased the available training opportunities, positions remain limited in many geographic regions and cannot accommodate the number of LMIC anesthesiologists interested in subspecialty training. There remains the concern that these external fellowship programs could promote medical migration, which affects medical care in many LMICs [56]. The ability to successfully retain locally trained anesthesiologists is a core component of increasing the quality of anesthesia care in LMICs. In addition to concerns of medical migration that may arise, subspecialty learning in a foreign medical environment with greater resources can limit the applicability of one's learning upon return to the home country. Unless the training program carries a heavy emphasis on resource building and program development (rather than pure medical knowledge and procedural expertise), an out-of-country trainee may return and be unable to apply what their subspeciality learning to the local context for a multitude of reasons, including lack of resources, leadership buy-in, and barriers to change current practices and processes. For instance, for regional anesthesia training, learning at an established program with a well-developed regional block room workflow might facilitate understanding of how to perform the relevant blocks but the training may not provide the necessary expertise of how to set up that block room workflow in a low-resource setting that does not currently have one.

In-context, in-country subspeciality training could address these issues and provide fellowship learning and subspecialty expertise while focusing heavily on process improvement and the leadership skills necessary to translate the medical knowledge in one's home context. However, the development of subspecialty training programs in LMICs is hampered mainly by a lack of local expertise and teaching in these subspecialties. With the recent focus on anesthesiology residency program development by certain societies (American Society of Anesthesiologists, Canadian Anesthesiologists' Society International Education Foundation, International Association for the Study of Pain, to name a few), the opportunity to subsequently use the educational infrastructure to develop subspecialty training programs has grown due to local desire for such training. The main challenges faced in developing these in-country fellowship programs in LMICs include funding, resources, obtaining dedicated fellowship time for trainees, and availability of expert teaching. If no local in-country subspeciality expert exists, a multi-institutional collaboration is commonly needed to provide the level of expert teaching necessary for a near-continuous presence during the fellowship time. Growing these multi-institutional collaborations to provide the necessary teaching expertise takes a considerable amount of time and effort since many institutions may not provide the funding or academic time to partake. The initial efforts of such in-country fellowships can focus on the development of a local expert who then can lead subsequent fellowship efforts with ideally less reliance on external teaching. The ultimate goal of such fellowship programs should be to not only become an expert in a particular subspecialty but also to understand how to apply that expertise to low-resource settings with an emphasis on program development, process improvement, and improving quality of care while under the constraint of limited resources.

Development of in-country regional anesthesia and acute pain medicine fellowship programs in LMICs represents a significant need in these countries in order to advance anesthesia care for local residents and provide local residency graduates with further education and expertise for their professional advancement. While pharmacologic perioperative analgesia can be limited due to certain drug availability and inadequate postoperative monitoring, regional anesthesia and peripheral nerve blocks can be performed in a cost-effective manner in many LMICs given the proliferation of ultrasound access and local anesthetic availability. While specialized block needles might not always be available in many LMIC settings, less expensive Tuohy needles can commonly be purchased with pre-existing supply chains (i.e. from same spinal needle supplier) and used for peripheral nerve blocks with already available syringes and intravenous tubing. The resultant avoidance of general anesthesia for many brachial plexus and lower extremity blocks can increase patient safety, improve perioperative analgesia, and decrease the need for perioperative opioids. While there is no perfect substitute for in-person, hands-on teaching, the newly available tele-ultrasound component of portable ultrasound devices can allow for hands-on, real-time, remote procedural teaching when gaps in in-person teaching occur during the fellowship year [57]. Lastly, the addition of required scholarly activity and quality improvement to these fellowship programs benefits the local anesthesia department and patient care by increasing scholarship and academic opportunities.

6 Key Points

With the increasing linguistic, cultural, and ethnic diversity worldwide, healthcare professionals need to be cognizant of pain disparities that can affect different populations. Healthcare professionals should aim to improve pain communication, public health education focused on pain management, and cultural competence to effectively treat pain in patients of various backgrounds.

Globally, substantial pain management disparities exist in LMICs and are associated with variability in medication/equipment availability and a paucity of healthcare professionals specifically trained in the provision of regional anesthesia and acute pain medicine. Regional anesthesia can provide safe, effective, and less costly analgesia and anesthesia with the appropriate resources. Therefore, it is imperative that anesthesia professionals in LMICs be trained in regional anesthesia and acute pain medicine to improve perioperative pain control and enhance public health.

References

1. Size M, Soyannwo OA, Justins DM. Pain management in developing countries. Anaesthesia. 2007;62(s1):38–43.
2. Lipnick MS, Dubowitz G, Wabule A. Regional Anesthesia in resource-constrained environments. In: Atlas of ultrasound-guided regional anesthesia. Elsevier, Inc.; 2019. p. 405–12.
3. Kovoor JG, Bacchi S, Stretton B, Lam L, Jiang M, Gupta AK, Maddern GJ. Language and gender barriers to pain control after general surgery. ANZ J Surg. 2022;93(1–2):104–7

4. Diamond LC, Reuland DS. Describing physician language fluency. JAMA. 2009;301(4):426.
5. Meara JG, Leather AJM, Hagander L, Alkire BC, Alonso N, Ameh EA, et al. Global surgery 2030: evidence and solutions for achieving health, welfare, and economic development. The Lancet. 2015;386(9993):569–624.
6. Jacob E, McCarthy KS, Sambuco G, Hockenberry M. Intensity, location, and quality of pain in Spanish-speaking children with cancer. Pediatr Nurs. 2008;34(1):45–52.
7. Schenker Y, Lo B, Ettinger KM, Fernandez A. Navigating language barriers under difficult circumstances. Ann Intern Med. 2008;149(4):264–9.
8. Jimenez N, Moreno G, Leng M, Buchwald D, Morales LS. Patient-reported quality of pain treatment and use of interpreters in Spanish-speaking patients hospitalized for obstetric and gynecological care. J Gen Intern Med. 2012;27(12):1602–8.
9. Mosher CE, Duhamel KN, Egert J, Smith MY. Self-efficacy for coping with cancer in a multiethnic sample of breast cancer patients: associations with barriers to pain management and distress. Clin J Pain. 2010;26(3):227–34.
10. Jimenez N, Jackson DL, Zhou C, Ayala NC, Ebel BE. Postoperative pain management in children, parental English proficiency, and access to interpretation. Hosp Pediatr. 2014;4(1):23–30.
11. Campbell CM, Edwards RR. Ethnic differences in pain and pain management. Pain Manag. 2012;2(3):219–30.
12. Ali PA, Watson R. Language barriers and their impact on provision of care to patients with limited English proficiency: nurses' perspectives. J Clin Nurs. 2018;27(5–6):e1152-60.
13. Guedj R, Marini M, Kossowsky J, Berde CB, Kimia AA, Fleegler EW. Racial and ethnic disparities in pain management of children with limb fractures or suspected appendicitis: a retrospective cross-sectional study. Front Pediatr. 2021;3:9.
14. Mills AM, Shofer FS, Boulis AK, Holena DN, Abbuhl SB. Racial disparity in analgesic treatment for ED patients with abdominal or back pain. Am J Emerg Med. 2011;29(7):752–6.
15. Anderson KO, Green CR, Payne R. Racial and ethnic disparities in pain: causes and consequences of unequal care. J Pain. 2009;10(12):1187–204.
16. Peacock S, Patel S. Cultural influences on pain. Rev Pain. 2008;1(2):6–9.
17. Cleeland CS. Pain and treatment of pain in minority patients with cancer: the eastern cooperative oncology group minority outpatient pain study. Ann Intern Med. 1997;127(9):813.
18. Morales ME, Yong RJ. Racial and ethnic disparities in the treatment of chronic pain. Pain Medicine. 2021;22(1):75–90.
19. Green CR, Anderson KO, Baker TA, Campbell LC, Decker S, Fillingim RB, et al. The unequal burden of pain: confronting racial and ethnic disparities in pain. Pain Medicine. 2003;4(3):277–94.
20. Mossey JM. Defining racial and ethnic disparities in pain management. Clin Orthop Relat Res. 2011;469(7):1859–70.
21. Nyirigira G, Wilson RA, VanDenKerkhof EG, Goldstein DH, Twagirumugabe T, Mahaffey R, et al. Barriers and facilitators to postoperative pain management in Rwanda from the perspective of health care providers: a contextualization of the theory of planned behavior. Can J Pain. 2018;2(1):87–102.
22. Morriss WW, Roques CJ. Pain management in low- and middle-income countries. BJA Educ. 2018;18(9):265–70.
23. Brennan F, Carr DB, Cousins M. Pain management: a fundamental human right. Anesth Analg. 2007;105(1):205–21.
24. Knaul FM, Farmer PE, Krakauer EL, De Lima L, Bhadelia A, Jiang Kwete X, et al. Alleviating the access abyss in palliative care and pain relief-an imperative of universal health coverage: the Lancet Commission report. Lancet. 2018;391(10128):1391–454.
25. Price R, Makasa E, Hollands M. World health assembly resolution WHA68.15: "strengthening emergency and essential surgical care and anesthesia as a component of universal health coverage"—Addressing the public health gaps arising from lack of safe, affordable and accessible surgical and anesthetic services. World J Surg. 2015;39(9):2115–25.

26. Quene T Mac, Bust L, Louw J, Mwandri M, Chu KM. Global surgery is an essential component of global health. Surgeon. 2022;20(1):9–15.
27. Bhadelia A, De Lima L, Arreola-Ornelas H, Kwete XJ, Rodriguez NM, Knaul FM. Solving the Global crisis in access to pain relief: lessons from country actions. Am J Public Health. 2019;109(1):58–60.
28. Vijayan R, Afshan G, Bashir K, Cardosa M, Chadha M, Chaudakshetrin P, et al. Tramadol: a valuable treatment for pain in Southeast Asian countries. J Pain Res. 2018;11:2567–75.
29. Anekar AA, Cascella M. WHO analgesic ladder. 2022.
30. Aweke Z, Seyoum F, Shitemaw T, Doba DN. Comparison of preemptive paracetamol, paracetamol-diclofenac & paracetamol-tramadol combination on postoperative pain after elective abdominal surgery under general anesthesia, Ethiopia: a randomized control trial study, 2018. BMC Anesthesiol. 2020;20(1):191.
31. Joshi GP, Onajin-Obembe B. The role of Ketamine in low- and middle-income countries. Anesth Analg. 2016;122(3):908–10.
32. Dong TT, Mellin-Olsen J, Gelb AW. Ketamine: a growing global health-care need. Br J Anaesth. 2015;115(4):491–3.
33. Jishun J, Mittelman M. Acupuncture: past, present, and future. Glob Adv Health Med. 2014;3(4):6–8.
34. Eshete MT, Baeumler PI, Siebeck M, Tesfaye M, Haileamlak A, Michael GG, et al. Quality of postoperative pain management in Ethiopia: a prospective longitudinal study. PLoS One. 2019;14(5): e0215563.
35. Faponle AF, Sayannwo OA, Ajayi IO. Post operative pain therapy: a survey of prescribing patterns and adequacy of analgesia in Ibadan, Nigeria. Cent Afr J Med. 2001;47(3).
36. Ariyo P, Trelles M, Helmand R, Amir Y, Hassani GH, Mftavyanka J, et al. Providing Anesthesia care in resource-limited settings. Anesthesiology. 2016;124(3):561–9.
37. Dohlman L, Kwikiriza A, Ehie O. Benefits and barriers to increasing regional anesthesia in resource-limited settings. Local Reg Anesth. 2020;13:147–58.
38. Ho M, Livingston P, Bould MD, Nyandwi JD, Nizeyimana F, Uwineza JB, et al. Barriers and facilitators to implementing a regional anesthesia service in a low-income country: a qualitative study. Pan Afr Med J. 2019;32.
39. Dohlman LE, Thakkar N, Jivanelli B, Pakala S, Brouillette MA. Regional anesthesia global health collaborations- a scoping review of current intervention methods. Curr Opin Anaesthesiol. 2022;35(5):647–53.
40. Mgbakor AC, Adou BE. Plea for greater use of spinal anaesthesia in developing countries. Trop Doct. 2012;42(1):49–51.
41. Okafor UV, Ezegwui HU, Ekwazi K. Trends of different forms of anaesthesia for caesarean section in South-eastern Nigeria. J Obstet Gynaecol (Lahore). 2009;29(5):392–5.
42. Sobhy S, Zamora J, Dharmarajah K, Arroyo-Manzano D, Wilson M, Navaratnarajah R, et al. Anaesthesia-related maternal mortality in low-income and middle-income countries: a systematic review and meta-analysis. Lancet Glob Health. 2016;4(5):e320-7.
43. Anderson RE, Ahn R, Nelson BD, Chavez J, de Redon E, Burke T. Defining the anesthesia gap for reproductive health procedures in resource-limited settings. Int J Gynecol Obstet. 2014;127(3):229–33.
44. Imarengiaye CO, Ande ABA. Demand and utilisation of labour analgesia service by Nigerian women. J Obstet Gynaecol (Lahore). 2006;26(2):130–2.
45. Olufolabi AJ, Atito-Narh E, Eshun M, Ross VH, Muir HA, Owen MD. Teaching Neuraxial Anesthesia techniques for obstetric care in a ghanaian referral hospital. Anesth Analg. 2015;120(6):1317–22.
46. Kodali BS, Jagannathan DK, Owen MD. Establishing an obstetric neuraxial service in low-resource areas. Int J Obstet Anesth. 2014;23(3):267–73.
47. Dyer RA, Reed AR, James MF. Obstetric anaesthesia in low-resource settings. Best Pract Res Clin Obstet Gynaecol. 2010;24(3):401–12.
48. Rukewe A, Fatiregun A. The use of regional anesthesia by anesthesiologists in Nigeria. Anesth Analg. 2010;110(1):243–4.

49. Rukewe A, Fatiregun A, Alonge TO. Orthopaedic anaesthesia for upper extremity procedures in a Nigerian hospital. Malawi Med J. 2014;26(3):90–2.
50. Schnittger T. Regional anaesthesia in developing countries. Anaesthesia. 2007;62(s1):44–7.
51. Hodges SC, Mijumbi C, Okello M, McCormick BA, Walker IA, Wilson IH. Anaesthesia services in developing countries: defining the problems. Anaesthesia. 2007;62(1):4–11.
52. Wilhelm TJ, Anemana S, Kyamanywa P, Rennie J, Post S, Freudenberg S. Anaesthesia for elective inguinal hernia repair in rural Ghana-appeal for local anaesthesia in resource-poor countries. Trop Doct. 2006;36(3):147–9.
53. Gathuya ZN. Pro: pediatric anesthesia training in developing countries is best achieved by selective out of country scholarships. Paediatr Anaesth. 2009;19(1):42–4.
54. Coté CJ, Cavallieri S, Ben Ammar MS, Bosenberg A, Jacob R. Pediatric anesthesia fellowship programs established through the World Federation of Societies of Anesthesiologists (WFSA): origins and perspectives. Int Anesthesiol Clin. 2010;48(2):47–57.
55. Walker IA. Con: pediatric anesthesia training in developing countries is best achieved by out of country scholarships. Paediatr Anaesth. 2009;19(1):45–9.
56. Botezat A, Ramos R. Physicians' brain drain-a gravity model of migration flows. Global Health. 2020;16(1):7.
57. Grubic N, Belliveau DJ, Herr JE, Nihal S, Wong SWS, Lam J, et al. Training of non-expert users using remotely delivered, point-of-care tele-ultrasound: a proof-of-concept study in 2 Canadian communities. Ultrasound Q. 2022.

Pain Management Considerations in Critical Care

Clare Hasken, Kenji Tanabe, and Sarah M. Alber

Abstract Pain management is an essential component of critical care medicine, and effective treatment improves short and long-term patient outcomes. At the forefront is the need for regular assessments of pain using validated tools, a few of which are validated for patients able to communicate, or alternative tools for patients who are unable to effectively communicate. With a recent recognition of harm resulting from heavy sedation and immobility, current trends in critical care have transitioned to the concept of "analgosedation." This treatment paradigm prioritizes the use of multimodal analgesia prior to the administration of sedating medications to facilitate early mobilization and participation with rehabilitation exercises. While the administration of opioids remains a common practice in the intensive care unit, multimodal anesthesia using non-opioid medications, as well as regional anesthetic techniques have demonstrated improved outcomes and, in some cases, a decreased incidence of chronic pain syndromes. The critically ill population provides several unique challenges to pain management that are discussed in this chapter.

Keywords Critical care · Numeric rating scale · Behavioral pain scale · Critical care pain observation tool · Analgosedation · Acetaminophen · Non-steroidal anti-inflammatory drugs · Neuropathic pain · Opioids · Ketamine · Lidocaine · Dexmedetomidine · Regional anesthesia · Epidural · Peripheral nerve block

---

C. Hasken
Department of Anesthesiology, University of Colorado, Aurora, Colorado, USA
e-mail: Clare.Hasken@cuanschutz.edu

K. Tanabe · S. M. Alber (✉)
University of Colorado, Aurora, Colorado, USA
e-mail: Sarah.Alber@cuanschutz.edu

K. Tanabe
e-mail: Kenji.Tanabe@cuanschutz.edu

A. Abd-Elsayed and K. Schroeder (eds.), *Perioperative Pain Management*,
https://doi.org/10.1007/978-3-031-67648-2_14

1 Introduction

Pain management is a fundamental human right and is an essential component of critical care medicine [1]. Pain in the critically ill patient is complex, and affects the vast majority of patients [2]. Pain may be acute, chronic, or acute-on-chronic in nature; it may arise from visceral, neuropathic, or somatic etiologies or may be a combination of these. Pain may be associated with underlying pathologies, post-surgical, and/or procedural as the result of the standard course of treatment in the intensive care unit. Most patients experience pain both at rest and with procedures [3]. Add to this the vast differences in the perception or tolerability of pain and it is evident that patients require an individualized approach for effective management.

Pain is common in the intensive care unit and increases with routine procedures performed in the critical care setting. Procedures associated with greatest intensity of pain include arterial line insertion, chest tube removal, wound drain removal, turning/repositioning, and tracheal suctioning [3]. The Europain Study evaluated the severity of pain associated with procedures in 3,851 patients in 192 intensive care units (ICUs) in 28 countries [4]. Patients were asked to rate the severity of pain induced by frequently performed ICU procedures on a Numeric Rating Scale of 0–10 (0 being no pain, 10 being the worst possible pain). Over 37% of patients in the study were receiving mechanical ventilation during the procedure. All procedures were associated with a significant increase in pain scores. The most painful procedures identified in this investigation were chest tube removal, wound drain removal and arterial line insertion. The least painful procedure was mobilization, and the most common procedure performed was turning. Patients with higher pre-procedure pain scores were more likely to report more severe pain during the procedure. Given the relatively low mortality of 10% in the patients participating in this study compared to the general ICU population, this may indicate an enrollment bias towards patients with less severe acute illness. However, this large international investigation highlights the ubiquity and importance of pain management in the critical care setting.

Healthcare professionals working in an intensive care setting may be hesitant to treat pain, particularly with opioid analgesics, as this population commonly develops altered pharmacokinetics and pharmacodynamics and an increased susceptibility to side effects including vasoplegia (and subsequently worsening end-organ dysfunction), respiratory depression, inhibition of cough and risk for development of pneumonia, constipation, and altered mentation[5]. Contrary to this traditional thought process, the adequate treatment of pain is more likely correlated with an improvement in short and long-term patient outcomes [4]. Acutely, inadequate pain management can result in hemodynamic alterations, hypoxia, decreased oxygen delivery to essential organ systems, increased myocardial work and catabolism, psychological stress, sleep disturbance with increased risk for development of delirium, and may limit participation with mobility and rehabilitation therapies [6]. Untreated pain contributes to immunosuppression, hypercoagulability, nosocomial infections, and the downstream development of anxiety, depression, and post-traumatic stress disorder [4]. Indeed, multiple studies have determined that adequate pain management is associated with improvements in several clinical variables including a decreased duration of mechanical ventilation, reduced agitation and sedation administration, ICU length of stay, and in-hospital mortality [2, 6]. With an increasing recognition of the importance of light sedation and early mobilization in patients on mechanical ventilation, adequate pain control is paramount in reducing sedative mediations and facilitating participation and performance during rehabilitation therapies [3, 6].

Clinical practice guidelines recommend that all critically ill patients be assessed for pain routinely using appropriate assessment tools [1, 6]. In this chapter, we review validated tools to assess pain and treatment strategies for this unique patient population.

2 Patient Population & Demographics

A 2017 population-based study by Halpern *et al.* evaluated the growth of critical care beds in the United States between 2000 and 2010, specifically comparing these trends with the age and utilization trends of critical care beds during that timeframe [7]. While the number of critical care beds increased, Medicaid beneficiaries used a larger proportion of critical care beds compared to Medicare beneficiaries. This delineation suggests a shift towards critical care treatment of a younger patient population, with likely decreased access to healthcare and subsequently poorly managed medical conditions, being treated in the ICU setting. This contrasts with the traditional "aging population" model [7]. Predictors of higher pain scores in the ICU setting include pre-existing anxiety or depression, younger age, female sex, non-white ethnicity, presence of comorbidities, the expectation of poor future quality of life, ICU length of stay, and patients with a history of prior surgery or trauma [3]. These findings suggest that pain will continue to be an important and pervasive component of critical care medicine in the future.

The makeup of patients in the critical care setting varies widely depending on the subspecialty focus of the ICU. Smaller or more rural ICUs may consist of a mix of critically ill patients with medical, surgical, or traumatic pathology. In larger hospitals, ICUs may be separated into specialized medical, oncologic, surgical, cardiothoracic, trauma, burn, and neurologic care. The patient populations of specialized ICUs have unique drivers of pain, different frequencies of routine procedures, and variable use of pain management strategies. This clinical diversity further emphasizes the need for thoughtful and individualized care for the critically ill patient.

3 Unique Considerations when Managing Pain for the Critically Ill

Multiple factors contribute to the complexity of managing pain in the critically ill patient, however at the forefront is a limited ability to effectively identify and assess pain. ICU patients frequently have communication barriers. Barriers may arise from intubation and mechanical ventilation, altered mental status, insomnia and exhaustion, or severe immobility and severity of illness altering the perception of pain. Multiple clinical practice guidelines have highlighted the importance of regular and standardized pain assessments [1–3, 6].

Family and friends can serve as proxies for patients unable to communicate. Proxies are valuable sources of information as resources of pain history, conveying the patient's wishes prior to becoming critically ill, and assisting with assessments of pain in the ICU. Pontillo *et al.* found that family proxies' estimated pain scores were closer predictors of 245 patients' self-reported pain scores than the nurses or physicians caring for them [8]. Notably, there was only a moderate level of agreement between patients and family.

Vitals signs should not be used as indicators of pain in the ICU [3, 6]. Vital sign alterations are affected by inotropes, vasopressors, catabolic or sepsis states and are not valid indicators of pain in the critically ill patient. However, vital sign changes should prompt clinicians to assess for the driver of the change, including performing an assessment for pain.

There are three generally accepted and validated tools to assess pain in the critical care setting that are recommended in the latest clinical practice guidelines [3]. The Numeric Rating Scale (NRS) is for patients who can communicate, and the Behavioral Pain Score (BPS) or Critical Care Pain Observation Tool (CPOT) is for use in patients with impaired communication. Self-reported pain is the gold standard for pain assessment in patients able to effectively communicate [3, 9]. The NRS can be used visually, orally, written, or with other electronic forms of communication, making it a useful assessment strategy in a wide variety of patient interactions, including those requiring mechanical ventilation. The NRS has superior sensitivity, negative predictive value, and accuracy compared to the verbal descriptor scale (no pain, mild pain, moderate pain, severe pain, extreme pain), and the visual analog (faces) scale [3].

For patients who are unable to communicate, for example with altered mental status or traumatic brain injury, two behavioral assessment tools have been validated. The Behavioral Pain Scale uses facial expressions, upper limb movements, and compliance with mechanical ventilation as indicators of pain [10]. The Critical Care Pain Observation Tool (CPOT) is similar, although it differentiates between intubated and non-intubated patients and additionally observes for the degree of muscle tension [11]. Both scales have been validated for use in critically ill patients who are unable to self-report pain scales [3, 9–11]. It is important to note that these scales have not been extensively studied in patients with delirium, although some smaller studies suggest CPOT may be more reliable in this setting [1, 9]. Rijkenberg *et al.* compared the BPS vs. CPOT in mechanically ventilated patients and found that CPOT was less likely to score for pain during procedures that were determined as not painful (oral care), potentially decreasing unnecessary sedation or opioid administration.

Delirium is common in the ICU, with a prevalence between 26 and 78% depending on the subspecialty type of the ICU [1]. Delirium is multifactorial, but may be triggered by untreated pain as well as analgesics, making the balance between these contradictory goals difficult. Studies validating pain assessment tools have specifically excluded delirious patients due to the similar symptoms of pain and delirium (particularly hyperactive delirium) [1, 3, 6], which unfortunately has left a significant proportion of the critical care population without strong evidence-based guidelines for pain management. As the importance of light sedation, early mobilization, and prevention of delirium become more recognized, routine assessment and adequate treatment of pain is essential and should be an area of focus and future study. Current guidelines recommend that pain be treated first with an analgesic instead of a sedative agent and have also introduced the concept of analgosedation, making pain intervention a priority over sedating medications [3]. Care of mechanically ventilated patients using this method is associated with reduced sedative requirements, decreased duration of mechanical ventilation, lower pain intensity and shorter length of ICU stay [3]. Importantly, this method was not associated with increased rates of hypotension, constipation, or opioid exposure [3].

4 Pharmacological Management of Pain

Both opioid and non-opioid medications are utilized in intensive care units globally for the management of pain. Some medications such as acetaminophen and non-steroidal anti-inflammatory drugs (NSAIDs) have been available for decades. Other medications, including ketamine and long-acting opioids, were more recently developed and are increasingly used for pain control in critically ill patients. Regional anesthetic techniques and non-pharmacological methods for pain management may be useful as adjuncts to decrease opioid use [12]. When assessing pain control in patients, one must consider the origin of the pain when choosing an analgesic agent or technique. For acute postoperative or traumatic pain, a regional versus systemic option for analgesia should be considered [12]. Endotracheal tube irritation or intermittent procedural discomfort may be best treated using short acting opioid medications or local anesthesia to minimize over-sedation and adequately treat pain [12]. For patients with a history of chronic pain, home regimens consisting of long-acting opioids and neuropathic pain medications may be most effective.

A group of international experts developed evidence-based guidelines for pain management in critically ill patients, which were revised and republished in 2018 [3]. Multiple expert groups have contributed to guidelines for analgesia in both pediatric and adult intensive care patients [3, 6]. However, these recommendations are often based on weak evidence or "expert consensus" for specific agents utilized in the ICU. An overview and summary of the current evidence for both pharmacological and non-pharmacological management of pain in the adult ICU patient are discussed below (Table 1).

Table 1 Summary of pharmacologic management of pain

Drug	Recommended dosing	Evidence
Acetaminophen	IV, PO, and PR: 1 g q6h for maximum of 4 g daily in patients with normal liver function	Recommended for routine use in ICU for analgesia; likely similar analgesic effect regardless of route of administration
NSAIDs	Ibuprofen, PO: 600 mg q6h Ketoprofen, PO and IV: 25 mg–50 mg q6–8 hr for maximum of 300 mg daily Ketorolac, IV and IM: 15–30 mg q6h PO: 10 mg q4–6h Only used for short term use (up to 5 days)	Not recommended for routine use in ICU for analgesia; additional RCTs needed particularly for COX-2 inhibitors Not recommended in patients with renal failure
Neuropathic medications	Gabapentin, PO: 300–1200 mg TID for maximum of 3600 mg daily Pregabalin, PO: 75–150 mg BID Carbamazepine, PO: 100 mg TID	Recommended for routine use in ICU for neuropathic pain; requires enteral access and has sedating side effects; further RCTs needed; very limited data regarding carbamazepine use in this setting
Opioids	Sufentanil, IV: 0.23–0.37 mcg/kg/hr Nalbuphine, IV: 0.15–0.17 mg/kg/hr Methadone, PO and IV: 5–15 mg q8h	Evidence from Ji *et al.* suggests sufentanil and nalbuphine are safe and effective in ICU patients at these doses; very limited data for dosing of all opioid agents in the ICU setting
Ketamine	IV: 0.1–0.5 mg/kg bolus followed by 0.12–0.36 mg/kg/hr infusion	Recommended as low dose bolus and infusion combination in conjunction with opioids; further evidence needed for exact dosing guidelines in ICU patients
Systemic lidocaine	IV: +/−1.5 mg/kg bolus followed by 1–2 mg/min infusion for up to 24 hours postoperatively	Strong evidence in postoperative colorectal surgery patients; no evidence to support its use outside of this population
Topical lidocaine	Patch: 5% lidocaine with 700 mg applied for 12 hours on and 12 hours off	Evidence is mixed; may provide benefit for post-thoracotomy patients as adjunct but additional evidence is needed

5 Acetaminophen

Acetaminophen is the most commonly used analgesic medication globally [13]. This drug acts as a cyclooxygenase inhibitor and additionally exhibits serotonergic effects [14]. There are numerous routes of administration–oral (PO), intravenous (IV) and per rectum (PR)—which makes acetaminophen an acceptable option for many critically ill patients. Randomized controlled trials to date have focused primarily on IV acetaminophen use in ICU patients, and the evidence suggests acetaminophen can effectively decrease pain severity[3, 14-16]. Furthermore, this medication may decrease opioid consumption, decrease mechanical ventilation time, and reduce sedation [3, 14]. Although most studies have evaluated the efficacy of IV acetaminophen, experts generalize this data to both PO and PR acetaminophen and recommend the use of acetaminophen as an adjunct for pain management in the ICU [3]. Studies suggest PO and PR administration are as effective for analgesia as IV administration and may decreases costs [16]. In critically ill patients, dose adjustment may be required in patients with liver dysfunction or altered intestinal absorption [3]. As with all medications in the setting of critical illness, careful assessment and dosing based on individual patient factors is essential.

6 Non-steroidal Anti-inflammatory Drugs

In the critical care setting, non-steroidal anti-inflammatory drugs (NSAIDs) also may be a useful adjunct for acute pain. These medications include cyclo-oxygenase 1 (COX-1) and cyclo-oxygenase 2 (COX-2) inhibitors, both of which inhibit prostaglandin synthesis [17]. Despite their analgesic effect, NSAIDs are associated with adverse effects such as platelet dysfunction, renal injury, and gastrointestinal irritation, which may cause harm to already critically ill patients [17]. However, in a randomized controlled trial for post-operative cardiac surgery patients, Hynninen *et al.* found no difference in change in creatinine from baseline in patients receiving NSAIDs versus placebo. While this study failed to demonstrate a difference in pain scores among patients treated with NSAIDs versus placebo, diclofenac and other NSAIDs may help reduce the need for additional pain medications [17]. In critically ill patients following major abdominal surgery, Oberhofer *et al.* found significant improvements in pain in the NSAID group with reduced nausea and vomiting side effects compared to the control group [18]. Importantly, there was no significant difference in bleeding in the NSAID group [18]. With somewhat mixed evidence and potential adverse effects, one expert task force [3] does not recommend the routine use of NSAIDs for analgesia in critically ill patients. Additional randomized controlled trials are needed to better understand the general efficacy and safety of NSAIDs in the ICU setting.

7 Neuropathic Pain Medications

In recent years, the use of pregabalin, gabapentin, and carbamazepine as perioperative and neuropathic pain analgesic agents has garnered significant attention. Both pregabalin and gabapentin have structures similar to gamma-aminobutyric acid (GABA) and bind voltage-gated calcium channels within the central nervous system. Their specific mechanism related to neuropathic pain control is poorly understood, but both drugs likely reduce glutamatergic activity and minimize the development of hyperalgesia [19, 20]. Carbamazepine, an antiepileptic drug, is involved in the inactivation of sodium channels, which leads to inhibition of high frequency neuronal activity at epileptic foci [19]. A similar mechanism may explain why carbamazepine demonstrates an analgesic effect at the site of a painful stimulus. Randomized controlled trials to date have focused on the use of these medications in Guillain-Barre syndrome patients in the ICU as well as patients undergoing cardiothoracic surgery. Pandey and colleagues determined gabapentin to have a superior analgesic effect compared to carbamazepine in Guillain-Barre patients admitted to the ICU for respiratory support [19, 21]. Gabapentin also reduced opioid requirements compared to placebo [21]. This reduction in neuropathic pain may be generalizable to other patient populations but further evidence is needed. In postoperative cardiothoracic surgery patients, pregabalin is associated with reduced opioid requirements and reduced pain scores at three months postoperatively in two randomized controlled trials [20, 22]. This suggests neuropathic pain medications may not only effectively treat acute pain, but they also may reduce the risk of developing chronic neuropathic pain. An expert international task force recommends the use of neuropathic pain medications in critically ill patients but notes enteral administration is required and not always feasible [3]. These medications are also associated with adverse sedating effects, which may expose patients to an elevated risk of additional complications [3].

8 Opioids

Nearly all opioids used for analgesia have mu opioid agonist properties with variability in onset, duration of action, and side effects. Common adverse effects include respiratory depression, nausea, vomiting, constipation, urinary retention, itching, and sedation, which can all be detrimental to the recovery of critically ill patients [23]. Opioids with adequate analgesic properties and minimal adverse effects are ideal for use in the ICU. Sufentanil and nalbuphine may provide an improved safety profile relative to other commonly used opioids such as fentanyl or morphine. Sufentanil, a mu agonist, is highly lipophilic with a fast onset and offset following IV administration. Nalbuphine produces analgesia through opioid agonist-antagonist effects on mu and kappa receptors in the central nervous system. Both of these opioids can be administered as a continuous infusion for analgesia. Nalbuphine has a ceiling effect on respiratory depression at doses greater than 30 mg per 70 kg [23]. This drug may offer a safer alternative to other opioid infusions and achieve adequate pain control with a lower risk of respiratory complications. An interesting study from Ji *et al.* demonstrated the safe and effective use of both nalbuphine and sufentanil for pain control in patients admitted to the ICU [23]. In their retrospective analysis, nalbuphine provided superior analgesia for patients age 60 years or younger, whereas sufentanil provided better analgesia for patients over the age of 60 years [23]. No patients experienced hypoxemia, hypotension, or bradycardia related to opioid administration. Use of these agents in the ICU setting is uncommon, and randomized controlled trials are needed to determine if nalbuphine and sufentanil are superior in efficacy or safety compared to other opioid agents.

The use of methadone in critically ill patients is growing, but evidence remains limited regarding appropriate patient selection, dosing, and duration of use. Methadone primarily acts as a mu opioid receptor agonist, N-methyl-D-aspartate (NMDA) receptor antagonist, and inhibitor of serotonin and norepinephrine reuptake [24]. This drug may assist with analgesia, as well as decrease mechanical ventilation time, reduce opioid withdrawal after prolonged sedation from a continuous opioid infusion, and improve delirium [24]. However, adverse effects including respiratory depression are still a risk with methadone. Additional studies are needed to guide the appropriate use of methadone for analgesia in critically ill patients.

Many ICU patients have baseline chronic pain conditions that make adequate pain control challenging during a critical illness or in the postoperative period. Patients with substantial baseline opioid tolerance require higher opioid dosing to achieve an appropriate comfort level when subjected to noxious stimuli. Unfortunately, these patients are often undertreated with opioids during hospital admission. This may be due to provider unfamiliarity or discomfort prescribing high dose opioid regimens, as well as difficulty quantifying baseline opioid requirements. The baseline opioid calculations can be particularly difficult for patients who abuse opioids and for whom baseline administration data is inconsistent [25]. Regardless of the etiology, opioid underdosing in these patients can lead to an increased hospital length of stay and worsened patient outcomes. Patients on chronic opioid therapy require their baseline morphine milligram equivalents in addition to additional short acting opioids for acute pain control [25]. Dosing of medications may need adjustments based on changes in hepatic and renal function from baseline, volume status, and mental status alterations in critically ill patients.

9 Ketamine

The use of ketamine as an analgesic alternative to opioids in critically ill patients is rapidly expanding. Ketamine acts primarily as an analgesic via NMDA receptor antagonism [26]. Potentially beneficial effects of ketamine in ICU patients include preservation of airway reflexes, increases in lung compliance, minimal respiratory depression, and reduction in respiratory complications [26]. However, ketamine may cause hallucinations or worsen delirium in critically ill patients [26]. One randomized controlled trial suggested a higher dose ketamine infusion (2 mg/kg/hr) can actually decrease the incidence of delirium in mechanically ventilated patients but may not improve outcomes such as opioid consumption, ventilator free days, ICU length of stay, or mortality [27]. Other studies have shown a reduction in opioid requirements for patients treated with ketamine [28, 29]. For analgesia, lower doses of ketamine as an IV bolus (0.1–0.3 mg/kg) or as an IV infusion (0.12–0.36 mg/kg/hr) have improved pain control with minimal adverse psychogenic effects [29]. The optimal dosing regimen is typically an IV bolus followed by an IV infusion for up to 48 hours [29]. The KAPT trial is a large randomized controlled trial currently underway aiming to evaluate the impact of ketamine on trauma patients in stepdown units and ICUs [30]. Results of this study may provide some clarity regarding appropriate patient selection, ketamine dosing, and duration of treatment for critically ill trauma patients. Current clinical practice guidelines recommend using low dose ketamine as a 0.5 mg/kg IV bolus followed by a 0.06-0.12 mg/kg/hr IV infusion in conjunction with opioids for postoperative ICU patients [3].

There are several studies that evaluated the use of ketamine in combination with local anesthetic for wound infiltration and regional blocks perioperatively [31, 32]. The evidence is mixed, but small randomized controlled trials have shown improved analgesia with ketamine plus local anesthetic infiltration compared to only local anesthetic infiltration for patients undergoing abdominal surgery [31, 32]. Further trials specific to critically ill patients are needed to assess the utility of ketamine for wound infiltration in the ICU setting.

10 Systemic Lidocaine

Most studies assessing systemic lidocaine use for perioperative analgesia are among colorectal patients and not specific to ICU patients. In multiple randomized controlled trials, systemic lidocaine decreased the duration of postoperative ileus, decreased hospital length of stay, and possibly reduced pain scores compared to alternative analgesic options for colorectal surgery patients[33–35]. One small randomized controlled trial demonstrated equivalent pain scores, postoperative return of bowel function, and hospital length of stay among patients receiving systemic lidocaine versus thoracic epidural analgesia following open colorectal surgery [36]. This suggests IV lidocaine administration is a reasonable analgesic alternative for patients unable to receive an epidural catheter for open colorectal surgeries. Regarding dosing of systemic lidocaine, the data is variable. Some studies included a bolus of IV lidocaine prior to starting the IV infusion, and others did not. Dosing ranged from 1 to 2 mg/min and duration ranged from only intraoperatively versus up to 24 hours postoperatively in these studies [33–35]. Outside of colorectal surgery patients, minimal evidence exists to support the use of systemic lidocaine for analgesia. In postoperative cardiac surgery patients, one randomized trial found no benefit in time to extubation, ICU length of stay, or hospital length of stay among patients receiving systemic lidocaine versus placebo infusion [37]. Although systemic lidocaine may be beneficial in certain ICU patients, few studies have specifically evaluated its use in critically ill patients. Additional large investigations are needed, but current evidence recommends the use of systemic lidocaine for up to 24 hours postoperatively in colorectal surgery patients admitted to the ICU.

11 Dexmedetomidine

With potential benefits as both a sedative and analgesic agent, dexmedetomidine has become a popular tool for analgosedation, typically administered as an infusion for patients in the intensive care unit. The primary focus of the literature in critically ill patients is in reducing or preventing delirium with the use of dexmedetomidine [38]. The use of dexmedetomidine for pain control in ICU patients remains sparse. As a centrally acting alpha-2 receptor agonist, dexmedetomidine reduces norepinephrine release and can lead to bradycardia, hypotension, and decreased cardiac output [38]. For critically ill patients with cardiovascular instability, the risks may outweigh the benefits for use as an analgesic. In the peripheral nervous system, dexmedetomidine also inhibits C-fibers and A alpha-fibers which can decrease pain[39]. Postoperative analgesic benefit has been shown via multiple routes of administration including intravenous, epidural, intrathecal, intra-articular, and as an adjunct to local anesthetics in nerve blocks [39]. Despite the promising data to date in the perioperative period, additional evidence in critically ill patients is needed to safely and effectively use dexmedetomidine as an analgesic.

12 Other Adjuncts

Evidence is variable regarding the use of lidocaine patches for analgesia in post-operative cardiothoracic surgery ICU patients [40, 41]. Fiorelli *et al.* found that lidocaine patches may reduce pain both at rest and with coughing, as well as reduce opioid requirements in these patients. However, Liu *et al.* found no difference in pain scores, ICU length of stay, or hospital length of stay for patients who received lidocaine patches. Perhaps in certain patient populations, such as those with chronic pain or with limited options for analgesia, utilizing a lidocaine patch may provide benefit as an adjunct to other therapies with minimal risk. However, additional evidence is needed to recommend routine use.

Cannabinoids have the potential to provide analgesia in conjunction with other methods. Narang *et al.* suggest cannabinoids can reduce pain scores and improve patient satisfaction in the outpatient chronic pain population but this has not been studied in ICU patients [42]. More evidence is needed prior to recommending their use in critically ill patients for analgesic purposes.

13 Regional Anesthesia Techniques

For critically ill patients, delirium and other complications can result from complex medication regimens and polypharmacy. Regional anesthesia including neuraxial blocks, peripheral nerve blocks, and truncal blocks can reduce the amount of systemic pain medications required for adequate pain control. Regional anesthetic techniques may reduce sedation requirements, thereby facilitating early mobilization, normal sleep and wake cycles, and meaningful interactions with family members and providers [12]. However, due to difficulty with positioning patients who require mechanical ventilation, with multiple lines and drains, skin edema, skin infections, hemodynamic instability, and coagulopathy, regional anesthesia techniques may be difficult to perform or even contraindicated in some critically ill patients [43]. Evidence supporting the use of regional anesthesia for analgesia in ICU patients is discussed below.

14 Neuraxial Anesthesia

Neuraxial techniques are commonly used in the ICU for pain control. For esophagectomy patients, thoracic epidural anesthesia (TEA) has been shown to reduce anastomotic leak rates and increase blood flow to the gastric conduit [44, 45]. TEA may also reduce mechanical ventilation time, reduce ICU length of stay, and decrease opioid requirements in esophagectomy patients [46]. For patients undergoing open nephrectomy, Capdevila *et al.* found that TEA significantly improved pain control and reduced opioid requirements compared to patients randomized to the morphine patient-controlled analgesia group [47]. Among patients undergoing elective abdominal aortic aneurysm repair, those who received general anesthesia with an epidural compared to general anesthesia without an epidural were less likely to require a surgical re-intervention at 30 days and less likely to develop bowel ischemia, respiratory complications, or renal failure requiring dialysis in a large retrospective analysis [48]. Among patients undergoing lung resection, TEA may reduce mortality and the risk of pulmonary complications [49]. For elective liver surgeries in the setting of cirrhosis, there may be increased risk of epidural hematoma even with normal coagulation profile due to thrombocytopenia and distended epidural veins [43]. Appropriate evaluation of risks and benefits of TEA in these patients is critical.

There is emerging evidence that patients undergoing cardiac surgery requiring full anticoagulation and cardiopulmonary bypass may also benefit from TEA. Landoni *et al.* performed a meta-analysis of 88,820 patients undergoing cardiac surgery with TEA in place. The group found a 1 in 3,552 incidence of epidural hematoma, which is approximately triple the risk in a non-cardiac surgery patient. However, they also determined the number needed to save a life was 70 cardiac surgery patients, which they suggest outweighs the risk of bleeding complications [50]. The meta-analysis further signaled a reduction in mechanical ventilation requirement and decreased incidence of myocardial infarction among patients with TEA. Although full anticoagulation on cardiopulmonary bypass has previously been considered a contraindication for neuraxial anesthesia, perhaps the benefits of analgesia and reduction in other morbidities should encourage anesthesiologists to reconsider this as an option for cardiac surgery patients.

Among patients with acute pancreatitis, there is strong evidence that TEA can improve patient analgesia and other recovery parameters [51, 52]. In animal models, TEA improves microcirculation to the pancreas due to splanchnic vasodilation from local sympathectomy [51, 52]. In these studies, TEA was associated with a decreased severity of pancreatitis on tissue exam and reduced mortality. In human patients, Al-Leswas *et al.* performed a meta-analysis of 726 patients with acute pancreatitis who received TEA [53]. Their analysis showed improvements in pain control, pancreatic perfusion, mechanical ventilation requirements, and mortality [53]. The patients who benefited most were those who received TEA early on in their hospital course. There were no major neurological complications related to TEA in this meta-analysis, suggesting TEA may not only provide significant analgesic benefit to patients with acute pancreatitis but is also safe and associated with reductions in morbidity and mortality.

Overall, neuraxial anesthesia is associated with additional benefits including improved coronary perfusion, reduced inflammation, improved intestinal perfusion and motility, and reduced respiratory complications [49]. Rodgers *et al.* performed a meta-analysis of randomized trials involving neuraxial versus non-neuraxial anesthesia and reported a reduction in thromboembolic events and transfusion requirements [54]. These implications may reduce ICU and hospital length of stay as patients are able to better mobilize and participate in rehabilitation postoperatively.

15 Other Regional Techniques

For patients in whom neuraxial anesthesia is contraindicated or for patients with localized extremity pain, alternative regional anesthesia techniques can assist with pain control in critically ill patients. Similar concerns including patient positioning, tissue edema, skin infection, hemodynamic instability, and safety of performing a block for a sedated patient should be carefully considered for truncal and peripheral blocks [43]. Assessments of neurovascular function during and after block placement may quickly identify or reduce complications such as nerve injury [43]. However, the benefits of decreased mechanical ventilation and sedation must be weighed against the potential consequences of undetected neurovascular injury. Conversations with the patient's family and multidisciplinary care team are essential to weigh these risks and benefits.

Thoracic surgery causes significant pain if not managed appropriately [55]. In addition to TEA, other regional techniques may provide similar analgesic benefits. A meta-analysis by Joshi *et al.* evaluated randomized controlled trials to compare the use of TEA, paravertebral blocks (PVB), intrathecal opioids, intercostal block, intrapleural anesthesia, and systemic pain medications for post-thoracotomy analgesia [55]. They found continuous PVB to be as effective as TEA for analgesic control but with a decreased risk of significant hypotension. Both TEA and PVB were superior to intrathecal and intercostal blocks. Systemic pain medications alone and intrapleural anesthesia were the least effective options for pain control [55].

Aside from postoperative chest wall pain, patients with traumatic rib fractures may also benefit from regional anesthesia. One small randomized controlled trial compared the use of continuous PVB and TEA for patients with three or more unilateral rib fractures [56]. Both options demonstrated similar analgesic effects, pulmonary complication incidence, opioid requirements, and ICU and hospital lengths of stay. More hypotension was noted in the TEA group, suggesting PVB may be a superior option for patients with hemodynamic instability [56]. In another randomized study, Elawamy *et al.* compared intermittent PVB and intermittent erector spinae plane (ESP) blocks for patients with multiple unilateral rib fractures and found no difference in pain reduction or time to opioid rescue request [57]. The investigators did not place continuous catheters but instead repeated single shot blocks as needed, so these results may not be generalizable to patients receiving continuous blocks. Alternatively, for interventions such as chest tube insertion, administering local anesthetic at the site or performing a single shot intercostal nerve block may provide analgesic benefit [43]. For any chest wall nerve block, there is a small risk of pneumothorax or rapid uptake of local anesthetic by intercostal vasculature [58].

For major abdominal surgery, alternatives to epidural anesthesia include transversus abdominus plane (TAP) blocks and rectus sheath blocks. TAP blocks can be helpful for analgesia at the level of T10 or below, but subcostal placement may provide higher coverage [43]. Patients undergoing surgeries including open cholecystectomy, hepatic resection, and cesarean section may benefit from TAP blocks. Rectus sheath blocks theoretically provide superior analgesia for vertical midline incisions of the upper and lower abdomen such as for an exploratory laparotomy [43]. Despite promising evidence that perioperative TAP and rectus sheath blocks can improve pain control, little is known regarding their use in critically ill patients. For open nephrectomy patients, Capdevila *et al.* found that continuous surgical site analgesia with catheters placed by the surgeons at the end of the case were equivalent to TEA for improved pain control and reduction in opioid consumption compared to patients randomized to systemic opioid analgesia [47]. Surgical site catheters were also associated with reduced pain at one month postoperatively, whereas TEA did not show this benefit [47].

For peripheral nerve blocks, a meta-analysis of 603 patients reported improved pain control at 24 hours, 48 hours, and 72 hours for all locations with continuous catheter infusions compared to those receiving only systemic opioids [59]. This analysis included both upper extremity and lower extremity nerve blocks [59]. Patients were more satisfied with analgesia in the nerve block group compared to the opioid group, and patients with blocks required less opioid for adequate analgesia [59]. Blocks can be performed for postoperative pain, traumatic injuries, and burn injuries with the same precautions as for perioperative block placement. For example, in patients with a tenuous respiratory status, an interscalene nerve block should be avoided due to ipsilateral phrenic nerve paralysis [43]. The use of peripheral nerve blocks in the ICU may in turn reduce ICU length of stay and hospital length of stay by improving patient mobility and participation in physical therapy [58]. However, peripheral nerve block administration specifically for critically ill patients requires additional consideration to determine patient selection, medication dosing, efficacy, and safety.

16 Non-pharmacological Options

From music therapy to virtual reality, non-pharmacological interventions for analgesia in the ICU vary widely depending on hospital resources and availability. Hypnosis, distraction, and virtual reality may provide some analgesic benefit [60]. Other options such as music therapy, listening to natural sounds, and emotional support can help improve critically ill patients' comfort. At advanced centers acupuncture, massage, or passive exercise are available for patients. In a scoping review by Sandvik *et al.*, evidence suggests that the most promising non-pharmacological interventions for analgesia in the ICU are acupuncture, hypnosis, and listening to natural sounds [60]. In a randomized trial specifically assessing the use of virtual reality and hypnosis for postoperative cardiac surgery patients in the ICU, Rousseaux *et al.* evaluated four modalities for their impact on recovery and analgesia—virtual reality, hypnosis, virtual reality plus hypnosis, and no intervention. All interventions showed a reduction in anxiety but no improvement in pain postoperatively [61]. There was no significant difference in opioid consumption between intervention groups [61]. Due to the limited evidence supporting the use of non-pharmacological interventions for analgesia, none of these interventions are currently recommended for routine use, and more data is needed to better understand the effects of each intervention. Availability of these modalities are limited by expense and local resources. However, these modalities may be useful in critically ill patients with limited analgesic options and may provide an additional method to alleviate anxiety and improve coping skills for pain [12].

17 The Multidisciplinary Approach to Pain Management in the ICU

The healthcare team in the ICU must balance the important need for pain management while simultaneously stabilizing and treating the critically ill patient, which requires forethought to counteract or limit the potential adverse effects associated with the administration of analgesic therapies. For this reason, pain management in the intensive care unit is a multidisciplinary challenge involving the multidisciplinary ICU team, the surgical team, and occasionally an expert acute pain team.

As one notable example, intensivists and surgeons often grapple with whether to place an epidural for patients with refractory pain who would otherwise benefit from aggressive anticoagulation. For critically ill patients with traumatic rib fractures, placement of an epidural is demonstrated in multiple studies to decrease pulmonary complications in specific patient populations [62, 63]. At the same time, patients with traumatic injuries develop hypercoagulability, with a conservative risk for development of deep venous thrombosis (DVT) of 7–12% [64]. The optimal prophylaxis for DVT in trauma patients is twice daily low molecular weight heparin. However, this thromboprophylaxis dose has been demonstrated to increase the risk of epidural hematoma and is not recommended with an indwelling epidural catheter according to the American Society of Regional Anesthesia and Pain Medicine guidelines [65]. Accordingly, an individualized and multidisciplinary decision must be made whether to prioritize optimal analgesia at the expense of less effective thromboprophylaxis. A similar multidisciplinary approach is required when considering neuraxial analgesia for patients with severe surgical pain after cardiac surgery, as this patient population commonly has postoperative coagulation deficits from cardiopulmonary bypass or may require anticoagulation for a mechanical valve replacement.

A similar collaborative approach is required to manage the hemodynamic effects of epidural analgesia in the immediate post-operative state. For large abdominal surgeries with fragile anastomoses such as a Whipple or esophagectomy, increased tissue edema and vasopressor use can threaten anastomosis viability [66–68]. Local anesthetic infused through thoracic epidurals causes an obligate sympathectomy, which can lead to increased fluid administration or vasopressor use to maintain adequate blood pressure. A balanced decision must thus be made between the surgical team, who have intricate knowledge of the patient's operative anatomy, and the multidisciplinary intensive care team, regarding the optimal dose and rate of the thoracic epidural.

Even the use of standard intravenous opioid analgesia requires careful consideration in certain critically ill patient populations, as is the case for liver transplant recipients hospitalized in the intensive care unit. Liver transplant recipients experience significant pain following surgery due to a large subcostal abdominal incision and prolonged surgical retraction [69]. Adequately treating this pain is important to allow for early liberation from the ventilator and sedation. However, nearly 25% of liver transplant patients experience early autograft dysfunction [70]. Since all opioids are hepatically metabolized, a liver transplant patient's circulating opioid level is intricately tied to graft function. Because neuraxial analgesia is rarely an option due to coagulopathy, the surgeons and ICU team must use their combined knowledge of the patient's pain level and predicted liver recovery in order to carefully dose opioids.

At many institutions, a dedicated acute pain service (APS) is available for consultation to assist with the management of challenging or refractory pain in the intensive care unit. This expert service is typically lead by an anesthesiologist who has undergone additional fellowship training in acute pain management, including regional procedures and novel pharmacologic approaches. Services offered by an

APS typically include neuraxial and regional interventions, guidance on adjunctive medical therapies such as intravenous ketamine and lidocaine infusions, and assistance managing patients with preexisting chronic pain. Multiple studies have corroborated the benefits of an APS for the management of post-operative patients, noting lower pain scores, improved patient satisfaction, and reduced post-operative opioid use [71, 72]. Since the APS has the ability to follow patients throughout their hospital stay, involving this expert team early in the intensive care hospitalization allows for continuity in pain management once the patient is stabilized.

18 Future Directions in Critical Care Pain Management

The large cohort of survivors of critical illness from the 2019 coronavirus pandemic has highlighted the need to address the significant psychological morbidity that is associated with surviving critical illness, for which the experience of pain plays a major role. One third of critical illness survivors experience chronic pain after discharge [73]. Additionally, one quarter of critical illness survivors experience post-traumatic stress disorder, with the memory of severe pain during an intensive care hospitalization significantly increasing this risk [74]. The physiologic mechanism for post-ICU chronic pain has not been fully elucidated, but is suspected to involve central sensitization from repeated noxious stimuli, similar to post-surgical chronic pain, as well as the impact of chronic inflammation on nociceptors [73]. Retrospective studies have identified risk factors for developing chronic pain following critical illness, including severe sepsis, high medical morbidity, and prolonged ICU length of stay [75–77]. Understanding that these risk factors generally align with the most critical subset of intensive care patients, exploring methods to mitigate the long-term risk of developing chronic pain in this population represents the next important frontier of analgesic therapy in the intensive care unit.

Two promising areas of research for the prevention of chronic pain following critical illness are "transitional pain clinics" and early mobilization. Transitional pain clinics are a multidisciplinary service provided to patients for three to six months following ICU discharge focused on preventing chronic pain [78]. The clinics provide psychological support and therapeutic education using a multi-disciplinary staff. They are modeled from similar clinics that have been established to successfully manage post-surgical pain [78]. Additionally, early physical therapy in the intensive care unit improves short-term quality of life and peripheral muscle strength [79, 80]. Given the interplay of mental health, chronic pain, and mobility, investigators are actively studying the benefits of early physical therapy to prevent chronic pain in critically ill patients.

19 Key Takeaways

- Pain is ubiquitous in critically ill patients and often multi-factorial. Pain in critically ill patients results from injuries, such as recent surgery or trauma, as well as routine intensive care procedures, such as repositioning and tracheal suctioning.
- Effective pain management in critically ill patients has been demonstrated to decrease the duration of mechanical ventilation and improve in-hospital mortality. Conversely, inadequate analgesia can have significant adverse consequences including increased myocardial demand and worsened delirium.
- Often critically ill patients cannot adequately communicate their pain due to pharmacologic sedation, delirium, or encephalopathy. For patients unable to communicate, clinical guidelines recommend using one of two validated tools—the Behavioral Pain Score (BPS) or the Critical Care Pain Observation Tool (CPOT).
- Unfortunately, neither the BPS nor the CPOT has been validated in critically ill patients with delirium, who comprise 26–78% of patients in intensive care units. For this patient population, clinical guidelines recommend using an "analgosedation" approach that prioritizes treatment of pain with an analgesic agent before employing sedative agents.
- Acetaminophen is a proven analgesic adjunct in critically ill patients with multiple modes of administration (oral, intravenous, per rectum). Its administration requires attention to enteric absorption and liver function.
- NSAIDs are not recommended for routine use in critically ill patients due to mixed evidence of efficacy and potential for adverse effects, including platelet dysfunction, kidney injury, and gastrointestinal irritation. However, they remain a helpful pain adjunct for the appropriate patient.
- Gabapentin, pregabalin, and carbamazepine are neuropathic pain medicines with a demonstrated opioid sparing effect in patients with Guillan-Barre syndrome and post-cardiothoracic surgery. These neuropathic pain medicines are recommended for use in critically ill patients, but notably require enteral administration.
- Opioids remain the mainstay of analgesia in critically ill patients, despite multiple adverse effects. Notably, patients on chronic opioid therapy require a dosing schedule that considers their baseline opioid regimen plus their requirement for acute pain. Methadone, sufentanil, and nalbuphine are emerging opioid therapies actively under study in critically ill patients.
- Ketamine is an NMDA antagonist that is rapidly growing as an analgesic agent for critically ill patients due to its opioid-sparing effect and lack of respiratory depression. Concerns remain about its potential to cause hallucinations and delirium, and the evidence on this topic is mixed.
- There is limited evidence to support the use of systemic lidocaine for analgesia in critically ill patients outside of the colorectal surgery population. Topical lidocaine patches have little downside and some evidence for reducing opioid requirements.
- Epidurals provide excellent analgesia in critically ill patients, with certain studies also demonstrating improved clinical outcomes in post-surgical patients and pancreatitis patients. The risk of epidural hematoma can be increased in patients

undergoing liver surgery due to complex coagulopathy and cardiac surgery patients receiving large heparin boluses for cardiopulmonary bypass. Viable alternatives to epidural analgesia include paravertebral blocks, erector spinae blocks, TAP blocks, and peripheral nerve blocks.

- Due to the adverse effects of epidurals and many analgesic medications, pain management in the intensive care unit is necessarily a multidisciplinary issue. Many institutions offer a dedicated acute pain service that provides assistance with regional procedures and medication management for refractory pain.
- Up to one third of patients discharged from the intensive care unit experience long-term chronic pain. In addition to effective analgesia, transitional pain clinics and early mobilization offer two promising strategies currently under investigation to mitigate the development of chronic pain in ICU survivors.

References

1. Phillips ML, Kuruvilla V, Bailey M. Implementation of the critical care pain observation tool increases the frequency of pain assessment for noncommunicative ICU patients. Aust Crit Care. 2019;32(5):367–72.
2. Rosenthal M, Grunow JJ, Spies CD, Mörgeli R, Paul N, Deffland M, et al. Critical care guidelines on pain, agitation and delirium management: which one to use? a systematic literature search and quality appraisal with AGREE II. J Crit Care. 2020;59:124–9.
3. Devlin JW, Skrobik Y, Gélinas C, Needham DM, Slooter AJC, Pandharipande PP, et al. Clinical practice guidelines for the prevention and management of pain, agitation/sedation, delirium, immobility, and sleep disruption in adult patients in the ICU. Crit Care Med. 2018;46(9):e825–73.
4. Puntillo KA, Max A, Timsit JF, Vignoud L, Chanques G, Robleda G, et al. Determinants of procedural pain intensity in the intensive care unit. The Europain® Study. Am J Respir Crit Care Med. 2014;189(1):39–47.
5. Chanques G, Jaber S, Barbotte E, Violet S, Sebbane M, Perrigault PF, et al. Impact of systematic evaluation of pain and agitation in an intensive care unit. Crit Care Med. 2006;34(6):1691–9.
6. Seo Y, Lee HJ, Ha EJ, Ha TS. 2021 KSCCM clinical practice guidelines for pain, agitation, delirium, immobility, and sleep disturbance in the intensive care unit. Acute Crit Care. 2022;37(1):1–25.
7. Halpern NA, Goldman DA, Tan KS, Pastores SM. Trends in critical care beds and use among population groups and medicare and medicaid beneficiaries in the United States: 2000–2010. Crit Care Med. 2016;44(8):1490–9.
8. Puntillo KA, Neuhaus J, Arai S, Paul SM, Gropper MA, Cohen NH, et al. Challenge of assessing symptoms in seriously ill intensive care unit patients: can proxy reporters help? Crit Care Med. 2012;40(10):2760–7.
9. Rijkenberg S, Stilma W, Endeman H, Bosman RJ, Oudemans-van Straaten HM. Pain measurement in mechanically ventilated critically ill patients: behavioral pain scale versus critical-care pain observation tool. J Crit Care. 2015;30(1):167–72.
10. Payen JF, Bru O, Bosson JL, Lagrasta A, Novel E, Deschaux I, et al. Assessing pain in critically ill sedated patients by using a behavioral pain scale. Crit Care Med. 2001;29(12):2258–63.
11. Gélinas C, Fortier M, Viens C, Fillion L, Puntillo K. Pain assessment and management in critically ill intubated patients: a retrospective study. Am J Crit Care. 2004;13(2):126–35.
12. Vincent JL, Shehabi Y, Walsh TS, Pandharipande PP, Ball JA, Spronk P, et al. Comfort and patient-centred care without excessive sedation: the eCASH concept. Intensive Care Med. 2016;42(6):962–71.

13. Ennis ZN, Dideriksen D, Vaegter HB, Handberg G, Pottegård A. Acetaminophen for chronic pain: a systematic review on efficacy. Basic Clin Pharmacol Toxicol. 2016;118(3):184–9.
14. Memis D, Inal MT, Kavalci G, Sezer A, Sut N. Intravenous paracetamol reduced the use of opioids, extubation time, and opioid-related adverse effects after major surgery in intensive care unit. J Crit Care. 2010;25(3):458–62.
15. Cattabriga I, Pacini D, Lamazza G, Talarico F, Di Bartolomeo R, Grillone G, et al. Intravenous paracetamol as adjunctive treatment for postoperative pain after cardiac surgery: a double blind randomized controlled trial. Eur J Cardiothorac Surg. 2007;32(3):527–31.
16. Tompkins DM, DiPasquale A, Segovia M, Cohn SM. Review of intravenous acetaminophen for analgesia in the postoperative setting. Am Surg. 2021;87(11):1809–22.
17. Hynninen MS, Cheng DC, Hossain I, Carroll J, Aumbhagavan SS, Yue R, et al. Non-steroidal anti-inflammatory drugs in treatment of postoperative pain after cardiac surgery. Can J Anaesth. 2000;47(12):1182–7.
18. Oberhofer D, Skok J, Nesek-Adam V. Intravenous ketoprofen in postoperative pain treatment after major abdominal surgery. World J Surg. 2005;29(4):446–9.
19. Pandey CK, Raza M, Tripathi M, Navkar DV, Kumar A, Singh UK. The comparative evaluation of gabapentin and carbamazepine for pain management in Guillain-Barré syndrome patients in the intensive care unit. Anesth Analg. 2005;101(1):220–5.
20. Gaber S, Saleh E, Elshaikh S, Reyad R, Elramly M, Mourad I, et al. Role of Perioperative Pregabalin in the Management of acute and chronic post-thoracotomy pain. Open Access Maced J Med Sci. 2019;7(12):1974–8.
21. Pandey CK, Bose N, Garg G, Singh N, Baronia A, Agarwal A, et al. Gabapentin for the treatment of pain in guillain-barré syndrome: a double-blinded, placebo-controlled, crossover study. Anesth Analg. 2002;95(6):1719–23.
22. Pesonen A, Suojaranta-Ylinen R, Hammarén E, Kontinen VK, Raivio P, Tarkkila P, et al. Pregabalin has an opioid-sparing effect in elderly patients after cardiac surgery: a randomized placebo-controlled trial. Br J Anaesth. 2011;106(6):873–81.
23. Ji K, Gong X, Luan T, Gao X, Zang B. Pain management of Nalbuphine and Sufentanil in patients admitted intensive care unit of different ages. BMC Emerg Med. 2022;22(1):50.
24. Elefritz JL, Murphy CV, Papadimos TJ, Lyaker MR. Methadone analgesia in the critically ill. J Crit Care. 2016;34:84–8.
25. Karamchandani K, Carr ZJ, Bonavia A, Tung A. Critical care pain management in patients affected by the opioid epidemic: a review. Ann Am Thorac Soc. 2018;15(9):1016–23.
26. Erstad BL, Patanwala AE. Ketamine for Analgosedation in critically ill patients. J Crit Care. 2016;35:145–9.
27. Perbet S, Verdonk F, Godet T, Jabaudon M, Chartier C, Cayot S, et al. Low doses of ketamine reduce delirium but not opiate consumption in mechanically ventilated and sedated ICU patients: a randomised double-blind control trial. Anaesth Crit Care Pain Med. 2018;37(6):589–95.
28. Chan K, Burry LD, Tse C, Wunsch H, De Castro C, Williamson DR. Impact of Ketamine on Analgosedative consumption in critically Ill patients: a systematic review and meta-analysis. Ann Pharmacother. 2022;56(10):1139–58.
29. Brown K, Tucker C. Ketamine for acute pain management and sedation. Crit Care Nurse. 2020;40(5):e26–32.
30. Puzio TJ, Klugh J, Wandling MW, Green C, Balogh J, Prater SJ, et al. Ketamine for acute pain after trauma: the KAPT randomized controlled trial. Trials. 2022;23(1):599.
31. Mohamed SA, Sayed DM, El Sherif FA, Abd El-Rahman AM. Effect of local wound infiltration with ketamine versus Dexmedetomidine on postoperative pain and stress after abdominal hysterectomy, a randomized trial. Eur J Pain. 2018;22(5):951–60.
32. Mansour RF, Afifi MA, Abdelghany MS. Transversus abdominis plane (TAP) block: a comparative study between Levobupivacaine versus Levobupivacaine plus Ketamine in Abdominoplasty. Pain Res Manag. 2021;2021:1762853.
33. Marret E, Rolin M, Beaussier M, Bonnet F. Meta-analysis of intravenous lidocaine and postoperative recovery after abdominal surgery. Br J Surg. 2008;95(11):1331–8.

34. Herroeder S, Pecher S, Schönherr ME, Kaulitz G, Hahnenkamp K, Friess H, et al. Systemic lidocaine shortens length of hospital stay after colorectal surgery: a double-blinded, randomized, placebo-controlled trial. Ann Surg. 2007;246(2):192–200.
35. Harvey KP, Adair JD, Isho M, Robinson R. Can intravenous lidocaine decrease postsurgical ileus and shorten hospital stay in elective bowel surgery? a pilot study and literature review. Am J Surg. 2009;198(2):231–6.
36. Swenson BR, Gottschalk A, Wells LT, Rowlingson JC, Thompson PW, Barclay M, et al. Intravenous lidocaine is as effective as epidural bupivacaine in reducing ileus duration, hospital stay, and pain after open colon resection: a randomized clinical trial. Reg Anesth Pain Med. 2010;35(4):370–6.
37. Insler SR, O'Connor M, Samonte AF, Bazaral MG. Lidocaine and the inhibition of postoperative pain in coronary artery bypass patients. J Cardiothorac Vasc Anesth. 1995;9(5):541–6.
38. Wujtewicz M, Maciejewski D, Misiołek H, Fijałkowska A, Gaszyński T, Knapik P, et al. Use of Dexmedetomidine in the adult intensive care unit. Anaesthesiol Intensive Ther. 2013;45(4):235–40.
39. Tang C, Xia Z. Dexmedetomidine in perioperative acute pain management: a non-opioid adjuvant analgesic. J Pain Res. 2017;10:1899–904.
40. Fiorelli A, Pace C, Cascone R, Carlucci A, De Ruberto E, Izzo AC, et al. Preventive skin analgesia with lidocaine patch for management of post-thoracotomy pain: results of a randomized, double blind, placebo controlled study. Thorac Cancer. 2019;10(4):631–41.
41. Liu M, Wai M, Nunez J. Topical Lidocaine patch for Postthoracotomy and Poststernotomy pain in Cardiothoracic intensive care unit adult patients. Crit Care Nurse. 2019;39(5):51–7.
42. Narang S, Gibson D, Wasan AD, Ross EL, Michna E, Nedeljkovic SS, et al. Efficacy of Dronabinol as an adjuvant treatment for chronic pain patients on opioid therapy. J Pain. 2008;9(3):254–64.
43. Rubio-Haro R, Morales-Sarabia J, Ferrer-Gomez C, de Andres J. Regional analgesia techniques for pain management in patients admitted to the intensive care unit. Minerva Anestesiol. 2019;85(10):1118–28.
44. Michelet P, Roch A, D'Journo XB, Blayac D, Barrau K, Papazian L, et al. Effect of thoracic epidural analgesia on gastric blood flow after Oesophagectomy. Acta Anaesthesiol Scand. 2007;51(5):587–94.
45. Michelet P, D'Journo XB, Roch A, Papazian L, Ragni J, Thomas P, et al. Perioperative risk factors for anastomotic leakage after Esophagectomy: influence of thoracic epidural analgesia. Chest. 2005;128(5):3461–6.
46. Heinrich S, Janitz K, Merkel S, Klein P, Schmidt J. Short- and long term effects of epidural analgesia on morbidity and mortality of Esophageal cancer surgery. Langenbecks Arch Surg. 2015;400(1):19–26.
47. Capdevila X, Moulard S, Plasse C, Peshaud JL, Molinari N, Dadure C, et al. Effectiveness of epidural analgesia, continuous surgical site analgesia, and patient-controlled analgesic morphine for postoperative pain management and hyperalgesia, rehabilitation, and health-related quality of life after open nephrectomy: a prospective, randomized. Controlled Study Anesth Analg. 2017;124(1):336–45.
48. Bardia A, Sood A, Mahmood F, Orhurhu V, Mueller A, Montealegre-Gallegos M, et al. Combined epidural-general anesthesia vs general anesthesia alone for elective abdominal aortic aneurysm repair. JAMA Surg. 2016;151(12):1116–23.
49. Freise H, Van Aken HK. Risks and benefits of thoracic epidural anaesthesia. Br J Anaesth. 2011;107(6):859–68.
50. Landoni G, Isella F, Greco M, Zangrillo A, Royse CF. Benefits and risks of epidural analgesia in cardiac surgery. Br J Anaesth. 2015;115(1):25–32.
51. Windisch O, Heidegger CP, Giraud R, Morel P, Bühler L. Thoracic epidural analgesia: a new approach for the treatment of acute pancreatitis? Crit Care. 2016;20(1):116.
52. Bachmann KA, Trepte CJ, Tomkötter L, Hinsch A, Stork J, Bergmann W, et al. Effects of thoracic epidural anesthesia on survival and microcirculation in severe acute pancreatitis: a randomized experimental trial. Crit Care. 2013;17(6):R281.

53. Al-Leswas D, Baxter N, Lim WB, Robertson F, Ratnayake B, Samanta J, et al. The safety and efficacy of epidural anaesthesia in acute pancreatitis: a systematic review and meta-analysis. HPB (Oxford). 2023;25(2):162–71.
54. Rodgers A, Walker N, Schug S, McKee A, Kehlet H, van Zundert A, et al. Reduction of postoperative mortality and morbidity with epidural or spinal anaesthesia: results from overview of randomised trials. BMJ. 2000;321(7275):1493.
55. Joshi GP, Bonnet F, Shah R, Wilkinson RC, Camu F, Fischer B, et al. A systematic review of randomized trials evaluating regional techniques for Postthoracotomy analgesia. Anesth Analg. 2008;107(3):1026–40.
56. Mohta M, Verma P, Saxena AK, Sethi AK, Tyagi A, Girotra G. Prospective, randomized comparison of continuous thoracic epidural and thoracic paravertebral infusion in patients with unilateral multiple fractured ribs–a pilot study. J Trauma. 2009;66(4):1096–101.
57. Elawamy A, Morsy MR, Ahmed MAY. Comparison of thoracic erector spinae plane block with thoracic paravertebral block for pain management in patients with unilateral multiple fractured ribs. Pain Physician. 2022;25(6):483–90.
58. De Pinto M, Dagal A, O'Donnell B, Stogicza A, Chiu S, Edwards WT. Regional anesthesia for management of acute pain in the intensive care unit. Int J Crit Illn Inj Sci. 2015;5(3):138–43.
59. Richman JM, Liu SS, Courpas G, Wong R, Rowlingson AJ, McGready J, et al. Does continuous peripheral nerve block provide superior pain control to opioids? A meta-analysis Anesth Analg. 2006;102(1):248–57.
60. Sandvik RK, Olsen BF, Rygh LJ, Moi AL. Pain relief from nonpharmacological interventions in the intensive care unit: a scoping review. J Clin Nurs. 2020;29(9–10):1488–98.
61. Rousseaux F, Dardenne N, Massion PB, Ledoux D, Bicego A, Donneau AF, et al. Virtual reality and hypnosis for anxiety and pain management in intensive care units: a prospective randomised trial among cardiac surgery patients. Eur J Anaesthesiol. 2022;39(1):58–66.
62. Bulger EM, Edwards T, Klotz P, Jurkovich GJ. Epidural analgesia improves outcome after multiple rib fractures. Surgery. 2004;136(2):426–30.
63. Carrier FM, Turgeon AF, Nicole PC, Trépanier CA, Fergusson DA, Thauvette D, et al. Effect of epidural analgesia in patients with traumatic rib fractures: a systematic review and meta-analysis of randomized controlled trials. Can J Anaesth. 2009;56(3):230–42.
64. Barrera LM, Perel P, Ker K, Cirocchi R, Farinella E, Morales Uribe CH. Thromboprophylaxis for trauma patients. Cochrane Database Syst Rev. 2013(3):CD008303.
65. Horlocker TT, Vandermeulen E, Kopp SL, Gogarten W, Leffert LR, Benzon HT. Regional anesthesia in the patient receiving antithrombotic or thrombolytic therapy: american society of regional anesthesia and pain medicine evidence-based guidelines (Fourth Edition). Reg Anesth Pain Med. 2018;43(3):263-309.
66. Han IW, Kim H, Heo J, Oh MG, Choi YS, Lee SE, et al. Excess intraoperative fluid volume administration is associated with pancreatic fistula after Pancreaticoduodenectomy: a retrospective multicenter study. Medicine (Baltimore). 2017;96(22): e6893.
67. Kubo Y, Tanaka K, Yamasaki M, Yamashita K, Makino T, Saito T, et al. The Impact of Perioperative Fluid Balance on Postoperative Complications after Esophagectomy for Esophageal Cancer. J Clin Med. 2022;11(11).
68. Theodorou D, Drimousis PG, Larentzakis A, Papalois A, Toutouzas KG, Katsaragakis S. The effects of vasopressors on perfusion of gastric graft after Esophagectomy. An experimental study J Gastrointest Surg. 2008;12(9):1497–501.
69. Milan Z. Analgesia after liver transplantation. World J Hepatol. 2015;7(21):2331–5.
70. Lee DD, Croome KP, Shalev JA, Musto KR, Sharma M, Keaveny AP, et al. Early allograft dysfunction after liver transplantation: an intermediate outcome measure for targeted improvements. Ann Hepatol. 2016;15(1):53–60.
71. Werner MU, Søholm L, Rotbøll-Nielsen P, Kehlet H. Does an acute pain service improve postoperative outcome? Anesth Analg. 2002;95(5):1361–72.
72. Said ET, Sztain JF, Abramson WB, Meineke MN, Furnish TJ, Schmidt UH, et al. A Dedicated acute pain service is associated with reduced postoperative opioid requirements in patients undergoing Cytoreductive surgery with Hyperthermic intraperitoneal chemotherapy. Anesth Analg. 2018;127(4):1044–50.

73. Pota V, Coppolino F, Barbarisi A, Passavanti MB, Aurilio C, Sansone P, et al. Pain in intensive care: a narrative review. Pain Ther. 2022;11(2):359–67.
74. Schelling G, Stoll C, Haller M, Briegel J, Manert W, Hummel T, et al. Health-related quality of life and posttraumatic stress disorder in survivors of the acute respiratory distress syndrome. Crit Care Med. 1998;26(4):651–9.
75. Battle CE, Lovett S, Hutchings H. Chronic pain in survivors of critical illness: a retrospective analysis of incidence and risk factors. Crit Care. 2013;17(3):R101.
76. Griffith DM, Salisbury LG, Lee RJ, Lone N, Merriweather JL, Walsh TS, et al. Determinants of health-related quality of life after ICU: importance of patient demographics, previous comorbidity, and severity of illness. Crit Care Med. 2018;46(4):594–601.
77. Boyle M, Murgo M, Adamson H, Gill J, Elliott D, Crawford M. The effect of chronic pain on health related quality of life amongst intensive care survivors. Aust Crit Care. 2004;17(3):104-6, 8-13.
78. Katz J, Weinrib A, Fashler SR, Katznelzon R, Shah BR, Ladak SS, et al. The Toronto general hospital transitional pain service: development and implementation of a multidisciplinary program to prevent chronic postsurgical pain. J Pain Res. 2015;8:695–702.
79. Kayambu G, Boots R, Paratz J. Physical therapy for the critically ill in the ICU: a systematic review and meta-analysis. Crit Care Med. 2013;41(6):1543–54.
80. Connolly B, O'Neill B, Salisbury L, Blackwood B, Group ERACIP. Physical rehabilitation interventions for adult patients during critical illness: an overview of systematic reviews. Thorax. 2016;71(10):881-90.

Psychological Considerations in Perioperative Acute Pain Management

John B. Silva

Abstract Psychology and pain are closely intertwined and have bidirectional effects on one another. Psychology affects the perception of pain in both positive and negative ways at the same time that pain can reduce quality of life to a point of creating psychological disorder. This chapter reviews the interplay of psychology and pain specifically in the perioperative environment. There is significant evidence to suggest that a variety of psychological conditions predispose patients to worse acute pain, with the most research identifying anxiety, depression and the thought process of catastrophizing as risk factors. Additionally, the treatment of acute pain in the perioperative period relies on the appropriate management and treatment of patient psychology by assessing risk factors for pain as well as employing pharmacologic and non-pharmacologic forms of treatment. Overall, the treatment of acute perioperative pain is a multidisciplinary endeavor with proper understanding and management of patient psychology playing a significant role.

Keywords Psychology · Pain · Acute pain · Anxiety · Depression · Catastrophizing

1 Psychology and Perioperative Pain Management

2 Introduction

Acute pain following surgery has been reported in as high as 86% of patients [1–4]. Evidence demonstrates that uncontrolled perioperative pain is associated with a demonstrable worsening of patient outcomes including opioid abuse, chronic pain

J. B. Silva (✉)
Department of Anesthesiology, University of Wisconsin, Madison, Wisconsin, USA
e-mail: jbsilva@wisc.edu

A. Abd-Elsayed and K. Schroeder (eds.), *Perioperative Pain Management*,
https://doi.org/10.1007/978-3-031-67648-2_15

development, delirium, increased hospital length of stay, decreased patient satisfaction, increased complications and increased cost [5–8]. Therefore, proper management of perioperative pain has become essential to optimal patient care and has increasingly been used as an indicator to judge the quality of intramural healthcare.

Pain itself can be subdivided into a four-part process of transduction, transmission, modulation and perception. The process begins with noxious stimuli being transduced into neural information via nociceptors. These signals are then transmitted from peripheral nerves to the central nervous system where the pain stimulus continues from one neuron to another and is modulated by input from descending facilitatory and inhibitory nerves, neurotransmitters and local signaling factors before terminating in the cerebral cortex. The final step is the act of perception where the signal is then integrated with cognitive, emotional and sensory characteristics. It is this last step that converts the process of nociception, a unidimensional biological process resulting from the stimulation of nerves that convey potential tissue damage, to pain, the subjective multidimensional experience contextualizing nociception.

The experience of pain is influenced by a variety of factors including genetics, prior experiences, sociocultural influences and psychological status [9]. Because of this, the relationship of nociception to pain is non-linear, with similar nociceptive inputs causing a spectrum of pain responses in different patients [10]. Additionally, the relationship of pain and psychology is bidirectional with increased pain leading to psychological dysfunction and psychological dysfunction being strongly associated with increased pain [9]. Studies assessing predictors of acute postoperative pain after surgery find psychological factors to be leading predictors of post-surgical pain and analgesic consumption [11, 12].

Perioperative pain management focuses on the management of acute pain which is classified as pain that lasts less than three months [13] and is primarily the result of an insult such as trauma, surgery or significant disease. Acute pain serves a useful biologic purpose and is limited to the resolution of the disease state. This is in contrast to chronic pain which lasts longer than three months, and is often related to altered activities of the neurologic system such as altered activity of peripheral nerve fibers or central pain related to abnormalities in the responsiveness to neural activity or psychological states. Chronic pain does not serve a biologic purpose, has no endpoint and often lasts longer than the time of healing. These differing characteristics lead to differences in treatment approaches with acute pain management focusing primarily on interrupting nociception. In contrast, chronic pain management has historically employed a multidisciplinary approach and involved more than one therapeutic modality [14]. Due to the classical difference in treatment approach, understanding and treating the psychology related to a patient's pain has classically resided in the purview of chronic pain treatment, however more and more research has shown that psychology plays an important role in acute pain as well.

3 Psychological Issues that Predispose Patients to Acute Pain

Anxiety

Anxiety is defined as an emotion characterized by an unpleasant state of inner turmoil in anticipation of a future threat [15]. Anxiety ranges from adaptive anxiety that allows for preparation for future challenges to pathological anxiety such as generalized anxiety disorder, panic disorder and phobias. The distinction between the two is typically diagnosed by symptoms of anxiety that are excessive, persisting for more than 6 months, causing dysfunction in various domains of life and inhibiting activities of daily living [15].

Anxiety has repeatedly been shown to be correlated and in some cases a predictor of acute postoperative pain after elective surgery across multiple studies and metanalyses [11, 12, 16, 17]. In fact, a metanalysis performed by Hui Yun et al. of 48 studies found anxiety to be the most commonly found predictive factor of postoperative pain. This relationship has been demonstrated across multiple subtypes of surgeries including gastrointestinal surgery [18–20], obstetrics and gynecologic surgery [21–23], thoracic surgery [24], breast surgery [25], spine surgery [26] and dental procedures [11]. Moreover, some studies have found direct correlations between anxiety and post-operative analgesic consumption [25, 27].

One important delineation when assessing anxiety is assessing trait versus state anxiety. State anxiety is a transient reaction to an adverse situation while trait anxiety is a more stable personality attribute in experiencing events [28]. Magnetic resonance imaging of the brain shows that these separate forms of anxiety are mapped differently in the human brain with trait anxiety related to structural configurations of the brain while state anxiety correlates with functional patterns of the brain [29]. Some studies have found state anxiety[18] to be a significant predictor of post-operative pain, while other have suggested that trait anxiety[30] is similarly associated with pain. It is unclear if either type of anxiety is a stronger predictor of post-operative acute pain, however it is important to understand the distinction and further study is required to assess which anxiety type is more strongly correlated with postoperative pain.

Depression

Depression is a common mood disorder affecting 4.4% of the world's population [31]. It generally revolves around feelings of sadness that lead to symptoms of fatigue, weight loss, feelings of worthlessness, anhedonia, insomnia, and difficulty concentrating. In severe cases, depression symptomology includes suicide and/or major effects on a patient's ability to function in society. The Diagnostic and Statistical

Manual of Mental Disorders Fifth Edition has multiple subtypes of depressive disorders that make up a spectrum from dysthymia to major depression with psychotic features, depending on the severity and duration of symptoms [32].

Pain and depression are frequently comorbid conditions, with an estimated 13% of the elderly population suffering simultaneously from the two conditions [33]. Pain and depression have bidirectional influences on one another with pain demonstrating an ability to decrease quality of life and increase the risk of depression[34]. Conversely, individuals who suffer from major depressive disorder are more likely to suffer from chronic pain[34]. This association is so closely intertwined that it is remarkably common for patients suffering from depression to present exclusively with physical symptoms including pain [35]. Evidence linking the perception of pain and depression symptomology continues to evolve. Some have theorized that depressed patients experience an altered perception of pain that may be manifested as a lower pain threshold [36], a higher threshold [37], with some studies demonstrating no difference [38].

An evaluation of depressed patient's undergoing laparoscopic cholecystectomy by De Cosmo et al. with self-rating questionnaire found that not only did depressed patients have higher pain indicators during the postoperative 24 hours, but regression analysis revealed that tramadol consumption could be predicted by preoperative depression[19]. An assessment of acute pain in the postoperative, post-labor, post-cesarean and dental setting performed by Barman et al. found a statistically significant and strong correlation between depression and acute pain across multiple clinical settings [39].

The bidirectional nature of the depression pain relationship was further demonstrated by Eisenach who found that severe acute postpartum pain led to a 2.5-3 fold increase in postpartum depression[40]. Another facet of this relationship is that sometimes the presence of pain has the additional negative effect of preventing the proper recognition and management of depression[41]. Given this tight relationship between depression and pain, it is clear that the appropriate approach to perioperative pain includes a simultaneous treatment of both.

Catastrophizing

Research into the relationship between psychology and acute pain is not limited to mood disorders. Specific cognitive processes have been evaluated with the thought process of catastrophizing having frequently been shown to be one of the most important predictors of post-operative acute pain. Catastrophizing is defined as an exaggerated negative orientation to aversive stimuli that involves rumination about painful sensations, magnification of threat value of the painful stimulus and perceived inability to control pain [42]. Catastrophizing is significantly correlated with mood and personality variables such as depression, fear of pain, coping strategies, and state and trait anxiety[18].

An analysis of 1490 patients found that one of the strongest predictors of moderate to intense post-operative pain was found in patients who held catastrophizing cognitions about the meaning of pain [12]. This relationship between pain catastrophizing and pain has been replicated in orthopaedic [43], gynecological [44], thoracic [45], and dental surgery/procedures [46]. A 2005 study by Granot demonstrated a strikingly and direct linear correlation between the pain catastrophizing scale and pain score.

A variety of theoretical conceptualizations have been proposed that seek to understand the cognitive process of pain catastrophizing[47]. The first is an attention bias in information processing that either focuses on sensory and affective pain information and amplifies it, or is unable to inhibit pain-related cognitions, to a point that interrupts ongoing mental processes [48]. There is also an appraisal theory where a potential stressor undergoes a primary appraisal as to whether or not it is a severely negative experience, and a secondary appraisal as to whether or not the person feels they can control it [49]. There is theorized to be a communal coping component where catastrophizing pain elicits behaviors that engender support from others [50]. This action and response can create a feedback loop that incentivizes further catastrophizing and exaggeration of pain responses. The final component is a neural component where pain catastrophizing repeatedly activates and reinforces certain brain regions implicated in the processing of pain signals in the spine and brain [49, 51].

4 Management of Psychology in the Perioperative Setting

Given the close and reciprocal relationship of psychology and acute pain, proper management and understanding of psychological conditions can theoretically lead to better pain control and better pain control can improve the psychological health of patients. Therefore, the remainder of this chapter addresses psychologically focused interventions that can improve acute pain.

Psychological Protective Factors

Research into the relationship between psychology and acute pain has focused predominantly on factors associated with worsened acute pain outcomes. Significantly less research has focused on identifying and analyzing potentially protective psychological factors. Bruce J et al. evaluated the concept of psychological robustness, a concept associated with higher values of dispositional optimism, lower values of trait anxiety, and decreased depression. Evaluation of this variable found that the presence of higher levels of psychological robustness predicted a lower incidence of chronic pain at 4 months in women undergoing breast cancer surgery [52].

More specifically, trait optimism has been found to improve post-operative pain outcomes. A systematic review of the effects of trait optimism in the post-operative recovery from coronary artery graft surgery found that optimism was associated with reduced pain after surgery and significant improvements in several categories of recovery, including reduced rehospitalization rate, complications, pain, improved quality of life, and enhanced rate of return to normal life and psychological status [53]. Notably, this relationship becomes more nuanced when evaluating optimistic pre-surgical expectations of post-operative outcomes. As a whole, the evidence strongly supports an association between optimistic expectations and positive psychosocial outcomes if expectations are based in reality. However, if preoperative optimism is unrealistic, this optimism can become a liability and lead to worse outcomes [54].

Another trait that has been shown to be beneficial in preventing acute post-operative pain is an individual's propensity to engage in adaptive health behaviors. A multicenter study performed by Andrawis J et al. evaluated patient activation, which is a measure of an individual's propensity to engage in adaptive health behaviors, and found that higher preoperative activation was associated with better pain relief, decreased pain symptoms, improved mental health and greater satisfaction after total joint arthroplasty [55]. A similar and related study evaluating self-efficacy, otherwise known as the conviction that one can successfully execute the behavior required to produce the outcomes desired, found that self-efficacy was found to be a significant preoperative predictor of functional ability but was unrelated to reports of postoperative pain[56].

Overall, there is a dearth of research into the psychological traits and cognitive thought processes that reduce post-operative acute pain, but what there is suggests that individuals who have a generally positive outlook and adaptability are the least likely to experience post-operative pain and most likely to recover better. Further research is needed to validate risk stratifying patients based on psychological factors as well as evaluate if there are any preoperative interventions that can improve these positive traits preoperatively.

Pre-operative Psychological Intervention

Analysis of the efficacy of psychological interventions on pain has primarily been done in the realm of chronic pain. Psychosocial interventions have been shown to be beneficial in the management of arthritis and cancer pain[57, 58]. Cognitive behavioral therapy has been shown to have beneficial effects on the pain experience [59], however more recent metanalyses have found the benefit to be small for reducing pain, disability and distress related to chronic pain (excluding headache) in adults [60]. Similarly, evaluations of mindfulness and its effect on musculoskeletal pain have found mixed results across a range of outcomes (pain, sleep quality, depression, quality of life, physical functioning, mindfulness) [61]. A Cochrane review of psychological interventions for chronic, non-specific low back pain found that psychological interventions are most effective and sustainable when delivered as part of a multidisciplinary approach that includes physiotherapy, pain education and behavioral therapy [62]. One difficulty associated with analyzing psychological interventions in the treatment or prevention of pain is the breadth of psychological interventions available and the variability in intervention implementation. It is difficult to make a definitive statement on the usefulness of psychological therapy in chronic pain management, but it seems likely that psychological interventions do have beneficial effects, however modest, and are best used as a component of a multidisciplinary approach[62].

A similar conclusion can be found when looking into the realm of perioperative pain management, however, given the significant difference in nature between chronic and perioperative pain, there are a host of other potential psychological interventions available. A Cochrane review that evaluated psychological interventions associated with reductions in needle-related procedural pain and distress in children and adolescents found evidence to support the efficacy of distraction, hypnosis, cognitive-behavioral therapy and breathing interventions [63]. Some hospitals are even testing out the effects of virtual reality interventions with mixed results [64, 65]. Psychoeducational preparation has also been shown to have positive outcomes [66]. Studies evaluating strategies to reduce patients' anxiety and pain prior to c-section found that patient familiarity with the cesarean section operation and operating room environment caused a decline in anxiety prior to c-section, reductions in pain scores after the operation, and enhanced hemodynamic stability [67, 68]. Recent metanalyses have suggested that psychological preparation may improve postoperative pain, behavioral recovery, and reduce hospital length of stay. Unfortunately, the evidence was insufficient to reach firm conclusions at this time [69].

Given the documented effects of pre-operative anxiety and catastrophizing thought processes, it stands to reason that pre-operative relaxation techniques may also have a beneficial effect. A randomized controlled trial evaluating the preoperative administration of quick, basic relaxation exercises in the setting arthroscopic shoulder repair showed that these patients experienced less postoperative pain and used appreciably lower opioid analgesic doses over the first 2 weeks following surgery [70]. However, this success has not been replicated in other contexts [71].

Much like chronic pain, given the modest gains of seemingly all interventions, post-operative acute pain will also require employment of a multidisciplinary approach across multiple treatment vectors. Employment of a multidisciplinary management team at Toronto General Hospital Transitional Pain Service that consists of pain physicians, advanced practice nurses, psychologists and physical therapists has shown promising results with another randomized control trial underway in several Ontario hospitals [72].

Pre-operative Pharmacological Interventions

There are a host of medications used in the perioperative setting that affect both pain and psychology in the perioperative setting. Given the significant overlap of the two, it can be difficult to discern what is being treated at any given time.

Opioids are a mainstay in the treatment of perioperative pain, the effectiveness of which is so well established that it doesn't require exploration. More recently, however, there has been exploration into the role of opioid peptides and their receptors (mu, delta and kappa) as novel targets for antidepressant therapy [73]. In fact, there is accumulating evidence from animal research models that the opioid system exerts highly distinct controls over mood-related processes with delta opioid receptor agonist and kappa mu receptor agonists shown to have promising antidepressant potential [74, 75]. Unfortunately, study into this area is limited by the high abuse potential of these drugs. Additionally, these studies have to be weighed against other studies that have shown that longer durations of opioid use are associated with new-onset depression[76].

Selective serotonin reuptake inhibitors and serotonin-norepinephrine reuptake inhibitors are a mainstay of depression treatment; however, less is known about their role as adjuncts for postoperative pain management. A metanalysis evaluating their use in standard perioperative care found a small reduction in both acute and chronic postoperative pain and opioid consumption, as well as a small improvement in patient satisfaction [77].

Again, given the documented effects of pre-operative anxiety and catastrophizing thought processes, it stands to reason that medications focused on treating pre-operative anxiety would have a beneficial effect. A study by Kain et al. found that patients treated with a benzodiazepine (midazolam) 30 minutes before surgery reported a greater reduction in postoperative pain throughout the first postoperative week and a greater decrease of anxiety through the first post-operative month [78]. Unfortunately, this finding was not found by the same study group one year later when evaluating preoperative treatment with lorazepam and midazolam for women undergoing abdominal hysterectomy [79]. Other anxiolytic medications have been evaluated including alpha-2 agonists (e.g., clonidine and dexmedetomidine) which resulted in a reduction in post-operative opioid consumption, pain intensity and nausea [80]. Gabapentin and pregabalin represent another pharmacologic class of agents possessing promise in reducing post-operative acute pain. At this time, mixed results limit the ability to make strong clinical recommendations [81–83].

5 Conclusions

Ultimately, surgical recovery is complicated and multifaceted as patients deal with pain, disability and multiple setbacks in the setting of an often-uncertain future. There will never be a single panacea that will solve perioperative acute pain in its entirety. However, what is clear is that psychology and pain are closely intertwined and psychology affects the perception of pain both positively and negatively. There is significant evidence to suggest that psychological conditions predispose patients to worse acute pain and that proper treatment of acute pain in the perioperative period includes the assessment, management and treatment of patient psychology. The benefits of this focus are likely to be modest and difficult to understand given the complex nature of psychology and the wide variety of potential interventions, however, what is clear is that the proper treatment of psychological derangements in an integral component of the multimodal and multidisciplinary management of perioperative pain.

Key Takeaways

- Psychology plays a significant role in the higher order perception and experience of pain.
- Severe pain can have a significant effect on psychology and reduce quality of life to a point that precipitates psychological dysfunction.
- Psychologic risk factors for severe acute pain after surgery include anxiety, depression, and the thought process of catastrophizing.
- There are a variety of pharmacologic and non-pharmacological psychological interventions that have shown some promise in the reduction of acute pain.
- The understanding and treatment of psychology and acute pain represents a significant component of the multimodal and multidisciplinary approach required to best treat acute pain.

References

1. Apfelbaum JL, Chen C, Mehta SS, Gan and TJ. Postoperative pain experience: results from a national survey suggest postoperative pain continues to be undermanaged. Anesth Analg. 2003 Aug;97(2):534–40.
2. Gan TJ, Habib AS, Miller TE, White W, Apfelbaum JL. Incidence, patient satisfaction, and perceptions of post-surgical pain: results from a US national survey. Curr Med Res Opin. 2014;30(1):149–60.
3. Buvanendran A, Fiala J, Patel KA, Golden AD, Moric M, Kroin JS. The incidence and severity of postoperative pain following inpatient surgery. Pain Med. 2015;16(12):2277–83.
4. Sommer M, de Rijke JM, van Kleef M, Kessels AGH, Peters ML, Geurts JWJM, et al. The prevalence of postoperative pain in a sample of 1490 surgical inpatients. Eur J Anaesthesiol. 2008;25(4):267–74.
5. Ranawat AS, Ranawat CS. Pain management and accelerated rehabilitation for total hip and total knee arthroplasty. J Arthroplasty. 2007;22(7):12–5.
6. van Boekel RLM, Warlé MC, Nielen RGC, Vissers KCP, van der Sande R, Bronkhorst EM, et al. Relationship between postoperative pain and overall 30-day complications in a broad surgical population. Ann Surg. 2019;269(5):856–65.
7. Gan TJ. Poorly controlled postoperative pain: prevalence, consequences, and prevention. J Pain Res. 2017;10:2287–98.

8. Hanley C, Ladha KS, Clarke HA, Cuthbertson BC, Wijeysundera DN. Association of postoperative complications with persistent post-surgical pain: a multicentre prospective cohort study. Br J Anaesth. 2022;128(2):311–20.
9. Gatchel RJ, Peng YB, Peters ML, Fuchs PN, Turk DC. The biopsychosocial approach to chronic pain: scientific advances and future directions. Psychol Bull. 2007;133(4):581–624.
10. Wiech K, Ploner M, Tracey I. Neurocognitive aspects of pain perception. Trends Cogn Sci. 2008;12(8):306–13.
11. Ip HYV, Abrishami A, Peng PWH, Wong J, Chung F. Predictors of postoperative pain and analgesic consumption. Anesthesiology. 2009;111(3):657–77.
12. Sommer M, de Rijke JM, van Kleef M, Kessels AGH, Peters ML, Geurts JW, et al. Predictors of acute postoperative pain after elective surgery. Clin J Pain. 2010;26(2):87–94.
13. Classification of chronic pain. Descriptions of chronic pain syndromes and definitions of pain terms. Prepared by the international association for the study of pain, Subcommittee on Taxonomy. Pain Suppl. 1986;3:S1–226.
14. Auvenshine RC. Acute versus chronic pain. Tex Dent J. 2000 Jul;117(7):14–20.
15. Chand SP, Marwaha R. Anxiety. 2022.
16. Coppes OJM, Yong RJ, Kaye AD, Urman RD. Patient and surgery-related predictors of acute postoperative pain. Curr Pain Headache Rep. 2020;24(4):12.
17. Vaughn F, Wichowski H, Bosworth G. Does preoperative anxiety level predict postoperative pain? AORN J. 2007;85(3):589–604.
18. Granot M, Ferber SG. The roles of pain catastrophizing and anxiety in the prediction of postoperative pain intensity. Clin J Pain. 2005;21(5):439–45.
19. De Cosmo G, Congedo E, Lai C, Primieri P, Dottarelli A, Aceto P. Preoperative psychologic and demographic predictors of pain perception and tramadol consumption using intravenous patient-controlled analgesia. Clin J Pain. 2008;24(5):399–405.
20. Aceto P, Lai C, Perilli V, Sacco T, Modesti C, Raffaelli M, et al. Factors affecting acute pain perception and analgesics consumption in patients undergoing bariatric surgery. Physiol Behav. 2016;1(163):1–6.
21. Pud D, Amit A. Anxiety as a predictor of pain magnitude following termination of first-trimester pregnancy. Pain Med. 2005;6(2):143–8.
22. Rudin A, Wölner-Hanssen P, Hellbom M, Werner MU. Prediction of post-operative pain after a laparoscopic tubal ligation procedure. Acta Anaesthesiol Scand. 2008;52(7):938–45.
23. Kain ZN, Sevarino F, Alexander GM, Pincus S, Mayes LC. Preoperative anxiety and postoperative pain in women undergoing hysterectomy. J Psychosom Res. 2000;49(6):417–22.
24. Bachiocco V, Morselli-Labate AM, Rusticali AG, Bragaglia R, Mastrorilli M, Carli G. Intensity, latency and duration of post-thoracotomy pain: relationship to personality traits. Funct Neurol. 1990;5(4):321–32.
25. Hosgor H, Coskunses FM, Tokuc B. Correlation between preoperative pressure pain assessments and anxiety and postoperative pain in impacted lower third molar surgery. J Korean Assoc Oral Maxillofac Surg. 2021;47(1):15–9.
26. Costelloe C, Burns S, Yong RJ, Kaye AD, Urman RD. An analysis of predictors of persistent postoperative pain in spine surgery. Curr Pain Headache Rep. 2020;24(4):11.
27. Pan PH, Coghill R, Houle TT, Seid MH, Lindel WM, Parker RL, et al. Multifactorial preoperative predictors for Postcesarean section pain and analgesic requirement. Anesthesiology. 2006;104(3):417–25.
28. State-Trait SS, Inventory A. In: Encyclopedia of personality and individual differences. Cham: Springer International Publishing; 2018. p. 1–3.
29. Saviola F, Pappaianni E, Monti A, Grecucci A, Jovicich J, De Pisapia N. Trait and state anxiety are mapped differently in the human brain. Sci Rep. 2020;10(1):11112.
30. Caumo W, Schmidt AP, Schneider CN, Bergmann J, Iwamoto CW, Adamatti LC, et al. Preoperative predictors of moderate to intense acute postoperative pain in patients undergoing abdominal surgery. Acta Anaesthesiol Scand. 2002;46(10):1265–71.
31. Depression and other common mental disorders: global health estimates. World Health organization. 2017.

32. Regier DA, Kuhl EA, Kupfer DJ. The DSM-5: classification and criteria changes. World Psychiatry. 2013;12(2):92–8.
33. Zis P, Daskalaki A, Bountouni I, Sykioti P, Varrassi G, Paladini A. Depression and chronic pain in the elderly: links and management challenges. Clin Interv Aging. 2017;12:709–20.
34. Jackson T, Chen H, Iezzi T, Yee M, Chen F. Prevalence and correlates of chronic pain in a random population study of adults in Chongqing. China Clin J Pain. 2014;30(4):346–52.
35. Stahl SM. Does depression hurt? J Clin Psychiatry. 2002;63(4):273–4.
36. Nitzan U, Hecht M, Braw Y, Maoz H, Levkovitz Y, Yarnitsky D, et al. Initial evaluation of pain intensity among depressed patients as a possible mediator between depression and pain complaints. Front Psychiatry. 2019;10:48.
37. Schwier C, Kliem A, Boettger MK, Bär KJ. Increased cold-pain thresholds in major depression. J Pain. 2010;11(3):287–90.
38. Hermesdorf M, Berger K, Baune BT, Wellmann J, Ruscheweyh R, Wersching H. Pain sensitivity in patients with major depression: differential effect of pain sensitivity measures, somatic cofactors, and disease characteristics. J Pain. 2016;17(5):606–16.
39. Barman D, Mishra S, Mishra J, Mahapatra P, Manjareeka M. association between depression and acute pain in adults attending a tertiary care hospital in Bhubaneswar. J Clin Diagn Res. 2015 Jul;9(7):CC08-11.
40. Eisenach JC, Pan PH, Smiley R, Lavand'homme P, Landau R, Houle TT. Severity of acute pain after childbirth, but not type of delivery, predicts persistent pain and postpartum depression. Pain. 2008 Nov 15;140(1):87–94.
41. Bair MJ, Robinson RL, Katon W, Kroenke K. Depression and pain comorbidity: a literature review. Arch Intern Med. 2003;163(20):2433–45.
42. Rosenstiel AK, Keefe FJ. The use of coping strategies in chronic low back pain patients: relationship to patient characteristics and current adjustment. Pain. 1983;17(1):33–44.
43. Riddle DL, Wade JB, Jiranek WA, Kong X. Preoperative pain catastrophizing predicts pain outcome after knee arthroplasty. Clin Orthop Relat Res. 2010;468(3):798–806.
44. Strulov L, Zimmer EZ, Granot M, Tamir A, Jakobi P, Lowenstein L. Pain catastrophizing, response to experimental heat stimuli, and post-Cesarean section pain. J Pain. 2007;8(3):273–9.
45. Bayman EO, Parekh KR, Keech J, Larson N, Vander Weg M, Brennan TJ. Preoperative patient expectations of postoperative pain are associated with moderate to severe acute pain after VATS. Pain Med. 2019;20(3):543–54.
46. Altan A, Akkoç S, Erdil A, Çolak S, Demir O, Altan H. Effects of pain catastrophizing and anxiety on analgesic use after surgical removal of impacted mandibular third molars. J Dent Anesth Pain Med. 2019;19(6):379–88.
47. Quartana PJ, Campbell CM, Edwards RR. Pain catastrophizing: a critical review. Expert Rev Neurother. 2009;9(5):745–58.
48. Eccleston C, Crombez G. Pain demands attention: a cognitive-affective model of the interruptive function of pain. Psychol Bull. 1999;125(3):356–66.
49. Sullivan MJL, Thorn B, Haythornthwaite JA, Keefe F, Martin M, Bradley LA, et al. Theoretical perspectives on the relation between catastrophizing and pain. Clin J Pain. 2001;17(1):52–64.
50. Keefe FJ, Lipkus I, Lefebvre JC, Hurwitz H, Clipp E, Smith J, et al. The social context of gastrointestinal cancer pain: a preliminary study examining the relation of patient pain catastrophizing to patient perceptions of social support and caregiver stress and negative responses. Pain. 2003;103(1–2):151–6.
51. Gracely RH, Geisser ME, Giesecke T, Grant MAB, Petzke F, Williams DA, et al. Pain catastrophizing and neural responses to pain among persons with fibromyalgia. Brain. 2004;127(Pt 4):835–43.
52. Bruce J, Thornton AJ, Powell R, Johnston M, Wells M, Heys SD, et al. Psychological, surgical, and sociodemographic predictors of pain outcomes after breast cancer surgery: a population-based cohort study. Pain. 2014;155(2):232–43.
53. Arsyi DH, Permana PBD, Karim RI, Abdurachman. The role of optimism in manifesting recovery outcomes after coronary artery bypass graft surgery: a systematic review. J Psychosom Res. 2022 Nov;162:111044.

54. Sweeny K, Andrews SE. Should patients be optimistic about surgery? Resolving a conflicted literature. Health Psychol Rev. 2017;11(4):374–86.
55. Andrawis J, Akhavan S, Chan V, Lehil M, Pong D, Bozic KJ. Higher preoperative patient activation associated with better patient-reported outcomes after total joint arthroplasty. Clin Orthop Relat Res. 2015;473(8):2688–97.
56. Wylde V, Dixon S, Blom AW. The role of preoperative self-efficacy in predicting outcome after total knee replacement. Musculoskeletal Care. 2012;10(2):110–8.
57. Dixon KE, Keefe FJ, Scipio CD, Perri LM, Abernethy AP. Psychological interventions for arthritis pain management in adults: a meta-analysis. Health Psychol. 2007;26(3):241–50.
58. Sheinfeld Gorin S, Krebs P, Badr H, Janke EA, Jim HSL, Spring B, et al. Meta-analysis of psychosocial interventions to reduce pain in patients with cancer. J Clin Oncol. 2012;30(5):539–47.
59. Morley S, Eccleston C, Williams A. Systematic review and meta-analysis of randomized controlled trials of cognitive behaviour therapy and behaviour therapy for chronic pain in adults, excluding headache. Pain. 1999;80(1–2):1–13.
60. Williams AC de C, Fisher E, Hearn L, Eccleston C. Psychological therapies for the management of chronic pain (excluding headache) in adults. Cochrane Database Syst Rev. 2020 Aug 12;8(8):CD007407.
61. Cardle P, Kumar S, Leach M, McEvoy M, Veziari Y. Mindfulness and Chronic Musculoskeletal pain: an umbrella review. J Multidiscip Healthc. 2023;16:515–33.
62. Ho EKY, Chen L, Simic M, Ashton-James CE, Comachio J, Wang DXM, et al. Psychological interventions for chronic, non-specific low back pain: systematic review with network meta-analysis. BMJ. 2022;30(376): e067718.
63. Birnie KA, Noel M, Chambers CT, Uman LS, Parker JA. Psychological interventions for needle-related procedural pain and distress in children and adolescents. Cochrane Database Syst Rev. 2018 Oct 4;10(10):CD005179.
64. Addab S, Hamdy R, Thorstad K, Le May S, Tsimicalis A. Use of virtual reality in managing paediatric procedural pain and anxiety: an integrative literature review. J Clin Nurs. 2022;31(21–22):3032–59.
65. Lambert V, Boylan P, Boran L, Hicks P, Kirubakaran R, Devane D, et al. Virtual reality distraction for acute pain in children. Cochrane Database Syst Rev. 2020;10(10):CD010686.
66. Johnston M, Vogele C. Benefits of psychological preparation for surgery: a meta-analysis. Ann Behav Med. 1993;15(4):245–56.
67. Eslami J, Hatami N, Amiri A, Akbarzadeh M. The potential beneficial effects of education and familiarity with Cesarean section procedure and the operating room environment on promotion of anxiety and pain intensity: a randomized controlled clinical trial. J Educ Health Promot. 2020;9:240.
68. Mostafayi M, Imani B, Zandi S, Jongi F. The effect of familiarization with preoperative care on anxiety and vital signs in the patient's Cesarean section: a randomized controlled trial. Eur J Midwifery. 2021;5:21.
69. Powell R, Scott NW, Manyande A, Bruce J, Vögele C, Byrne-Davis LMT, et al. Psychological preparation and postoperative outcomes for adults undergoing surgery under general anaesthesia. Cochrane Database Syst Rev. 2016;2016(5):CD008646.
70. Weekes DG, Campbell RE, Wicks ED, Hadley CJ, Chaudhry ZS, Carter AH, et al. Do relaxation exercises decrease pain after arthroscopic rotator cuff repair? a randomized controlled trial. Clin Orthop Relat Res. 2021;479(5):870–84.
71. Gavin M, Litt M, Khan A, Onyiuke H, Kozol R. A prospective, randomized trial of cognitive intervention for postoperative pain. Am Surg. 2006;72(5):414–8.
72. Katz J, Weinrib AZ, Clarke H. Chronic postsurgical pain: from risk factor identification to multidisciplinary management at the Toronto General Hospital transitional pain service. Can J Pain. 2019;3(2):49–58.
73. Berrocoso E, Sánchez-Blázquez P, Garzón J, Mico JA. Opiates as antidepressants. Curr Pharm Des. 2009;15(14):1612–22.

74. Lutz PE, Kieffer BL. Opioid receptors: distinct roles in mood disorders. Trends Neurosci. 2013;36(3):195–206.
75. Browne CA, Lucki I. Targeting opioid dysregulation in depression for the development of novel therapeutics. Pharmacol Ther. 2019;201:51–76.
76. Salas J, Scherrer JF, Schneider FD, Sullivan MD, Bucholz KK, Burroughs T, et al. New-onset depression following stable, slow, and rapid rate of prescription opioid dose escalation. Pain. 2017;158(2):306–12.
77. Wang L, Tobe J, Au E, Tran C, Jomy J, Oparin Y, et al. Selective serotonin reuptake inhibitors and serotonin-norepinephrine reuptake inhibitors as adjuncts for postoperative pain management: systematic review and meta-analysis of randomised controlled trials. Br J Anaesth. 2022;128(1):118–34.
78. Kain ZN, Sevarino F, Pincus S, Alexander GM, Wang SM, Ayoub C, et al. Attenuation of the preoperative stress response with midazolam: effects on postoperative outcomes. Anesthesiology. 2000;93(1):141–7.
79. Kain ZN, Sevarino FB, Rinder C, Pincus S, Alexander GM, Ivy M, et al. Preoperative anxiolysis and postoperative recovery in women undergoing abdominal hysterectomy. Anesthesiology. 2001;94(3):415–22.
80. Blaudszun G, Lysakowski C, Elia N, Tramèr MR. Effect of perioperative systemic α2 agonists on postoperative morphine consumption and pain intensity: systematic review and meta-analysis of randomized controlled trials. Anesthesiology. 2012;116(6):1312–22.
81. Adegboye KA, Kolawole IK, Bolaji BO, Suleiman ZA, Adegboye MB. Post-operative Analgesic and opioid-sparing effect of a single-dose pre-operative oral Pregabalin in gynaecological surgeries. J West Afr Coll Surg. 2022;12(3):1–7.
82. Hu J, Huang D, Li M, Wu C, Zhang J. Effects of a single dose of preoperative Pregabalin and gabapentin for acute postoperative pain: a network meta-analysis of randomized controlled trials. J Pain Res. 2018;11:2633–43.
83. Ni J, Jiang J, Mao S, Sun RF. Pregabalin does not decrease acute pain or postoperative nausea and vomiting after hysterectomy: a meta-analysis. J Int Med Res. 2020;48(12):300060520954720.

Pain Management in Children

Leah Margalit Winters Webb, Erin Adams, Billy McElroy, Ashley Reid, and Kim M. Strupp

Abstract Until the 1980s, it was a widely held belief that premature infants and newborns did not feel pain. In the decades since, research supports that these patients do, in fact, feel pain and moreover that there are deleterious effects of poorly controlled or untreated pain in patients from newborn to adolescence. Pain assessment and treatment in the pediatric population is complicated by changes in mental, emotional, behavioral, and physical development and physiology that vary with age. This chapter broadly covers considerations and techniques for assessing and treating pediatric pain, while highlighting differences in the pediatric population compared to adults.

Keywords Pediatrics · Pain management · Pain · Anesthesia and Analgesia · Regional Anesthesia

L. M. W. Webb (✉) · E. Adams · B. McElroy · K. M. Strupp
Division of Pediatric Anesthesiology, Department of Anesthesiology, University of Colorado/Children's Hospital Colorado, Aurora, USA
e-mail: Leah.Webb@childrenscolorado.org

E. Adams
e-mail: erin.adams@childrenscolorado.org

B. McElroy
e-mail: billy.mcelroy@childrenscolorado.org

K. M. Strupp
e-mail: kim.strupp@childrenscolorado.org

A. Reid
Department of Pediatric Pharmacy Services, Children's Hospital Colorado, Aurora, USA
e-mail: ashley.reid@childrenscolorado.org

A. Abd-Elsayed and K. Schroeder (eds.), *Perioperative Pain Management*,
https://doi.org/10.1007/978-3-031-67648-2_16

1 Introduction

This chapter will focus on the fundamentals of pediatric pain management—its own multi-book topic—by highlighting both the differences between children and adults and the special considerations specific to pediatric pain. While the definition of pain is the same in pediatrics and adults, pediatric pain assessment and treatment are affected by developmental, physiologic, and anatomic variations with age. For example, pathways for distinguishing and processing nociceptive and non-nociceptive stimuli are not fully developed at birth, such that neonates, especially those born prematurely, experience pain differently from adults and can suffer worse pain, due to enhanced excitability with reduced inhibitory neurotransmission [1]. Distinguishing factors in pediatric pain do not stop here. Below, the topics of pediatric pharmacokinetics and pharmacodynamics, pain assessment, and pain treatment—from pharmacologic to interventional to integrative—and complications will be addressed.

2 Developmental Pharmacokinetics and Pharmacodynamics

Children have variable drug pharmacokinetics and pharmacodynamics that affect appropriate medication administration. Dosing is generally based on body weight, body surface area, age, or a combination thereof. Volume of distribution, drug clearance, and other pharmacodynamic factors—all of which change with age—influence ideal medication regimens [2]. Body composition, renal function, and liver function vary as the body ages, contributing to the changing medication pharmacokinetics as children progress from neonate to adult.

Pediatric dosing guidelines are largely extrapolated from adult studies due to a lack of targeted studies in children, with 70–90% of medications used in the US pediatric population being considered "off-label" [3]. While vital to caring for pediatric patients, off-label use puts children at risk for adverse effects and over- and underdosing [3]. Health care professionals are hampered by limited evidence to support drug choice and dose selection [3].

Many factors affect gastro-enteral transit time in children and therefore absorption, onset of action and duration, bioavailability, and drug binding. Infants have higher gastric pH due to decreased acid production leading to increased absorption of acid labile medications and reduced absorption of drugs requiring acid for absorption [4]. Bacterial colonization of the colon occurs in the first days of life. Over the first year of life the gut microbiome changes significantly, affecting bacteria-produced enzymes in the gut that can alter bioavailability [4]. In the first week of life, gastric emptying time is significantly prolonged and continues to be delayed and irregular until six to eight months of age. Relative to adults, transit time remains reduced in older infants (even up to age three) such that onset of action may be faster with shorter duration of action of medications [4, 5]. Infants have reduced drug-metabolizing enzymes and drug transporters in the gut that increase to levels at or above adult activity in the first few years of life [6].

Body composition affects drug distribution. In infants and children, increased body water composition increases volume of distribution for water soluble medications, leading to a longer half-life and potentially higher milligram per kilogram (mg/kg) dosing [4, 6]. Adipose tissue can serve as a reservoir for lipophilic medications, which particularly impacts the obese population. Further, in obese patients, water-soluble medications (like morphine) have more free-drug available, thus dosing should be based on ideal body weight [4]. Protein binding can affect free or unbound drug. For example, reduced protein levels in neonates and infants leads to increased free drug availability and larger volumes of distribution for highly protein-bound drugs [4]. Particularly salient to pain management is the decreased production of alpha-1-acid glycoprotein in infants; consequently, highly protein-bound local anesthetics have increased levels of free, unbound drug and thus more availability of active drug [4]. Adult binding is reached by about 1 year of age.

Most drug metabolism is reduced at birth and this decrement is related to underdeveloped drug metabolizing enzymes, transporters, and elimination pathways. Cytochrome 2C9 activity is very low to absent at birth, exceeds adult activity during childhood, and then returns to adult activity around 10 years of age [5]. Functional genetic polymorphisms exist that impact its activity, such that some medications (including hydrocodone, codeine, and tramadol) are not reliably metabolized [5]. Cytochrome 3A4 activity is very low at birth but rapidly develops in the first month of life [5]. Further, the kidneys, critical for drug elimination, are immature in both structure and function at birth, when they receive only 5%–6% of cardiac output (as compared to 15%–25% in adults) via renal blood flow, which increases during the first year of life [5].

3 Pain Assessment

Pain is a dynamic process that arises from, and is greatly influenced by, multifactorial components including sensation, cognition, developmental maturity, behavior, emotion, and culture. Pain is defined by the expression of a discomforting sensory and emotional experience. The experience of pain is subjective, being built on one's perspective of an unpleasant sensation, in the context of the above biopsychosocial factors, and therefore can be difficult to effectively assess and treat.

The goal of pain assessment is to acquire information about the location, quality, and intensity of discomfort. Multiple tools have been developed and validated to assess pain in children, taking into consideration development based on age with varying verbal or mental capabilities. Self-reporting tools are ideal for characterizing the patient's expression of pain; however, they are not applicable to patients who are non-verbal, cognitively impaired, critically ill, or otherwise unable to respond given their medical requirements. In these patients, clinicians can assess for physiologic responses to pain (heart rate and blood pressure trends), as well as for behavioral changes in response to discomfort (facial expression, crying, and body positioning). A non-exhaustive list of validated self-report and observational pain scales can be found in Table 1.

These pain assessment tools are useful in scoring an experience that is otherwise highly subjective to the patient experiencing it. Clinicians, however, must understand that these scales are influenced by the child's ability to apply it to their situation. Pain may be underestimated and/or poorly differentiated from agitation, delirium, and even patient frustration and understanding. These scales do not fully consider patients with chronic pain, who may experience normalization of vital signs and altered mental or behavioral understanding of their situation (such as catastrophizing). As a result, the scoring may not accurately reflect their pain states. Also, parents play a significant role in pediatric pain management since they are often highly involved in the recognition and treatment of their child's pain. Consequently, parental education and involvement are essential to children's pain treatment plans.

Regarding pain assessment after anesthesia and surgery, it may be challenging to distinguish between pain and emergence agitation or delirium (EA/ED) in the pediatric recovery room; yet, ensuring adequate pain control in a child exhibiting EA/ED is crucial. Scoring systems such as the Pediatric Anesthesia Emergence Delirium Scale (PAEDS) have been shown to be valid and reliable in detecting emergence delirium [7] and can help in distinguishing EA/ED from pain. EA/ED occurs more commonly with sevoflurane or desflurane anesthesia and is theorized to occur due

Table 1 Recommended sample list of pain assessment tools that have been validated for use in children. Please reference Manworren [73] for a comprehensive list and details.

Acronym	Patient Age	Reference	Notes
Behavioral			
N-PASS	Premature infants 23–40 weeks gestational age	Hummel [74]	N-PASS = Neonatal Pain, Agitation, and Sedation Scale
NIPS	Pre-term to term infants	Lawrence [75]	NIPS = Neonatal Infant Pain Scale
CRIES	Neonate	Ahn [76]	CRIES = crying, requires oxygen, increased vital signs, expression, and sleeplessness
COMFORT Behavior Scale	Neonate to 3 years	Van Dijk [77]	For patients in intensive care units
rFLACC	4 to 19 years	Malviya [78]	rFLACC = revised Faces, Legs, Activity, Cry, and Consolability Observational Tool; for patients with intellectual disabilities
Self-report			
FPS-R	4 to 12 years	Hicks [79]	FPS-R = Faces Pain Scale-Revised
NRS	8 years and up		NRS = Numeric Rating Scale; 0 (no pain) to 10 (worst possible pain) point scale; can be assessed verbally

to rapid awakening in a strange environment with the faster offset of these volatile anesthetics [8]. Children demonstrating symptoms of EA/ED appear in a dissociated state and exhibit inconsolability, thrashing, and incoherence, which could otherwise be interpreted as pain.

4 Multimodal Pain Treatment: Pharmacologic, Interventional, Non-pharmacologic

Untreated pain can deleteriously affect children by altering neurocognition, psychosocial interaction, somatosensory processing, and executive functioning [9, 10], highlighting the critical need for efficacious pain treatment. Moreover, stress and pain early in life can lead to lifelong changes in pain processing and modulation. These patients are not only prone to amplified, recurrent, and/or chronic pain but also an increased risk of developing disease in other organ systems [10]. Minor procedural pain (like that associated with venipuncture, injections, and intravenous and bladder catheterization) is often associated with anxiety, and treating both factors is critical to reducing the sequelae of painful experiences in children and preventing resistance to future healthcare resource utilization [10, 11].

Multimodal pain therapy in infants and children, just as in adults, is important for effective treatment of pain and associated stressors [12–14]. (See Table 2 for simplified medication dosing regimens, as exhaustive regimens are too lengthy for review in this chapter.) A comprehensive multimodal plan includes pharmacologic interventions, as well as procedures (including regional anesthesia) and nonpharmacologic adjuncts [12, 13]. Mechanism of action is the same across patients and thus not mentioned in this chapter.

5 Pharmacologic Therapies: Nonopioid and Opioid Medications

Nonopioid Medications

Acetaminophen is a commonly used, nonopioid analgesic that can be administered orally, rectally, and intravenously. It has a wide safety margin and can be used without significant concerns in most pediatric patients. Acetaminophen must be dosed appropriately, considering age and weight, given its association with hepatic necrosis; it is often avoided in patients with decreased liver function [15].

Nonsteroidal analgesics, or nonsteroidal anti-inflammatory drugs (NSAIDs), are often first choice medications in the treatment of pain. NSAIDs are frequently administered as adjuvant therapy to reduce opioid use; however, nonsteroidals have a ceiling

Table 2 Suggested dosing for commonly used medications in pediatric pain management. (Non-exhaustive list, which uses dosing recommendations from Lexicomp® [77], unless otherwise noted.)

Neuraxial Medication Dosing					
Local Anesthetic: Spinal Anesthetic Blockade (SAB) adapted from Kokki [64]					
Bupivacaine 0.75%: max 20 mg [80]			Ropivacaine 0.75%: max 20 mg [80]		
Weight (kg)	*Dose (mg/kg)*	*Duration (min)*	*Weight (kg)*	*Dose (mg/kg)*	*Duration (min)*
<5	0.3–1	65–90	<5	0.5–1	45–80 min
6–10	0.4–0.5	75	6–10	0.5	90 min
11–20	0.3–0.4	80	11–20	0.5	90 min
>20	0.25–0.3	>85	>20	0.5	105 min
Local Anesthetic: Epidural Anesthesia (EA) and Peripheral Nerve Catheter(PNC)					
Infusion	*Starting Dose (mg/kg/hr)*	*Maximum Dose (mg/kg/hr), upper limit 28 mg/hr*			
Bupivacaine	0.2	0.5			
Ropivacaine	0.2	0.5			
Chloroprocaine	2	6			
Loading Dose	*Epidural (mg/kg)*	*Peripheral Nerve Catheter (mg/kg)*			
Ropivacaine	0.3–0.5, max 10–20 cc	0.1–0.5$^{¤}$			
Bupivacaine	0.3–0.5, max 10–20 cc	0.1–0.5$^{¤}$			
Adjuvants adapted from Anderson [81]					
Additive	*SAB Dose* (mcg/kg)	*EA Dose* (mcg/kg)	*Effect*	*Side Effect*	
Epinephrine	3–4	1–5 mcg/ml	D§	None	
Clonidine	0.5–1	0.5–2	D§, A	H, S	
Fentanyl*	0.25–0.5	0.2–1	A‡	N, V, P, S, RD$^{¥}$	

(continued)

Table 2 (continued)

Neuraxial Medication Dosing				
Morphine*	3–10*	10–30*	A	N, V, P, S, RD[¥], U
Hydromorphone	1–4	3–5	A	N, V, P, S, RD[¥], U

Pain Medications

Nonopioid	*Route*	*Dose (mg/kg/dose)*	*Frequency*	*Notes: Dose adjustments may be required for hepatic or renal impairment*
Acetaminophen (age >2 years)	PO IV PR	10–15 10–15 20–25 (load 40)	Q4–6H	1. Under 2: limit to 7.5–15 mg/kg Q6H; max 60 mg/kg/day. 2. Max daily dose: < 50 kg = 3,750 mg; >50 kg = 4,000 mg.
Ibuprofen[š]	PO	4–10	Q6–8H	1. Max single dose 600 mg. 2. Max daily dose 2,400 mg.
Naproxen[š]	PO	5–7	Q8–12H	1. Max daily dose 600–1000 mg. 2. Usual adult dose 250–500 mg Q12H.
Celecoxib[š] (≥ 2 years)	PO	≥ 10 kg: 50 mg ≥ 25 kg: 100 mg	BID BID	1. Max daily dose 200 mg.
Ketorolac[š, o]	PO IV IM	1 0.5 mg 1	Q6–8H Q6–8H Q6–8H	1. Max duration 5 days. 2. Max oral dose age 2–16 years 40 mg/day. 3. Max IV dose <50 kg 15 mg, ≥ 50 kg 30 mg.
Gabapentin	PO	5	TID (at max)	1. Start 300 mg (max) QHS, increase to BID day 2, then TID day 3. 2. Usual dose range 8–35 mg/kg/day split TID; max daily dose 3,600 mg.

(continued)

Table 2 (continued)

Neuraxial Medication Dosing				
Pregabalin	PO	25–150 mg	QD or BID	1. 25 mg QD or 50–150 mg/day in 2–3 doses. 2. Can increase weekly by 25–150 mg increments to 300–600 divided mg/day. 3. Convert from gabapentin with 6:1 ratio (gabapentin:pregabalin).
Dronabinol (≥ 6 years)	PO	2.5–5 mg/m2/dose	Q3–4H	1. Dosing for chemo-induced nausea and vomiting (CINV)—off-label for pain control. 2. Single doses 2.5–10 mg.
Nabilone (≥ 3 years)	PO	<18 kg: 0.5 mg ≥ 18–30 kg: 1 mg >30 kg: 1 mg	BID BID TID	1. Dosing for CINV—off-label for pain control.
Infusion	*Route*	*Dose (mg/kg/hr)*		*Notes*
Ketamine	IV	0.025–0.5		1. Infusion dosing based on authors' hospital guidelines. 2. Consider max dose of 30 mg/hr.
Dexmedetomidine	IV	0.5–2 mcg/kg/hr		1. Requires continuous monitoring. 2. Watch for bradycardia and hypotension.
Lidocaine	IV	0.5–2		1. Requires continuous monitoring. 2. Availability of serum lidocaine level monitoring desirable.
Opioid	*Route*	*Dose (mg/kg/dose)*	*Frequency*	*Notes: ≥ 50 kg use adult dosing.*

(continued)

Table 2 (continued)

Neuraxial Medication Dosing				
Oxycodone (IR)	PO	≤ 6 months: 0.025–0.05 >6 months and <50 kg: 0.1–0.2	Q6H Q4–6H	1. Can be immediate release (IR) or extended (ER). 2. Do not start ER before patient is on stable IR dosing. 3. Conversion to ER should involve pain management specialist.
Tramadol (≥ 12 years)	PO	1–2	Q4–6H	1. Max single dose 100 mg. 2. Max daily dose 400 mg.
Morphine	PO (IR) IV/SC Infusion	≤ 6 months: 0.08–0.1 >6 months and <50 kg: 0.15–0.3 ≤ 6 months: 0.025–0.05 >6 months and <50 kg: 0.05–0.1 ≤ 6 months: 0.008–0.02 mg/kg/hr >6 months and <50 kg: 0.01–0.04 mg/kg/hr	Q3–4H Q3–4H Q2–4H Q2–4H Continuous Continuous	1. Use caution in patients with sleep apnea or other respiratory compromise. 2. Frequency of IV/SC in infants <3 months Q4–6H. 3. Dose-reduce in patients with renal impairment due to active metabolite build up. 4. Continuous or prolonged doses require weaning. 5. Conversion to ER should involve pain management specialist.
Fentanyl	IV Infusion Patch	<50 kg: 0.5–1 mcg/kg/dose <50 kg: 0.5–2.5 mcg/kg/hr 12.5–300 mcg/hr	Q1–2H Continuous Q72H	1. Continuous infusion may require weaning based on duration. 2. Patch for opioid tolerant on >60 mg MME daily and initiation should involve pain management specialist. 3. Patch should not be titrated more than Q3–6Days.

(continued)

Table 2 (continued)

Neuraxial Medication Dosing				
Hydromorphone	PO IV Infusion	>6 months and >10 kg: 0.03–0.06 <50 kg: 0.03–0.08 >6 months and >10 kg: 0.005–0.015 <50 kg: 0.015 >6 months and >10 kg: 0.003–0.005 mg/kg/hr <50 kg: 0.003–0.005 mg/kg/hr	Q4H Q3–4H Q3–6H Q3–6H Continuous Continuous	1. Usual adult PO dose is 2–4 mg, max 8 mg. 2. Max initial infusion rate in patients <50 kg is 0.2 mg/hr.
Methadone	PO IV	≤ 6 months: 0.025–0.05 >6 months and <50 kg: 0.1–0.2 ≤ 6 months: 0.025 >6 months and <50 kg: 0.1	Once Once Once Once	1. Can prolong QT interval; baseline ECG recommended. 2. Many metabolic interferences—check interactions with other medications for dose adjustments. 3. Repeat dosing useful in opioid tolerant patients using graded conversions under guidance of pain management expert; caution in opioid naïve patients.
Butorphanol (≥ 18 years)	IM IV IN	1–4 mg 0.5–2 mg 1 mg	Q3–4H Q3–4H Q3–4H	1. Use is off-label in patients <18 years with defined pediatric regimen.
Naloxone	IV/IM/SC/IO IN	<5 years and ≤ 20 kg: 0.1 ≥ 5 years and >20 kg: 2 mg/dose 4–8 mg	Q2–3 min Q2–3 min Q2–3 min	1. Table dosing is for opioid overdose. 2. Reversal of respiratory depression: 0.001–0.005 mg/kg/dose, up to 2 mg/dose, Q2 min. 3. Pruritus: infusion at 0.25–2 mcg/kg/hr; higher doses may reverse pain control.

(continued)

Table 2 (continued)

Neuraxial Medication Dosing				
Naltrexone (low-dose) [82]	PO	1–5 mg	QD	1. Low-dose naltrexone (LDN) defined by <5 mg daily. 2. Use of LDN in chronic pain supported by emerging data.
Nalbuphine	IV/IM/SC	0.05–0.2	Q3–6H	1. Max single dose 20 mg. 2. Max daily dose 160 mg.
Buprenorphine	IM/IV Transdermal	2–12 years: 2–6 mcg/kg/dose >12: 0.3 mg ≥ 18 years: start 5 mcg/hr	Q4–8H Q6–8H Q7D	1. IV administration should be via slow push. 2. IV/IM doses are for acute pain. 3. Transdermal patch is off-label in pediatrics; titration is beyond scope of this chapter.
PCA/NCA/CCA (dosing for patients <50 kg)	*Basal (mg/kg/hr)*	*Demand (mg/kg/dose)*	*Lockout (minutes)*	*Notes*
Morphine	0–0.03	0.01–0.03	6–8	1. Demand dose is delivered by nurse or caregiver for NCA/CCA. 2. Lockout on NCA/CCA is usually 30 minutes. 3. For children and adolescents ≥ 50 kg, use adult PCA dosing guidelines. 4. Clinician boluses can be administered and are usually twice the demand dose with lockout averaging 1–2 hours.
Fentanyl	0–0.5 mcg/kg/hr	0.2–0.5 mcg/kg/dose	5–15	
Hydromorphone	0–0.004	0.003–0.004	6–10	

§ Increased: with epinephrine in neonates and with clonidine in both neonates and adolescents [64].
‡ Lipophilic opioids may improve CA density but do not increase analgesic duration [45].
¥Especially with higher dose opioids (intrathecal fentanyl >1 mcg/kg or morphine >5 mcg/kg) [64].
* Maximum dose: fentanyl SAB = 25–50 mcg; fentanyl CA=50 mcg; morphine SAB=250 mcg [81].
¤Maximum dose: for single shot or loading PNC depends on patient weight, age, and number of blocks.
šNSAIDs may require dose reduction for renal impairment.
°Ketorolac dosing varies significantly with age/weight.

effect and are not always sufficient when used by themselves [16]. Special considerations should be made when using NSAIDs in infants less than six months of age, as well as those patients with concerns for kidney dysfunction, given the increased risk of developing acute kidney injury [16]. Topical NSAIDs, like diclofenac, may be an option for those in whom systemic administration is contraindicated or in the treatment of musculoskeletal pain.

Antidepressants including selective serotonin and combined serotonin and norepinephrine reuptake inhibitors (SSRIs and SNRIs) and tricyclics are becoming a core treatment of neuropathic and other chronic pain states. Mood stabilizers—for example duloxetine, which is an SNRI—can therefore be utilized to decrease the reuptake of serotonin and norepinephrine, leading to improved pain pathway inhibition and pain control [17]. Furthermore, these medications are useful for managing anxiety and depression, which frequently coincide and interplay with chronic pain states [17].

Gabapentinoids, which include gabapentin and pregabalin, have a long-standing history in the treatment of chronic and neuropathic pain in adults and can be used to successfully treat pain in children. Neuropathic and chronic pain in children can be associated with or caused by numerous etiologies not limited to injury, surgery, phantom limb pain, cancer and chemotherapy, and chronic illnesses [18]. Gabapentinoids are some of the most frequently used medications for pain control in these pain states [18].

The use of cannabis and its derivatives for pain management, and other indications, has exploded in recent years, particularly with increased legalization of medical and recreational use [19, 20]. While the adult literature supports several indications, including management of a variety of pain syndromes [19, 21], data supporting the use of cannabinoids in the pediatric population has been limited mostly to treatment of chemotherapy-induced nausea and vomiting (CINV) and seizures/epilepsy [19, 20]. Presently, nabilone and dronabinol are the only regulated synthetic cannabinoids available [19, 20], and both have dosing guidelines (Table 2) for pediatric patients. There are case reports of cannabis successfully treating pain conditions in pediatric patients [20], but there is a paucity of evidence detailing efficacy and safety [19, 20].

However, there is strong evidence for the importance of the endocannabinoid system in brain development, with the perinatal and adolescent periods being particularly vulnerable; the sequelae of pediatric marijuana exposure during these periods is linked with far-reaching effects on neurocognition, psychiatric disease, addiction, and even epigenetics [19, 20, 22, 23]. Because cannabinoid metabolism is complex, with significant inhibitory effects on the cytochrome P450 pathway, drug interactions are another important consideration in their use [19, 21]. Further studies are needed to elucidate whether there is a role for cannabis in the treatment of pediatric pain and provide guidelines for safe administration.

Nonopioid intravenous infusions, such as ketamine (an NMDA-receptor antagonist), dexmedetomidine (an alpha-agonist), and lidocaine (a local anesthetic with NMDA-receptor antagonism) are effective in the pediatric population [24]. Despite ketamine's common use in the pediatric population, consideration should be paid to conflicting evidence about neurotoxicity versus neuroprotection in brain development of young patients, especially under the age of three years [25]. Dexmedetomidine is recently purported to have properties protective of the brain and other organs, which perhaps increases its utility in pediatric pain management [26, 27]. Infusions in pediatric patients require weight-based dosing (Table 2) to avoid under- or overdosing.

Opioid Medications

Opioid medications are a mainstay of pain treatment in pediatric patients because of efficacy and relative safety, but opioid administration is not without risk and controversy [5, 13, 14]. Pediatric opioid dosing (Table 2) is usually weight- and/or age-based and administration can be considerably different in pediatric patients compared to adults. Patient-controlled analgesia (PCA) use is prevalent with the inclusion of nurse- and caregiver-controlled analgesia (NCA and CCA) utilized for patients without the developmental or neurocognitive abilities to self-administer analgesic doses [13, 28–31]. Continuous opioid infusions are commonly used in pediatric pain management, despite evidence contrary to that in adults, showing non-superior pain control and increased adverse events [13, 30, 31]. Continuous cardiorespiratory monitoring is mandatory while administering intravenous opioids [30, 31]. Capnography may enhance the safety of administration of opioid medications but presents challenges in pediatric patients [32].

While most opioid formulations are safe to administer to children, there are special considerations for pediatric patients [5]. Route of administration—oral, intravenous, intranasal, transdermal, subcutaneous, intrathecal, and rectal—is impacted by pharmacodynamics, pharmacokinetics, and even pharmacogenetics [5]. Naloxone should be dispensed to high-risk pediatric patients in case of accidental overdose [14]. Methadone is safe and efficacious in children; it requires monitoring due to the risk of QT prolongation and metabolic effects with drug interactions [13]. Codeine has a black box warning for pediatric administration due to the potential for fatal overdose in rapid metabolizers [5, 33]; further, its unreliable metabolism makes it an undesirable choice [5, 13]. Tramadol should not be administered to children under the age of twelve due to similar concerns about ultrarapid metabolizers and overdose [5, 33]. Use of meperidine is not recommended in infants and children due to its side effect profile and the availability of safer alternatives [5]. Transdermal patches have also been used with success in children and may be a consideration when other routes of administration are challenging [5, 34]. Mixed agonist-antagonists (nalbuphine, butorphanol, and buprenorphine) and pure antagonists (naltrexone) have also been used to treat a variety of pain conditions [5, 34].

Consideration must be given to common complications of opioid therapy including constipation, nausea/vomiting, pruritis, respiratory depression, urinary retention, and sedation, in addition to tolerance, dependence, and withdrawal [13]. Naloxone can be used to treat many opioid-related side effects, including overdose

[14]. Nalbuphine is effective for pain control with fewer side effects [5, 35] and is used to treat opioid-induced side effects, with particular efficacy in treating opioid-induced pruritis and urinary retention [35, 36]. The risk of opioid exposure leading to abuse increases significantly in adolescence and early adulthood. Therefore, practices that promote opioid stewardship, such as proper prescribing and disposal of opioids, are vital to curbing the opioid epidemic [13, 14]. While they are not without complications and side effects, opioids remain a commonly used, safe, and efficacious treatment for pediatric pain, when administered properly and thoughtfully with appropriate patient education [13, 14].

Opioid dosing conversion tables, whether in pediatrics or adults, should be used as a rough guide, considering that tables are largely based on single dose studies in the adult population and without consideration for each medication's steady state concentration. One should always complete the math associated with opioid conversions, including a dose reduction when needed for incomplete cross-tolerance. Assessment of the patient's condition and clinical judgement should ultimately determine the final dose calculation and desired regimen. An example of an online automated opioid conversion calculator can be found at https://globalrph.com/medcalcs/opioid-pain-management-converter-advanced/.

6 Interventional Pain Therapy: Regional Anesthesia, Complications, and Imaging

Regional Anesthesia

Though frequently questioned, the safety and efficacy of pediatric nerve block performance, even in anesthetized children, has been demonstrated by several large studies [37–40]. However, pediatric local anesthetic dosing should be weight-based (Table 2) and further decreased in infants less than six months old, who have decreased levels of protein, specifically alpha-1-acid glycoprotein. Because local anesthetics are highly protein-bound, more unbound (active) local anesthetic is present in young infants, requiring decreased dosing compared even to older children [41]. While techniques for performance of neuraxial, especially thoracic and lumbar epidural, and peripheral nerve blockade in the pediatric population are similar to adults, anatomic and physiologic considerations differ in pediatrics.

Awareness of anatomic landmark differences is paramount when performing neuraxial anesthesia in neonates and children. The adult spinal cord and dural sac commonly terminate around L1/2 and S2, respectively, whereas spinal cord and dural termination in infants is around L3 and S3/4, respectively [42]. In addition, the distance to the epidural space is very small compared to adults, typically about 1mm per kg in infants older than six months [43].

The infant neuraxis differs from adults physiologically in that infants have nearly twice the volume of cerebrospinal fluid and have increased spinal cord blood flow with higher uptake of drugs from the subarachnoid space [41]. As such, spinal blockade in infants has a shorter duration of action with requirement for increased local anesthetic dose [41]. See Table 2 for weight-based spinal dosing.

Caudal epidural anesthesia (CEA) remains one of the most commonly performed nerve blocks in children. CEA has typically been performed via a landmark-based approach with identification of the sacral cornua guiding access to the epidural space through the sacral hiatus. Ultrasound use for CEA has been shown to increase the accuracy of block placement and likely increase block success [44]. Dosing of CEA is based on level of desired coverage, with 0.5 ml/kg covering the sacral dermatomes, 1ml/kg covering the lumbar dermatomes, and 1.25 ml/kg covering thoracic dermatomes [45]. In the setting of CEA, local anesthetics frequently require dilution to achieve higher dermatomal spread and avoid exceeding weight-based dosing limits. The maximum dosing for CEA is less than 25 ml, restricting its use for thoracic coverage in older children [46].

Continuous neuraxial and peripheral nerve infusions can be used in pediatric patients, keeping in mind that these patients are more sensitive to local anesthetics and have age-dependent metabolism and clearance [4]. Studies of continuous local infusions of ropivacaine and bupivacaine in the pediatric population have shown that infusion rates to a maximum dose of 0.5 mg/kg/hour can be safely used [47]. A typical starting dose for these infusions is 0.2 mg/kg/hour and slow titration, and careful monitoring for signs of local anesthetic systemic toxicity (LAST), maximizes the ability to safely achieve pain control. Ropivacaine has been shown to be safer in pediatrics, when compared to bupivacaine, given its decreased cardiotoxicity and decreased plasma accumulation during an infusion [48, 49]. Consider chloroprocaine infusions for infants less than six months of age or less than eight kg in weight, as immature renal and hepatic function can lead to decreased clearance of amide local anesthetics and decreased volume of local anesthetic at therapeutic doses may not allow for adequate spread within the epidural space to provide coverage. See epidural adjuvant dosing in Table 2.

Growing demand for improved outpatient pain control that minimizes opioids and other medications has enhanced the popularity of ambulatory nerve catheter infusions. Multiple factors require consideration when running home catheter programs: (a) patient selection (healthy, cooperative); (b) reliable families who express comfort with managing the catheter and its requirements; and (c) the establishment of a home catheter service with resources, protocols, and personnel to manage outpatients with infusions. Complications are typically minor, such as leaking or early dislodgement, and education is essential in the success of these catheters [50].

Regional Anesthesia Complications

Though the incidence of complications in pediatric regional anesthesia is rare, as evidenced by the large studies mentioned above, they do occur. Special considerations apply to complications including local anesthetic systemic toxicity (LAST), catheter dislodgement, neurologic complications, and postdural puncture headache.

One of the rare, yet most serious complications of regional and neuraxial anesthesia in children is LAST. Children have both a relatively increased cardiac output and systemic uptake of local anesthetics, putting them at increased risk for toxicity [8]. Since anesthesiologists perform much of pediatric regional and neuraxial anesthesia/analgesia while the patient is under general anesthesia, patients do not exhibit the typical symptoms of LAST (headache, somnolence, vertigo, perioral or lingual paresthesia). Rather the clinician must watch for signs of toxicity including muscle rigidity, unexplained hypoxemia, tachycardia, dysrhythmias, or cardiovascular collapse [8]. Because early warning signs may be masked by general anesthesia, cardiovascular collapse may be the presenting sign [51]. Monitoring with an electrocardiogram (ECG) is essential, as peaked T waves are one of the earlier signs of LAST; further, T wave change on ECG (not heart or blood pressure change like adults) is the most sensitive marker for positive test dose in children [52]. A test dose should contain 0.5 mcg/kg epinephrine, up to 15 mcg (adult dose). Management must be quick and cognitive aids such as the Society for Pediatric Anesthesia's Pedi Crisis (https://pedsanesthesia.org/pedi-crisis-app/) can help ensure complete and effective management. To treat LAST, administer intralipid 20% as a bolus (1.5 ml/kg intravenous over one minute, repeat every three to five minutes until hemodynamically stable), followed by an intralipid infusion for at least ten minutes after the patient is hemodynamically stable (0.25 mL/kg/min, increase as needed to 0.5 mL/kg/min). Ensure that epinephrine dosing is decreased (1 microgram/kg intravenous/intraosseous as needed) compared to the cardiac arrest dose. Treat seizures with midazolam (0.05-0.1 mg/kg intravenous), not propofol, which will worsen hemodynamic collapse. Additionally, avoid vasopressin, calcium channel blockers, and beta blockers. LAST may recur four to six hours after the initial event, so patient monitoring must continue through this period [53].

An additional complication that occurs in pediatric regional and neuraxial analgesia is catheter dislodgement, which is a leading factor in epidural analgesic failure [54]. Unlike in adult patients, replacing an epidural or regional catheter in children may require general anesthesia or deep sedation, making the replacement of a dislodged catheter very challenging and potentially forcing a change in pain management modality. Catheters in pediatric patients have the propensity to leak, and leakage or sweating can cause the dressing to loosen or fall off, risking exposure of the insertion site. Measures like the use of Dermabond® at the insertion site and Mastisol® Liquid Adhesive to help secure the transparent occlusive dressing (Tegaderm™) are helpful to prevent displacement of the dressings and decrease leaking [55]. Using consistent securement, including subcutaneous tunneling and/or suturing where appropriate, and education may decrease rates of catheter dislodgement [55, 56].

Neurologic complications in pediatric patients are rare. A recent review of over 100,000 blocks by the Pediatric Regional Anesthesia Network (PRAN) found a rate of 2.4 in 10,000 cases [40]. Most of the complications were sensory and resolved within weeks to months, with no permanent deficits noted [40]. If a patient develops sensory or motor deficits after regional or neuraxial anesthesia, it is essential to ensure rapid assessment (history and physical exam), diagnosis, and treatment. For peripheral nerve injuries, consultation with neurology and early imaging are essential when motor deficits are present [57, 58]. Neurophysiologic tests including electromyography and nerve conduction studies can help to localize the site of nerve injury, though it may not be possible to distinguish whether the injury resulted from anesthesia or surgery [58]. These studies also offer prognostic information depending on the degree of injury. Most injuries improve with physical therapy [57].

In pediatric patients, post-dural puncture headaches (PDPH) may occur as a complication of neuraxial anesthesia/analgesia or as a complication of diagnostic lumbar puncture, especially when performed with a large gauge cutting needle. PDPH in children exhibits similar symptoms to adults [59]. The majority of PDPH resolve within a week with conservative management and symptomatic treatment with medications (methylxanthines, gabapentin, cosyntropin, and/or hydrocortisone) and minor interventions (greater occipital nerve blocks and sphenopalatine blocks) [60–63].

Conservative therapy (as above) should be considered first line for pediatric patients with PDPH, but epidural blood patch (EBP) may be required when conservative therapy fails. Children may not tolerate or be eligible for an EBP, since general anesthesia or deep sedation are often required for pediatric patients to tolerate the invasive procedure; thus, it is utilized less commonly in children compared to adults. Performance of an EBP is the same as in adults with the following caveats: a. if awake, the injection should cease if the child describes pressure or discomfort in the back; b. if anesthetized, no more than 0.3 ml/kg or 20 mL of blood should be injected [64]. Two hospitals in Finland described their experience in performing 42 EBPs in 41 children over a ten-year period. Five patients were aged 3–12 years and the remaining 36 patients were aged 13–18 years. The initial success rate of EBP was 90%, with permanent relief in 85%. There was no correlation with the volume of blood injected and the efficacy of EBP [64].

Imaging in Children

A discussion of pediatric regional anesthesia is not complete without considering risks and benefits of imaging modalities in children. The use of ultrasound (US) is now a mainstay of acute pain and regional anesthesia clinical practice, and it is critical to pediatric anesthesia for its role in improving safety and providing diagnostic imaging. US enhances safety in the following ways: a. avoids radiation exposure to vulnerable patients, many of whom may require further medical radiation exposure in their lives; b. enhances safety margin for patients receiving regional anesthesia, most of whom are under general anesthesia where typical safety warnings—like paresthesia—are masked; and c. allows for targeted placement of local anesthetic in a population where volume is limited by lower toxic doses and landmark techniques carry increased risk due to anatomical variations based on changes in patient age and size [65, 66]. US is increasingly utilized in aiding pediatric neuraxial anesthesia, especially caudal epidural anesthesia (CEA), which is the most common pediatric regional anesthesia technique. CEA historically relied solely on landmark palpation, but recent studies show the usefulness of US for confirmation of proper local anesthetic placement [44]. Unossified bones in the pediatric skeleton and decreased adipose tissue allow US imaging to be highly reliable and effective in children and enhance its diagnostic utility [65]. For example, while MRI remains the gold standard for spine imaging, improvements in US quality have increased its use in evaluating pediatric spine anomalies, such that US is the first line modality for spinal cord screening in neonates and young infants [67].

According to the United States Food and Drug Association, pediatric patients are more sensitive to cancer risk per unit dose of ionizing radiation, requiring careful consideration of x-ray use in this population. In addition, pediatric patients have a longer expected lifetime, increasing the chance of cancer developing from radiation during their life. Therefore, it is important to consult the age-appropriate radiation settings for equipment and consider whether radiation exposure is truly necessary for patient care. Consequently, while an epidurogram is useful for confirmation of correct epidural or caudal catheter placement in anesthetized patients [68], widespread use is limited due to logistical restraints, including time, radiation exposure, and the general efficacy of ultrasound for the same indication.

Nonpharmacologic Pain Management

Though medication administration is an important component of pain therapy, evidence supports the use of non-pharmacologic adjuncts for reducing pain and anxiety, while increasing children's coping and resiliency [11, 12, 69]. Studied interventions include music, art, and animal therapy, acupuncture and acupressure, hypnosis, child life specialists, pain psychology (e.g. guided-imagery, deep breathing, biofeedback), physical therapy, use of transcutaneous electrical nerve stimulation (TENS) unit, virtual reality, distraction, breastfeeding, comfort holds, and sucrose [11, 12, 69].

Chronic Pain

Chronic pain, generally defined as pain lasting longer than three months, is a significant problem in the pediatric population. According to a systematic review by King et al from 2011, pediatric chronic pain is prevalent in specific conditions with the following ranges: "headache: 8–83%; abdominal pain: 4–53%; back pain: 14–24%; musculoskeletal pain: 4–40%; multiple pains: 4–49%; other pains: 5–88%" [70]. The prevalence of chronic pain is higher in those with female gender, lower socioeconomic status, and increasing age [70]. Patients can experience pain from a vast number of conditions including illness or injury; complex regional pain syndrome;

and numerous medical conditions such as Sickle Cell Disease, Hypermobile Ehlers Danlos Syndrome, Juvenile Idiopathic Arthritis, and Epidermolysis Bullosa. Chronic pain is complex—resulting from an interplay of many variables from neurons and spinal cord pathways to neurotransmitters to psychosocial and behavioral factors and more—and, can lead to the development of intensified pain signaling through central sensitization or hyperexcitability and wind-up phenomena leading to poorly controlled pain [71]. Chronic pain decreases children's quality of life and functional status [70–72]. Children with chronic pain are benefited by a multidisciplinary care model that includes psychologists, physical therapists, and the use of multimodal pain pharmacology and procedural intervention [72]. Treatment, therefore, is primarily directed at patients' functional improvements in day-to-day skills and needs, in addition to the reduction of pain [72].

Key Takeaways

1. Medication dosing and management in pediatrics is often off-label and is age- and weight-dependent based on physiologic changes associated with age and size.
2. Validated pediatric-specific pain assessment tools are necessary to account for developmental roadblocks to solely using verbal assessment tools.
3. Anatomic and physiologic considerations specific to infants and children require careful consideration when placing and dosing regional anesthetics.
4. Effects of medications on brain development in children and adolescents must be weighed against the necessity of their use in pain management, especially given the negative effects of poorly treated or uncontrolled pain.
5. Multimodal therapy is effective in treating both acute and chronic pain in the pediatric population.

References

1. Pattinson D, Fitzgerald M. The neurobiology of infant pain: development of excitatory and inhibitory neurotransmission in the spinal dorsal horn. Reg Anesth Pain Med. 2004;29(1):36–44.
2. Anderson BJ, McKee AD, Holford NH. Size, myths and the clinical pharmacokinetics of analgesia in paediatric patients. Clin Pharmacokinet. 1997;33(5):313–27.
3. Bazzano AT, Mangione-Smith R, Schonlau M, Suttorp MJ, Brook RH. Off-label prescribing to children in the United States outpatient setting. Acad Pediatr. 2009;9(2):81–8.
4. Kearns GL, Abdel-Rahman SM, Alander SW, Blowey DL, Leeder JS, Kauffman RE. Developmental pharmacology–drug disposition, action, and therapy in infants and children. N Engl J Med. 2003;349(12):1157–67.
5. Thigpen JC, Odle BL, Harirforoosh S. Opioids: a review of pharmacokinetics and pharmacodynamics in neonates, infants, and children. Eur J Drug Metab Pharmacokinet. 2019;44(5):591–609.
6. Mooij MG, Nies AT, Knibbe CA, Schaeffeler E, Tibboel D, Schwab M, et al. Development of human membrane transporters: drug disposition and pharmacogenetics. Clin Pharmacokinet. 2016;55(5):507–24.

7. Sikich N, Lerman J. Development and psychometric evaluation of the pediatric anesthesia emergence delirium scale. Anesthesiology. 2004;100(5):1138–45.
8. Davis PJ, Cladis FP. Smith's anesthesia for infants and children. Ninth edition. ed. St. Louis, Missouri: Elsevier; 2017. xviii, 1399
9. Hall RW, Anand KJ. Pain management in newborns. Clin Perinatol. 2014;41(4):895–924.
10. Walker SM. Long-term effects of neonatal pain. Semin Fetal Neonatal Med. 2019;24(4): 101005.
11. Committee ECPG, Liaisons: EBoD, Methodologist:, Liaisons: S, Staff: A. Clinical practice guideline: needle-related or minor procedural pain in pediatric patients. J Emerg Nurs. 2019;45(4):437.e1-.e32.
12. Friedrichsdorf SJ. Multimodal pediatric pain management (part 2). Pain Management. 2017;7(3):161–6.
13. Yaster M, Reid AL, Cohen MN, Monitto CL. Opioids in the management of acute Pediatric pain: an update in a time of crisis. Clin J Pain. 2019;35(6):487–96.
14. Yaster M, McNaull PP, Davis PJ. The opioid epidemic in pediatrics: a 2020 update. Curr Opin Anaesthesiol. 2020;33(3):327–34.
15. Jóźwiak-Bebenista M, Nowak JZ. Paracetamol: mechanism of action, applications and safety concern. Acta Pol Pharm. 2014;71(1):11–23.
16. Cooney MF. Pain management in children: NSAID use in the perioperative and emergency department settings. Paediatr Drugs. 2021;23(4):361–72.
17. Skånland SS, Cieślar-Pobuda A. Off-label uses of drugs for depression. Eur J Pharmacol. 2019;865: 172732.
18. Howard RF, Wiener S, Walker SM. Neuropathic pain in children. Arch Dis Child. 2014;99(1):84–9.
19. Dharmapuri S, Miller K, Klein JD. Marijuana and the pediatric population. Pediatrics. 2020;146(2).
20. Wong SS, Wilens TE. Medical Cannabinoids in children and adolescents: a systematic review. Pediatrics. 2017;140(5).
21. Mlost J, Bryk M, Starowicz K. Cannabidiol for pain treatment: focus on pharmacology and mechanism of action. Int J Mol Sci. 2020;21(22).
22. Bara A, Ferland JN, Rompala G, Szutorisz H, Hurd YL. Cannabis and synaptic reprogramming of the developing brain. Nat Rev Neurosci. 2021;22(7):423–38.
23. Lubman DI, Cheetham A, Yücel M. Cannabis and adolescent brain development. Pharmacol Ther. 2015;148:1–16.
24. Boric K, Dosenovic S, Jelicic Kadic A, Batinic M, Cavar M, Urlic M, et al. Interventions for postoperative pain in children: an overview of systematic reviews. Pediatric Anesthesia. 2017;27(9):893–904.
25. Yan J, Jiang H. Dual effects of ketamine: neurotoxicity versus neuroprotection in anesthesia for the developing brain. J Neurosurg Anesthesiol. 2014;26(2):155–60.
26. Unchiti K, Leurcharusmee P, Samerchua A, Pipanmekaporn T, Chattipakorn N, Chattipakorn SC. The potential role of Dexmedetomidine on neuroprotection and its possible mechanisms: evidence from in vitro and in vivo studies. Eur J Neurosci. 2021;54(9):7006–47.
27. Liaquat Z, Xu X, Zilundu PLM, Fu R, Zhou L. The Current role of Dexmedetomidine as Neuroprotective agent: an updated review. Brain Sci. 2021;11(7).
28. Czarnecki ML, Ferrise AS, Jastrowski Mano KE, Garwood MM, Sharp M, Davies H, et al. Parent/nurse-controlled analgesia for children with developmental delay. Clin J Pain. 2008;24(9):817–24.
29. Donado C, Solodiuk J, Rangel SJ, Nelson CP, Heeney MM, Mahan ST, et al. Patient-and nurse-controlled Analgesia: 22-year Experience in a Pediatric hospital. Hosp Pediatr. 2019;9(2):129–33.
30. Hayes J, Dowling JJ, Peliowski A, Crawford MW, Johnston B. Patient-controlled analgesia plus background opioid infusion for postoperative pain in children: a systematic review and meta-analysis of randomized trials. Anesth Analg. 2016;123(4):991–1003.

31. Lehr VT, BeVier P. Patient-controlled analgesia for the pediatric patient. Orthop Nurs. 2003;22(4):298-304; quiz 5-6.
32. Miller KM, Kim AY, Yaster M, Kudchadkar SR, White E, Fackler J, et al. Long-term tolerability of capnography and respiratory inductance plethysmography for respiratory monitoring in pediatric patients treated with patient-controlled analgesia. Paediatr Anaesth. 2015;25(10):1054–9.
33. FDA restricts use of prescription codeine pain and cough medicines and tramadol pain medicines in children; recommends against use in breastfeeding women, (2017).
34. Haupt TS, Smyth M, Gregoire MC. A scoping review of transdermal buprenorphine use for non-surgical pain in the Pediatric population. Cureus. 2019;11(10): e5954.
35. Larsen D, Maani CV. Nalbuphine. 2022. In: StatPearls [Internet]. Treasure Island, FL: StatPearls Publishing LLC. Available from: https://www.ncbi.nlm.nih.gov/books/NBK534283/
36. Reiter PD, Clevenger AC. Nalbuphine reduces opioid-associated urinary retention in Pediatric patients. Pediatr Crit Care Med. 2019;20(5):e240–4.
37. Giaufré E, Dalens B, Gombert A. Epidemiology and morbidity of regional anesthesia in children: a one-year prospective survey of the French-Language society of Pediatric Anesthesiologists. Anesth Analg. 1996;83(5):904–12.
38. Polaner DM, Taenzer AH, Walker BJ, Bosenberg A, Krane EJ, Suresh S, et al. Pediatric regional anesthesia network (PRAN): a multi-institutional study of the use and incidence of complications of Pediatric regional anesthesia. Anesth Analg. 2012;115(6):1353–64.
39. Taenzer AH, Walker BJ, Bosenberg AT, Martin L, Suresh S, Polaner DM, et al. Asleep versus awake: does it matter?: Pediatric regional block complications by patient state: a report from the pediatric Regional anesthesia Network. Reg Anesth Pain Med. 2014;39(4):279–83.
40. Walker BJ, Long JB, Sathyamoorthy M, Birstler J, Wolf C, Bosenberg AT, et al. Complications in pediatric regional anesthesia: An analysis of more than 100,000 blocks from the pediatric regional anesthesia network. Anesthesiology. 2018;129(4):721–32.
41. Suresh S, Ecoffey C, Bosenberg A, Lonnqvist PA, de Oliveira GS, de Leon Casasola O, et al. The European society of regional anaesthesia and pain Therapy/American Society of regional anesthesia and pain medicine recommendations on local anesthetics and Adjuvants Dosage in pediatric regional anesthesia. Reg Anesth Pain Med. 2018;43(2):211–6.
42. Van Schoor AN, Bosman MC, Bosenberg AT. Descriptive study of the differences in the level of the conus medullaris in four different age groups. Clin Anat. 2015;28(5):638–44.
43. De Jose Maria B, Tielens L, Roberts S. Pediatric Epidural and spinal anesthesia and analgesia: New York school of anesthesia; 2023 [Available from: https://www.nysora.com/topics/sub-specialties/pediatric-anesthesia/pediatric-epidural-spinal-anesthesia-analgesia/
44. Adler AC, Belon CA, Guffey DM, Minard CG, Patel NV, Chandrakantan A. Real-time ultrasound improves accuracy of caudal block in children. Anesth Analg. 2020;130(4):1002–7.
45. Wiegele M, Marhofer P, Lönnqvist PA. Caudal epidural blocks in paediatric patients: a review and practical considerations. Br J Anaesth. 2019;122(4):509–17.
46. Jöhr M, Berger TM. Caudal blocks. Paediatr Anaesth. 2012;22(1):44–50.
47. Berde CB. Convulsions associated with pediatric regional anesthesia. Anesth Analg. 1992;75(2):164–6.
48. Bösenberg AT, Thomas J, Cronje L, Lopez T, Crean PM, Gustafsson U, et al. Pharmacokinetics and efficacy of ropivacaine for continuous epidural infusion in neonates and infants. Paediatr Anaesth. 2005;15(9):739–49.
49. Graf BM, Abraham I, Eberbach N, Kunst G, Stowe DF, Martin E. Differences in cardiotoxicity of bupivacaine and Ropivacaine are the result of physicochemical and Stereoselective properties. Anesthesiology. 2002;96(6):1427–34.
50. Gable A, Burrier C, Stevens J, Wrona S, Klingele K, Bhalla T, et al. Home peripheral nerve catheters: the first 24 months of experience at a children's hospital. J Pain Res. 2016;9:1067–72.
51. Gunter JB. Benefit and risks of local anesthetics in infants and children. Paediatr Drugs. 2002;4(10):649–72.
52. Coté CJ, Lerman J, Anderson B, Suresh S, Polaner D. Regional anesthesia. In: A practice of anesthesia for infants and children. Philadelphia, PA: Elsevier; 2019.

53. Anesthesia SfP. Pedi Crisis 2.0. https://pedsanesthesia.org/wp-content/uploads/2020/01/SPA PediCrisisChecklistsJan2020.pdf; 2018.
54. Motamed C, Farhat F, Rémérand F, Stéphanazzi J, Laplanche A, Jayr C. An analysis of post-operative epidural analgesia failure by computed tomography Epidurography. Anesth Analg. 2006;103(4):1026–32.
55. Webb L, Bielsky A, Strupp K. Reducing early epidural dislodgement with standardized securement. SPPM News. 2019.
56. Aram L, Krane EJ, Kozloski LJ, Yaster M. Tunneled epidural catheters for prolonged analgesia in pediatric patients. Anesth Analg. 2001;92(6):1432–8.
57. O'Flaherty D, McCartney CJL, Ng SC. Nerve injury after peripheral nerve blockade-current understanding and guidelines. BJA Educ. 2018;18(12):384–90.
58. Hewson DW, Bedforth NM, Hardman JG. Peripheral nerve injury arising in anaesthesia practice. Anaesthesia. 2018;73(Suppl 1):51–60.
59. Bezov D, Lipton RB, Ashina S. Post-dural puncture headache: part I diagnosis, epidemiology, etiology, and pathophysiology. Headache. 2010;50(7):1144–52.
60. Niraj G, Critchley P. Management and outcomes of persistent headache after accidental dural puncture in the obstetric population: a 9-year prospective audit. Headache. 2023;63(1):71–8.
61. Patel R, Urits I, Orhurhu V, Orhurhu MS, Peck J, Ohuabunwa E, et al. A comprehensive update on the treatment and management of postdural puncture headache. Curr Pain Headache Rep. 2020;24(6):24.
62. Bezov D, Ashina S, Lipton R. Post-dural puncture headache: part II–prevention, management, and prognosis. Headache. 2010;50(9):1482–98.
63. Basurto Ona X, Osorio D, Bonfill Cosp X. Drug therapy for treating post-dural puncture headache. Cochrane Database Syst Rev. 2015;2015(7):CD007887.
64. Kokki H. Spinal blocks. Paediatr Anaesth. 2012;22(1):56–64.
65. Barbuto L, Di Serafino M, Della Vecchia N, Rea G, Esposito F, Vezzali N, et al. Pediatric musculoskeletal ultrasound: a pictorial essay. J Ultrasound. 2019;22(4):491–502.
66. Tsui BC, Suresh S. Ultrasound imaging for regional anesthesia in infants, children, and adolescents: a review of current literature and its application in the practice of Neuraxial blocks. Anesthesiology. 2010;112(3):719–28.
67. Rees MA, Squires JH, Coley BD, Hoehne B, Ho ML. Ultrasound of congenital spine anomalies. Pediatr Radiol. 2021;51(13):2442–57.
68. Taenzer AH, Clark C, Kovarik WD. Experience with 724 Epidurograms for epidural catheter placement in pediatric anesthesia. Reg Anesth Pain Med. 2010;35(5):432–5.
69. Gaglani A, Gross T. Pediatric pain management. Emerg Med Clin North Am. 2018;36(2):323–34.
70. King S, Chambers CT, Huguet A, MacNevin RC, McGrath PJ, Parker L, et al. The epidemiology of chronic pain in children and adolescents revisited: a systematic review. Pain. 2011;152(12):2729–38.
71. Pas R, Ickmans K, Van Oosterwijck S, Van der Cruyssen K, Foubert A, Leysen L, et al. Hyperexcitability of the central nervous system in children with chronic pain: a systematic review. Pain Med. 2018;19(12):2504–14.
72. Rabin J, Brown M, Alexander S. Update in the treatment of chronic pain within pediatric patients. Curr Probl Pediatr Adolesc Health Care. 2017;47(7):167–72.
73. Manworren RC, Stinson J. Pediatric pain measurement, assessment, and evaluation. Semin Pediatr Neurol. 2016;23(3):189–200.
74. Hummel P, Puchalski M, Creech SD, Weiss MG. Clinical reliability and validity of the N-PASS: neonatal pain, agitation and sedation scale with prolonged pain. J Perinatol. 2008;28(1):55–60.
75. Lawrence J, Alcock D, McGrath P, Kay J, MacMurray SB, Dulberg C. The development of a tool to assess neonatal pain. Neonatal Netw. 1993;12(6):59–66.
76. Ahn Y, Jun Y. Measurement of pain-like response to various NICU stimulants for high-risk infants. Early Hum Dev. 2007;83(4):255–62.
77. van Dijk M, de Boer JB, Koot HM, Tibboel D, Passchier J, Duivenvoorden HJ. The reliability and validity of the comfort scale as a postoperative pain instrument in 0 to 3-year-old infants. Pain. 2000;84(2–3):367–77.

78. Malviya S, Voepel-Lewis T, Burke C, Merkel S, Tait AR. The revised FLACC observational pain tool: improved reliability and validity for pain assessment in children with cognitive impairment. Paediatr Anaesth. 2006;16(3):258–65.
79. Hicks CL, von Baeyer CL, Spafford PA, van Korlaar I, Goodenough B. The faces pain scale-revised: toward a common metric in pediatric pain measurement. Pain. 2001;93(2):173–83.
80. *Spinal Anesthesia*: *NYSORA, Inc.*; 2022 [Available from: https://www.nysora.com/techniques/neuraxial-and-perineuraxial-techniques/spinal-anesthesia/
81. Anderson C. Adjuvants in regional and Neuraxial anesthesia: An update: society of pediatric anesthesia; 2013 [Available from: https://www2.pedsanesthesia.org/meetings/2013winter/syllabus/submissions/sig-pain/CAnderson.pdf
82. Soin A. Management of pediatric complex regional pain syndrome with low-dose Naltrexone. Am Soc Intervent Pain Phys. 2019;5(3):109–13.

Perioperative Analgesia for a Patient Going for Spine Surgery

Michael Louis Ma and Vivian Ip

Abstract Spinal surgery is frequently complicated by significant acute postoperative pain. Suboptimal pain management can lead to persistent post surgical and chronic pain. There are multiple avenues to perioperatively manage pain including non-pharmacological, pharmacological and interventional. To optimize the patient experience, clinicians must strive to incorporate and individualize analgesic regimes, taking into account all phases of perioperative care. Novel modalities such as cryotherapy and neuromodulation require further investigation.

Keywords Spinal surgery · Spine · Pain management · Acute on chronic pain · Neuropathic pain · Multimodal analgesia · Opioids · Regional anesthesia

1 Introduction

In this chapter, we will explore the perioperative pain management of patients undergoing spinal surgery. Main areas of focus will be the challenges observed in this cohort, current treatment modalities, and future developments.

The Struggle

It is estimated that every year "900,000 American and 30,000 Canadian adults undergo spine surgery" [1]. A retrospective cohort study of 2491 adult patients undergoing lumbar fusion found that 12.8% of opioid naïve patients became long term

M. L. Ma
Department of Anesthesia and Pain Medicine, University of Alberta Hospital, Edmonton, AB, Canada

V. Ip (✉)
Department of Anesthesia, Perioperative and Pain Medicine, University of Calgary, Calgary, Canada
e-mail: hip@ualberta.ca

A. Abd-Elsayed and K. Schroeder (eds.), *Perioperative Pain Management*,
https://doi.org/10.1007/978-3-031-67648-2_17

opioid users and that 77.1% of long-term preoperative opioid users continued with their chronic opioid use [2]. A major contributor to this prolonged requirement for opioid use may be persistent post-surgical pain. Persistent post-surgical pain occurs in 10–40% of patients undergoing lumbar spine surgery and is associated with a 50% escalation in healthcare costs [3]. An American 2-year longitudinal cohort study found that 70% of lumbar fusion patients incurred $9 million in additional medical claim payments, averaging $9383 per patient, which included pain management interventions and the need for long term analgesia [4]. The optimization of perioperative pain management for patients undergoing spinal surgery is crucial but remains beset by many challenges. The surgery itself requires major disruption of various tissue types and the patient cohort is one often suffering with pre-existing chronic pain treated with preoperative multimodal analgesia and habitual opioid use.

The Surgery

There are four major indications for spinal surgery which include decompression of the spinal cord or nerve roots, correction of spinal deformity, excision of tumour, and stabilization following trauma [5]. Excluding minimally invasive procedures, spinal surgery involves the extensive disruption of subcutaneous tissue, ligaments and bone to correct these pathologies [6]. Laminectomies, discectomies, spinal fusions, instrumentations, scoliosis corrections, and spinal tumor excision are just some of the common spinal surgeries performed [6]. Significant postoperative pain is routinely associated with complex spine surgery involving the thoracolumbar regions with instrumentation, surgery for scoliosis, or laminectomies at three or more levels associated with an elevated risk of pain symptomology [7]. This severe postoperative pain is particularly worse within the first three postoperative days. Surgical factors that increase the chance of postoperative chronic opioid use include lumbar fusion of 4 or more levels and extended intraoperative times [8]. While these surgical procedures are known to be uniquely painful, there is an increased interest in shortening hospital length of stay or conversion to ambulatory procedures that requires attention to pain management and analgesic treatment that limits the need for opioid analgesics.

The Patient

A high percentage of patients requiring elective spinal surgery suffer with pre-existing neuropathic and/or chronic pain. These pathologies are notoriously difficult to treat. As a result, they often preoperatively utilize a wide range of multimodal analgesics that may include opioids. Some patients may have an opioid use disorder and or 'recreational drug use' such as cannabis, in the form of Tetrahydrocannabinol (THC) oil.

Older populations who may be suffering from disc degeneration and or arthritic pathology frequently have other associated comorbidities which further complicate analgesic management. Cardiac, renal and liver dysfunction, and polypharmacy may further impact efforts to optimize pain management.

Psychological components of catastrophization, anxiety and depression, as well as other predicting factors including female gender, preoperative opioid use, and pain sensitivity contribute to challenging pain management in this population [9]. Therefore, one of the most important factors in planning perioperative analgesia is aligning expectations for postoperative pain control with patients in the pre-operative setting.

2 Treatment Modalities

Analgesic management for patients undergoing spinal surgery is multifaceted. One must consider pharmacological, non-pharmacological and interventional methods and how these modalities might be leveraged at various periods during the patient's perioperative experience.

Non-pharmacological

- Education

In the preoperative phase, it is crucial to obtain a thorough history of current and previous efforts at analgesic management, outline the analgesic options available for the upcoming procedure, manage the patient's analgesic expectations and address concerns surrounding their upcoming surgery. When the clinician can explore the patient's beliefs and align their analgesic goals with what is realistic for them before surgery, effective progression to functional aims in the postoperative period will be more attainable. As discussed earlier, anxiety may be a significant contributing factor to analgesic management. Often it is possible to alleviate this apprehension with an empathetic discussion and teaching. A systematic review on the effect of pre-emptive and preventive psychoeducation on postoperative pain control concluded that there was strong evidence suggesting a mismatch between pain expectation and physical sensation can develop in patients who are not fully informed about postoperative pain [10]. Further to this, patients who opted out of procedural pain education experienced more frequent uncontrolled pain and longer hospital stays [10]. Horn et al. also found that preoperative anxiety and pain catastrophizing had negative effects on recovery and concluded that "an open and sympathetic discussion between providers and patients is crucial for optimal satisfaction and maximum recovery." [10].

- Physical Interventions

The use of acupuncture and acupressure as analgesic adjuncts in spinal surgery patients has demonstrated variable results. A systematic review and meta-analysis of 5 randomized controlled trials (RCTs) studying acupuncture for acute postoperative pain in patients undergoing back surgery concluded that there was limited evidence supporting acupuncture treatment in this cohort [11]. However, a recent retrospective study investigating patients given either meperidine, PCA or acupuncture for post-operative lumbar spinal surgeries found acupuncture to be non-inferior to the other 2 arms when included as a component of a multimodal analgesic regimen [12].

- Behavioural Interventions

Perioperative multimodal rehabilitation that includes preoperative education/ prehabilitation and early postoperative mobilization is an important interventional component of postoperative pain control. Exercise therapy with cognitive behavioural training is emerging as a useful technique to decrease postoperative disability and pain. A systematic review with meta-analysis of rehabilitation strategies in patients undergoing lumbar fusion surgery reviewed 18 RCTs and found promising evidence that multimodal rehabilitation and exercise therapy were effective in improving outcomes like decreasing disability and pain-related fear [13].

Pharmacological

Multimodal analgesia has become a widespread strategy when it comes to acute pain management. The overall aim is to target multiple pain receptors to optimally decrease pain scores and opioid requirements.

- Acetaminophen

Acetaminophen is one of the most commonly used analgesics for the treatment of mild to moderate pain. Acetaminophen acts centrally with inhibitory effects on cyclooxygenase (COX) isoenzymes as well as serotonergic effects [14]. A dose of 15 mg per kilogram is the standard with a maximum administration of 4 g over a 24 h period. Acetaminophen is metabolized in the liver primarily via conjugation to sulfate and glucuronide conjugates later excreted in the urine. Caution and dose adjustments may be necessary when patients display significant hepatic impairment, particularly transaminitis, or hepatic disease. Evidence supporting the use of acetaminophen in spine patients is, unfortunately, scarce. However, acetaminophen is considered low risk and is typically recommended as part of a multimodal analgesic approach for a wide array of surgical procedures. The PROcedure-SPECific Pain ManagemenT (PROSPECT) collaboration recommends acetaminophen as a valuable addition to multimodal spinal surgery analgesic regimens [7]. The faster onset of intravenous administration compared to the enteral route may be beneficial in the immediate postoperative phase but widespread utilization may be limited secondary to cost disparities that exist between the different routes of administration.

- Non-steroidal Anti-inflammatory Drugs (NSAIDs)

Non-steroidal anti-inflammatory drugs (NSAIDs) are another commonly used analgesic for the treatment of mild to moderate pain. This class of medication acts by inhibiting the COX 1 and 2 enzymes centrally and peripherally, preventing the production of prostaglandins and decreasing the inflammatory response. Contraindications to NSAIDs include renal dysfunction, gastrointestinal inflammation or bleeding, coagulopathy and heart failure.

NSAID use has been shown to be an effective opioid sparing technique in spinal surgery. A meta-analysis of 8 RCTs of NSAID use in lumbar spine surgery concluded that NSAIDs were effective in reducing visual analogue scores compared to placebo, particularly in the COX-2 selective group [15]. Another meta-analysis of 17 double-blinded RCTs found that patients who were administered NSAIDs in spinal surgery had significantly lower pain scores and less opioid consumption [16].

- Opioids

Opioids are the most common analgesic treatment for the treatment of spinal surgery pain in the perioperative phase of care. This class of analgesics targets μ opioid receptors both peripherally and centrally. Side effects of opioid administration include nausea and vomiting, respiratory depression, constipation, sedation, dizziness, pruritus, dependency and tolerance. Opioid metabolism is primarily by the CYP450 system in the liver with subsequent renal excretion of metabolites. Preoperative opioid use is associated with an increased incidence of prolonged postoperative opioid requirements and worsened surgical outcomes [17]. There has been a movement to reduce or eliminate pre-operative opioid administration to improve perioperative μ opioid receptor sensitivity and improve efforts at pain management [18]. However, care must be taken to avoid withdrawal and these dose alterations may be challenging to implement without the guidance of a dedicated healthcare clinician, especially in the community setting. The use of buprenorphine is becoming an increasingly common component of medication treatment of opioid use disorder (MOUD). It is a partial mu-receptor agonist that acts centrally and is used as a substitute for full opioid agonists with the aim of safely reducing opioid cravings and withdrawal symptoms. Guidelines that detail the management of patients on preexisting buprenorphine recommend the continuation of the same dose of buprenorphine preoperatively, although the dosage postoperatively can be divided into twice or three times per day to maximize analgesic efficacy [19]. Patients on buprenorphine can be prescribed additional opioid postoperatively for optimal pain control and these patients often require robust multimodal analgesia regimens, especially if the spine surgery is complex.

Similar to buprenorphine use, patients on preoperative methadone should continue their normal prescription throughout their perioperative experience. Methadone is a potent mu-receptor agonist with secondary N-methyl-D-aspartate (NMDA) receptor inhibition that inhibits ascending pain pathways. Methadone dosing can be complicated by a long elimination half-life of 33–46 h. Methadone also has a prolonged duration of action, as such, the practicalities of its regular use with regards to titration for acute postoperative pain maybe challenging. Despite this, a 2017 RCT of 120 patients undergoing spinal fusion surgery were either administered methadone or hydromorphone intraoperatively [20]. The patients in the methadone group required less opioids, had lower pain scores and displayed improved patient satisfaction [20].

All patients with an opioid-use-disorder will be expected to require an increased amount of opioid postoperatively and experience prolonged hospital admissions secondary to difficulties associated with analgesic management. The opioid dose at discharge should be returned to baseline or a weaning plan should be made available that details a gradual opioid reduction back to baseline. Therefore, institutions with transitional pain services will be advantageous for patients with significant baseline opioid requirements [21].

- Gabapentinoids

Gabapentinoids were originally indicated as anticonvulsants but have now become a component of neuropathic and chronic pain management regimens. Their use has crept into the acute postoperative pain realm; however, this is an off-label indication. The mechanism of action of these medications is central binding to the alpha-2-delta subunits of voltage dependent calcium channels leading to inhibition of excitatory neurotransmitter release. Gabapentin is dosed enterally 900–2400 mg per day divided into 3 doses. Pregabalin is first dosed at 75–150 mg 2 times per day or 50–100 mg 3 times per day, titrated as needed to a maximum of 600 mg per day. Common side effects seen in this group of medications include dizziness, drowsiness, ataxia, weight gain, abuse, and respiratory depression in the setting of overdose. Particular caution should be used in the elderly and patients with renal dysfunction. Concurrent use of opioids and benzodiazepines may also be associated with an increased incidence of significant sedation and respiratory depression.

The evidence supporting the analgesic benefit of gabapentinoids in postoperative patients has been inconsistent [22, 23]. A meta-analysis of 16 clinical trials found that gabapentinoids were associated with decreased pain scores and cumulative morphine use up to 48 h following surgery [24]. Contrary to this, other recent studies have found that gabapentinoids in other surgical cohorts lack opioid sparing effects and are associated with an increased risk of opioid overdose and opioid-related adverse effects, especially postoperative pulmonary complications [25, 26]. The use of gabapentinoids for postoperative analgesia in spinal surgery requires a careful benefit risk analysis, especially in elderly patients who are susceptible to side effects such as drowsiness. The PROSPECT working group do not recommend routine use in complex spinal surgical patients [7].

- Ketamine

Ketamine is a valuable and potent addition to multimodal analgesic armamentariums that can be utilized throughout the perioperative continuum. It is a NMDA receptor antagonist and dissociative anesthetic that might be particularly useful in opioid tolerant patients. Side effects of this medication include nausea and vomiting, disorientation, confusion, sedation, dysphoria, dizziness, hallucinations, hypertension and tachycardia. Subanesthetic bolus doses of 0.1–0.3 mg/kg can be given either intra or postoperatively to augment analgesia and minimize opioid requirements. Ketamine can also be delivered as an intraoperative infusion of 0.1–1 mg/kg/h with many institutions implementing protocols that allow for infusions on the ward postoperatively. An example of our institutional protocol for postoperative ward infusions can be found in Table 1.

The evidence supporting the perioperative analgesic use of ketamine for patients undergoing spine surgery is reassuring. A recent systematic review and meta-analysis of 30 RCTs which included 1865 elective spine surgery patients found significantly lower opioid consumption and pain intensity with no increased adverse events experienced by patients who were administered low-dose ketamine perioperatively up to 48 h [27]. These positive results were not observed for the pediatric cohort in this meta-analysis [27]. Despite this finding, a 2022 meta-analysis of 5 RCTs examining ketamine use in adolescent idiopathic scoliosis patients undergoing fusion surgery concluded that intra and postoperative use of continuous low dose ketamine significantly decreased opioid requirements within the first 48 h after surgery [28].

Ketamine is often an analgesic included in multimodal strategies to combat pain in opioid-dependent patients. A RCT of the analgesic effects of intraoperative ketamine use on opiate-dependent patients with a history of chronic pain showed a significant reduction in morphine consumption up to 48 h and at 6 weeks postoperatively [29]. It was also found that pain intensity was significantly lower in the PACU and at 6 weeks with no differences in opioid related adverse events [29]. There is evidence

Table 1 An example of a ketamine infusion protocol for adults

Ketamine 250 mg in NaCl 0.9% 250 mL (1 mg/mL) infusion 0.1 mg/kg/h × Weight in kg, intravenous, continuous Use the actual body weight up to a maximum weight of 100 kg Maximum 0.4mg/kg/hr
Notify Most responsible Health Practitioner Respiratory Rate less than 8 breaths per minute Other: Sedation level of 4
Vital Signs—Protocol for duration of infusion and 8 h post discontinuation of Low-Dose Ketamine Infusion for Analgesia Monitor as follows: Every 15 min for 1 h, every 2 h for 4 h, then every 4 h for duration of infusion and 8 h post discontinuation of infusion. Repeat monitoring sequence with any rate increase of the low-dose ketamine infusion for analgesia
Nursing Communication—Notify Pain Notify Acute Pain Service/Pain Consultant for all problems and orders related to pain, sedation, nausea and vomiting, and pruritus
Nursing Communication—Notify Agitation Notify Acute Pain Service/Pain Consultant if patient continues to experience agitation/psychotomimetic effects despite administration of benzodiazepine and reduction of ketamine infusion
Maintain IV Access Maintain Intravenous Access for duration of therapy and for 8–12 h post discontinuation of Low-Dose Ketamine Infusion for Analgesia

that ketamine administration may not be as efficacious in opiate-naïve spinal surgery patients [8]. A RCT of adults undergoing multilevel spine surgery in a mixed cohort of opioid naïve and dependent patients either given multimodal analgesia, including ketamine, compared to opioid only analgesia showed no difference in Quality of Recovery scores up to 48 h postoperatively [22].

- Lidocaine Infusions

Intravenous (IV) lidocaine infusions have been used perioperatively as an opioid sparing analgesic. This amide local anesthetic (LA) mainly acts by blocking voltage gated sodium channels. Secondary target sites of action include inhibiting calcium and potassium channels. Lidocaine is metabolised the P450 enzyme system in the liver. It would be prudent to caution use or reduce dosage in patients with cardiac, liver or renal dysfunction as well as in the elderly. Regular monitoring for local anesthetic systemic toxicity should be observed, especially during infusions continuing more than 24 h [30, 31]. Lidocaine infusions should not concurrently be used with other local anesthetic infusions such as nerve block catheter infusions and 20% lipid emulsion should be easily accessible [31].

There is a wide variability in IV lidocaine dosing administration reported in the literature. Various protocols outline bolus doses of 1–2 mg/kg over 10 min with or without a continuous infusion at 1–3 mg/kg/h intraoperatively and/or postoperatively. The proposed mechanism of lidocaine analgesia is through reductions in inflammation supports delivery at various timepoints within the perioperative period. The efficacy of intravenous lidocaine administration beyond 24 h postoperatively, however, is questionable.

A 2021 international consensus statement on the use of intravenous lidocaine for postoperative pain considers this form of analgesia as "high risk" [31]. Some of the recommendations listed as best practice safety considerations include informed patient consent before use, considering toxic plasma lidocaine concentrations as > 5 mcg/ml, utilizing ideal body weight for dosing calculations, avoiding use in patients < 40 kg, avoiding doses in excess of 120 mg/h, limiting loading bolus dosing to no more than 1.5 mg/kg, and limiting ongoing infusions to a maximum of 1.5 mg/kg/h and less than 24 h use [31].

A 2022 systematic review and meta-analysis of 8 RCTs examining the effectiveness of perioperative intravenous lidocaine administration in patients undergoing spine surgery found pain scores were significantly decreased up to 24 h in adult and pediatric cohorts but up to 48 h specifically in adult populations [32]. Opioid requirements and hospital length of stay were also reduced in the same review [32]. In all 8 studies, an initial bolus was administered along with an occasional continuous infusion running into the postoperative period [32].

Interventional

- Neuraxial

Spinal surgery is still preferentially performed under general anesthesia; however, with advancements in minimally invasive and endoscopic spine surgery, neuraxial techniques have become increasingly feasible. There are many advantages associated with the use of neuraxial anesthesia as a sole technique or as an analgesic adjunct to general anesthesia. These advantages include shorter operative times, cost savings, and superior analgesia. In addition, decreased pulmonary complications, cognitive dysfunction, thrombotic events, and intraoperative blood loss have all been reported with the use of neuraxial anesthesia [8, 33].

When compared to general anesthesia, the benefits of a neuraxial anesthetic for lumbar and some lower thoracic spine surgeries are that the patient experiences less nausea and vomiting, has improved hemodynamic stability, experiences decreased surgical bleeding and need for transfusion, is able to position themselves comfortably intraoperatively (theoretically reducing the risk of stretch/pressure injuries), realizes improved perioperative pain control, and avoids the risks associated with airway instrumentation and general anesthesia [8, 34]. Disadvantages of neuraxial anesthesia for spine surgery include limited anesthetic duration of non-catheter based techniques, non-ubiquitous availability, lack of airway protection in a prone patient, the frequent need for sedation in a prone patient, and coughing/patient movement that might be substantially magnified under the surgical microscope [34]. A recent scoping review of the literature studying regional anesthetic techniques for spinal surgery found that bupivacaine was the most frequently utilized local anesthetic [33]. Advantages of isobaric bupivacaine administration include decreased cephalad local anesthetic spread and block extension while in the prone position [8]. Spinal anesthetic adjuncts including fentanyl and epinephrine may be useful when prolongation of surgical anesthesia is required [8].

Epidural techniques in spinal surgery have been used less as a replacement for general anesthesia for a number of reasons. Despite the benefits outlined above, it's analgesic effects can be inconsistent and large volumes of local anesthetic in the epidural space obstructs the surgical field [34]. In addition, inadvertent dural punctures can produce difficult postdural puncture headache management conundrums in patients recovering from recent spinal surgery. Epidural and combined spinal-epidural placements for spinal surgeries were observed to use a range of amide local anaesthetics including lidocaine, bupivacaine or ropivacaine [33]. Adjuncts ranged from a variety of opioids to dexmedetomidine and methylprednisolone [33]. It should be noted that surgically placed epidural catheters have been utilized for the provision of postoperative analgesia although practice has not been widespread [35].

- Nerve Blocks

Multiple regional anesthetic blocks have been shown to decrease opioid requirements and pain scores following spinal surgery. These blocks are frequently placed prior to surgery and are generally used as an analgesic adjunct and not as a replacement for general anesthesia.

- Erector Spinae Plane Blocks

The use of erector spinae plane blocks for postoperative analgesia following spine surgery makes conceptual sense as this block has a well-defined mechanism for anesthetizing the dorsal rami of the thoracolumbar spinal nerves [33]. Advantages of erector spinae plane blocks include surgical procedural versatility and relative ease associated with block placement. Erector spinae place blocks can be performed as a single injection or as a continuous catheter insertion, although the latter may be logistically challenging given the proximity to the surgical field. Under ultrasound guidance, the paraspinal fascial plane block is typically carried out using an in-plane technique, targeting the plane between the erector spinae muscle and the transverse process. A large volume (15–20 ml) of local anesthetic is deposited bilaterally and spread in a cranial to caudal direction achieves a multi-dermatomal block (Fig. 1).

- Thoracolumbar Interfascial Plane Block

The thoracolumbar interfascial plane (TLIP) block targets the medial branch of the thoracolumbar dorsal rami as it passes between the multifidus and longissimus thoracis fascial plane components of the erector spinae muscle (Fig. 2) [36]. Needle insertion is typically with an in-plane technique and 20 ml of local anesthetic is

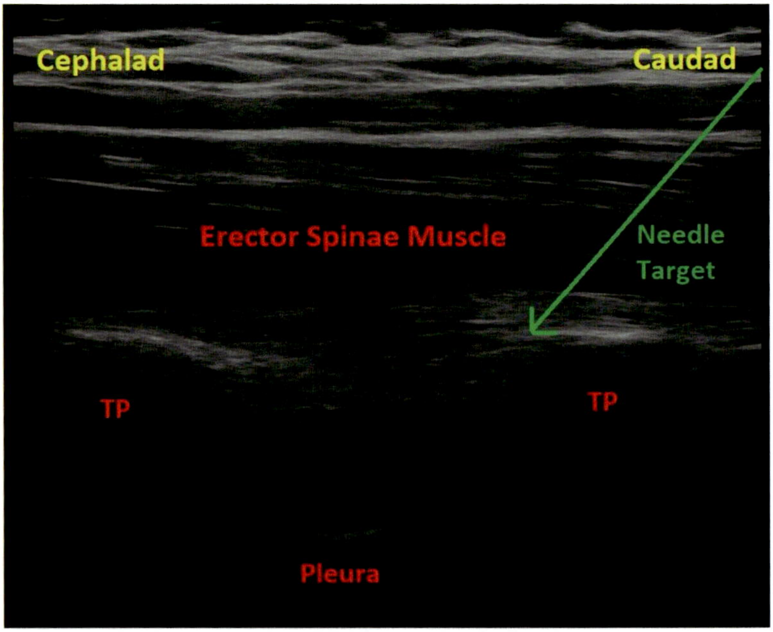

Fig. 1 Erector spinae plane block—TP (Transverse Process)

deposited between these planes with cranial to caudal spread, blocking 2–3 spinal levels in either direction from the point of injection. The block is performed bilaterally for a complete block covering the midline either as a single-shot or continuous block. A recent meta-analysis of 17 RCTs for lumbar spine surgeries showed moderate quality evidence that TLIP blocks reduce PONV, total analgesic consumption and pain scores up to 24 h [37]. However, further robust RCTs are warranted to examine its efficacy.

- Multifidus Cervices Plane block

A block aimed at supplying analgesia for the cervical spine is the multifidus cervices plane block (Fig. 3). This block was first described in a 2017 case report where it was described as an analgesic strategy for patients undergoing a cervical laminoplasty [38]. It is similar to the TLIP block, however it targets the cervical dorsal rami via local anesthetic deposition within the fascial plane between the multifidus cervicis and semispinalis cervicis muscles at the C5 level. Ohgoshi et al. described using 20ml of 0.375% ropivacaine [38]. Further high quality research is required to recommend regular use.

- Superficial Cervical Plexus Block

Patients undergoing cervical surgery with an anterior approach may benefit from administration of a superficial cervical plexus (SCP) block (Fig. 4). This nerve block targets the SCP formed by the ventral rami of C1–4 and can be performed under ultrasound guidance or landmark technique to provide analgesia to the anterolateral

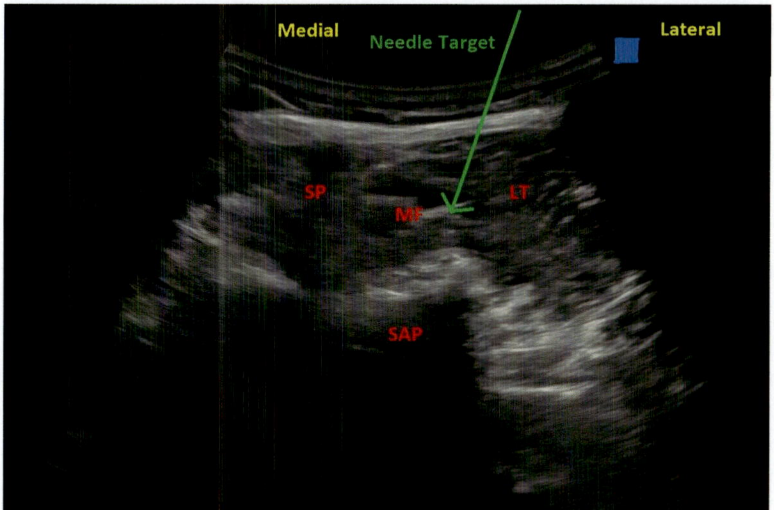

Fig. 2 Thoracolumbar Interfascial Plane block—SP (Spinous Process), SAP (Superior Articular Process), MF (Multifidus), LT (Longissimus Thoracis)

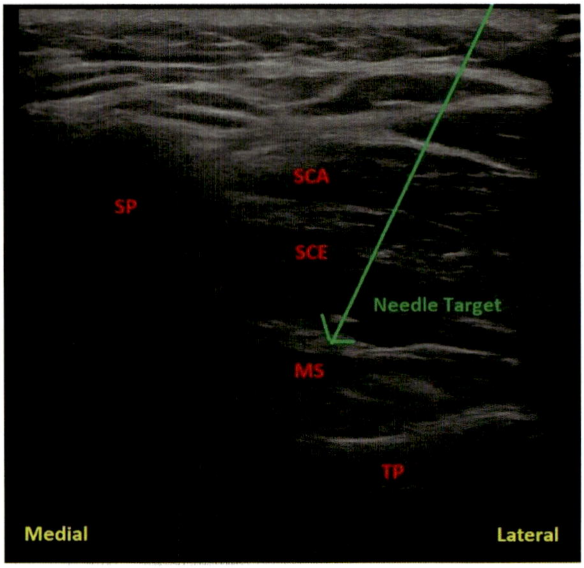

Fig. 3 Multifidus Cervices Plane block—SP (Spinous Process), MS (Multifidus Cervicis Muscle), SCE (Semispinalis Cervicis Muscles), SCA (Semispinalis Capitis Muscle)

aspect of the neck. The aim is to deposit 10–15 ml of local anesthetic in the fascial layer under the posterior/lateral border of sternocleidomastoid at the C5 level, above the pre-vertebral fascia. A common complication of this procedure is phrenic nerve blockade, especially if local anesthetic is deposited below the pre-vertebral fascia, causing unilateral diaphragmatic paralysis. A RCT of patients undergoing anterior cervical discectomy and fusion surgery found that patients who had SCP blocks performed after induction compared to those who had not been blocked, had a higher global quality of recovery questionnaire (QoR) score, but failed to show a difference in 24 h opioid consumption or realize earlier discharge [39]. Mulcahy et al. are in the process of carrying out a randomized placebo-controlled trial investigating the use of bilateral SCP blocks on patients undergoing anterior cervical spine surgery [40].

3 Future Developments

Optimal analgesic management for patients undergoing spinal surgeries is rapidly evolving. Secondary to multiple analgesic challenges encountered in the management of these patients, innovative approaches are being continuously developed and optimal analgesic management may not yet be determined. Cryotherapy and cryo-compression may ultimately play a role in treating acute postoperative pain following spine surgery [41, 42]. Neuromodulation might represent another significant area which could be further explored. The individualized care package consisting of a transitional pain service is an area for investigation, however, a lack of funding and specialized healthcare allies forming a collaborative team may pose a challenge.

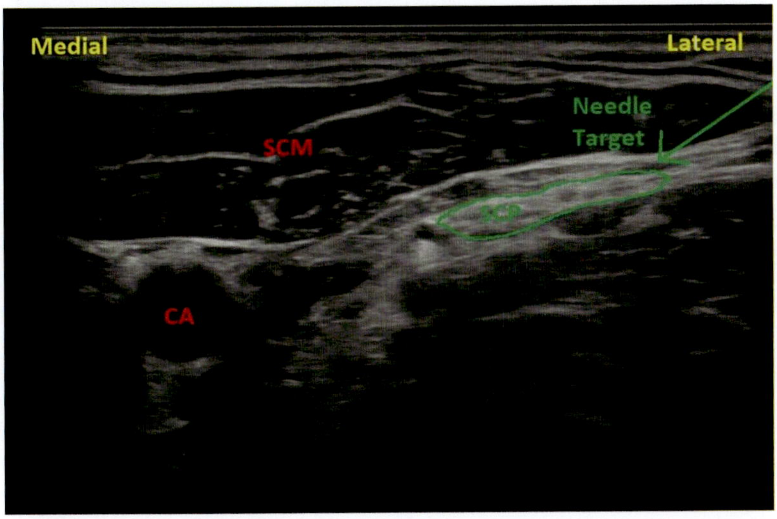

Fig. 4 Superficial Cervical Plexus Block—SCM (Sternocleidomastoid Muscle), SCP (Superficial Cervical Plexus), CA (Carotid Artery)

4 Conclusion

The nature of spinal surgery and the characteristics of those who require these surgeries frequently coalesce to produce challenges when attempting to deliver effective postoperative analgesia. Multiple factors require consideration when balancing the risks and benefits of analgesic requirements for this patient cohort. Multimodal pharmacological regimens may not be a panacea for complex spinal patients but the perioperative implementation of individualized non-pharmacological, pharmacological and regional anesthetic techniques can help multidisciplinary teams deliver the best results for these patients.

Key Takeaways of the Chapter

1. Pain control for patients undergoing spine surgery can be challenging as these patients may have pre-existing chronic pain and/or opioid tolerance.
2. Preoperative education and alignment of goals of pain management is important for successful postoperative course.
3. Multimodal individualized care involving multidisciplinary care is necessary.
4. Regional anesthesia techniques are good analgesic adjuncts to reduce opioid consumption and should not be overlooked.
5. Alternative modalities such as acupuncture and behavioral interventions for pain management should also be considered.

References

1. Cram P, Landon BE, Matelski J, Ling V, Perruccio AV, Paterson JM, et al. Utilization and outcomes for spine surgery in the United States and Canada. Spine. 2019;44(19):1371–80.
2. Deyo RA, Hallvik SE, Hildebran C, Marino M, O'Kane N, Carson J, et al. Use of prescription opioids before and after an operation for chronic pain (lumbar fusion surgery). Pain. 2018;159(6):1147–54.
3. Davin SA, Savage J, Thompson NR, Schuster A, Darnall BD. Transforming standard of care for spine surgery: integration of an online single-session behavioral pain management class for perioperative optimization. Front Pain Res. 2022;3:1–8.
4. Mino DE, Munterich JE, Castel LD. Lumbar fusion surgery for degenerative conditions is associated with significant resource and narcotic use 2 years postoperatively in the commercially insured: a medical and pharmacy claims study. J Spine Surg. 2017;3(2):141–8.
5. Prout J, Jones T, Martin D. Advanced training in anaesthesia the essential curriculum. Oxford: Oxford University Press; 2014.
6. Bajwa SJS, Haldar R. Pain management following spinal surgeries: an appraisal of the available options. J Craniovertebral Junction Spine. 2015;6:105–10.
7. Waelkens P, Alsabbagh E, Sauter A, Joshi GP, Beloeil H. Pain management after complex spine surgery: a systematic review and procedure-specific postoperative pain management recommendations. Eur J Anaesthesiol. 2021;38:985–94.
8. Prabhakar NK, Chadwick AL, Nwaneshiudu C, Aggarwal A, Salmasi V, Lii TR, et al. Management of postoperative pain in patients following spine surgery: a narrative review. Int J General Med. 2022;15:4535–49.
9. Ip HYV, Abrishami A, Peng PWH, Wong J, Chung F. Predictors of postoperative pain and analgesic consumption: a qualitative systematic review. Anesthesiology. 2009;111(3):657–77.
10. Horn A, Kaneshiro K, Tsui BCH. Preemptive and preventive pain psychoeducation and its potential application as a multimodal perioperative pain control option: a systematic review. Anesth Analg. 2020;130(3):559–73.
11. Cho YH, Kim CK, Heo KH, Lee MS, Ha IH, Son DW, et al. Acupuncture for acute postoperative pain after back surgery: a systematic review and meta-analysis of randomized controlled trials. Pain Pract: Official J World Inst Pain. 2015;15(3):279–91.
12. Chen BA, Deng WC, Chen MY. Acupuncture for pain control after degenerative lumbar spine surgery. Eur J Med Res. 2022;27(1):167–75.
13. Bogaert L, Thys T, Depreitere B, Dankaerts W, Amerijckx C, Wambeke PV, et al. Rehabilitation to improve outcomes of lumbar fusion surgery: a systematic review with meta-analysis. Eur Spine J. 2022;31(6):1525–45.

14. Kaye AD, Granier AL, Garcia AJ, Carlson SF, Fuller MC, Haroldson AR, et al. Non-opioid perioperative pain strategies for the clinician: a narrative review. Pain Ther. 2020;9(1):25–39.
15. Zhang Z, Xu H, Zhang Y, Li W, Yang Y, Han T, et al. Nonsteroidal anti-inflammatory drugs for postoperative pain control after lumbar spine surgery: a meta-analysis of randomized controlled trials. J Clin Anesth. 2017;43:84–9.
16. Jirarattanaphochai K, Jung S. Nonsteroidal antiinflammatory drugs for postoperative pain management after lumbar spine surgery: a meta-analysis of randomized controlled trials. J Neurosurg Spine. 2008;9(1):22–31.
17. Wang M, Harrop J, Bisson E, Dhall S, Dimar J, Mohamed B, et al. Congress of neurological surgeons systematic review and evidence-based guidelines for perioperative spine: preoperative opioid evaluation. Neurosurgery. 2021;89(Suppl1):S1–8.
18. McAnally H. Rationale for and approach to preoperative opioid weaning: a preoperative optimization protocol. Perioper Med (London, England). 2017;6(19).
19. Kohan L, Potru S, Barreveld A, Sprintz M, Lane O, Aryal A, et al. Buprenorphine management in the perioperative period: educational review and recommendations from a multisociety expert panel. Regional Anesth Pain Med 2021:1–20
20. Murphy G, Szokol JW, Avram MJ, Greenberg SB, Shear TD, Deshur MA, et al. Clinical effectiveness and safety of intraoperative methadone in patients undergoing posterior spinal fusion surgery: a randomized, double-blinded, controlled trial. Anesthesiology. 2017;126:822–33.
21. Mikhaeil J, Ayoo K, Clarke H, Wasowicz M, Huang A. Review of the transitional pain service as a method of postoperative opioid weaning and a service aimed at minimizing the risk of chronic post-surgical pain. Anaesthesiology Intens Ther. 2020;52(2):148–53.
22. Maheshwari K, Avitsian R, Sessler DI, Makarova NSM, Tanios M, et al. Multimodal analgesic regimen for spine surgery. Anesthesiology 2020;132:992–1002.
23. Farhat B, Ip V, Sondekoppam RV. Curb your enthusiasm: should gabapentinoids be a routine component of multimodal analgesia? ASRA News. 2022;47.
24. Liu B, Liu R, Wang L. A meta-analysis of the preoperative use of gabapentinoids for the treatment of acute postoperative pain following spinal surgery. Medicine (Baltimore). 2017;96(37):1–11.
25. McGauvran M, Ohnuma T, Raghunathan K, Krishnamoorthy V, Johnson S, Lo T, et al. Association between gabapentinoids and postoperative pulmonary complications in patients undergoing thoracic surgery. J Cardiothorac Vasc Anesth. 2022;36:2295–302.
26. Bykov K, Bateman BT, Franklin JM, Vine SM, Patorno E. Assoication of Gabapentinoids with the risk of opioid-related adverse events in surgical patients in the United States. JAMA Network Open. 2020;3(12).
27. Zhou L, Yang H, Hai Y, Cheng Y. Perioperative low-dose ketamine for postoperative pain management in spine surgery: a systematic review and meta-analysis of randomized controlled trials. Pain Res Manage. 2022.
28. Mariscal G, Morales J, Perez S, Rubio-Belmar PA, Bovea-Marco M, Bas JL, et al. Meta-analysis of the efficacy of ketamine in postoperative pain control in adolescent idiopathic scoliosis patients undergoing spinal fusion. Eur Spine J. 2022;31(12):3492–9.
29. Loftus RW, Yeager MP, Clark JA, Brown JR, Abdu WA, Sengupta DK, et al. Intraoperative ketamine reduces perioperative opiate consumption in opiate-dependent patients with chronic back pain undergoing back surgery. Anesthesiology. 2010;113(3):639–49.
30. Eipe N, Gupta S, Penning J. Intravenous lidocaine for acute pain: an evidence-based clinical update. BJA Educ. 2016;16(9):292–8.
31. Foo I, Macfarlane A, Srivastava D, Bhaskar A, Barker H, Knaggs R, et al. The use of intravenous lidocaine for postoperative pain and recovery: international consensus statement on efficacy and safety. Anesthesia. 2021;76(2):238–50.
32. Licina A, Silvers A. Perioperative intravenous lidocaine infusion for postoperative analgesia in patients undergoing surgery of the spine: systematic review and meta-analysis. Pain Med. 2022;23(1):45–56.

33. Eochagain AN, Singleton BN, Moorthy A, Buggy DJ. Regional and neuraxial anaesthesia techniques for spinal surgery: a scoping review. Br J Anaesth. 2022;129(4):598–611.
34. Garg B, Ahuja K, Sharan AD. Regional anesthesia for spine surgery. J Am Acad Orthop Surg. 2022;30(17):809–19.
35. Turner A, Lee J, Mitchell R, Berman J, Edge G, Fennelly M. The efficacy of surgically placed epidural catheters for analgesia after posterior spinal surgery. Anaesthesia. 2000;55(4):370–3.
36. Hand WR, Taylor JM, Harvey NR, Epperson TI, Gunselman RJ, Bolin ED, et al. Thoracolumbar interfascial plane (TLIP) block: a pilot study in volunteers. Can J Anesth. 2015;62:1196–200.
37. Long G, Liu C, Liang T, Zhan X. The efficacy of thoracolumbar interfascial plane block for lumbar spinal surgeries: a systematic review and meta-analysis. J Orthop Surg Res. 2023;18(1):318–30.
38. Ohgoshi Y, Izawa H, Kori S, Matsukawa M. Multifidus cervicis plane block is effective for cervical spine surgery. Can J Anesth. 2017;64:329–30.
39. Mariappan R, Mehta J, Massicotte E, Nagappa M, Manninen P, Venkatraghavan L. Effect of superficial cervical plexus block on postoperative quality of recovery after anterior cervical discectomy and fusion: a randomized controlled trial. Can J Anesth. 2015;62:883–90.
40. Mulcahy MJ, Elalingam T, Jang K, D'Souza M, Tait M. Bilateral cervical plexus block for anterior cervical spine surgery: study protocol for a randomised placebo-controlled trial. Trials. 2021;22(1):424.
41. Murata K, Yoshimoto M, Takebayashi T, Ida K, Nakano K, Yamashita T. Effect of cryotherapy after spine surgery. Asian Spine J. 2014;8(6):753–8.
42. Nabiyev V, Ayhan S, Adhikari P, Cetin E, Palaoglu S, Acaroglu R. Cryo-compression therapy after elective spinal surgery for pain management: a cross-sectional study with historical control. Neurospine. 2018;15(4):348–52.

Perioperative Considerations for Palliative and Terminally Ill Patients

Lara India

Abstract Pain related to serious illness, especially cancer, is a common complaint amongst patients with terminal illness or receiving palliative care. Anesthesiologists must carefully consider how to control these patients' intra- and postoperative pain due to their complex pre-existing pain management regimens and potential contraindications to certain adjuvant pain medications. Understanding the patient's baseline opioid use and how to convert it to appropriate intravenous formulations is crucial. Additionally, anesthesiologists should recognize that terminally ill patients are susceptible to non-physical types of pain, which may emerge or worsen during the perioperative period. It is essential for anesthesiologists to be familiar with non-pharmacological interventions to address these different facets of a patient's total pain.

Keywords Palliative care · Cancer pain · Total pain · Opioid conversions · Goals of care

1 Introduction

Palliative care is a clinical approach that aims to improve quality of life metrics for patients facing serious illnesses, regardless of whether the illness is terminal or life-prolonging treatments are offered concurrently [1]. While the development of palliative care in the United States historically focused on symptom management and end-of-life care specifically for cancer patients, a patient with any serious illness may benefit from palliative care.

This chapter will largely focus on perioperative considerations for palliative care patients with cancer-related pain, given its prevalence and the high number of cancer patients encountered by anesthesiologists in the perioperative setting. According to the National Cancer Institute, there were 1.8 million new cancer diagnoses in 2020

L. India (✉)
Anesthesiology and Hospice and Palliative Medicine, Medical College of Wisconsin, Milwaukee, USA
e-mail: lindia@mcw.edu

A. Abd-Elsayed and K. Schroeder (eds.), *Perioperative Pain Management*,
https://doi.org/10.1007/978-3-031-67648-2_18

[2], and cancer survival rates continue to increase, with an estimated 22 million cancer survivors in the United States predicted by 2030 [3]. It is important to note that nearly 40% of all cancer patients report moderate-to-severe pain at some point, which may persist even after curative treatment [4]. Therefore, it is essential for anesthesiologists to understand the unique perioperative considerations encountered when caring for patients receiving palliative care and seeking to provide effective pain management and improve the patient's overall quality of life.

2 Case Presentation

Mrs. Arnold is an 83 kg, 54-year-old female, who was diagnosed with breast cancer two years ago. She works full-time in the toddler room at a daycare center. She lives alone and takes pride in driving herself to appointments. Unfortunately, her disease has progressed despite multiple rounds of chemotherapy, resulting in bony and liver metastases that cause constant pain currently managed by her palliative care doctor. She also developed chemotherapy-induced peripheral neuropathy approximately one year ago.

During her last visit to her palliative care doctor one month ago, Mrs. Arnold's extended-release morphine was increased to 45 mg every 12 h. She is also prescribed oxycodone 20 mg every 4 h as needed, usually requiring two or three doses daily, and pregabalin 150 mg twice daily. Mrs. Arnold is now presenting for surgical fixation of a pathologic left femur fracture.

3 Palliative Approaches to Symptom Management

Pain

Managing physical pain requires distinguishing whether it is nociceptive, visceral, or neuropathic. Due to its nociceptive and progressive nature, cancer pain management heavily relies on the use of opioids. The World Health Organization (WHO) analgesic ladder is a commonly followed algorithm for cancer pain management [5]. Non-opioid adjuvants like acetaminophen or non-steroidal anti-inflammatory drugs (NSAIDs) are used to treat mild pain at the first step of the ladder. However, these medications have certain limitations in the context of cancer pain management. For instance, acetaminophen should be used cautiously in patients with risk factors for hepatic toxicity and in the immunocompromised population as it can mask fever, an early warning sign of infection [6]. Furthermore, preclinical studies suggested that concomitant use of NSAIDs and immune checkpoint inhibitors may worsen patient outcomes; however, the clinical effect may not be significant [7].

Short-acting opioids, such as immediate-release morphine or oxycodone, are used for moderate cancer-related pain. To achieve adequate pain control, oncologists or palliative care doctors will frequently initiate short-acting opioid therapy and then assess the average opioid amount required in a 24 h period. The total oral morphine equivalents (OME) used in the course of this trial is then used to determine a starting dose of long-acting opioid. Both the short- and long-acting opioids are then titrated further as needed.

Currently, muscle relaxants are not included in the WHO analgesic ladder or other national guidelines for treatment of cancer-related pain [5, 6], and thus they do not have a large role in cancer pain management unless imaging specifically suggests irritation of a muscle group by tumor involvement. Antiepileptics like pregabalin or gabapentin, and SNRIs may be used to treat chemotherapy-induced peripheral neuropathy [6].

Patients receiving outpatient palliative care have frequent contact with their health-care team, and their pain management regimen is typically titrated over the course of weeks or months. Therefore, the majority of patients treated by an anesthesiologist will have been stable on their short- and long-acting opioids for some weeks. This regimen stability is particularly important when considering acutely painful injuries that may cause patients to present for a surgical intervention, such as repair of a pathologic fracture. A patient's pre-existing pain management regimen is intended to meet their baseline pain management requirements. As such, long-acting and short-acting opioids should be continued in the perioperative period at equipotent doses. Although patients may undergo procedures expected to result in an acute decrease in pain (such as vertebroplasty or fracture fixation), their baseline pain is not expected to decrease as their underlying disease remains unchanged.

Dyspnea

Anesthesiologists should be familiar with palliative strategies for managing dyspnea, in addition to pain management. Chronic dyspnea is a common symptom in illnesses such as COPD, heart failure, cancer, and ESRD, and refers to the sensation of breathlessness over several weeks. After optimizing the underlying illness and implementing non-pharmacological measures, opioids or benzodiazepines may be prescribed to manage residual dyspnea. While opioids were historically used for dyspnea management exclusively in patients with comfort-focused goals of care, this practice is evolving. Patients managed by palliative care services may benefit from dyspnea therapies and receive low-dose, long-acting opioids regardless of their goals of care [8]. Managing chronic dyspnea in the perioperative period can be challenging, as the anesthesiologist must balance treating the patient's baseline dyspnea and postoperative pain while ensuring adequate respiratory drive for extubation at the conclusion of the procedure. Long-acting opioids prescribed for this indication should be continued throughout the perioperative period. Short-acting opioids and benzodiazepines are intended to relieve acute dyspnea and do not provide lasting relief. Therefore, their continuation in the perioperative period is subject to the anesthesiologist's discretion.

4 Total Pain in Serious and Terminal Illness

Patients with serious or terminal illness may experience pain from causes beyond nociception. This concept is known as total pain, which considers physical, psychological, social, and spiritual factors that together contribute to a patient's overall pain experience. Dame Cicely Saunders, the founder of the modern hospice movement, developed this concept. While physical pain is often the primary focus of clinicians, neglecting the spiritual, social, and psychological components may lead to overmedication or unnecessary suffering [9].

Spiritual pain may manifest as feelings of despair or hopelessness regarding the meaninglessness of life. Patients may feel disconnected from their spiritual community or abandoned by God. Anesthesiologists may observe signs of spiritual pain such as patients excessively worrying about death in the perioperative setting. Social pain refers to the feeling of becoming a burden on loved ones and society, as well as grieving the loss of roles or tasks that had previously defined the patient's identity and self-worth. Anesthesiologist may notice signs of social pain including expressions of concern regarding the degree of necessary physical and occupational rehabilitation, the expected time to recovery, and the anticipated level of physical function in the postoperative phase of care.

Patients with serious or terminal illness may develop new anxiety related to the uncertainty of their medical condition, which contributes to their psychological pain. This anxiety may be compounded by the stress and uncertainty of surgery, making psychological pain a condition frequently encountered by anesthesiologists. Manifestations of psychological pain include nervousness, restlessness, tearfulness, the demonstration of a withdrawn affect, or expressions of generalized fear of surgery and the future. In certain situations, preoperative anxiety can negatively affect patient outcomes and therefore should be addressed prior to surgery [10].

Recognizing and addressing spiritual and social pain with appropriate interventions can help to reduce patient suffering. These feelings are more easily identified during a longer visit, such as a preoperative clinic appointment, though the observant anesthesiologist may also notice them in the immediate preoperative setting. Providing additional support, as discussed later in this chapter, may alleviate non-nociceptive sources of pain and distress, thereby reducing the amount of pharmacological intervention a patient requires [11].

5 Case Considerations

When Mrs. Arnold is met by the anesthesiologist in the preoperative holding area, she is very upset. She shares that the pain in her left leg is excruciating. Although she took an extra dose of extended-release morphine in the middle of the night, the pain remained too severe, leading her to the emergency room. She has also taken her oxycodone every four hours for the past two days. After concluding the preoperative assessment and offering reassurances that she will receive further pain management, the anesthesiologist asks if she has any additional questions. Mrs. Arnold has several, including how long it will be before she can walk again, return to work, and resume chemotherapy.

The anesthesiologist must approach both the physical and the non-physical aspects of Mrs. Arnold's pain. Injuries that threaten a patient's mobility pose a significant risk for social pain. Mrs. Arnold works a physically demanding job, and she may be distressed over whether she can continue to work. More broadly, she may be anxious about whether she can care for herself independently at home. Both these concerns impact her role in her societal structure and her sense of dignity. If such worries are identified in the immediate preoperative setting, the anesthesiologist should inform the surgical team, who can plan appropriate interventions after surgery. If the patient had presented to the preoperative clinic, then the anesthesiologist could have partnered with the patient, their caregiver(s), the surgical team, and social workers to ensure that Mrs. Arnold was appropriately placed in a rehabilitation center after surgery and that she had access to other necessary support services, such as a psychologist or transportation to oncology appointments.

Mrs. Arnold is also likely experiencing psychological pain. Her questions at the end of the interview demonstrate her concern about the uncertainty of her medical situation. The psychological pain related to her metastatic cancer may be compounded by the anxiety associated with the perioperative period. Suppose significant psychological distress is identified in the preoperative clinic. In that case, anesthesiologists may recommend further preoperative education or referral to a psychologist. Additional interventions such as music therapy, acupuncture, and hypnosis may also reduce perioperative anxiety although further investigation is needed [10]. Anesthesiologists may use benzodiazepines to treat the psychological pain associated with surgery; however, it is important to recognize the risk of postoperative delirium associated with benzodiazepine use, particularly in elderly and frail patients [12].

Spiritual pain may become evident when patients use language around God and prayer in the immediate preoperative setting. Anesthesiologists should feel comfortable being present for patient-led prayers and may even choose to participate in said prayer. If available, it is also appropriate to ask chaplaincy to visit patients in the preoperative holding area. However, there is no indication in Mrs. Arnold's interview that she is experiencing significant spiritual pain.

Developing an appropriate plan to manage Mrs. Arnold's physical pain involves considering several factors. One essential aspect is calculating her baseline preoperative opioid use, which can aid in achieving adequate pain control both during and after surgery. Mrs. Arnold reported taking her extended-release morphine as prescribed, except for a one-time additional dose she took yesterday. This isolated occurrence is not sufficient to alter her average OME and can therefore be disregarded when determining her baseline opioid use. However, any longer-term deviations from her prescribed opioid regimen must be considered. The situation is less clear when considering her recent increase in oxycodone intake, from two-to-three tablets per day to six per day, due to pain from the acute fracture. Because of the short-term nature of this opioid increase in response to an acute injury, many clinicians would exclude this change from the patient's OME calculation. However, if increased short-acting opioid use persists for several days to weeks, it should be included in the daily OME calculation. The anesthesiologist may gain valuable information through exploring how well oxycodone 20mg controlled her pain and using that feedback to guide opioid dosing during and after surgery.

To determine Mrs. Arnold's average opioid use, her total daily OME needs to be calculated. This is shown in Table 1. Table 2 then shows a set of equipotent opioids commonly used in anesthesia practice. It is important to note that individual patients may have varying responses to different opioids, and any conversions should be done with a dose reduction factor, usually between 25 and 50%. Dose reductions are performed for patient safety, due in part to the incomplete understanding of relative opioid potencies and individual genetic variation in drug metabolism [13]. Based on the calculations, Mrs. Arnold requires a total daily OME of 180. An effective perioperative pain management plan will ensure that she receives her OME through a combination of oral and IV medications. Additional medication for intra- and postoperative pain management can then be planned accordingly.

Table 1 Calculation of Mrs. Arnold's baseline oral morphine equivalents

Opioid	Route of administration	Daily total dose	Conversion ratio to oral morphine	OME (mg)
Extended-release morphine	Oral	90 mg (45 mg twice daily)	N/A	90
Oxycodone	Oral	60 mg (20 mg three times daily)	3:2	90

Table 2 Equipotent doses of select short-acting oral opioids and select IV opioids commonly used in anesthesia practice

Opioid	Equipotent oral dose (mg)	Equipotent IV dose (mg)
Morphine	30	10
Codeine	130	75
Fentanyl	–	0.1
Hydromorphone	7.5	1.5
Oxycodone	20	–

If Mrs. Arnold has missed her extended-release morphine dose, then she should either receive the missed dose or an equipotent dose of another opioid prior to proceeding to surgery. Depending on her current pain level, an additional dose of her home oxycodone or an equipotent dose of an IV opioid may also be considered before surgery.

6 Additional Analgesic Options

Multimodal analgesia is recommended in the perioperative period, which includes the use of adjuvant medications such as acetaminophen or NSAIDs in addition to opioids. While long-term use of these medications is often avoided in certain patient populations, they are generally tolerable for short-term use surrounding surgery. Furthermore, patients on high doses of opioids at baseline may also benefit from IV ketamine during and after surgery.

Depending on the timing of the patient's presentation and their specific serious illness, interventional pain management procedures may be considered before undergoing surgery. For example, patients with certain abdominal cancers such as pancreatic cancer may derive benefit from a celiac plexus block. This procedure may reduce pre-procedure opioid use, thus assisting in greater postoperative pain control.

7 Risk of Opioid Misuse

Although patients receiving palliative or hospice care have definitive reasons for experiencing pain, they are still at risk for developing opioid use disorder. Additionally, the issue of diversion of hospice-prescribed opioids is not yet fully researched [14]. Anesthesiologists may become aware of these issues based on their observations of a patient's response to perioperative opioids. For example, if a patient's pain is not effectively managed with a calculated opioid dose based on their OME, it may signal an opioid use disorder. Conversely, if a dose is overly sedating, it may indicate that the patient is not taking the prescribed opioids themselves. Such concerns should be discussed with the patient's palliative care doctor for further assessment and management.

8 Additional Roles for the Anesthesiologist

In addition to providing excellence in pain management, anesthesiologists are poised to ensure that patients who are terminally ill or receiving palliative care receive goal-concordant care in the perioperative period. While these patients often discuss their goals of care and set treatment limitations with other clinicians in various settings, the unique nature of the perioperative period requires additional conversations. Such conversations may include a patient's preferences on resuscitation, emphasizing the aspects of the perioperative period that promote successful resuscitation compared to resuscitation in any other setting.

In addition to resuscitation preferences, anesthesiologists may also verify any other treatment preferences expressed in a patient's advance directive, such as a living will or healthcare power of attorney document. If a patient does not have an advance directive on file prior to surgery, the anesthesiologist should at least confirm the designation of a surrogate decision maker, in the event that the patient loses the capacity for medical decision-making in the postoperative period.

The anesthesiologist's role in these patients' care may continue to expand, as more work is conducted on the optimization of frailty, nutrition, and physical function.

Key Takeaway Points

- Opioid therapy, including both short- and long-acting formulations, is essential to managing moderate-to-severe cancer pain.
- Anesthesiologists must thoroughly understand the patient's baseline opioid use to ensure effective perioperative pain control.
- Thoughtful conversions of oral opioid doses to IV formulations enables improved intraoperative pain management.
- Patients who are terminally ill or receiving palliative care are also at risk for non-physical pain complaints, including spiritual, social, and psychological pain. These components may arise during the perioperative period, necessitating the anesthesiologist to address and treat these aspects of pain.

References

1. World Health Organization. Palliative care. 2021. https://www.who.int/news-room/fact-sheets/detail/palliative-care. Accessed 20 March 2023.
2. National Cancer Institute. Cancer Statistics. 2022. https://www.cancer.gov/about-cancer/understanding/statistics. Accessed 20 Mar 2023.
3. Miller KD, Nogueira L, Mariotto AB, et al. Cancer treatment and survivorship statistics. CA Cancer J Clin. 2019;69(5):363–85.
4. van den Beuken-van Everdingen MH, Hochstenbach LM, et al. Update on prevalence of pain in patients with cancer: systematic review and meta-analysis. J Pain Symptom Manage. 2016;51(6):1070–90.
5. World Health Organization. 2019. https://www.who.int/publications/i/item/9789241550390. Accessed 22 Mar 2023
6. Swarm RA, Paice JA, Anghelescu DL et al. Adult cancer pain, version 3.2019, NCCN clinical practice guidelines in oncology. J Natl Compr Canc Netw. 2019;17(8):977–1007
7. Zhang Y, Chen H, Chen S, et al. The effect of concomitant use of statins, NSAIDs, low-dose aspirin, metformin and beta-blockers on outcomes in patients receiving immune checkpoint inhibitors: a systematic review and meta-analysis. Oncoimmunology. 2021;10(1):1957605.
8. Crombeen AM, Lilly EJ. Management of dyspnea in palliative care. Curr Oncol. 2020;27(3):142–5.

9. Wood J. Cicely Saunders, 'Total pain' and emotional evidence at the end of life. Med Humanit. 2022;48(4):411–20.
10. Stamenkovic DM, Rancic NK, Latas MB, et al. Preoperative anxiety and implications on postoperative recovery: what can we do to change our history. Minerva Anestesiol. 2018;84(11):1307–17.
11. Singh P, Arya A, Singh MK, et al. Effect of spiritual music on old-age patients undergoing lower limb surgery under spinal anesthesia. Anesth Essays Res. 2022;16(2):208–12.
12. Friedrich S, Reis S, Meybohm P, et al. Preoperative anxiety. Curr Opin Anaesthesiol. 2022;35(6):674–8.
13. Fine PG, Portenoy RK. Establishing "Best practices" for opioid rotation. J Pain Symptom Manage. 2009;38(3):418–25.
14. Cagle JG, McPherson ML, Frey JJ, et al. Estimates of medication diversion in hospice. JAMA. 2020;323(6):566–8.

Perioperative Management of Opioid Tolerant Patients

Lady Christine Ong Sio, Shuchita Garg, and Adil Qarni

Abstract The increase in worldwide prescription opioid use has resulted in a parallel increase in the need to consider the analgesic management of patients who are opioid-tolerant. Opioids provide effective analgesia; however, effective utilization can be limited by opioid-related adverse events and abuse potential. The use of multimodal analgesic therapy has been recommended by numerous societies and entails the concurrent perioperative utilization of multiple pharmacologic and/or non-pharmacologic agents with different mechanisms of action. The perioperative period represents a vulnerable time for opioid tolerant patients due to the risk of undertreatment of pain, risk of opioid withdrawal and relapse, not to mention the fear of possible adverse judgment by providers. This chapter presents current recommendations in the perioperative management of opioid tolerant patients. While the management of these patients may be challenging, leveraging, multimodal therapies and multi-disciplinary planning and strategies remain essential components of optimized perioperative analgesia.

Keywords Opioid tolerance · Opioid use disorder · Perioperative period · Multimodal analgesia · Chronic pain

L. C. Ong Sio (✉)
Department of Anesthesiology and Perioperative Medicine, University of Louisville, Louisville, KY, USA
e-mail: ladychristine.ongsio@uoflhealth.org

S. Garg · A. Qarni
Department of Anesthesia and Chronic Pain Division, University of Cincinnati, Cincinnati, OH, USA
e-mail: gargsh@ucmail.uc.edu

A. Qarni
e-mail: qarniam@ucmail.uc.edu

A. Abd-Elsayed and K. Schroeder (eds.), *Perioperative Pain Management*,
https://doi.org/10.1007/978-3-031-67648-2_19

1 Introduction

Opioid use disorder pertains to a pattern of opioid use that is associated with physical, mental, social, and legal problems [1]. It is a treatable chronic disorder characterized by remission and recurrence due to loss of control of opioid use, compulsive use, and continued use despite harms [2]. It is a chronic and relapsing disorder of the brain caused by repeated exposure to exogenous opioids [3]. The development of opioid tolerance, dependence, and addiction are manifestations of brain changes resulting from chronic opioid abuse.

Data from the Centers for Disease Control and Prevention demonstrates that the increase in opioid prescriptions that began in the 1990s was associated with a concurrent increase in the occurrence of drug-related overdose and death. Between the years 1999 and 2020, more than 263,000 people died in the United States due to overdoses from prescription opioids, and the mortality rate for this cause of death increased by five times during that period [4]. In 2021, 106,699 inclusive overdose deaths occurred, resulting in an age-adjusted rate of 32.4 per 100,000 standard population. The rate of drug overdose deaths involving synthetic opioids other than methadone increased 22%, while the rate of deaths involving heroin declined 32% between 2020 and 2021. From 2020 through 2021, the rate of drug overdose deaths increased for deaths involving cocaine and those involving psychostimulants with abuse potential [5].

Opioid tolerance may be a consequence of prescribed use of pain medications or illicit use. The term opioid tolerance is characterized by a reduced response to an opioid analgesic and manifests by the need to use increasing doses to achieve the desired effect. Tolerance occurs because brain cells with opioid receptors become less responsive to opioid stimulation, i.e., more opioid is needed to stimulate the ventral tegmental area brain cells of the mesolimbic reward system to release the same amount of dopamine in the nucleus accumbens [6]. Tolerance to the analgesic and euphoric effects develops quickly, while tolerance to respiratory depression develops more slowly [7].

Opioid dependence is defined by the presence of withdrawal symptoms in the absence of opioid use or use in reduced amounts. Withdrawal symptoms include piloerection, chills, diarrhea, nausea, vomiting, muscle aches, and insomnia, and can vary in severity and duration in each person. Opioid addiction, as defined by the Diagnostic and Statistical Manual of Mental Disorders V, is characterized by pronounced craving and drug-related perseveration, with an absence of inhibitory control over efforts to refrain from drug use in the setting of compulsive and harmful use.

2 Preoperative Evaluation

Obtaining a comprehensive pain history well in advance of surgery aids in the identification of opioid tolerance and facilitates perioperative planning. This history should evaluate concomitant comorbidities such as anxiety, depression, and substance use or abuse in the past. It is also important to consider that patients may deliberately omit or fail to declare a history of opioid use or those with current opioid addiction struggles may give a false history in the presence of parents, family, or friends. The clinical importance associated with identifying these patients is highlighted in their increased risk of prolonged postoperative opioid use, worse clinical outcomes, increased pain, and diverse postoperative complications [8].

In the perioperative setting, patients who are opioid-tolerant can fall into one of three categories: First are patients who are maintained on large doses of opioids for the treatment of chronic non-malignant or malignant pain. Second are patients who have opioid addiction and are actively misusing opioids, with or without other illicit substances. Third are those who have a previous history of substance use disorders and are on medication-assisted treatment (MAT) to simultaneously dampen cravings for opioids and diminish the risk of relapse [9].

It is important to acknowledge that the acute management of perioperative pain in opioid tolerant patients is challenging. This subset of patients may report higher pain scores than the average patient, and their pain is often poorly managed in the hospital setting. The mechanism involved in this difference in symptomatic pain control is multifactorial and includes the interrelation between psychologic, physiologic, and physical alterations that happen in individuals exposed to long-term opioid administration [10]. The goals of perioperative treatment in these patients are to prevent opioid withdrawal, provide effective analgesia, and ensure continuity of care after discharge [11].

Long-term preoperative opioid use is associated with a higher risk of both short- and long-term adverse postoperative outcomes, including increased rates of surgical infection and revision surgery, higher readmission rates, longer hospital stay, and higher medical costs after surgery. Identifying those patients already exposed to opioid analgesics is a core tenet of perioperative analgesic management. Fortunately, several tools can be used to help identify these patients and screen for substance use disorders. For patients on long term opioid therapy or with a history of substance abuse, tools such as the ORT (Opioid Risk Tool), DIRE (Diagnosis, Intractability, Risk, Efficacy) score, and SOAPP (Screener and Opioid Assessment for Patients and Pain) may be used [12, 13].

In addition to obtaining a comprehensive preoperative history and physical examination, thorough discussions, counseling, and expectation settings are important. The patient's concerns and overall expectations should be considered as a component of analgesic planning and in the development of a treatment approach. A reassuring discussion is essential in reducing stress and fear of pain during the perioperative period.

3 Challenges in the Management of Opioid Tolerant Patients

Opioid tolerant patients have higher pain scores than non-opioid tolerant patients and oftentimes require higher doses of opioids. Undertreatment of pain can lead to opioid-seeking behavior, and the patient can be perceived as 'manipulative' and 'non-cooperative' [11].

The Food and Drug Administration defines a patient as opioid tolerant if, for at least 1 week, the patient has been receiving oral morphine 60 mg/day, transdermal fentanyl 25 mcg/hour, oral oxycodone 30 mg/day, oral hydromorphone 8 mg/day, oral oxymorphone 25 mg/day, or an equianalgesic dose of any other opioid [14].

Besides opioid tolerance, the risk of respiratory events, immune suppression, and opioid-induced hyperalgesia can impact post-operative outcomes. Evidence suggests that patients with a history of opioid tolerance may also be at increased risk for the development of surgical site and periprosthetic infections, revision surgeries, prolonged hospital stay, unplanned hospital readmission, non-home discharge, and postoperative emergency room visits. Each of these adverse events has the binary effect of worsening patient outcomes and increasing healthcare costs [12].

Another subset of patients at risk for poor perioperative pain control are those who are in remission from an opioid use disorder and are not being maintained on partial mu receptor agonist or antagonist therapeutics. These patients do not generally exhibit signs and symptoms of opioid dependence but are still susceptible to triggers and relapse. Whenever possible, regional anesthesia and/or peripheral nerve blocks should be used in these patients to minimize pain and subsequent opioid requirements, along with adjunct medications, to reduce the need for opioid medications. Opioid analgesics should be given at the lowest possible effective dose and for a limited period. Close follow-up of these patients is important to prevent the re-development of use disorder pathologies.

4 Perioperative Pain Management Considerations (Fig. 1)

Oral Opioids

In general, when significant pain after surgery is anticipated, patients should be advised to take their usual dose of oral opioid on the morning of surgery, with preoperative administration of daily maintenance or baseline opioid dose occurring before the induction of anesthesia [15]. If patients are unable to take medications by mouth, they can be given an equivalent dose via the intravenous route. Calculating intravenous opioid replacement dosing is often done by determining the total 24-h dose of the current oral opioid regimen by converting to oral morphine equivalent dose (MED) using equianalgesic tables. Finally, the calculated oral MED can be converted to parenteral morphine by using the conversion 3:1 oral: parenteral morphine ratio.

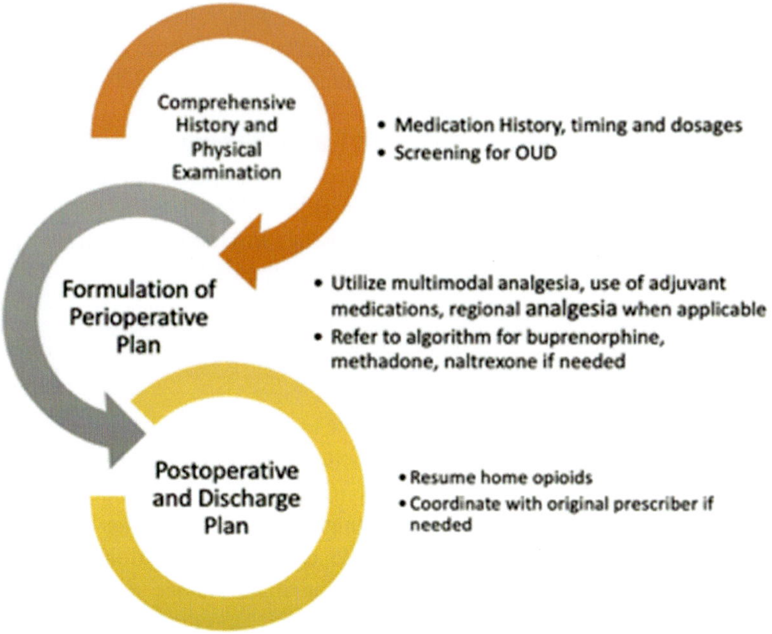

Fig. 1 Approach to perioperative management of patients with OUD

Transdermal Opioids

Transdermal fentanyl patches should be maintained intra-operatively to ensure maintenance of baseline opioid requirement. The presence of an external heat source, however, can potentially increase cutaneous perfusion and subsequently increase fentanyl absorption and lead to overdose [16]. In the case of major surgery, it is preferable to remove the fentanyl patch and administer an equipotent morphine dose as a substitute [9, 15]. In most cases, it is prudent to coordinate with the surgical team to ensure that fentanyl patches are reapplied following the conclusion of the surgical procedure.

5 Intravenous Opioids

Despite a recent impetus to decrease intravenous opioid administration, patient-controlled analgesia in the postoperative period can often be effectively utilized in the management of acute pain in opioid tolerant patients. It allows for individual dose titration and decreases staff workload. It may be challenging to determine the optimal dose in opioid-tolerant patients, but it is recommended to consider the patient's usual daily 24-h opioid requirements when calculating effective dosing regimens.

Equianalgesic tables can be used to help calculate equivalent doses of an alternative opioid but should be used with caution. When considering an opioid rotation, it is recommended to reduce the calculated equianalgesic dose by 30 to 50% to allow for incomplete cross-tolerance [11].

Once the patient is ready to be converted back to an oral opioid formulation, a useful guide is to identify the intravenous opioid consumption in the previous 24 h and convert to an equivalent oral dose. As a rule of thumb, fifty percent of this calculated dose is given as sustained-release dosing, and the remaining fifty percent can be divided into 4 to 6 divided doses throughout the day.

Methadone

Differing expert opinions exist on the preferred management of patients on MAT scheduled for elective surgery. In general, patients who can tolerate oral medications should be advised to continue oral methadone on the morning of surgery and throughout the perioperative period. If unable to do so, methadone can be given parenterally, at a dose half to two-thirds of the maintenance dose, divided into two to four doses throughout the day [9, 15, 17]. If parenteral methadone is not available, methadone can be converted to morphine, however, this is challenging as the half-life of methadone is very long (15–40 h). The challenges associated with methadone conversions suggest that the inclusion of a dedicated pain service may confer perioperative safety benefits.

Buprenorphine

Patients on buprenorphine often require higher doses of opioids or express higher pain scores following surgical procedures. The etiology for these differences is related to buprenorphine acting as a partial mu-agonist with a high affinity for opioid receptors that outcompetes full opioid agonists. In OUD maintenance programs, buprenorphine is often dosed once a day or three times a week at a higher dose. Available buprenorphine formulations include sublingual, buccal, transdermal, subdermal, or injectable. Buprenorphine may be administered in isolation or may be a component of a formulation that includes naloxone. Several strategies exist to address the perioperative management of patients on buprenorphine presenting or recovering from elective surgical procedures. One option is to continue buprenorphine and use a different opioid for analgesia. The use of opioids with a high affinity for the opioid receptor (i.e. fentanyl derivatives and hydromorphone) may be used and titrated to the desired effect. It should be considered that higher doses of opioid agonists may be necessary to provide analgesia in the setting of buprenorphine [15, 18, 19]. Buprenorphine dosing modifications may also provide effective perioperative pain relief. For example, increasing dosing to three times daily or increasing the daily dose to 24–32 mg daily may greatly enhance the analgesia provided through buprenorphine administration.

Naltrexone

Naltrexone is an opioid antagonist that is used to prevent relapse in patients with a history of alcohol abuse and in the treatment of fibromyalgia pain disorders. It competitively binds to opioid receptors, causing reduced sensitivity to opioids and can precipitate withdrawal symptoms in patients with a history of opioid dependency. Naltrexone is available in oral and injectable forms and should be discontinued at least 24–72 h prior to planned surgical procedures if opioid-based anesthesia is planned [15]. The recommendation for injectable naltrexone is to postpone elective surgery for 30 days following the last injection. Daily oral naltrexone should be discontinued 72 h before surgery [20–22].

Regional Anesthesia

Neuraxial and peripheral nerve blocks are widely used techniques that are frequently utilized to manage acute perioperative pain. For example, the use of brachial plexus blocks and catheter techniques can be utilized as either the sole anesthetic during surgery or for postoperative pain control in the setting of significant shoulder or arm surgery. Thoracic paravertebral blocks, erector spinae blocks, transversus abdominis plane blocks and catheters can be used for truncal surgeries. Neuraxial techniques such as spinal and epidural are safe and effective for lower extremity procedures. With an improved understanding of anatomy and ultrasound technology, there is an ever-expanding scope of surgical procedures that might benefit from regional anesthesia and the thoughtful application of these techniques should be strongly considered in patients with a history of opioid use or abuse.

Adjuvant Medications

Non-opioid adjuvant medications can be combined with opioids to improve pain control and potentially decrease opioid consumption. The use of non-steroidal anti-inflammatory drugs and acetaminophen should be strongly considered unless otherwise contraindicated.

Acetaminophen inhibits prostaglandin synthesis in the central nervous system, leading to inhibition of inflammation in the peripheral nervous system. It is available in oral, intravenous, or rectal forms.

Gabapentinoids such as gabapentin and pregabalin are antiseizure medications with analgesic and anxiolytic properties [20]. These medications are believed to act as inhibitors of voltage-gated calcium channels. There is no consensus that exists for optimal dosing and caution should be exercised in patients who are elderly or otherwise at risk for sedation and respiratory depression.

Clonidine and dexmedetomidine are alpha-2 adrenergic agonists that have analgesic properties and have been used to reduce perioperative pain. Clonidine is particularly useful as a component of an analgesic program aimed at preventing opioid withdrawal symptoms and may have efficacy comparable to buprenorphine [23].

Opioid antagonists (naloxone and naltrexone) as well as mixed agonist-antagonist types of opioids (nalbuphine, pentazocine, butorphanol), should be used with tremendous caution in patients on chronic opioid therapy because these drugs can precipitate acute opioid withdrawal.

Non-pharmacologic Therapies

A multi-disciplinary pain approach consisting of non-opioid and non-pharmacologic modalities is helpful in managing opioid-tolerant patients. Not only does it help decrease postoperative pain, but it also limits opioid dose requirements and subsequently reduce opioid-related side effects. Non-pharmacological treatments include cognitive behavioral therapy, mindfulness training, relaxation strategies and phone applications, physical therapy, peer, and family support. Other support groups such as narcotics anonymous may also be helpful. Acupuncture and topical analgesics, such as ice, can be beneficial [24].

6 Conclusion

Perioperative pain management in the setting of preoperative opioid use or abuse, introduces tremendous analgesic management complexity and is associated with a significant potential to impact recovery outcomes well beyond the immediate postoperative period. These patients should be monitored not only for achievement of analgesic milestones but also for signs of withdrawal and cravings that might be associated with dangerous use or misuse of opioids. If a perioperative interruption in baseline opioid administration does occur, there needs to be communication with the patient's outpatient opioid prescriber such that arrangements could be done to restart medications. Difficulties encountered with these multifaceted management strategies highlight why it is most frequently prudent to continue baseline opioid dosing throughout the postoperative period and supplement with additional analgesics as needed. Finally, a multidisciplinary team approach and evidence-based treatment strategy are critical to safely manage opioid tolerant patients in the perioperative arena and ensure adequate analgesia while reducing the risk of relapse.

Key Takeaways

1. Early identification of opioid-tolerant patients undergoing surgery is an essential component of successful perioperative care and management.
2. The goals of perioperative treatment are to prevent opioid withdrawal, provide effective analgesia, and ensure continuity of care post-discharge.
3. A multi-disciplinary team approach is important to safely manage opioid tolerant patients and at the same time, ensure adequate analgesia while avoiding relapse.

References

1. Blanco C, Volkow ND. Management of opioid use disorder in the USA: present status and future directions. Lancet. 2019;393(10182):1760–72.
2. Taylor JL, Samet JH. Opioid use disorder. Ann Intern Med. 2022;175(1):ITC1–ITC16.
3. Herlinger K, Lingford-Hughes A. Opioid use disorder and the brain: a clinical perspective. Addiction. 2022;117(2):495–505.
4. Centers for Disease Control. Media release 2017.
5. Spencer MR, Miniño AM, Warner M. Drug overdose deaths in the United States, 2001–2021. NCHS Data Brief. 2022;457:1–8.
6. Kosten TR, George TP. The neurobiology of opioid dependence: implications for treatment. Sci Pract Perspect. 2002;1(1):13–20.
7. Volkow ND, McLellan AT. Opioid abuse in chronic pain—misconceptions and mitigation strategies. N Engl J Med. 2016;374(13):1253–63.
8. Hah JM, et al. Factors associated with opioid use in a cohort of patients presenting for surgery. Pain Res Treat. 2015;2015: 829696.
9. Rajput K, Vadivelu N. Acute pain management of chronic pain patients in ambulatory surgery centers. Curr Pain Headache Rep. 2021;25:1–12.
10. Henshaw DS, Turner JD, Khanna AK. Opioid abuse and perioperative care: a new medical disease. Curr Opin Anaesthesiol. 2022;35(3):401–8.
11. Simpson G, Jackson M. Perioperative management of opioid-tolerant patients. BJA Educ. 2016;17(4):124–8.
12. Quinlan J, et al. Preoperative opioid use: a modifiable risk factor for poor postoperative outcomes. Br J Anaesth. 2021;127(3):327–31.
13. Macintyre PE, et al. Current Issues in the use of opioids for the management of postoperative pain: a review. JAMA Surg. 2022;157(2):158–66.
14. Adesoye A, Duncan N. Acute pain management in patients with opioid tolerance. US Pharmacist. 2017;42(3):28–32.
15. Coluzzi F, et al. The challenge of perioperative pain management in opioid-tolerant patients. Ther Clin Risk Manag. 2017;13:1163–73.
16. Frölich MA, Giannotti A, Modell JH. Opioid overdose in a patient using a fentanyl patch during treatment with a warming blanket. Anesth Analg. 2001;93(3):647–8.
17. Sritapan Y, Clifford S, Bautista A. Perioperative management of patients on buprenorphine and methadone: a narrative review. Balkan Med J. 2020;37(5):247–52.
18. March 18, 2022. Available from: https://www.cdc.gov/opioids/basics/epidemic.html

19. Kohan L, et al. Buprenorphine management in the perioperative period: educational review and recommendations from a multisociety expert panel. Reg Anesth Pain Med. 2021;46(10):840–59.
20. Aroke EN, et al. A practical approach to acute postoperative pain management in chronic pain patients. J Perianesth Nurs. 2020;35(6):564–73.
21. Harrison TKMD, et al. Perioperative considerations for the patient with opioid use disorder on buprenorphine, methadone, or naltrexone maintenance therapy. Anesthesiol Clin. 2018;36(3):345–59.
22. Ward EN, Quaye AN, Wilens TE. Opioid use disorders: perioperative management of a special population. Anesth Analg. 2018;127(2):539–47.
23. Jain N, et al. Efficacy of buprenorphine and clonidine in opioid detoxification: a hospital- based study. Indian J Psychiatry. 2018;60(3):292–9.
24. Barreveld AM, et al. Caring for our patients with opioid use disorder in the perioperative period: a guide for the anesthesiologist. Anesth Analg. 2023;137(3):488–507.

Perioperative Care of the Opioid-Tolerant Patient

Nathan J. Rudin

Abstract Surgical patients who chronically use opioids pose unique challenges for anesthesia and perioperative pain management. This chapter provides recommendations for optimal perioperative pain care in the opioid-tolerant patient, including attention to special cases such as patients taking buprenorphine for opioid use disorder or receiving intrathecal opioids for pain management. Clinicians can maximize safety and efficacy using a combination of non-opioid medications, regional blocks, and nonpharmacologic strategies. Treatment should be tailored to the specific needs of each patient.

Keywords Surgical anesthesia · Perioperative · Pain management · Opioids · Opioid use disorder · Buprenorphine · Intrathecal drug delivery · Regional anesthesia · Tolerance · Dependence

1 Introduction

Clinicians will commonly encounter opioid-tolerant patients who need surgery. Opioid use for chronic non-cancer pain is declining but still substantial, opioids remain a primary treatment for cancer-related pain, and the use of illicit opioids is on the rise. Early identification of opioid-tolerant surgical patients is vital to ensure appropriate care before, during and after surgery.

Treating the opioid-tolerant surgical patient can be challenging. Too much additional perioperative opioid may increase the risk of morbidity, and postoperative pain control can be difficult to attain; insufficient perioperative analgesia raises the risk

The original version of this chapter has been revised. The Chapter title has been corrected. A correction to this chapter can be found at
https://doi.org/10.1007/978-3-031-67648-2_45

N. J. Rudin (✉)
Division of Rehabilitation Medicine, Department of Orthopedics and Rehabilitation, School of Medicine and Public Health, University of Wisconsin, Madison, WI, USA
e-mail: rudin@rehab.wisc.edu

A. Abd-Elsayed and K. Schroeder (eds.), *Perioperative Pain Management*,
https://doi.org/10.1007/978-3-031-67648-2_20

of other harms. Patients using intrathecal opioids for pain treatment pose special challenges, as do those with opioid use disorder. The latter, especially if they are taking opioid agonist-antagonists (usually buprenorphine) for medication-assisted treatment, may require special measures to mitigate acute opioid withdrawal.

In this chapter we synthesize the best available evidence for perioperative pain management in opioid-tolerant individuals. Thoughtful care planning and management will result in effective, compassionate, and safe treatment.

2 Opioid Tolerance and Surgery

In practice, perioperative management of the opioid-tolerant patient varies widely because of competing concerns and preferences.

- *Patients taking chronic opioids may have worse surgical outcomes.* Joint arthroplasty patients on chronic opioids have lower preoperative function and higher pain, lower postoperative function and satisfaction [1], longer lengths of stay, higher revision rates, and higher medical costs [2] than those not taking opioids. Opioid-tolerant patients were twice as likely to be re-hospitalized following major abdominal surgery [3], and perioperative opioids were associated with worse outcomes and higher costs [4]. Preoperative opioid use was associated with a higher risk of wound infection after multilevel lumbar fusion [5]. In general, patients on chronic opioids report higher postsurgical pain and demonstrate slower pain resolution [6]. These concerns have led to recommendations that chronic opioids be tapered and, where possible, discontinued prior to elective surgery.
- *Aggressive opioid dose reduction may itself lead to significant morbidity.* Long-term opioid tolerance may represent a persistent neural adaptation requiring extended periods to reverse [7]. Rapid tapering can result in uncontrolled pain, disruptions of sleep and appetite, and the opioid withdrawal syndrome, leading to an increase in physiological stress [8, 9]. Stressed patients have suboptimal surgical outcomes [10]. For these reasons, some authorities recommend maintaining the preoperative opioid dose, or higher if indicated for additional relief, during the perioperative period [11–13].

Faced with these conflicting concerns, the clinician is best served by using a common-sense, evidence-driven approach to perioperative pain management, adjusting the treatment plan to meet the needs and circumstances of each patient. The focus should remain on the primary goal of effective anesthesia and analgesia with the lowest possible risk and morbidity.

The key principles of perioperative pain management are:

1. Perioperative pain management should be unique for each patient.
2. Where possible, the management plan begins well before surgery.
3. The plan must be flexible enough to change as circumstances demand.

3 Steps for Perioperative Pain Management

1. **Perform a thorough perioperative pain evaluation** [13–15].

   a. *Diagnose pain conditions.* Understand causes of pain both related and unrelated to the planned surgery.
   b. *Understand the patient's preoperative medication regimen and stratify risk.* Ascertain doses of opioids and other medications, as well as drug allergies/intolerances. Risk stratification method schemes include the Perioperative Quality Initiative (POQI)'s "O-NET+" [15], the ORBIT instrument [16] and the RIOSORD scale [17].
   c. *Determine psychological comorbidities* which may affect the patient's ability to cope with surgery and changes to the regimen.
   d. *Understand the patient's support network.* Educating family and caregivers can improve adoption of and adherence to pain care goals.
   e. Solicit the patient's concerns and questions about surgery and pain management.

2. **Educate the patient and family before surgery**. Education ideally takes place well before the day of surgery, often during a preoperative evaluation visit [14, 18].

   a. *Explain the surgery thoroughly* as per standard informed consent methods.
   b. *Define perioperative pain management goals and explain available pain care tools.* A thorough understanding of the pain care plan mitigates anxiety while helping patients and families plan ahead before surgery occurs.
   c. *Elicit agreement on pain management goals and medication plan.* Achieving shared expectations and patient buy-in before surgery facilitates better pain care and improves outcomes.

   a. *Aim for a minimum effective dose rather than opioid cessation.* Lower preoperative opioid doses are preferable, especially for patients on higher doses, to minimize potential morbidity. However, the approach to opioid dosing must be individualized to the patient. Routine preoperative opioid tapering, especially to zero, without appropriate alternative treatment is not recommended [19, 20]. While a zero preoperative opioid dose may be desirable, it is not necessarily realistic or achievable; in many individuals it is necessary to settle for the lowest possible dose that still preserves comfort and function. Flexibility in the optimization plan is therefore required.
   b. *Combine opioid weaning with non-opioid strategies.* Careful preoperative opioid reduction can be accomplished given adequate time, use of behavioral and non-opioid techniques (leveraging the biopsychosocial model of pain), and clear establishment of expectations. For individuals with a higher risk of opioid-related adverse events, consider consulting a pain specialist for assistance with the pain care plan. Multidisciplinary centers for perioperative

pain management, when available, provide ideal environments for successful preoperative opioid reduction [20, 21].

c. *Make and share a plan for postoperative management.* If the planned surgery is intended to address the pain condition being treated with opioids, a postoperative opioid tapering plan should be discussed and outlined before surgery.

3. **Optimize mood and coping skills where needed**. Individuals at higher risk for opioid-related morbidity can receive mindfulness-based or other stress management training before surgery to enhance pain coping; if in-person sessions are not available, extensive resources are available on websites and smartphone applications. Group-based or individual health psychology interventions can also improve and strengthen pain coping skills. Psychiatric evaluation and treatment, and broader psychotherapy, may be necessary for patients in severe emotional distress [15, 22]. Preoperative ("prehabilitation") programs incorporating stress reduction are associated with significant surgical cost savings and improved outcomes [10].
4. **Individualize the treatment plan, using non-opioid and low-opioid strategies where possible**. The primary goal of treatment is achievement of effective anesthesia and analgesia with minimal risk and morbidity. A rational prescribing approach, using multimodal anesthesia and analgesia, is paramount [22].

   a. *Make sure pain is controlled.* Reduction of opioids must not be allowed to result in undertreatment of perioperative pain, which is associated with delirium, surgical and cardiopulmonary complications, deconditioning, development of chronic pain, relapse in patients with substance abuse disorders, and reduced quality of life [19].
   b. *Maintain preoperative opioid dose.* For those who continue to take opioids preoperatively, the immediate preoperative daily opioid dose (or its equivalent in potency) should be maintained during surgery and early recovery. Opioid withdrawal must not be allowed to occur.
   c. *Use non-opioid agents where possible.* Non-opioid agents should be used during anesthesia and for postoperative anesthesia. Where postoperative opioids are required, the minimum effective dose should be used to minimize the risk of opioid-induced hyperalgesia[23] or other adverse events.
   d. *Limit postoperative opioids to the minimum necessary.* Patients should be transitioned to non-opioid analgesics as soon as possible after surgery. Opioid-tolerant patients should be rapidly returned to their preoperative baseline opioid dose. When surgery is intended to address the pain condition being treated with opioids, postoperative tapering can begin once surgical recovery is well underway.

4 Opioid-Sparing Anesthesia and Analgesia Techniques

Numerous non-opioid agents are available for intraoperative and postoperative use. They can be quite useful, both alone and in combination, for anesthesia and pain management. They must be used cautiously, as all have significant potential for side effects and drug-drug interactions, and all have therapeutic ceilings [24]. Definitive combinations and dosages of these agents in multimodal anesthesia have not yet been determined, but the skilled anesthesiologist can apply these agents judiciously, with or without opioids, to provide satisfactory anesthesia and effective postoperative pain control [25–29].

Fully opioid-free anesthesia (OFA) is a desirable goal in the opioid-tolerant patient, but the science of OFA remains in its early stages. Currently available evidence for OFA is of variable quality. The best available meta-analyses suggest that OFA is not inferior to regimens which include opioids [22], but which patients and surgeries are most suitable for OFA has not yet been determined.

We here briefly summarize common non-opioid agents for perioperative pain management. The choice of agent must be individualized, taking patient-specific variables into account. The reader is directed to the growing literature on opioid-sparing and opioid-free anesthesia for the latest evidence and recommendations.

a. **Preoperative regional and local anesthetic techniques** reduce intraoperative and postoperative opioid use [30]. Targeted regional nerve blocks, epidural anesthetics, perineural catheters, and/or anesthetic infiltration at incision sites can significantly reduce postoperative pain.
b. **Nonsteroidal anti-inflammatory drugs (NSAIDs)** may be useful in some perioperative settings, especially given the putative role of the cyclooxygenase-2 (COX-2) enzyme in central nociceptive processing [31]. Limited preoperative use of COX-2 inhibiting NSAIDs reduces opioid need in patients undergoing total knee arthroplasty [32] and spinal fusion [24]. Conventional non-selective NSAIDs can reduce postoperative opioid requirements [33]. Some authorities advise against the routine preoperative use of a COX-2 inhibitor [34]. Recent large studies show no increased risk of postoperative hemorrhage or renal injury with the judicious perioperative use of NSAIDs [35].
c. **Propofol** is a common and effective non-opioid agent for anesthesia induction and maintenance and is a valuable tool for anesthesia where patients are at elevated risk for opioid-related adverse events [36].
d. **Dexmedetomidine** is an adrenergic alpha-2_A agonist with sedative and mild analgesic effects and is commonly employed for procedural sedation. It is a key element of many OFA regimens, which show promise for better quality of recovery and fewer side effects in multiple surgical settings [37–40].
e. **Ketamine** has proven efficacy in acute pain care. Subanesthetic ketamine infusions may be helpful perioperatively in opioid-tolerant patients [41]. Evidence that ketamine decreases perioperative opioid use is limited. It may work best for this purpose in opioid-tolerant patients [42].

f. **Intravenous lidocaine** significantly reduces postoperative pain in multiple settings [43], and may reduce postoperative opioid need [44]. It may reduce persistent postsurgical pain, but evidence is limited [45, 46]. Topical lidocaine patches may be helpful for the treatment of cutaneous dysesthesia but are not effective for acute wound pain management [47].
g. **Gabapentin and pregabalin** are commonly used perioperatively to reduce postsurgical pain and opioid use. There is evidence for decreased analgesic use when gabapentin is administered preoperatively [48], but the effect is modest; gabapentin may promote postoperative opioid cessation [49]. Perioperative pregabalin can reduce opioid use but is associated with significant sedation [50]. The safety of these drugs is decreased when coadministered with opioids, as the combination increases the risk of respiratory depression and death, likely through reversal of respiratory tolerance to opioids [51].
h. **Acetaminophen** is now available intravenously, though this dosage form is expensive relative to oral/rectal formulations. Perioperative IV acetaminophen reduces opioid use after lumbar disc surgery [52] and pancreaticoduodenectomy [53] but not after hip fracture [54].
i. **Other agents** employed to reduce or avoid perioperative opioid administration include corticosteroids, magnesium and beta-blockers.

5 Special Case: Patients Using Buprenorphine

Buprenorphine is a partial μ-opioid receptor agonist and a κ and Δ receptor antagonist. It has high affinity for the μ opioid receptor with slow dissociation. High doses of conventional opioids are required to displace buprenorphine from the μ receptor. Buprenorphine use poses unique challenges to perioperative management of the opioid-tolerant patient.

Buprenorphine is frequently prescribed in oral or sublingual form for the treatment of opioid use disorder, and occasionally for chronic pain (or where opioid use disorder and pain coexist). Transdermal preparations are available at considerably lower potency for the treatment of chronic pain. Transdermal buprenorphine does not significantly interfere with perioperative pain management [55], but higher-dose buprenorphine results in a high perioperative opioid requirement to compete with buprenorphine's binding to the μ receptor.

For patients taking buprenorphine for opioid use disorder, current evidence argues for perioperatively maintaining patients on the regular home buprenorphine dose to reduce the risk of postoperative relapse into opioid abuse [56]. Non-opioid drugs and regional anesthetic techniques should be maximized. Dose reduction is not generally necessary; reduction to 16 mg/d or below before surgery may be helpful if postoperative need for opioids is anticipated [57]. Where opioids are required to treat moderate to severe postoperative pain, short-acting opioids with high affinity for the μ receptor (usually hydromorphone) should be employed under close monitoring, and consulting the hospital's acute pain service is recommended. Close postoperative follow-up with the buprenorphine prescriber is vital [55].

6 Special Case: Patients with Intrathecal Opioid Delivery Systems

Implanted intrathecal drug delivery pumps may be used to deliver opioid analgesics for the treatment of chronic cancer or noncancer pain. Advantages of intrathecal delivery include targeting of the painful body region by intrathecal catheter positioning, the ability to use low drug concentrations and thus minimize systemic side effects, and automation of dosing. Other medications commonly used in intrathecal pumps include baclofen (for spasticity management), clonidine and bupivacaine (for analgesia), and ziconotide (for treatment of neuropathic pain). Interrogation of a programmable intrathecal pump is relatively simple, but pump programming and changing the intrathecal drug require experienced personnel.

Evidence is limited, but for patients receiving intrathecal opioids, it appears that in most circumstances, the clinician can maintain the baseline intrathecal drug regimen unchanged. Case reports have documented the successful perioperative use of standard patient-controlled analgesia, epidural anesthesia, and oral opioid regimens in individuals using intrathecal opioids [58]. In one cohort study, surgical patients on intrathecal opioids had identical outcomes to matched controls but did require more opioid postoperatively, suggesting tolerance [59]. Evidence regarding the effects of other intrathecal agents on surgical anesthesia is lacking.

Abrupt cessation of an intrathecal drug regimen can cause severe complications. If a pump contains clonidine and/or baclofen, abrupt discontinuation can result in life-threatening symptoms. Pain specialist consultation is recommended whenever concerns about intrathecal therapy arise.

7 Conclusion

With thoughtful, individualized and multimodal care, opioid-tolerant patients can be taken safely through surgery while effectively managing their pain. We have herein summarized best practices, tools and techniques to help clinicians and patients achieve this goal.

Key Takeaways

1. Safe, effective, and compassionate perioperative pain management is possible for opioid-tolerant patients and should be considered the standard of care.

2. Effective management requires comprehensive patient evaluation, preoperative education and goal setting. Baseline opioid doses should be reduced where possible but do not insist on a zero dose for all patients.
3. Use non-opioid and opioid-sparing techniques wherever possible during and after surgery.
4. Limit postoperative opioids to the minimum necessary.

References

1. Morris BJ, Sciascia AD, Jacobs CA, Edwards TB. Preoperative opioid use associated with worse outcomes after anatomic shoulder arthroplasty. J Shoulder Elbow Surg. 2016;25:619–23.
2. Blevins Peratikos M, Weeks HL, Pisansky AJB, Yong RJ, Stringer EA. Effect of preoperative opioid use on adverse outcomes, medical spending, and persistent opioid use following elective total joint arthroplasty in the United States: a large retrospective cohort study of administrative claims data. Pain Med. 2020;21:521–31.
3. Owodunni OP, Zaman MH, Ighani M, et al. Opioid tolerance impacts compliance with enhanced recovery pathway after major abdominal surgery. Surgery. 2019;166:1055–60.
4. Cron DC, Englesbe MJ, Bolton CJ, et al. Preoperative opioid use is independently associated with increased costs and worse outcomes after major abdominal surgery. Ann Surg. 2017;265:695–701.
5. Pirkle S, Reddy S, Bhattacharjee S, Shi LL, Lee MJ. Chronic opioid use is associated with surgical site infection after lumbar fusion. Spine (Phila Pa 1976). 2020;45:837–42.
6. Chapman CR, Davis J, Donaldson GW, Naylor J, Winchester D. Postoperative pain trajectories in chronic pain patients undergoing surgery: the effects of chronic opioid pharmacotherapy on acute pain. J Pain. 2011;12:1240–6.
7. Mitra S, Sinatra RS. Perioperative management of acute pain in the opioid-dependent patient. Anesthesiology. 2004;101:212–27.
8. Joshi GP, Ogunnaike BO. Consequences of inadequate postoperative pain relief and chronic persistent postoperative pain. Anesthesiol Clin North Am. 2005;23:21–36.
9. Mark TL, Parish W. Opioid medication discontinuation and risk of adverse opioid-related health care events. J Subst Abuse Treat. 2019;103:58–63.
10. Howard R, Yin YS, McCandless L, Wang S, Englesbe M, Machado-Aranda D. Taking control of your surgery: impact of a prehabilitation program on major abdominal surgery. J Am Coll Surg. 2019;228:72–80.
11. Grancaric N, Lee W, Scanlon M. Postoperative analgesia in the chronic pain patient. Otolaryngol Clin North Am. 2020;53:843–52.
12. Group AMD. Prescribing opioids for postoperative pain—supplemental guidance. 2018. Available from: https://www.agencymeddirectors.wa.gov/Files/FinalSupBreeAMDGPostopPain091318wcover.pdf.
13. Dykstra KM. Perioperative pain management in the opioid-tolerant patient with chronic pain: an evidence-based practice project. J Perianesth Nurs. 2012;27:385–92.
14. Devin CJ, Lee DS, Armaghani SJ, et al. Approach to pain management in chronic opioid users undergoing orthopaedic surgery. J Am Acad Orthop Surg. 2014;22:614–22.
15. Edwards DA, Hedrick TL, Jayaram J, et al. American society for enhanced recovery and perioperative quality initiative joint consensus statement on perioperative management of patients on preoperative opioid therapy. Anesth Analg. 2019;129:553–66.
16. Larance B, Bruno R, Lintzeris N, et al. Development of a brief tool for monitoring aberrant behaviours among patients receiving long-term opioid therapy: the opioid-related behaviours in treatment (ORBIT) scale. Drug Alcohol Depend. 2016;159:42–52.

17. Zedler BK, Saunders WB, Joyce AR, Vick CC, Murrelle EL. Validation of a screening risk index for serious prescription opioid-induced respiratory depression or overdose in a US commercial health plan claims database. Pain Med. 2018;19:68–78.
18. Doan LV, Blitz J. Preoperative assessment and management of patients with pain and anxiety disorders. Curr Anesthesiol Rep. 2020;10:28–34.
19. Dickerson DM, Mariano ER, Szokol JW et al. Multiorganizational consensus to define guiding principles for perioperative pain management in patients with chronic pain, preoperative opioid tolerance, or substance use disorder. Reg Anesth Pain Med. 2023;rapm-2023.
20. McAnally H. Rationale for and approach to preoperative opioid weaning: a preoperative optimization protocol. Perioper Med (London). 2017;6:19.
21. Gulur P, Nelli AH. The opioid-tolerant patient: opioid optimization. J Arthroplasty. 2020;35:S50–2.
22. Adams TJ, Aljohani DM, Forget P. Perioperative opioids: a narrative review contextualising new avenues to improve prescribing. Br J Anaesth. 2023S0007-0912(23)00124.
23. Colvin LA, Bull F, Hales TG. Perioperative opioid analgesia-when is enough too much? A review of opioid-induced tolerance and hyperalgesia. Lancet. 2019;393:1558–68.
24. Shanthanna H, Ladha KS, Kehlet H, Joshi GP. Perioperative opioid administration. Anesthesiology. 2021;134:645–59.
25. Eisenbraun A, Schroeder D, Schaff HV, Martin E, Wittwer ED. Single-center retrospective comparison of opioid-based and multimodal analgesic regimens in adult cardiac surgery. J Cardiothorac Vasc Anesth. 2023S1053-0770(23)00168.
26. Haffner M, Saiz AM, Nathe R, et al. Preoperative multimodal analgesia decreases 24-hour postoperative narcotic consumption in elective spinal fusion patients. Spine J. 2019;19:1753–63.
27. Nassif GJ, Miller TE. Evolving the management of acute perioperative pain towards opioid free protocols: a narrative review. Curr Med Res Opin. 2019;35:2129–36.
28. O'Neill A, Lirk P. Multimodal analgesia. Anesthesiol Clin. 2022;40:455–68.
29. Stone A, Roberts A, de Boer HD, Kaye AD, Fawcett WJ, Urman RD. Recommendations for managing opioid-tolerant surgical patients within enhanced recovery pathways. Curr Pain Headache Rep. 2020;24:28.
30. Cardwell TW, Zabala V, Mineo J, Ochner CN. The effects of perioperative peripheral nerve blocks on peri- and postoperative opioid use and pain management. Am Surg. 2022;88:2842–50.
31. Martin F, Fletcher D, Chauvin M, Bouhassira D. Constitutive cyclooxygenase-2 is involved in central nociceptive processes in humans. Anesthesiology. 2007;106:1013–8.
32. Buvanendran A, Kroin JS, Tuman KJ, et al. Effects of perioperative administration of a selective cyclooxygenase 2 inhibitor on pain management and recovery of function after knee replacement: a randomized controlled trial. JAMA. 2003;290:2411–8.
33. Martinez L, Ekman E, Nakhla N. Perioperative opioid-sparing strategies: utility of conventional NSAIDs in adults. Clin Ther. 2019;41:2612–28.
34. Joshi GP. Rational multimodal analgesia for perioperative pain management. Curr Pain Headache Rep. 2023
35. Warinner C, Parker LF, Shapiro F, Jowett N. Evidence-based perioperative opioid-sparing techniques during the United States opioid crisis. Curr Opin Otolaryngol Head Neck Surg. 2023;31:231–7.
36. Ameiro RJ, Neves SS, Oliveira RP, Marques BB, Ferreira PC. Perioperative challenges of heroin addiction: a case report of opioid-free anesthesia in tongue carcinoma excision with free-flap reconstruction. Cureus. 2023;15: e41195.
37. Choi H, Song JY, Oh EJ, Chae MS, Yu S, Moon YE. The effect of opioid-free anesthesia on the quality of recovery after gynecological laparoscopy: a prospective randomized controlled trial. J Pain Res. 2022;15:2197–209.
38. Zhou F, Cui Y, Cao L, Opioid-Free AWG. The effect of opioid-free anaesthesia on the quality of recovery after endoscopic sinus surgery: a multicentre randomised controlled trial. Eur J Anaesthesiol. 2023;40:542–51.

39. Liu Y, Liang F, Liu X, Shao X, Jiang N, Gan X. Dexmedetomidine reduces perioperative opioid consumption and postoperative pain intensity in neurosurgery: a meta-analysis. J Neurosurg Anesthesiol. 2018;30:146–55.
40. Ahmed SA, Abdelghany MS, Afandy ME. The effect of opioid-free anesthesia on the post-operative opioid consumption in laparoscopic bariatric surgeries: a randomized controlled double-blind study. J Opioid Manag. 2022;18:47–56.
41. Schwenk ES, Viscusi ER, Buvanendran A, et al. Consensus guidelines on the use of intravenous ketamine infusions for acute pain management from the American Society of Regional Anesthesia and Pain Medicine, the American Academy of Pain Medicine, and the American Society of Anesthesiologists. Reg Anesth Pain Med. 2018;43:456–66.
42. Meyer-Frießem CH, Lipke E, Weibel S, et al. Perioperative ketamine for postoperative pain management in patients with preoperative opioid intake: a systematic review and meta-analysis. J Clin Anesth. 2022;78: 110652.
43. Chu R, Umukoro N, Greer T, et al. Intravenous lidocaine infusion for the management of early postoperative pain: a comprehensive review of controlled trials. Psychopharmacol Bull. 2020;50:216–59.
44. Ahn E, Kang H, Choi GJ, et al. Intravenous lidocaine for effective pain relief after a laparoscopic colectomy: a prospective, randomized, double-blind, placebo-controlled study. Int Surg. 2015;100:394–401.
45. Chang YC, Liu CL, Liu TP, Yang PS, Chen MJ, Cheng SP. Effect of perioperative intravenous lidocaine infusion on acute and chronic pain after breast surgery: a meta-analysis of randomized controlled trials. Pain Pract. 2016
46. Doleman B, Mathiesen O, Sutton AJ, Cooper NJ, Lund JN, Williams JP. Non-opioid analgesics for the prevention of chronic postsurgical pain: a systematic review and network meta-analysis. Br J Anaesth. 2023;130:719–28.
47. Shi W, Ren YF, Chen JF, Ye X. Efficacy and safety of lidocaine patch in the management of acute postoperative wound pain: a comprehensive systematic review and meta-analysis of randomized controlled trials. Adv Wound Care (New Rochelle). 2023;12:453–66.
48. Nir RR, Nahman-Averbuch H, Moont R, Sprecher E, Yarnitsky D. Preoperative preemptive drug administration for acute postoperative pain: a systematic review and meta-analysis. Eur J Pain. 2016;20:1025–43.
49. Hah J, Mackey SC, Schmidt P, et al. Effect of perioperative gabapentin on postoperative pain resolution and opioid cessation in a mixed surgical cohort: a randomized clinical trial. JAMA Surg. 2018;153:303–11.
50. Kaye AD, Cornett EM, Helander E, et al. An update on nonopioids: intravenous or oral analgesics for perioperative pain management. Anesthesiol Clin. 2017;35:e55–71.
51. Tambon M, Montarnal B, Lepetit M, Lapeyre-Mestre M. Non-opioid antinociceptive drugs: risk of respiratory depression and death related to concomitant use of gabapentinoids in addition to opioids. Expert Opin Drug Saf. 2023;22:183–94.
52. Yin F, Wang XH, Liu F. Effect of intravenous paracetamol on opioid consumption in multimodal analgesia after lumbar disc surgery: a meta-analysis of randomized controlled trials. Front Pharmacol. 2022;13: 860106.
53. Hirano K, Igarashi T, Murotani K et al. Efficacy and feasibility of scheduled intravenous acetaminophen administration after pancreatoduodenectomy: a propensity score-matched study. Surg Today. 2023
54. Stone AB, Iban YC, Zhong H, et al. Opioid sparing effects of intravenous and oral acetaminophen in hip fracture patients: a population-based study. J Clin Anesth. 2023;86: 111074.
55. Anderson TA, Quaye ANA, Ward EN, Wilens TE, Hilliard PE, Brummett CM. To stop or not, that is the question: acute pain management for the patient on chronic buprenorphine. Anesthesiology. 2017;126:1180–6.
56. Goel A, Azargive S, Weissman JS, et al. Perioperative Pain and Addiction Interdisciplinary Network (PAIN) clinical practice advisory for perioperative management of buprenorphine: results of a modified Delphi process. Br J Anaesth. 2019;123:e333–42.

57. Selvamani BJ, Kral L, Swaran Singh T. Perioperative management of patients on buprenorphine for opioid use disorder. ASRA Pain Med News. 2022;47.
58. Grider JS, Brown RE, Colclough GW. Perioperative management of patients with an intrathecal drug delivery system for chronic pain. Anesth Analg. 2008;107:1393–6.
59. D'Souza RS, Warner MA, Olatoye OO, et al. Perioperative opioid consumption and clinical outcomes in surgical patients with a pre-existing opioid-based intrathecal drug delivery system. Anesth Analg. 2022;134:35–43.

Opioid Agonists and Perioperative Management of Patients on Maintenance Therapy

Sherief Boss, Thomas Bielawiec, Michael Gwede, Bhuvaneswari Sandeep Ram, and Dalia H. Elmofty

Abstract Opioids are commonly used analgesic agents. They bind to specific receptors found throughout the body exerting agonistic, antagonistic, or mixed (partial agonistic) response. Opioids are associated with addiction potential due to activation of reward centers and can cause opioid use disorder (OUD). Methadone, Buprenorphine, and Naltrexone are medications used to treat OUD commonly known as maintenance therapy. Due to the increasing number of patients presenting to the perioperative arena on maintenance therapy, it is imperative for physicians to be familiar with the complexity involved in managing patients with OUD. This chapter reviews the literature on opioid agonists and the perioperative management of patients with OUD on maintenance therapies.

Keywords Opioids · Opioid use disorder · Perioperative pain management · Methadone · Buprenorphine · Naltrexone

1 Opioids

Introduction

Opioids are a class of drugs which are primarily used for analgesia with additional applications as anesthetics, antitussives, and antidiarrheal agents. "Opioid" is an umbrella term referring to both natural, semi-synthetic, and synthetic drug variants [1]. "Opiate" refers to the naturally-produced subset of opiates that include morphine, heroin, and codeine [1]. These natural substances were first derived from opium which is a dark resin present in poppy seeds. Opiates are all structurally like morphine. The term "narcotic" is typically used to describe substances with morphine-like activity [1].

S. Boss · T. Bielawiec · M. Gwede · B. S. Ram · D. H. Elmofty (✉)
University of Chicago, Chicago, USA
e-mail: delmofty@bsd.uchicago.edu

A. Abd-Elsayed and K. Schroeder (eds.), *Perioperative Pain Management*,
https://doi.org/10.1007/978-3-031-67648-2_21

Opioids can be divided into several groups based on the response elicited when the substance is bound to an opioid receptor: opioid receptor agonists, opioid receptor antagonists, or partial agonists. Opioid receptor agonists activate opioid receptors leading to the primary analgesic effect. Examples of opioids agonists include oxycodone, morphine, and fentanyl. In contrast, opioid receptor antagonists inhibit opioid receptors and can further prevent opiate agonists from acting on these receptors. Opioid receptor antagonists include pentazocine, butorphanol, and nalbuphine. Opioid receptor partial agonists display agonist and antagonist effect. They have less effect at the receptor than full agonists and can be used to mitigate or antagonize the action of full agonists. Buprenorphine is an example of an opioid partial agonists [1, 2].

There are also endogenous substances which carry morphine-like activity. These have been classified as three families of neuropeptides: enkephalins, endorphins, and dynorphins [1]. Each of these groups are distinguished from one another by their precursor polypeptides: pro-enkephalin, pro-opiomelanocortin, and prodynorphin. They each have a unique anatomical distribution. While several other morphine-like molecules have been found in mammalian brains, it is not currently clear if these are endogenous substances are derived from dietary intake [1].

2 Mechanisms of Action

Opioids act by binding to specific receptors found throughout the body, exerting agonistic, antagonistic, or mixed (partial agonistic) response. There are three widely accepted opioid receptor types, each designated by a Greek symbol: mu (μ), kappa (κ), and delta (δ). In additional, the opioid receptor-like receptor-1 (ORL-1) also known as the Nociception Opioid Receptor (NOP) receptor is often included in the opioid receptor family due to its structural similarity [1]. These opioid receptors work by coupling to inhibitory G proteins. When an endogenous opioid or opioid agonist binds to these receptors, the inhibitory g-protein leads to an inhibition of enzyme adenylyl cyclase which leads to a downstream reduction of cyclic adenosine monophosphate (cAMP) and activation of phospholipase C. The g-protein leads to inhibition of voltage-gated calcium influx channels and activation of K+ efflux channels that results in membrane hyperpolarization. These changes cause a decrease in neurotransmission of excitatory neurotransmitters such as acetylcholine and substance P from the nociceptive neuron involved leading to the opiate effect of analgesia [1].

Opioid receptors are primarily found in the central nervous system at the dorsal horn of the spinal cord and can be augmented through both neuraxial and systemic administration. They have also been found in the peripheral nervous system and binding can augment the somatic and autonomic nervous system [1].

3 Pharmacookinetics and Pharmacoodynamics

Most opioids go through first pass metabolism in the liver before entering the systemic circulation. This can lead to a decrease in the amount of bioavailable metabolites. The liver produces specific enzymes that aid in the metabolism of the opioids. Phase 1 metabolism, otherwise known as the modification reaction, involves the cytochrome P450 enzymes and results in oxidation or hydrolysis [3]. Phase 2 metabolism, or the conjugate reaction, conjugates the drugs with hydrophilic substances as sulfate, glucuronic acid, glycine, or glutathione. This creates highly hydrophilic products that can be easily excreted [3]. Some opioids are processed into inactive and active metabolites as summarized in Table 1 [3–6].

Opioids metabolisms differ from one individual to another based on the age, ethnicity and sex as described in Table 2 [3]. Half-life of a drug is the time it takes for the amount of the drug's active substance in the body to reduce by half. This can vary from a few hours to a few days. The half-life of Morphine is 2–3.5 h, Hydromorphone 2–3 h, Oxycodone 2–3 h, Fentanyl 3.7 h, Buprenorphine 3–5 h, and Methadone 24 h [7].

Table 1 Opioids and Metabolites

Opioid	Inactive metabolites	Active metabolites with pharmacological opioids	Active metabolites with non-pharmacological opioids
Morphine	Normorphine	Hydromorphone	Morphine 3- glucuronide Morphine 6-glucuronide
Hydromorphone	Minor metabolites	None	Morphine 3- glucuronide
Hydrocodone	Norhydrocodone	Hydromorphone	None
Codeine	Norcodeine	Hydrocodone Morphine	None
Oxycodone	None	Oxymorphone	Noroxycodone
Oxymorphone	Oxymorphone 3-glucuronide	None	6-Hydroxy-oxymorphone
Fentanyl	Norfentanyl	None	None
Tramadol	Nortramadol	None	O-desmethyltramadol
Methadone	2-Ethylidene-1, 5dimethyl-3, 3-diphenylpyrolidine 2-Ethyl-5-Methyl-3, 3-Diphenylpyroline	None	None
Heroin	Normorphine	Morphine	6-Monoacetylmorphine

Table 2 Opioid metabolism based on age, sex, ethnicity, and hepatic or renal impairment

Opioid	Age	Sex	Ethnicity	Hepatic impairment	Renal impairment
Morphine	Clearance may be reduced in older patients	No effect	Chinese patients have higher clearance of morphine	Dose adjustment recommended	Dose adjustment recommended
Codeine	Caution recommended in older patients	No effect	CYP2D6 allelic variants may alter metabolism more common in population of Asian or African Descent	Dose adjustment recommended	Dose adjustment recommended
Hydrocodone	Caution recommended in older patients	No effect	CYP2D6 allelic variants may alter metabolism more common in population of Asian or African Descent	Most frequently administered in combination with acetaminophen, liver function monitoring is advised during treatment in patient with hepatic impairment	Most frequently administered in combination with acetaminophen, renal function monitoring is advised during treatment in patient with severe renal impairment
Oxycodone	Concentration normally higher in older patients	Concentration 25% higher in women than men	No effect	Dose adjustment recommended	Dose adjustment recommended
Methadone	Dose adjustment may be necessary in older patients	No effect	No Effect	Dose adjustment recommended in patients with severe impairment	Dose adjustment recommended in patients with severe impairment
Tramadol	Effects of age on pharmacokinetics have not been studied	No effect	No Effect	Pharmacokinetics is severely altered in patients with severe hepatic impairments	Pharmacokinetics is severely altered in patients with severe renal impairments
Fentanyl	Clearance may be reduced in older patients	No effect	No Effect	Dose adjustment may not be necessary in patient with hepatic impairment	Dose adjustment may not be necessary in patient with renal impairment

(continued)

Table 2 (continued)

Opioid	Age	Sex	Ethnicity	Hepatic impairment	Renal impairment
Hydromorphone	No effect	Concentration maximum (C-max) 25% higher in women than in men with similar area under plasma concentration	No Effect	Dose adjustment recommended	Dose adjustment recommended
Oxymorphone	Steady state concentration, 40% higher in patients > 65	Concentration same in men and women after controlling body weight	No Effect	Contraindicated in patient with moderate or severe hepatic impairment	Dose adjustment recommended

4 Indications for Use

Opioids are mainly used as analgesics but some opioids, such as codeine, are indicated for use as an antitussive [8, 9]. Diphenoxylate and Loperamide are used in the treatment of diarrhea. There is strong evidence for the benefit of opioids in treatment of acute and subacute pain but there is a lack of evidence of the benefit of opioids in the chronic pain management specially in non-cancer related pain [10–13].

5 Effects on Organ Systems

Cardiovascular

The cardiovascular system is least effected by opioids with minimal effects on chronotropy, inotropy, dromotropy, and lusitropy. The effect is variable depending on the opioid administered. Most opiates have a neutral to negative chronotropic effect caused by vagal nerve stimulation leading to a bradycardic response [14]. This can explain the hemodynamic depressive effect noted with administration of opioids. While opioids do not have a profound effect on most functional dynamics of the heart, the bradycardic effect can lead to a decrease in blood pressure by reducing cardiac output (C0) as CO = stroke volume (SV) x heart rate (HR). Opioids cause vasodilation of peripheral arteries and veins. The primary analgesic effect of opioids causes a decrease in sympathetic tone which further contributes to the decrease in blood pressure. Meperidine is an exception as its administration leads to increased chronotropy due to its structural similarity to atropine. Meperidine decreases inotropy when given in large doses. With meperidine, while heart rate may increase, the decrease in inotropy, loss of tone, and increased vasodilation, leads to a net decrease in blood pressure [15]. Histamine release is noted with the administration of certain opioids when given intravenous such morphine and meperidine and leads to vasodilation. This effect can be countered by decreasing the dose or rate of administration along with pre-treating via antihistamine agents [16]. These effects do not cause significant shifts in cardiovascular function. But in patients with significant comorbidities, these factors should be considered, particularly in the perioperative setting as these patients are are exposed to additional medications that can cause cardiovascular instability. Care must be taken when crafting an anesthetic plan [17].

Respiratory

Opioids primarily affect the respiratory system by decreasing respiratory drive and ventilation. Opioids bind to mu receptors at respiratory neurons in the brainstem via the pre-botzinger complex which is responsible for generating respiratory rhythm in the pons [18, 19]. This binding results in the blockade of carbon dioxide (CO_2) chemoreceptors in the medulla and an increase of the arterial carbon dioxide partial pressure ($PaCO_2$). This leads to a right and downward shift of the CO_2 response curve [20]. These changes blunt the ventilatory response to increased levels of $PaCO_2$ as well as increases the apneic threshold and put patients at risk of opioid-induced respiratory failure. The apneic threshold is described as the level of $PaCO_2$ at which apnea is tolerated. Given these respiratory changes, patients with comorbidities that lead to baseline chronic CO_2 retention, such as obesity and obstructive sleep apnea, are at a higher risk of clinically significant respiratory depression when treated with opioids. These effects can be mitigated by judicious titration of opiates and close monitoring. Respiratory rate is particularly affected and makes this an ideal marker for respiratory compromise and overdose in patients receiving opioids [19].

Opioids have additional effects on respiratory physiology. Large doses of fentanyl can lead to profound chest wall, diaphragmatic, and airway rigidity due to the binding of central and peripheral muscle receptors [21]. This phenomenon is known as fentanyl-induced chest wall rigidity or wooden chest syndrome and can be life-threatening. Administration of neuromuscular blockade agents is the most appropriate treatment. Certain opioids also have additional indirect respiratory effects beyond the direct depression caused by mu receptor binding. Morphine and meperidine both lead to significant histamine release, which can lead to bronchospasm [16].

Given that mu receptor binding is the primary mediator of respiratory depression, drugs with more pronounced action on alternative receptors have been hypothesized to be safer for patients who are at risk of respiratory depression [19]. Active research is being performed into the selective blocking or downregulating receptors at these sites to reduce the respiratory side effects of opiate administration [19].

Cerebral

When adjusted for changes in $PaCO_2$, opioids cause a reduction in cerebral blood flow and cerebral O_2 consumption [22]. Intracranial pressure (ICP) is not significantly affected by opioid administration in healthy patients. There can be a small physiological increase that is typically blunted by autoregulation mechanisms [23].

Opioids have little to no effect on EEG. It was previously thought that large doses of opiates could produce or mimic seizures, but this was attributed to the motor manifestations of muscle rigidity, with no associated EEG changes during episodes [24]. This explains the lack of reliable amnesia with opioid administration. Administration of large opioid doses have been associated with a degree of slow brain wave activity, however the significance of this is unclear [24]. The exception to this is seen with meperidine as it has been associated with EEG effects and potential for seizure [16].

Endocrine and Reproductive

Opioids act on the hypothalamus by inhibiting pulsatile gonadotropin releasing hormone (GnRH) release that leads to a reduction in adrenocorticotropic hormone (ACTH) and growth hormone (GH) release, and in turn cortisol secretion [25]. Opioids administered prior to incision can reduce the surgical stress response. Reducing the surgical stress response has been correlated with improved post-surgical outcomes and decreased morbidity [26]. The dose needed to suppress these neuroendocrine markers has been reported as doses as high as > 50 mg/kg [21].

Chronic opioid use is linked to hypogonadism via inhibition of the gonadal axis of the hypothalamus. Hyperprolactinemia is associated with chronic opioid use causing GnRH suppression and further hypogonadism. Testosterone levels can decrease causing sexual dysfunction and gynecomastia in men and menstrual irregularity in women [27].

Opioid receptors have been found in reproductive tissue including the granulosa cells in the ovarian follicle, the oocyte, endometrial tissue, and somatic and germ cells of the testis. Research suggests that these receptors and endogenous opioids affect the maturation of oocytes and sperm production in women and men respectively [27]. These endogenous pathways have been the target of reproductive related treatment, for example the opiate antagonist naltrexone has been prescribed to target conditions like amenorrhea, polycystic ovarian disease, and male sexual dysfunction/infertility [27].

Opioid receptors have been found in pancreatic tissue. Increased levels of endogenous opioid β-endorphin have been noted in response to low blood glucose levels. Studies have shown that intravenous administration of opioids lead to insulin suppression at pancreatic beta cells and potentially induce hyperglycemia [28]. Paradoxically, patients with baseline hyperglycemia, opioid stimulation has been seen to lower blood glucose levels [29]. The clinical significance and mechanisms of these glucose modulating effects is an active area of research.

Gastrointestinal

Opioids have an inhibitory effect on gastrointestinal function that is mediated by direct binding of opioid receptors at peripheral receptors in the gut. This leads to decreased peristalsis and motility causing severe constipation [30]. Opioids delay gastric emptying and predispose patients to vomiting and aspiration [31]. Opioids cause contractions at the sphincter of Oddi triggering biliary colic and spasms mimicking choledocholithiasis [32]. There is an association between opioids and the incidence of acute pancreatitis secondary to long-term opioid-induced contractions and associated ductal dilation. Patients taking chronic opioids experience these side effects despite displaying tolerance to other opiate effects. This is due to the peripheral action of opiates at the enteric nerves of the colon [32]. Opioid antagonists that act on peripheral opioid receptors such as methylnaltrexone and naltrexone are used to mitigate these side effects [32].

Immunological

Immune cells secrete endogenous opioids that act peripherally at opioid receptors. The association between opioids and immunosuppression is an active area of research with mixed findings. Some research has shown chronic opioid use has been associated with decreased expression of genes that mediate antiviral and other immune responses in the body while other studies have found an upregulation of immune system responses with opioid therapy [33]. Exogenous opioids impair the function of several immune cells such as macrophages, natural killer cells, and t-cells that disrupt the gut microbiome [33]. Studies have shown a link between opioids administered with general anesthesia for cancer surgery and recurrence of cancer possibly through a similar immune modulation mechanism [33]. Some clinicians advocate for the use of regional anesthesia and other opiate sparing techniques for patients with cancer.

6 Maintenance Therapy and Perioperative Pain Management

Introduction

3.4% (9.5 million) individuals aged 26 older were reported to misuse opioids. [34] 2.7 million were diagnosed with OUD [34]. According to the American Psychiatric Association, OUD is a chronic problematic pattern of opioid use leading to behavioral changes and problems or distress [34]. Initiatives by the Secretary of Health and Human Services have been set forth to improve treatment and recovery services for patients who suffer from OUD. Although still underutilized, effective medications exist to aid in the treatment of OUD. As services expand, patients on maintenance therapies will be encountered in the perioperative setting and require unique pain management considerations. Patients on maintenance therapy perioperatively are at an above average risk of having poorly controlled postoperative pain leading to longer hospital course [35, 36]. Physicians may also carry a stigma towards patient that suffer from OUD [37]. Many providers share misconceptions and fears regarding managing these patients. There are reported concerns for over-prescribing and further contributing to their OUD along with apprehensions for physical dependence, opioid induced tolerance, hyperalgesia, withdrawal, and pseudo-addiction behaviors [38].

There are many clinical challenges that can present in a patient on maintenance therapy. Opioid tolerance can develop in patients with chronic exposure to opioids and is defined as a physiological state where an increased dose of opioid is required to provide an analgesic effect. Tolerance can lead to a decreased effect on analgesia, sedation, respiratory depression, anti-diuresis, emetic and hypotensive effects but typically spares constipation, miosis, and convulsions [39]. Tolerance can be variable by patient and depend on the drug used, dosage administered, length of time on a drug, and individual genetic factors [39]. The pathophysiology behind tolerance it thought to be due to upregulation of metabolism, desensitization of receptor signaling, downregulation of receptors, and via the adjustments in compensatory circuits that regulate nociception and mood [39]. Tolerance can abate with reduction in dosing or cessation of the opioid.

Patients exhibiting opioid tolerance require higher doses of opioids or alternative means of pain control in the perioperative setting. Tolerance should be distinguished from addiction and pseudo-addiction. Addiction is a chronic medical disease that incorporates neurobiological, physiological, psychosocial, genetic, and environmental components that creates a dysfunction in brain circuitry and exhibits impaired control of drug use and cravings with use of substances despite damaging consequences [40]. Pseudo-addiction is term which describes behavioral symptoms of addiction but in patients receiving inadequate doses of opioids for pain [40].

Tolerance should be distinguished from opioid induced hyperalgesia (OIH). OIH results in a generalized hypersensitive state to painful stimuli where opioid therapy causes an exacerbation in pain sensation rather than relief [41]. While increasing the dosage of opioids in a tolerant individual will improve pain, it will aggravate the pain in OIH. Opioid cessation or de-escalation is necessary to relieve hyperalgesia, in conjunction with other treatment strategies to address the pain. Symptoms of hyperalgesia might continue for months. The distinction between tolerance and OIH can be quite complex. Clinicians often increase doses to address suspected tolerance which in turn aid in the evolution of OIH. The diagnosis can be confounded by the progression of the disease process or misdiagnosed as a stress response or anxious state. There are many complex mechanisms in play that lead to tolerance and OIH. These includes changes occurring in the central nociceptive descending pathways by the rostral ventral medulla, microglial activation, N-methyl-D-aspartate (NMDA) receptor upregulation, non-central signal pathway changes, inflammation, purinergic signaling, epigenetics, and neuropeptides [41, 42]. While variable in clinical presentation, the pain associated with OIH is typically more diffuse and less defined, involving areas other than those initially involved in patients' pain complaints [42]. Increasing the opioid dose worsens the pain. Non-opioid analgesia should be utilized to treat OIH. Potential options include ketamine, alpha-2 adrenoreceptor agonists, regional analgesia, antidepressant therapy, anticonvulsant agents, or anti-inflammatories. Opioid rotation should be considered [42].

7 Maintenance Therapies

Maintenance therapy involves using a long-acting opioid agonist (i.e. methadone), partial agonist (i.e. buprenorphine), or antagonist (i.e. naltrexone) to assist individuals in abstaining from illicit substances or improper use of prescription opioids [40]. Patients on maintenance therapy, in contrast to total abstinence, are more likely to stay in treatment. They are less likely to relapse or overdose, be exposed to infectious disease, or participate in criminal activity [40, 43]. Although methadone and buprenorphine work on similar receptors as other opioids, they help eliminate withdrawal symptoms and relieve drug cravings [43]. Naltrexone limits the reward effect from opioids by blocking activation of certain receptors [43].

Methadone

Methadone is a μ- receptor agonist. Its racemic mixture of D- and L- methadone isomers block monoaminergic reuptake and NMDA receptors. It has been used since the 1940s in maintenance therapies. Methadone can be administered via the subcutaneous, oral, intravenous, and rectal routes with good bioavailability without formation of active metabolites [44]. The medication is relatively low cost and works to suppress withdrawal symptoms and relieve drug cravings. For most opioid-dependent patients, it does not create a sensation of euphoria and allows normal daily functioning. Methadone has a long half-life of 24–60 h [7, 44]. The combination of opioid and non-opioid receptor properties of methadone is useful in the treatment of complex pain and is often used in cancer pain, opioid tolerance, or OIH. A Cochrane database review compared methadone maintenance to placebo maintenance or other non-pharmacological therapy for opioid dependance and found that methadone was more effective in retaining patients in treatment and suppressed heroin use [44]. Maintenance therapy with methadone is initiated with 50–100 mg/day daily dosing. Given methadone's highly variable pharmacokinetics, individuals beginning therapy should be closely observed for adverse events. Methadone is metabolized by CYP2B6 and CYP3A4 isoforms in the liver [3]. Caution should be used in patients with hepatic dysfunction or with medications altering hepatic metabolism. Methadone can prolong the QTC interval. EKG monitoring is recommended. A thorough review of the patient's medication history should be conducted to avoid drug-drug interactions with other medications that can prolong the QTC interval [44].

Buprenorphine

Buprenorphine is a long acting phenanthrene derivative, full μ- receptor agonist for analgesia, partial μ- receptor agonist for respiratory depression, and κ- and δ-opioid receptor antagonist [45]. It is a mixed agonist-antagonist [45]. It has effects on the ORL-1 receptor and may contribute to an anti-hyperalgesia effect but its full contribution is still being investigated [45]. Buprenorphine has a ceiling effect for respiratory depression and analgesia but can be altered when other sedating medications are given. Buprenorphine reduces withdrawal symptoms and cravings, and its partial agonist effect minimizes euphoria [45]. The drug has a slow onset of action and a long half-life because of its delayed dissociation from receptors. This property may contribute to its mild withdrawal-like effects with cessation. A Cochrane database review found similar effectiveness between buprenorphine and methadone. It was suggested that doses of at least 16 mg/day be administered [45]. The drug has a high affinity for opioid receptors making it more challenging for other opioid agonists to bind. Higher doses of opioids are required when co-administered with buprenorphine. Administrating buprenorphine to a patient taking opioids may precipitate withdrawal as it antagonizes the action of μ- receptor agonists. Buprenorphine can be administered orally but has 10–15% bioavailability due to first-pass liver metabolism. Sublingual administration improves the bioavailability and buccal films provide over 50% availability [45]. It can also be administered via transdermal, intravenous (IV), or intramuscular (IM) route. The drug is metabolized by the CYP450 3A4 system into nonactive and active (norbuprenorphine) metabolites. Caution should be used in patients with liver disease or with medications affecting CYP3A4, as norbuprenorphine is more potent in its effects on respiratory depression. Other adverse effects include anxiety, nightmares, and hallucinations [45]. Buprenorphine is available in combination with naloxone to decrease illicit use. Naloxone is a potent μ- receptor antagonist with weak affinity at the κ- and δ-sites. While this medication is primarily administered IV, IM or intra-nasally in cases of suspected opioid overdose, it is also used in low dose to treat itching, vomiting, or nausea in patients receiving epidural or IV opioids.

Naltrexone

Naltrexone is used in opioid and alcohol addiction maintenance programs. The drug is a μ- receptor antagonist with weaker antagonism also at the κ- and δ-sites [46]. The medication is administered orally but can be given IM. Given its long duration of action, it serves to block the effects of the abused substance and limits reinforcing pathways [46]. Its clinical effectiveness has been debated. The medication is pharmacologically effective but often suffers from poor adherence and retention in real world settings [47]. Extended-release formulations that are injected monthly may improve adherence. Studies have shown promising effectiveness with abstinence, treatment retention, and reduction in cravings [48–50]. Buprenorphine-naloxone and extended-release naltrexone combinations were both similarly effective in treating OUD once detoxification was achieved [51]. Side effects associated with naltrexone include gastrointestinal irritation, headaches, and anxiety. It is important that patients are fully detoxified prior to initiating opioid antagonist therapy because they precipitate withdrawal-like symptoms.

8 Perioperative Management of Pateint's with Opioid Use Disorder

The perioperative phase is often a challenging time for patients with OUD because it is associated with fear of judgement and stigma that may result in a failure to seek medical care [52]. These patients report difficulties in controlling perioperative pain due to decreased tolerance to pain, increased perception of pain, and baseline chronic pain conditions [53, 54].

The preoperative evaluation is critical in guiding pain management. Patients should have consultation with a pain specialist or the preoperative anesthesia clinic prior to elective surgery to formulate an individualized pain management plan. Communication with the provider managing the patient's maintenance therapy is imperative. Obtaining a thorough pain history, medication history, and assessment of their current state regarding their psychiatric and substance use disorders is recommended. Urine toxicology screen may be indicated. Current medication use should be verified using prescription monitoring programs [55–59]. Screening questionnaires can be used to determine the degree of catastrophizing or anxiousness related to surgery. The opioid risk tool can assist in identifying patient at high risk of opioid misuse [60–62].

Patients with a history of OUD in remission are also at a high risk for relapse during the perioperative setting. The anxiety associated with surgery and concerns regarding the management of postoperative pain are significant stressor.

Clinicians treating these patients have concerns regarding unsupervised access to opioids that can trigger relapse but are also worried about undertreating postoperative pain that can trigger relapse as well [63–66]. Consulting the acute pain service can introduce alternative options include regional analgesia and non-opioid therapies to manage postoperative pain [67].

It is important to educating the patient and the family about the risks of opioid use and relapse. Clinicians should prescribe the minimally required dose and provide a weaning plan for opioid therapy. The patient and family should be educated regarding safe disposal of the unused pills, identify a responsible person to supervise intake, and assess for side effects from opioid therapy [60]. Patients should be discharged with naloxone to decrease the risk of opioid overdose. Patients should have a follow-up visit scheduled with the provider managing their maintenance therapy upon discharge. The in-patient team should directly communicate with the provider regarding the discharge pain management plan.

9 Management of Patients on Methadone Treatent

Patients should continue their outpatient regimen of methadone during hospitalization [68, 69]. The dose should be confirmed from the opioid treatment program managing the therapy. Patient's daily dose of methadone will not be sufficient to control their postoperative pain. [68, 69] Guidelines published on managing postoperative pain for patients on methadone therapy recommend the use of non-pharmacological interventions (peripheral, neuraxial or regional analgesia) and non-opioid pharmacological medications depending on the severity of the surgery [69]. Partial-agonist opioid analgesics (buprenorphine and butorphanol) are absolute contraindication because they will trigger withdrawal symptoms [69].

10 Mangement of Patients on Buprenorphine-Naloxone Treatment

Multiple papers have been published on the acute pain management for patients receiving buprenorphine [69–71]. Earlier guidelines recommended stopping buprenorphine 2–5 days before an elective surgery and replace it with opioid agonist in higher doses and supplementing with non-opioid analgesics and regional anesthesia procedures [72, 73]. Several healthcare systems have published protocols for the management of acute pain in patients receiving buprenorphine illustrated in Table 3 [60, 73–75].

A multi-society expert panel published recommendations in 2021 recommending buprenorphine therapy not be routinely discontinued in the perioperative setting in efforts to reduce the risk of OUD recurrence. They also recommended that buprenorphine therapy can be initiated in patient with untreated OUD and acute pain in the perioperative setting to reduce the risk of death from overdose [75]. They reported that effective analgesia can be obtained with concomitant use of full mu agonists in patient receiving buprenorphine therapy but also recommended the use of additional non-opioid and non-pharmacological therapy [75].

Buprenorphine is a reasonable and recommended alternative to methadone for managing pregnant women with UOD [40]. There is insufficient evidence on the safety of combination buprenorphine/naloxone during pregnancy [40]. The American Society of Addiction Medicine practice guidelines recommend continuing buprenorphine for pregnant women before elective cesarean section to decrease the chances of fetal opioid withdrawal [40, 76].

One study found that pregnant women on buprenorphine therapy had similar intrapartum pain and analgesic needs during labor, but experience more postpartum pain and require 47% more opioid analgesic following cesarean delivery [77].

Table 3 Protocols for Pain Management in Patients taking Buprenorphine-Naloxone

Patients taking buprenorphine-naloxone with mild pain	Patient taking buprenorphine-naloxone with moderate to severe pain
(a) Boston Medical Center	
1. Continue bup-nx and contact prescribing provider a. Consider dividing bup-nx dose to a q6–8 h scheduling regimen b. Consider increasing bup-nx dose 2. Consider adding NSAIDs and acetaminophen 3. Consider adding short-acting opioid analgesics	1. Hold bup-nx on the day of the surgery 2. Give single-dose ER/LA opioid before the surgery and continue ER/LA to manage baseline pain control 3. Use PCA with no basal dose or IR/SA opioid therapy for breakthrough pain 4. Return to bup-nx provider within a week for consideration to reinduce bup-nx
(b) University of Michigan Health System	
1. Continue Bup-nx and contact prescribing provider a. If off Bup-nx > 5 days, treat with opioid if indicated 2. Consider adding NSAIDs or Acetaminophen	1. Cancel elective surgery 2. Coordinate with bup-nx provider to stop bup-nx $\geq$ 5 d, transition to short-acting opioids before surgery 3. If off bup-nx $\geq$ 5 d, use opioid therapy for pain 4. Consider adjunct pain therapy (acetaminophen, NSAIDs, gabapentin/pregabalin, alpha-2 agonist, or ketamine infusion) 5. Consider regional anesthesia 6. Return to bup-nx provider for reinduction
(c) University of Kentucky Healthcare System	
1. Continue bup-nx and contact prescribing provider a. Consider dividing bup-nx dose every 6–8 h scheduling regimen b. If off bup-nx, consider short course of opioid therapy if indicated 2. Consider adjunct therapy (acetaminophen/NSAIDs)	1. Continue bup-nx and contact prescribing provider 2. Consider acute pain consult for PCA or regional analgesia 3. Close observation to assess analgesia 4. Continue opioid therapy for postoperative pain after discharge

Bup-nx Buprenorphine-naloxone, *NSAIDs* non-steroidal anti-inflammatories, *ER/LA* extended release/long-acting, *PCA* patient controlled analgesia, *IR/SA* immediate release/short acting)

11 OUD for Patients on Injectable Naltrexone

There is no standardized approach on managing perioperative pain in patients on injectable naltrexone. The plan should be discussed with the patient and prescriber prior to elective surgery or procedure. The possibility of managing the pain with opioids needs to be balanced against the risk of the patient relapsing. If the decision is made to stop naltrexone, it is recommended to arrange the surgery at least 4 weeks from the last injectable dose of extended-release form and 72 h from the last oral dose [78]. A degree of resistance to opioid analgesics is expected, although increased sensitivity is also possible. These patients should be closely monitored while on opioid therapy. In the event of emergency surgery or if the decision is made to operate while the patient is taking his naltrexone, it is recommended to use a higher dose of non-opioid analgesics. Non-steroidal anti-inflammatory drugs, acetaminophen, ketamine, or regional anesthesia should be considered [78–81]. Some animal studies have suggested that opioid receptor blockade with naltrexone can be overcome with higher doses of opioids [81]. It is recommended to consult the Acute Pain Service to help manage the perioperative pain in this patient population.

Key Points

- Patients with OUD on maintenance therapy are at high risk for uncontrolled postoperative pain.
- Patients with OUD on maintenance therapy who are at risk for increased postoperative pain may benefit from consultation by a pain medicine or acute pain specialists.
- Multimodal analgesia with regional techniques when feasible should be the cornerstone of management while applying individualized tailoring of analgesic regimen based on the type of maintenance therapy.
- Upon discharge, patients with OUD on maintenance therapy should have appropriate follow-up with treating physician and given a taper plan for postoperative opioid therapy.

References

1. Mozayani A, Raymon L. eds. Handbook of drug interactions: a clinical and forensic guide. Springer Science & Business Media; 2011. p. 159–91
2. Nafziger AN, Barkin RL. Opioid therapy in acute and chronic pain. J Clin Pharmacol. 2018;58(9):1111–22.
3. Smith HS. Opioid Metabolism. Mayo Clin. 2009;84(7):613–24.
4. Cone EJ, Heit HA, Caplan YH, Gourlay D. Evidence of morphine metabolism to hydromorphone in pain patients chronically treated with morphine. J Anal Toxicol. 2006;30(1):1–5.
5. Cone EJ, Caplan YH, Moser F, Robert T, Black D. Evidence that morphine is metabolized to hydromorphone but not to oxymorphone. J Anal Toxicol. 2008;32(4):319–23.
6. Oyler JM, Cone EJ, Joseph J, Huestis MA. Identification of Hydrocodone in Human Urine Following Controlled Codeine Administration. J Anal Toxicol. 2000;24(7):530–5.
7. Inturrisi CE. Pharmacology of analgesia: basic principles. Cancer Pain Assess Manag Second Ed 2009;167–79.
8. Elliott K, Kest B, Man A, Kao B, Inturrisi CE. N-methyl-d-aspartate (NMDA) receptors, mu and kappa opioid tolerance, and perspectives on new analgesic drug development. Neuropsychopharmacology. 1995;13(4):347–56.
9. Berlin CM, McCarver-May DG. Use of codeine-and dextromethorpan-containing cough remedies in children. Pediatrics. 1997;99(6):919–21.
10. Noble M, Treadwell JR, Tregear SJ, Coates VH, Wiffen PJ, Akafomo C, Schoelles KM, Chou R. Long-term opioid management for chronic noncancer pain. Cochrane Database Syst Rev. 2010;2010(1).

11. Eisenberg E, McNicol ED, Carr DB. Opioids for neuropathic pain. Cochrane Database Syst Rev. 2006;2006(3).
12. da Costa BR, Nüesch E, Kasteler R, Husni E, Welch V, Rutjes AWS, et al. Oral or transdermal opioids for osteoarthritis of the knee or hip. Cochrane Database Syst Rev. 2014;2014(9).
13. Chaparro LE, Furlan AD, Deshpande A, Mailis-Gagnon A, Atlas S, Turk DC. Opioids compared to placebo or other treatments for chronic low-back pain. Cochrane Database Syst Rev. 2013;2013(8).
14. Maslov LN, Lishmanov YB, Barzakh EI, Lasukova TV, Rice KK, Oeltgen PR. Negative inotropic and chronotropic effects of δ-opioid receptor antagonists are mediated via non-opioid receptors. Bull Exp Biol Med. 2006;141(4):420–3.
15. Chen A, Ashburn MA. Cardiac effects of opioid therapy. Pain Med. 2015;16(suppl_1):S27–31.
16. Baldo BA, Pham NH. Histamine-releasing and allergenic properties of opioid analgesic drugs: resolving the two. Anaesth Intensive Care. 2012;40(2):216–35.
17. Martin JA, Campbell A, Killip T, Kotz M, Krantz MJ, Kreek MJ, et al. QT interval screening in methadone maintenance treatment: Report of a SAMHSA expert panel. J Addict Dis. 2011;30(4):283–306.
18. Bachmutsky I, Wei XP, Kish E, Yackle K. Opioids depress breathing through two small brainstem sites. Elife 2020;9.
19. Palkovic B, Marchenko V, Zuperku EJ, Stuth EAE, Stucke AG. Multi-level regulation of opioid-induced respiratory depression. Physiology. 2020;35(6):391.
20. Boom M, Niesters M, Sarton E, Aarts L, W. Smith T, Dahan A. Non-analgesic effects of opioids: opioid-induced respiratory depression. Curr Pharm Des 2012;18(37):5994–6004.
21. Çoruh B, Tonelli MR, Park DR. Fentanyl-induced chest wall rigidity. Chest. 2013;143(4):1145–6.
22. Wiener J, McIntyre A, Janzen S, Mirkowski M, MacKenzie HM, Teasell R. Opioids and cerebral physiology in the acute management of traumatic brain injury: a systematic review. 2019;33(5):559–66.
23. Schregel W, Schaefermeyer H, Sihle-Wissel M, Klein R. Transcranial doppler sonography during isoflurane/N2O anaesthesia and surgery: flow velocity, "vessel area" and "volume flow." Can J Anaesth. 1994;41(7):607–12.
24. Manninen PH. Opioids and seizures. Can J Anaesth. 1997;44(5):463–6.
25. de Vries F, Bruin M, Lobatto DJ, Dekkers OM, Schoones JW, van Furth WR, et al. Opioids and their endocrine effects: a systematic review and meta-analysis. J Clin Endocrinol Metab. 2020;105(3):1020–9.
26. Kehlet H. The surgical stress response: should it be prevented? Can J Surg. 1991;34(6)L 565–7.
27. Seeber B, Böttcher B, D'Costa E, Wildt L. Opioids and reproduction. Vitam Horm. 2019;111:247–79.
28. Qian TL, Wang XH, Liu S, Ma L, Lu Y. Fentanyl inhibits glucose-stimulated insulin release from beta-cells in rat pancreatic islets. World J Gastroenterol. 2009;15(33):4163–9.
29. Koekkoek LL, van der Gun LL, Serlie MJ, la Fleur SE. The clash of two epidemics: the relationship between opioids and glucose metabolism. Curr Diab Rep. 2022;22(7):301.
30. Galligan JJ, Sternini C. Insights into the role of opioid receptors in the GI tract: experimental evidence and therapeutic relevance. Handb Exp Pharmacol. 2017;239:363.
31. Murphy DB, Sutton JA, Prescott LF, Murphy MB. Opioid-induced delay in gastric emptying a peripheral mechanism in humans. Anesthesiology. 1997;87(4):765–70.
32. Imam MZ, Kuo A, Ghassabian S, Smith MT. Progress in understanding mechanisms of opioid-induced gastrointestinal adverse effects and respiratory depression. Neuropharmacology. 2018;131:238–55.
33. Karagiannis TT, Cleary JP, Gok B, Henderson AJ, Martin NG, Yajima M, et al. Single cell transcriptomics reveals opioid usage evokes widespread suppression of antiviral gene program. Nat Commun. 2020;11(1).
34. Abuse S. Key substance use and mental health indicators in the United States: results from the 2019 National Survey on Drug Use and Health.

35. Malik KM, Imani F, Beckerly R, Chovatiya R. Risk of opioid use disorder from exposure to opioids in the perioperative period: a systematic review. Anesthesiol Pain Med. 2020;10(1):101339.
36. Rapp SE, Ready LB, Nessly ML. Acute pain management in patients with prior opioid consumption: a case-controlled retrospective review. Pain. 1995;61(2):195–201.
37. Stone EM, Kennedy-Hendricks A, Barry CL, Bachhuber MA, McGinty EE. The role of stigma in U.S. primary care physicians' treatment of opioid use disorder. Drug Alcohol Depend 2021; 221:108627.
38. Coluzzi F, Bifulco F, Cuomo A, Dauri M, Leonardi C, Melotti RM, et al. The challenge of perioperative pain management in opioid-tolerant patients. Ther Clin Risk Manag [Internet]. 2017;13:1163.
39. Cahill CM, Walwyn W, Taylor AMW, Pradhan AAA, Evans CJ. Allostatic mechanisms of opioid tolerance beyond desensitization and downregulation. Trends Pharmacol Sci. 2016;37(11):963.
40. Kampman K, Jarvis M. American Society of Addiction Medicine (ASAM) national practice guideline for the use of medications in the treatment of addiction involving opioid use. J Addict Med. 2015;9(5):358.
41. Mercadante S, Arcuri E, Santoni A. Opioid-induced tolerance and hyperalgesia. CNS Drugs. 2019;33(10):943–55.
42. Wilson SH, Hellman KM, James D, Adler AC, Chandrakantan A. Mechanisms, diagnosis, prevention and management of perioperative opioid-induced hyperalgesia. Pain Manag. 2021;11(4):405.
43. Wakeman SE, Larochelle MR, Ameli O, Chaisson CE, McPheeters JT, Crown WH, et al. Comparative effectiveness of different treatment pathways for opioid use disorder. JAMA Netw Open. 2020;3(2):e1920622–e1920622.
44. Mattick RP, Breen C, Kimber J, Davoli M. Methadone maintenance therapy versus no opioid replacement therapy for opioid dependence. Cochrane Database Syst Rev. 2009.
45. Mattick RP, Breen C, Kimber J, Davoli M. Buprenorphine maintenance versus placebo or methadone maintenance for opioid dependence. Cochrane Database Syst Rev. 2014(2).
46. DeMartini KS, Foster DW, Corbin WR, Fucito LM, Romano D, Leeman RF, et al. Drinking goals and goal attainment in a naltrexone trial for young adult heavy drinkers. J Consult Clin Psychol. 2018;86(9):765.
47. Minozzi S, Amato L, Vecchi S, Davoli M, Kirchmayer U, Verster A. Oral naltrexone maintenance treatment for opioid dependence. Cochrane Database Syst Rev. 2011(4).
48. Krupitsky E, Nunes EV, Ling W, Illeperuma A, Gastfriend DR, Silverman BL. Injectable extended-release naltrexone for opioid dependence: a double-blind, placebo-controlled, multicenter randomized trial. Lancet. 2011;377(9776):1506–13.
49. Syed YY, Keating GM. Extended-release intramuscular naltrexone (VIVITROL®): a review of its use in the prevention of relapse to opioid dependence in detoxified patients. CNS Drugs. 2013;27(10):851–61.
50. Krupitsky E, Nunes EV, Ling W, Gastfriend DR, Memisoglu A, Silverman BL. Injectable extended-release naltrexone (XR-NTX) for opioid dependence: long-term safety and effectiveness. Addiction. 2013;108(9):1628–37.
51. Lee JD, Nunes EV., MPA PN, Bailey GL, Brigham GS, Cohen AJ, et al. NIDA Clinical Trials Network CTN-0051, extended-release naltrexone vs. buprenorphine for opioid treatment (X:BOT): study design and rationale. Contemp Clin Trials [Internet]. 2016 Sep 1 [cited 2023 Jun 19];50:253. Available from: /pmc/articles/PMC5416469/
52. Matthews S. Self-stigma and addiction. In: The stigma of addiction: an essential guide. Cham: Springer International Publishing; 2019 Jan 10. p. 5–32
53. Wachholtz A, Gonzalez G. Co-morbid pain and opioid addiction: long term effect of opioid maintenance on acute pain. Drug Alcohol Depend. 2014;145:143–9.
54. Compton P, Charuvastra VC, Ling W. Pain intolerance in opioid-maintained former opiate addicts: effect of long-acting maintenance agent. Drug Alcohol Depend. 2001;63(2):139–46.

55. Apfelbaum JL, Connis RT, Nickinovich DG, Pasternak LR, Arens JF, Caplan RA, Fleisher LA, Flowerdew R, Gold BS, Mayhew JF, Rice LJ. Practice advisory for preanesthesia evaluation: an updated report by the American Society of Anesthesiologists Task Force on Preanesthesia Evaluation. Anesthesiology. 2012;116(3):522–38.
56. American Society of Anesthesiologists Task Force on Acute Pain Management. Practice guidelines for acute pain management in the perioperative setting: an updated report by the American Society of Anesthesiologists Task Force on Acute Pain Management. Anesthesiology. 2012;116(2):248–73.
57. Bush K, Kivlahan DR, McDonell MB, Fihn SD, Bradley KA. The AUDIT alcohol consumption questions (AUDIT-C): an effective brief screening test for problem drinking. Ambulatory Care Quality Improvement Project (ACQUIP). Alcohol Use Disorders Identification Test. Arch Intern Med. 1998;158(16):1789–95.
58. Spitzer RL, Kroenke K, Williams JBW, Löwe B. A brief measure for assessing generalized anxiety disorder: the GAD-7. Arch Intern Med. 2006;166(10):1092–7.
59. Smith PC, Schmidt SM, Allensworth-Davies D, Saitz R. A single-question screening test for drug use in primary care. Arch Intern Med. 2010;170(13):1155–60.
60. Ward EN, Quaye ANA, Wilens TE. Opioid use disorders: Perioperative management of a special population. Anesth Analg. 2018;127(2):539–47.
61. Webster LR, Webster RM. Predicting aberrant behaviors in opioid-treated patients: preliminary validation of the Opioid Risk Tool. Pain Med. 2005;6(6):432–42.
62. Sullivan MJL, Bishop SR, Pivik J. The pain catastrophizing scale: development and validation. Psychol Assess. 1995;7(4):524–32.
63. Koob GF, Volkow ND. Neurobiology of addiction: a neurocircuitry analysis. The lancet Psychiatry. 2016;3(8):760–73.
64. Volkow ND, Koob GF, McLellan AT. Neurobiologic advances from the brain disease model of addiction. N Engl J Med. 2016;374(4):363–71.
65. Tsui JI, Lira MC, Cheng DM, Winter MR, Alford DP, Liebschutz JM, et al. Chronic pain, craving, and illicit opioid use among patients receiving opioid agonist therapy. Drug Alcohol Depend. 2016;166:26–31.
66. Larson MJ, Paasche-Orlow M, Cheng DM, Lloyd-Travaglini C, Saitz R, Samet JH. Persistent pain is associated with substance use after detoxification: a prospective cohort analysis. Addiction. 2007;102(5):752–60.
67. Stromer W, Michaeli K, Sandner-Kiesling A. Perioperative pain therapy in opioid abuse. Eur J Anaesthesiol. 2013;30(2):55–64.
68. Peng PWH, Tumber PS, Gourlay D. Review article: Perioperative pain management of patients on methadone therapy. Can J Anesth. 2005;52(5):513–23.
69. Alford DP, Compton P, Samet JH. Acute pain management for patients receiving maintenance methadone or buprenorphine therapy. Ann Intern Med. 2006;144(2):127.
70. Sen S, Arulkumar S, Cornett EM, Gayle JA, Flower RR, Fox CJ, et al. New pain management options for the surgical patient on methadone and buprenorphine. Curr Pain Headache Rep. 2016;20(3):1–8.
71. Anthony Anderson T, Quaye ANA, Nalan Ward E, Wilens TE, Hilliard PE, Brummett CM. To stop or not, that is the question: acute pain management for the patient on chronic buprenorphine. Anesthesiology. 2017;126(6):1180.
72. Wenzel JT, Schwenk ES, Baratta JL, Viscusi ER. Managing opioid-tolerant patients in the perioperative surgical home. Anesthesiol Clin. 2016;34(2):287–301.
73. Bryson EO. The perioperative management of patients maintained on medications used to manage opioid addiction. Curr Opin Anaesthesiol. 2014;27(3):359–64.
74. Stern EE. Buprenorphine and the anesthesia considerations: a literature review. 2015. Available from: http://dune.une.edu/na_capstones
75. Kohan L, Potru S, Barreveld AM, Sprintz M, Lane O, Aryal A, Emerick T, Dopp A, Chhay S, Viscusi E. Buprenorphine management in the perioperative period: educational review and recommendations from a multisociety expert panel. Reg Anesth Pain Med. 2021;46(10):840–59.

76. Jones HE, Kaltenbach K, Heil SH, Stine SM, Coyle MG, Arria AM, et al. Neonatal abstinence syndrome after methadone or buprenorphine exposure. N Engl J Med. 2010;363(24):2320.
77. Meyer M, Paranya G, Keefer Norris A, Howard D. Intrapartum and postpartum analgesia for women maintained on buprenorphine during pregnancy. Eur J Pain. 2010;14(9):939–43.
78. Vickers AP, Jolly A. Naltrexone and problems in pain management: how to manage acute pain in people taking an opioid antagonist. BMJ Br Med J. 2006;332(7534):132.
79. Lesscher HMB, Bailey A, Burbach JPH, Van Ree JM, Kitchen I, Gerrits MAFM. Receptor-selective changes in μ-, δ- and κ-opioid receptors after chronic naltrexone treatment in mice. Eur J Neurosci. 2003;17(5):1006–12.
80. Fishman M. Precipitated withdrawal during maintenance opioid blockade with extended-release naltrexone. Addiction. 2008;103(8):1399–401.
81. Dean RL, Todtenkopf MS, Deaver DR, Arastu MF, Dong N, Reitano K, et al. Overriding the blockade of antinociceptive actions of opioids in rats treated with extended-release naltrexone. Pharmacol Biochem Behav. 2008;89(4):515–22.

Perioperative Pain Management of Patients Presenting for Cardiac Surgery

Eric R. Simon, Michelle Kuei, and Patrick Meyer

Abstract Pain following cardiac surgery is often severe and the consequences of undertreatment may result in significant complications in both the immediate and extended postoperative period. Improved postoperative pain control may substantially shorten hospital length of stay, decrease postoperative ventilation requirements, reduce postoperative complications, and improve patient satisfaction. In patients presenting for cardiac surgery, multidisciplinary and multimodal approaches that include oral and intravenous analgesics and regional anesthetic techniques represent techniques worthy of substantial consideration.

Keywords Cardiac surgery · Postoperative pain · Chronic pain · Regional anesthesia · Analgesics

1 Introduction

Death from cardiovascular disease remains the most common cause of worldwide mortality and many cardiovascular diseases require surgical intervention to provide definitive treatment. Pain after cardiac surgery is common, and despite multiple analgesic strategies that might provide substantial relief, is frequently moderate or severe in intensity. Uncontrolled pain following cardiac surgery may lead to significant complications for the patient in the immediate and extended postoperative period. Efforts to provide adequate pain control in patients requiring cardiac surgery should be a high priority for the entire perioperative care team and multidisciplinary

E. R. Simon (✉) · P. Meyer
School of Medicine and Public Health, University of Wisconsin, Madison, WI, USA
e-mail: esimon2@wisc.edu

P. Meyer
e-mail: psmeyer@wisc.edu

M. Kuei
Boulder Valley Anesthesiology, Boulder, CO, USA
e-mail: mkuei@bvapllc.com

A. Abd-Elsayed and K. Schroeder (eds.), *Perioperative Pain Management*,
https://doi.org/10.1007/978-3-031-67648-2_22

and multimodal approaches are more likely to provide meaningful perioperative analgesia.

2 Most Common Conditions in Adults Requiring Cardiac Surgery

Coronary artery bypass grafting (CABG) and heart valve surgeries are the most commonly performed procedures in cardiac surgical patients across the world [1]. Dramatic advancements in surgical skills and anesthetic techniques have allowed for increasingly complex surgeries in older patients with a multitude of comorbidities [2]. Historically, these procedures have always been performed through a midline sternotomy or a thoracotomy incision. However, efforts to minimize the postoperative pain experienced by cardiac surgical patients have resulted in the development of minimally invasive techniques including mini-sternotomy, mini-thoracotomy, and fully endoscopic surgery via port sites.

3 Acute Postoperative Pain

Pain after cardiac surgery is multifactorial and may be of musculoskeletal, visceral, or neuropathic origin. Most commonly, postoperative pain originates from myofascial structures such as muscle, bone, tendon, and ligament that are disrupted during sternotomy and surgical dissection. Additionally, sternal retraction may result in fractured ribs, dislocation of the costochondral junction, or costochondritis [3]. Other causes of musculoskeletal postoperative pain in the cardiac surgical patient include surgical positioning injuries or ancillary procedures requiring additional incisions, such as saphenous vein harvest or axillary artery cutdown [4].

Visceral cardiac pain is transmitted to the central nervous system via the vagus nerve, cervical sympathetic chain, and upper-thoracic sympathetic ganglia. Neuropathic pain after cardiac surgery is attributed to traumatization of the intercostal nerves that occurs when the intercostal space is opened. Postoperative pleural drains can intensify visceral pain originating from the parietal pleura through intercostal and phrenic nerve innervation [5]. Dissection of the internal mammary artery can induce an irritative state and neuritis that can cause significant pain following coronary artery bypass surgery [6].

The severity of pain after cardiac surgery is significant, with 30–75% of patients reporting at least moderate acute pain following these surgical procedures [4]. Postoperative pain is most severe during the first 24–48 h and generally decreases by postoperative day three [1]. A detailed analysis of pain evolution following cardiac surgery demonstrates that pain perception transitions from incisional, thoracic pain immediately after surgery to musculoskeletal pain elsewhere. Common sources of delayed pain complaints are numerous but include lower extremity pain after saphenous vein harvest or back pain related to positioning and prolonged procedures [4]. The median duration of pain following coronary artery bypass surgery is five days and is extended to six days for patients who underwent valve surgery [7]. Optimal pain management should consider the specific cause, location, and timing of pain foci to maximize successful outcomes in the cardiac surgical patient.

Risk factors for acute pain after cardiac surgery vary depending on the specific study, but generally include location and extent of the incision (thoracotomy), younger age (< 60 years), and prolonged surgery (> 2 h) [8]. Other studies have associated the use of cardiopulmonary bypass with slightly higher pain levels, potentially attributed to the induction of the systemic inflammatory response syndrome [9]. Additionally, some studies suggest that women report higher pain intensities and a significantly higher number of painful areas compared to men after cardiac surgery [10, 11]. Elevated preoperative anxiety has been shown to increase the sensation of pain in the postoperative period [12, 13], more so in men than women [14]. The effects of ethnic, cultural, and socioeconomic factors on the perception of postoperative pain have been demonstrated in some preliminary studies but warrant further investigation [15].

Patients undergoing cardiac surgery pose specific pain management challenges during the postoperative period due to a variety of both patient and procedural factors. Pain assessment is the first important step in effective treatment. However, it may be difficult for providers to assess pain following cardiac surgery secondary to ongoing intubation and sedation [16]. Postoperative delirium is common and may compound difficulties associated with pain assessment and treatment. Fortunately, a variety of patient assessment tools have been recently developed that serve to aid in the evaluation of postoperative pain, agitation, and delirium in intensive care unit (ICU) patients, and many of these have been specifically validated in the cardiac surgery population [17].

Additionally, patient beliefs about expected pain intensity and pain management may impact the efficacy of management by the postoperative care team. In a study of 564 patients scheduled for cardiac surgery, Cogan et al. showed that a considerable number of patients had negative misconceptions related to the treatment of pain after surgery that likely led to suboptimal treatment and possibly worse outcomes [18]. The authors concluded that there is an absolute necessity to provide pain education to patients undergoing cardiac surgery as this may improve patient expectations, satisfaction, and postoperative outcomes.

Physiological pain is one of the main defense mechanisms of the human body. Postoperative pain, however, is a consequence of a planned traumatic injury and therefore does not play a role in warning and defense. Instead, it leads to the development of a number of adverse pathophysiological processes instigated by nociceptor stimulation [19]. Of particular concern is the effect of pain on the respiratory system. Pain leads to reflex muscular tension and splinting, impairing the patient's ability to breathe leading to shortness of breath and a reduction in tidal volume, vital capacity, functional residual capacity, and pulmonary compliance [20]. Pain also impairs the ability to expectorate secretions that accumulate in the bronchial tree resulting in atelectasis, hypoxemia, and pneumonia [21].

Uncontrolled pain after cardiac surgery also results in activation of the sympathetic nervous system leading to increased heart rate, heart contractility, and blood pressure, all of which increase the risk of myocardial ischemia. Elevated circulating catecholamines increase the risk of arrhythmias such as atrial fibrillation. Poorly controlled pain results in reductions in peripheral blood flow and venous stasis, which predisposes the patient to the development of deep vein thrombosis particularly in the setting of postoperative immobilization. Activation of the sympathetic nervous system also impairs the mobility of the gastrointestinal tract and bladder, potentially leading to urinary retention, constipation, and ileus [22].

Detrimental changes in the endocrine system also occur [23]. There are increased circulating levels of cortisol, antidiuretic hormone, corticotropic hormone, renin, angiotensin, and aldosterone. Conversely, there are decreased circulating levels of insulin which leads to a catabolic state. Prolonged nociceptive stimulation can lead to suppression of the patient's immune system, increasing the risk of infections and impairing wound healing. Finally, severe uncontrolled pain has detrimental psychological effects for the patient, leading to anxiety, depression, and sleep disorders [24].

4 Chronic Pain After Cardiac Surgery

Pain after cardiac surgery may persist long enough that it loses its warning function and transitions into a pathologic state of chronic postoperative pain. Chronic pain most often arises following traumatic or inflammatory nerve injury which then establishes a neuropathic pain phenotype [25]. Diagnostic criteria for chronic pain typically include at least 3–6 months of consistent pain symptomology and pain of adequate severity to significantly impact a patient's quality of life [26]. Chronic pain after cardiac surgery is often underappreciated, as 21–55% of patients develop chronic pain syndromes following cardiac surgery [3, 27]. Higher levels of acute pain following cardiac surgery are associated with a 3.5-fold increased likelihood of chronic postoperative pain development [3]. Other risk factors for chronic postoperative pain development include depression, psychological vulnerability, high levels of stress, more extensive surgery, and prolonged surgery [28].

5 Pharmacologic Methods of Pain Control After Cardiac Surgery

Over the past decade, the emergence of enhanced recovery after surgery (ERAS) for cardiac surgery programs has prompted care teams to explore unique options for the management of postoperative pain in place of high-dose opioid administration. This section will explore pharmacological modalities that may be utilized to assist with pain control in the cardiac surgery patient.

Opioids

High dose opioids have historically been utilized in cardiac surgery patients to provide perioperative analgesia and intraoperative anesthesia. Although opioids have no analgesic ceiling effect, their use is mainly limited by the accumulation of side effects that are encountered with dose escalations. These side effects include somnolence, respiratory depression, hypotension, urinary retention, nausea and slowed gastrointestinal transport which can result in constipation and postoperative ileus. In cardiac surgery patients, the judicious use of opioids is necessary to avoid excess sedation and prolonged intubation [29]. Nonopioid analgesic adjuncts are important to minimize opioid use and enhance recovery following cardiac surgery and their use represents the focus of the remainder of this section.

Acetaminophen

Acetaminophen produces its analgesic effect by inhibiting central prostaglandin synthesis [30]. Although this medication has some similarities to a non-steroidal anti-inflammatory agent, acetaminophen is not felt to have an adverse effect on platelets or gastric mucosa [31, 32]. The perioperative analgesic effect of acetaminophen has been demonstrated in numerous randomized controlled trials and meta-analyses. In cardiac surgery, acetaminophen has been shown to reduce perioperative opioid use and improve overall pain scores [33]. When utilized in combination with other sedatives in older adults following cardiac surgery, a randomized controlled trial demonstrated a decreased postoperative opioid requirement and a lower incidence of in-hospital delirium in those patients who received scheduled acetaminophen along with their sedative regimen [34]. Acetaminophen can be administered orally, rectally, or intravenously. The daily dose of acetaminophen is generally limited to 3000–4000 mg per day to decrease hepatotoxicity risk.

Non-steroidal Anti-inflammatory Drugs

Nonsteroidal anti-inflammatory drugs (NSAIDs) are a class of medication used widely for their analgesic, antipyretic and anti-inflammatory effects. The mechanism of action of NSAIDs is via inhibition of the enzyme cyclooxygenase. This inhibition can impair production of thromboxanes, prostaglandins and prostacyclins, which together account for their analgesic efficacy as well as their side effects. Well known side effects include an increased risk of gastric mucosal damage, renal dysfunction, adverse cardiovascular events and hematologic effects secondary to antiplatelet activity [35]. NSAIDs are generally avoided following cardiac surgery in the United States due to the Food and Drug Administration (FDA) black box warning describing the potential for NSAIDs to induce adverse cardiovascular events, including myocardial infarction, cardiac arrest, stroke and pulmonary embolism [36–38]. NSAID use following cardiac surgery has also been associated with postoperative renal dysfunction [39]. Despite these concerns, the use of NSAIDs following cardiac surgery may represent an appropriate analgesic adjunct in select patients [40]. Patients with normal renal function and at low risk of perioperative kidney injury and those in whom there is a low bleeding risk may represent reasonable candidates for judicious NSAID therapy.

Gabapentinoids

The gabapentinoid drugs gabapentin and pregabalin are believed to exert their modulation of pain via blockade of a subunit of voltage-gated calcium channels. Gabapentinoids depress excitatory input onto dorsal horn neurons, stimulate descending inhibition, and have anti-inflammatory actions via incompletely understood mechanisms [41, 42]. Known side effects of these medications include sedation, respiratory depression, dizziness, and visual disturbances which can be more pronounced in the setting of renal dysfunction. Multiple studies evaluating the analgesic impact of perioperative administration of gabapentinoid drugs have shown conflicting results. A large meta-analysis of 281 randomized controlled trials comparing gabapentinoids with controls demonstrated no clinically meaningful difference in acute, subacute or chronic pain [43]. In coronary artery bypass grafting surgery, Menda et al. found significantly lower pain scores, opioid requirements and postoperative nausea and vomiting in patients who received gabapentin 600 mg preoperatively compared to placebo. However, the gabapentin group required longer postoperative ventilation and more patients were found to be overly sedated [44]. In another randomized controlled trial evaluating gabapentinoid administration in CABG patients, pregabalin administration failed to reduce opioid requirements despite reducing postoperative pain scores [45]. Interestingly, there may be a role for the use of pregabalin to reduce the prevalence of persistent postsurgical pain after cardiac surgery [46]. Gabapentinoids appear to have potential as a non-opioid adjunct, but optimal dosing regimens must be evaluated further to maximize analgesia and minimize side effects. The FDA has issued a warning for respiratory depression when these medications are utilized along with other central nervous system depressants such as opioids. There is currently insufficient evidence to recommend widespread utilization in cardiac surgery patients for postoperative pain control [47].

Ketamine

Ketamine is a noncompetitive N-methyl-D-aspartate (NMDA) and glutamate receptor antagonist that can be utilized as a dissociative anesthetic. When used in subanesthetic doses, it can serve as an analgesic adjunct that reduces opiate-induced hyperalgesia and improves pain control [48]. The most common side-effects include dizziness, drowsiness, confusion, and hallucinations that become more common at higher doses. In cardiac surgery patients, a ketamine infusion has been shown to result in a diminished opioid requirement and improved patient satisfaction despite not altering pain scores [49]. Nesher et al. similarly demonstrated that postoperative ketamine infusions were associated with a reduction in postoperative opioid requirements in patients who underwent thoracotomy, including minimally invasive CABG [50]. There is evidence that an intraoperative infusion of ketamine during cardiac surgery may attenuate the surgical stress response following cardiopulmonary bypass with several clinical trials showing decreased inflammatory biomarkers in patients receiving ketamine [51]. There is some evidence that intraoperative ketamine administration may be associated with a lower incidence of postoperative delirium [52], but this effect has not been consistently demonstrated in other major surgeries [53]. The potential benefits, relative absence of frequent serious side effects, and hemodynamic stability associated with ketamine administration has resulted in a significant increase in the use of this analgesic adjunct in cardiac surgery patients.

Dexmedetomidine

Dexmedetomidine is a highly selective alpha-2 adrenergic receptor agonist that is associated with sedative and analgesic effects. Clinical attributes associated with dexmedetomidine infusions include sedation, sympatholysis, analgesia, anxiolysis and maintenance of respiratory function. The widespread effects of dexmedetomidine can be attributed to the diverse and well-distributed sites of action in the body. Most of the analgesic effects relevant to dexmedetomidine administration occur via its agonist activity on alpha-2 adrenergic receptors in the spinal cord, which reduces transmission of nociceptive signals [54]. A systematic review of twelve clinical trials evaluating the clinical effect of dexmedetomidine on pain following cardiothoracic surgery supports routine administration secondary to observed reductions in postoperative pain and analgesic requirements for up to 24 h following surgery

[55]. Several other studies have shown a wide spectrum of beneficial effects associated with dexmedetomidine administration in cardiac surgery patients, including a decrease in postoperative mortality and delirium [56], as well as a reduction in ICU length of stay [57]. Other studies have found no difference in the rate of delirium or ICU length of stay when dexmedetomidine or propofol were used for postoperative sedation but did demonstrate decreased opioid requirements in patients receiving dexmedetomidine [34]. Given its ability to act as a sedative and potent analgesic, dexmedetomidine certainly has a role in the perioperative care of cardiac surgery patients.

Steroids

Surgery causes tissue injury and induces both a local and systemic inflammatory response. Corticosteroids have been found to possess analgesic benefits following surgery, likely due to their potent anti-inflammatory and immunosuppressive effects. Steroid use in noncardiac surgery has been extensively studied, with a large meta-analysis of randomized controlled trials demonstrating dexamethasone doses more than 0.1 mg/kg to be an effective adjunct to reduce postoperative pain and opioid consumptions following surgery [58]. The degree of analgesic benefit associated with perioperative steroid administration appears to vary by surgery type and appears to be most effective in orthopedic, oral and ear, nose and throat (ENT) surgery [59]. Randomized controlled trial data has previously demonstrated that two intraoperative doses of 250 mg of methylprednisolone did not improve postoperative analgesia after cardiac surgery [60]. Common concerns regarding steroid administration include a theoretical increased infection risk profile, impaired wound healing or an increased risk of gastrointestinal bleeding secondary to immune and inflammatory modulating properties. Currently, the best evidence supporting the safety of prophylactic corticosteroid administration on adult cardiac surgery outcomes is provided by two large randomized-controlled trials which found no difference in mortality or major morbidity [61]. Further investigation into the analgesic impact of different doses and types of steroids in cardiac surgery patients is warranted to guide future use as an analgesic adjunct.

Magnesium

Magnesium has been found to have antinociceptive properties, largely through its antagonist action at the N-methyl-d-aspartate (NMDA) receptor [62]. Given the significant role of NMDA receptors in pain transduction, many studies have evaluated this agent for a potential role in providing perioperative analgesia. In cardiac surgery, a randomized study found a bolus dose and subsequent continuous infusion of magnesium gluconate decreased remifentanil consumption without serious side effects following on-pump cardiac surgery [63]. Another study demonstrated a decreased time to extubation and decreased postoperative pain scores with magnesium sulfate administration during elective CABG surgery [64]. These studies demonstrate promise for magnesium as a non-opioid analgesic, but further high-quality studies are necessary to draw firm conclusions.

Intravenous Lidocaine

Perioperative infusions of intravenous lidocaine have been shown to improve pain control after certain types of surgery. The mechanism of action for intravenous lidocaine in improving perioperative pain control is complex and still being fully elucidated but is felt to be related to its ability to attenuate the proinflammatory effects of surgery rather than its effect on sodium channels [65]. Lidocaine infusions utilized for abdominal surgery have been found to reduce pain scores and postoperative opioid requirements [66]. Doses greater than or equal to 2 mg/kg/h were associated with decreased pain scores and opioid consumption in the first 24 h, however smaller doses were not. There is evidence that perioperative lidocaine administration may decrease the duration of ileus and decrease the incidence of postoperative nausea and vomiting [67]. In addition, toxicity related to the use of perioperative lidocaine infusions appears to be exceedingly rare [68]. The data for the use of perioperative lidocaine infusions in the setting of cardiac surgery is not as supportive. Insler et al. found no difference in pain scores or opioid consumption in cardiac surgery patients receiving an intraoperative lidocaine infusion [69]. However, Wang et al. did demonstrate a lower incidence of postoperative cognitive dysfunction in cardiac surgery patients receiving an intraoperative lidocaine infusion [70]. Based on this limited data, perioperative lidocaine infusions are not currently recommended for analgesia in cardiac surgery patients. Given the positive data in other surgical populations, further study may help define a role for this adjunct in the future in the cardiac surgery patient.

6 Regional Techniques

Multimodal analgesia techniques with regional anesthesia are becoming increasingly popular for ERAS to improve patient outcomes and satisfaction. Historically, regional techniques in cardiac surgery consisted of thoracic epidurals, paravertebral blocks, and intercostal blocks. However, with the introduction of and increased availability of ultrasound imaging, there are various fascial plane blocks that may now represent reasonable analgesic options for cardiac surgeries.

Thoracic Wall Innervation

Understanding the anatomy of the thoracic wall and its innervation is crucial to understanding the regional interventions available for the cardiac surgery patient. The thoracic wall is primarily innervated by the intercostal nerves, which derive from the anterior rami of spinal nerves T1-11. The intercostal nerves run between adjacent ribs. The anterior ramus of T12 is a subcostal nerve because it enters the abdominal wall [71, 72]. The typical intercostal nerve traverses laterally behind the sympathetic trunk, entering the intercostal space between the parietal pleura and intercostal membrane. In the costal groove, it runs with the intercostal vessels. Near the midaxillary line, the lateral cutaneous branches emerge. The lateral cutaneous branch pierces through the muscles of the lateral thoracic wall to divide into anterior and posterior branches and innervate the skin of the lateral thoracic wall. Near the sternum, the intercostal nerves cross anterior to the internal thoracic artery to become anterior cutaneous branches. The anterior cutaneous branch is the terminal branch. It divides into medial and lateral branches to supply sensory innervation to the skin of the anterior thoracic wall [71, 72].

Thoracic Epidural Analgesia

Thoracic epidural analgesia (TEA) has been considered the gold standard for postoperative pain management after thoracic surgeries. Epidural analgesia can also be beneficial for cardiac surgery. However, utilization is controversial due to the theoretical increased risk of epidural hematoma and consequent neurologic damage associated with full systemic heparinization for cardiopulmonary bypass. There is also a risk of hypotension from the sympathectomy that may compromise cardiac perfusion. Sympathectomy and resulting afterload reduction may be specifically contraindicated in patients with severe aortic stenosis or hypertrophic cardiomyopathy. Despite concerns, epidural analgesia may reduce the risk of postoperative complications, such as pneumonia, respiratory failure, myocardial infarction, renal injury, arrhythmias, decrease mechanical ventilation time, and decrease the amount of time that patients spend in the ICU. Epidural analgesia may also attenuate the surgical inflammatory response and provide cardioprotective effects by increasing myocardial oxygen availability and decreasing myocardial oxygen consumption due to the sympathectomy [73, 74].

In a 2019 Cochrane review, it was concluded that thoracic epidural analgesia does not change the risk of mortality or pneumonia compared to systemic analgesia in cardiac surgery [73]. Epidural analgesia may decrease the risk of myocardial infarction, respiratory depression, and atrial arrhythmias, reduce the duration of tracheal intubation, and decrease pain scores at 6, 24, 48, and 72 h following surgery. Epidural analgesia may increase the risk of hypotension and the need for vasopressor boluses, but there is no difference in vasopressor infusions. No increased risk for epidural hematoma was found, however, there were not enough participants to sufficiently evaluate the risk of hematoma formation following epidural catheter placement. The American Society of Regional Anesthesia and Pain Medicine (ASRA) guidelines are limited by insufficient available data to determine the increased risk of neuraxial hematoma formation encountered when using neuraxial techniques with full anticoagulation required for cardiac surgery. Perioperative anticoagulation guidelines provided by ASRA are intended to apply to neuraxial and deep blocks including paravertebral blocks [73].

Paravertebral Block

The thoracic paravertebral space is located on either side of the vertebral column. The anterolateral boundary is formed by the parietal pleura, the base is formed by the vertebral body, intervertebral disc, and the intervertebral foramen, and the posterior boundary is formed by the transverse process and superior costotransverse ligament. A paravertebral block (PVB) produces an ipsilateral motor, sensory, and sympathetic nerve block by anesthetizing the intercostal nerves in the paravertebral space, as well as local anesthetic extension into the intercostal space laterally and epidural space medially [75].

There are various ultrasound-guided PVB techniques, including transverse or sagittal transducer orientation and in-plane or out-of-plane approaches. In general, the needle will be directed between adjacent transverse processes and traverse the superior costotransverse ligament with anterior deflection of the parietal pleura observed when local anesthetic is injected into the paravertebral space. The block level should be near the dermatome for the incision and either multiple levels or a single injection of a larger volume of local anesthetic can be performed to cover the desired area of analgesia [75].

PVBs may be beneficial for minimally invasive procedures, thoracotomy incisions as well as midline sternotomy incisions given the location of neural blockade. Complications following paravertebral blockade include vascular puncture, hypotension, pleural puncture, pneumothorax, inadvertent epidural or spinal anesthesia, and local anesthetic systemic toxicity (LAST). PVBs are considered a deep block and are therefore subject to the same anticoagulation guidelines as those that exist for epidural catheter placement [75].

There are limited studies evaluating the role of PVBs in cardiac surgery. The few studies that are available have demonstrated that bilateral PVBs can be effective and safe. The use of PVBs can facilitate early extubation and decrease opioid usage [76–78]. They have been shown to reduce pain scores, decrease intraoperative opioid use, facilitate extubation, and provide similar analgesia to epidurals [79]. Studies have also shown that PVBs can decrease the incidence of nausea, vomiting, hypotension, and urinary retention [80, 81]. PVBs are becoming more popular for minimally invasive cardiac surgery through a thoracotomy or video-assisted thoracoscopic approach.

Pectoralis I and II Blocks

Pectoralis I (Pecs I) nerve block involves depositing local anesthetic between the pectoralis major and pectoralis minor muscles to block the lateral and medial pectoral nerves, which innervate the pectoralis muscles. Pectoralis II (Pecs II) nerve blocks involves depositing local anesthetic between the pectoralis muscles and a second injection between the pectoralis minor and serratus anterior muscles. Pecs II blocks the pectoral nerves, upper intercostal (3–6) nerves, as well as the intercostobrachial, thoracodorsal and long thoracic nerves.

These nerve blocks are performed in-plane with needle trajectory medial to lateral. The ultrasound transducer is positioned sagittal with an inferolateral angle at the midclavicular area. The transducer is then moved laterally to obtain the appropriate images. Pecs I is performed at the level of ribs 2–3. The first injection of Pecs II is similar to Pecs I, while the second injection is at the anterior axillary line at the level of the fourth rib [82].

Pecs I use is limited and primarily for more superficial, anterior chest wall surgeries that include disruption of the pectoralis muscles (i.e. placement of a submuscular ICD). Pecs II is more useful in the setting of cardiac procedures and may be utilized to provide analgesia for anterolateral chest surgeries, such as breast surgery, subcutaneous implantable cardiac defibrillators (SICD), video assisted thoracoscopic surgery (VATS), and anterior thoracotomies. Pecs blocks do not anesthetize anterior cutaneous branches and therefore may be better indicated for antero-lateral incisions and procedures. Complications are rare but include pneumothorax, infection, vascular puncture, and local anesthetic systemic toxicity [82].

There have been limited studies on Pecs blocks in the setting of cardiac surgery. These blocks are performed in a supine position so they can be useful as rescue blocks in patients who have limited mobility secondary to lines, chest tubes, and mechanical ventilation. A study of 40 patients undergoing coronary artery bypass grafting or valve surgeries via midline sternotomy found that bilateral Pecs II blocks helped with early extubation, improved pain scores at rest and with cough, and improved incentive spirometry flow rates compared with no Pecs blocks [81, 83].

Serratus Anterior Plane Block

The serratus anterior plane (SAP) block can be performed superficially or deep to the serratus anterior muscle to anesthetize the anterolateral chest wall (T2–9 dermatomes). This block targets the lateral cutaneous branches of the thoracic intercostal nerves as well as intercostobrachial, long thoracic, and thoracodorsal nerves. At the level of the fifth rib, the superficial plane is formed by the anterior aspect of the serratus anterior muscle and the posterior aspect of the latissimus dorsi muscle. The deep plane is formed by the posterior aspect of the serratus anterior muscle and the external intercostal muscles and ribs [84].

The SAP block is performed at the level of the fifth rib around the midaxillary line. The transducer is oriented in the coronal plane and tilted posteriorly to identify the latissimus dorsi lying superficial to the serratus anterior muscle. An in-plane technique is used with anterior to posterior needle trajectory and local anesthetic can be injected above or below the serratus anterior muscle [84].

Common indications for the SAP block include lateral rib fractures, VATS, thoracotomy, SICD placement, and breast surgery. Complications are rare but include pneumothorax in addition to other known complications inherent to regional techniques [84].

This block spares the midline chest area; thus, no studies have been performed for sternotomies. Two studies have shown that this block can be safe and efficacious in cardiac device implantation [81]. Several studies found that this block can reduce pain scores and opioid consumption for minimally invasive cardiac surgery [85–87].

Erector Spinae Plane Block

The erector spinae plane (ESP) block is a paraspinal fascial plane block where local anesthetic is injected between the erector spinae muscle and thoracic transverse processes. The mechanism of action is not fully understood. It blocks the dorsal and ventral rami of the thoracic spinal nerves for multi-dermatomal sensory block of anterior, posterior, and lateral thoracic walls. Local anesthetic may also diffuse into the paravertebral and epidural spaces [88].

The ESP block can be performed at either a single level or multiple levels for adequate analgesic coverage. The block spreads over multiple vertebral levels and therefore a single injection of a large volume of local anesthetic may provide diffuse analgesia. The ultrasound transducer is placed in a paramedian sagittal orientation and moved laterally until transverse processes are visible. Usually an in-plane approach is used with local anesthetic injected below the erector spinae muscle to effectively "lift" this muscle off the transverse processes below [88].

This block can be used for a wide variety of surgical procedures in the anterior, posterior, and lateral thoracic areas. Complications are rare, but include pleural puncture, pneumothorax, and other complications associated with regional techniques [88].

ESP blocks are not well studied in cardiac surgery, but have been shown to decrease opioid consumption, pain scores, duration of time in the ICU, and time to extubation [89–91]. One prospective study of 50 patients demonstrated that ESP blocks were comparable to TEA with regard to postoperative pain scores, incentive spirometry, and ventilator and ICU duration [92].

Pectointercostal Fascial Plane Block and Transverse Thoracic Muscle Plane Block

The pectointercostal fascial plane block (PIFB) involves injecting local anesthetic between the pectoralis major muscle and internal intercostal muscles to block the anterior cutaneous branches of the intercostal nerves. The transverse thoracic muscle plane (TTP) block is a deeper version of the PIFB with the injection of local anesthetic occurring between the internal intercostal and transverse thoracic muscles. These blocks target the T2-6 dermatomal distribution in a unilateral fashion meaning that bilateral blocks would be required to provide sternotomy analgesia [93, 94].

The PIFB is usually performed with an in-plane needle approach with the ultrasound transducer in a parasagittal orientation 1–2 cm lateral to the sternum. The local anesthetic is deposited between the pectoralis major and intercostal muscles. The TTP utilizes the same approach, except the local anesthetic is deposited deeper between the internal intercostal and transverse thoracic muscles. The injections usually occur at the level of the fourth or fifth rib [94].

Both blocks can be helpful for midline chest surgeries including thymectomies, sternotomies, and cardiac device implantation [93]. Complications are rare, but include injury to the internal thoracic artery, pneumothorax, and pericardial puncture. The PIFB is potentially safer than the TTP because it is a more superficial block.

Several studies have demonstrated that PIFBs decrease pain scores, opioid consumption, time to extubation, ICU duration, and hospital length of stay after cardiac surgery [95–99]. Several studies have also shown TTP blocks result in decreased opioid consumption, pain scores, time to extubation, ICU duration, and hospital length of stay after cardiac surgery [100–102]. A prospective study comparing PIFB to TTP blocks showed that they have similar efficacy and that pain scores and morphine consumption were similar for the two interventions in the first 24 h following cardiac surgery [103].

In general, studies on fascial plane blocks are limited in cardiac surgery but have been shown to have promising results. Fascial plane blocks have advantages over neuraxial blocks because they have a better safety profile, particularly in the setting of anticoagulation, are associated with hemodynamic stability, and can be performed under general anesthesia with most in a supine position. More randomized controlled trials are needed to effectively compare the various fascial plane blocks as well as continuous versus single shot blocks in both minimally invasive and open cardiac surgeries.

7 Conclusion

The push for fast-track and ERAS protocols for the postoperative management of the typical cardiac surgical patient has emphasized the need for aggressive pain management. Similar to noncardiac surgery, effective perioperative pain control can improve patient morbidity and mortality after cardiac surgery. Each member of the care team can make a significant contribution towards this effort, from preoperative education to prevention to assessment and treatment. In addition to standard multimodal management using oral and intravenous medications, the recent development of novel regional anesthesia techniques necessitates their inclusion in the perioperative management of the cardiac surgical patient.

References

1. Zubrzycki M, Liebold A, Skrabal C, et al. Assessment and pathophysiology of pain in cardiac surgery. J Pain Res. 2018;11:1599–611.
2. Doenst T, Essa Y, Jacoub K, et al. Cardiac surgery 2016 reviewed. Clin Res Cardiol. 2017;106(11):851–67.
3. Cogan J. Pain management after cardiac surgery. Semin Cardiothorac Vasc Anesth. 2010;14(3):201–4.
4. Bigeleisen PE, Goehner N. Novel approaches in pain management in cardiac surgery. Curr Opin Anaesthesiol. 2015;28(1):89–94.
5. Gerner P. Postthoracotomy pain management problems. Anesthesiol Clin. 2008;26(2):355–67.
6. Markman PL, Rowland MA, Leong JY, et al. Skeletonized internal thoracic artery harvesting reduces chest wall dysesthesia after coronary bypass surgery. J Thorac Cardiovasc Surg. 2010;139:674–9.
7. Reimer-Kent J. From theory to practice: preventing pain after cardiac surgery. Am J Crit Care. 2003;12(2):136–43.
8. Sommer M, de Rijke JM, van Kleef M, et al. The prevalence of postoperative pain in a sample of 1490 surgical inpatients. Eur J Anaesthesiol. 2008;25(4):267–74.
9. Träger K, Fritzler D, Fischer G, et al. Treatment of post-cardiopulmonary bypass SIRS by hemoadsorption: a case series. Int J Artif Organs. 2016;39(3):141–6.
10. Gerbershagen HJ, Pogatzki-Zahn E, Aduckathil S, et al. Procedure-specific risk factor analysis for the development of severe postoperative pain. Anesthesiology. 2014;120(5):1237–45.
11. Mueller XM, Tinguely F, Tevaearai HT, Revelly JP, Chioléro R, von Segesser LK. Pain location, distribution, and intensity after cardiac surgery. Chest. 2000;118(2):391–6.
12. Nelson F, Zimmerman L, Barnason S, Nieveen J, Schmaderer M. The relationship and influence of anxiety on postoperative pain in the coronary artery bypass graft patient. J Pain Symptom Manage. 1998;15(2):102–9.
13. Greszta E, Siemińska MJ. [Relationship of preoperative anxiety-state and anxiety-trait in patients qualified for coronary artery bypass graft surgery to the perception of postoperative pain and other pain complaints]. *Ann Acad Med Stetin.* 2008;54(1):157–63. Polish.
14. Thibodeau MA, Welch PG, Katz J, Asmundson GJ. Pain-related anxiety influences pain perception differently in men and women: a quantitative sensory test across thermal pain modalities. Pain. 2013;154(3):419–26.
15. Tan EC, Lim Y, Teo YY, Goh R, Law HY, Sia AT. Ethnic differences in pain perception and patient-controlled analgesia usage for postoperative pain. J Pain. 2008;9:849–55.
16. Stites M. Pain management observational pain scales in critically ill adults. Crit Care Nurse. 2013;33:68–79.
17. Linde S, Badger J, Roy N, et al. Re-evaluation of the critical care pain observation tool in intubated adults after cardiac surgery. Am J Crit Care. 2013;22:491–7.
18. Cogan J, Ouimette M, Vargas-Schaffer G, et al. Patient attitudes and beliefs regarding pain medication after cardiac surgery: barriers to adequate pain management. Pain Manag Nurs. 2014;15:574–9.

19. Offner KA, Loop T. Pathophysiology and epidemiology of pain in thoracic surgery. Anasthesiol Intensivmed Notfallmed Schmerzther. 2012;47(9):568–75.
20. Roncada G, Dendale P, Linsen L, Hendrikx M, Hansen D. Reduction in pulmonary function after CABG surgery is related to postoperative inflammation and hypercortisolemia. Int J Clin Exp Med. 2015;8(7):10938–46.
21. Milgrom LB, Brooks JA, Qi R. Pain levels experienced with activities after cardiac surgery. Am J Crit Care. 2004;13(2):116–25.
22. Liu SS, Wu CL, Cl W. Effect of postoperative analgesia on major postoperative complications: a systematic update of the evidence. Anesth Analg. 2007;104(3):689–702.
23. Schultz CH, Rivers EP, Feldkamp CS, et al. A characterization of hypothalamic-pituitary-adrenal axis function during and after human cardiac arrest. Crit Care Med. 1993;21(9):1339–47.
24. Swarm RA, Karanikolas M, Kalauokalani D. Pain treatment in the perioperative period. Curr Probl Surg. 2001;38(11):835–920.
25. Jayakumar S, Borrelli M, Milan Z, Kunst G, Whitaker D. Optimising pain management protocols following cardiac surgery: a protocol for a national quality improvement study. Int J Surg Protoc. 2019;14:1–8.
26. Werner MU, Kongsgaard UEI. Defining persistent post-surgical pain: is an update required? Br J Anaesth. 2014;113(1):1–4.
27. Lahtinen P, Kokki H, Hynynen M. Pain after cardiac surgery: a prospective cohort study of 1-year incidence and intensity. Anesthesiology. 2006;105(4):794–800.
28. Kehlet H, Jensen TS, Woolf CJ. Persistent postsurgical pain: risk factors and prevention. Lancet. 2006;367:1618–25.
29. White PF, Kehlet H, Neal JM, Schricker T, Carr DB, Carli F. Fast-track surgery study group. The role of the anesthesiologist in fast-track surgery: from multimodal analgesia to perioperative medical care. Anesth Analg. 2007;104(6):1380–96.
30. Graham GG, Scott KF. Mechanism of action of paracetamol. Am J Ther. 2005;12(1):46–55.
31. Mielke CH Jr. Comparative effects of aspirin and acetaminophen on hemostasis. Arch Intern Med. 1981;141(3 Spec No):305–10.
32. Hoftiezer JW, O'Laughlin JC, Ivey KJ. Effects of 24 hours of aspirin, Bufferin, paracetamol and placebo on normal human gastroduodenal mucosa. Gut J. 1982;23(8):692–7.
33. Jelacic S, Bollag L, Bowdle A, Rivat C, Cain KC, Richebe P. Intravenous acetaminophen as an adjunct analgesic in cardiac surgery reduces opioid consumption but not opioid-related adverse effects: a randomized controlled trial. J Cardiothorac Vasc Anesth. 2016;30(4):997–1004.
34. Subramaniam B, Shankar P, Shaefi S, et al. Effect of intravenous acetaminophen vs placebo combined with propofol or dexmedetomidine on postoperative delirium among older patients following cardiac surgery: the DEXACET randomized clinical trial. JAMA. 2019;321(7):686–96.
35. Ghlichloo I, Gerriets V. Nonsteroidal Anti-inflammatory Drugs (NSAIDs). In: StatPearls. Treasure Island (FL): StatPearls Publishing; 2022.
36. Nussmeier NA, Whelton AA, Brown MT, et al. Complications of the COX-2 inhibitors parecoxib and valdecoxib after cardiac surgery. N Engl J Med. 2005;352(11):1081–91.
37. Gislason GH, Jacobsen S, Rasmussen JN, et al. Risk of death or reinfarction associated with the use of selective cyclooxygenase-2 inhibitors and nonselective nonsteroidal antiinflammatory drugs after acute myocardial infarction. Circulation. 2006;113(25):2906–13.
38. US Food and Drug Administration. FDA Drug Safety Communication: FDA strengthens warning that non-aspirin nonsteroidal anti-inflammatory drugs (NSAIDs) can cause heart attacks or strokes. 2015. Available at https://www.fda.gov/drugs/drugsafety/ucm451800.htm
39. Qazi SM, Sindby EJ, Nørgaard MA. Ibuprofen—a safe analgesic during cardiac surgery recovery? a randomized controlled trial. J Cardiovasc Thorac Res. 2015;7(4):141–8.
40. Kulik A, Bykov K, Choudhry NK, Bateman BT. Non-steroidal anti-inflammatory drug administration after coronary artery bypass surgery: utilization persists despite the boxed warning. Pharmacoepidemiol Drug Saf. 2015;24(6):647–53.

41. Hayashida K, DeGoes S, Curry R, Eisenach JC. Gabapentin activates spinal noradrenergic activity in rats and humans and reduces hypersensitivity after surgery. Anesthesiology. 2007;106(3):557–62.
42. Chincholkar M. Analgesic mechanisms of gabapentinoids and effects in experimental pain models: a narrative review. Br J Anaesth. 2018;120(6):1315–34.
43. Verret M, Lauzier F, Zarychanski R, et al. Perioperative use of Gabapentinoids for the management of postoperative acute pain: a systematic review and meta-analysis [published correction appears in Anesthesiology. 2020 Aug 21]. Anesthesiology 2020;133(2):265–79.
44. Menda F, Köner O, Sayın M, Ergenoğlu M, Küçükaksu S, Aykaç B. Effects of single-dose gabapentin on postoperative pain and morphine consumption after cardiac surgery. J Cardiothorac Vasc Anesth. 2010;24(5):808–13.
45. Ziyaeifard M, Mehrabanian MJ, Faritus SZ, et al. Premedication with oral pregabalin for the prevention of acute postsurgical pain in coronary artery bypass surgery. Anesth Pain Med. 2015;5(1):e24837.
46. Anwar S, Cooper J, Rahman J, Sharma C, Langford R. Prolonged perioperative use of pregabalin and ketamine to prevent persistent pain after cardiac surgery. Anesthesiology. 2019;131(1):119–31.
47. Maitra S, Baidya DK, Bhattacharjee S, Som A. Gabapentina e pregabalina no período perioperatório em cirurgia cardíaca: uma revisão sistemática e metanálise [Perioperative gabapentin and pregabalin in cardiac surgery: a systematic review and meta-analysis]. Rev Bras Anestesiol. 2017;67(3):294–304.
48. Rosenbaum SB, Gupta V, Patel P, Palacios JL. Ketamine. In: StatPearls. Treasure Island (FL): StatPearls Publishing; 2022.
49. Lahtinen P, Kokki H, Hakala T, Hynynen M. S(+)-ketamine as an analgesic adjunct reduces opioid consumption after cardiac surgery. Anesth Analg. 2004;99(5):1295–301.
50. Nesher N, Ekstein MP, Paz Y, Marouani N, Chazan S, Weinbroum AA. Morphine with adjuvant ketamine vs higher dose of morphine alone for immediate postthoracotomy analgesia. Chest. 2009;136(1):245–52.
51. Mazzeffi M, Johnson K, Paciullo C. Ketamine in adult cardiac surgery and the cardiac surgery Intensive care unit: an evidence-based clinical review. Ann Card Anaesth. 2015;18(2):202–9.
52. Hudetz JA, Patterson KM, Iqbal Z, et al. Ketamine attenuates delirium after cardiac surgery with cardiopulmonary bypass. J Cardiothorac Vasc Anesth. 2009;23(5):651–7.
53. Avidan MS, Maybrier HR, Abdallah AB, et al. Intraoperative ketamine for prevention of postoperative delirium or pain after major surgery in older adults: an international, multicentre, double-blind, randomised clinical trial [published correction appears in Lancet. 2017;390(10091):230. Lancet. 2017;390(10091):267–75.
54. Kaur M, Singh PM. Current role of dexmedetomidine in clinical anesthesia and intensive care. Anesth Essays Res. 2011;5(2):128–33.
55. Habibi V, Kiabi FH, Sharifi H. The effect of dexmedetomidine on the acute pain after cardiothoracic surgeries: a systematic review. Braz J Cardiovasc Surg. 2018;33:404–17.
56. Ji F, Li Z, Nguyen H, et al. Perioperative dexmedetomidine improves outcomes of cardiac surgery. Circulation. 2013;127(15):1576–84.
57. Wang G, Niu J, Li Z, Lv H, Cai H. The efficacy and safety of dexmedetomidine in cardiac surgery patients: a systematic review and meta-analysis. PLoS ONE. 2018;13(9):e0202620.
58. De Oliveira GS, Jr AMD, Benzon HT, McCarthy RJ. Perioperative single dose systemic dexamethasone for postoperative pain: a meta-analysis of randomized controlled trials. Anesthesiology. 2011;115(3):575–88.
59. Myles PS, Corcoran T. Benefits and risks of dexamethasone in noncardiac surgery. Anesthesiology. 2021;135(5):895–903.
60. Turan A, Belley-Cote EP, Vincent J, et al. Methylprednisolone does not reduce persistent pain after cardiac surgery. Anesthesiology. 2015;123(6):1404–10.
61. Dieleman JM, Nierich AP, Rosseel PM, et al. Intraoperative high-dose dexamethasone for cardiac surgery: a randomized controlled trial. JAMA. 2012;308(17):1761–7.
62. Shin HJ, Na HS, Do SH. Magnesium and pain. Nutrients. 2020;12(8):2184.

63. Steinlechner B, Dworschak M, Birkenberg B, et al. Magnesium moderately decreases remifentanil dosage required for pain management after cardiac surgery. Br J Anaesth. 2006;96(4):444–9.
64. Ferasatkish R, Dabbagh A, Alavi M, et al. Effect of magnesium sulfate on extubation time and acute pain in coronary artery bypass surgery. Acta Anaesthesiol Scand. 2008;52:1348–52.
65. Dunn LK, Durieux ME. Perioperative use of intravenous lidocaine. Anesthesiology. 2017;126(4):729–37.
66. Kranke P, Jokinen J, Pace NL, et al. Continuous intravenous perioperative lidocaine infusion for postoperative pain and recovery. Cochrane Database Syst Rev. 2015;7:CD009642.
67. Marret E, Rolin M, Beaussier M, Bonnet F. Meta-analysis of intravenous lidocaine and postoperative recovery after abdominal surgery. Br J Surg. 2008;95(11):1331–8.
68. Vigneault L, Turgeon AF, Côté D, et al. Perioperative intravenous lidocaine infusion for postoperative pain control: a meta-analysis of randomized controlled trials. Can J Anaesth. 2011;58(1):22–37.
69. Insler SR, O'Connor M, Samonte AF, Bazaral MG. Lidocaine and the inhibition of postoperative pain in coronary artery bypass patients. J Cardiothorac Vasc Anesth. 1995;9(5):541–6.
70. Wang D, Wu X, Li J, Xiao F, Liu X, Meng M. The effect of lidocaine on early postoperative cognitive dysfunction after coronary artery bypass surgery. Anesth Analg. 2002;95(5):1134–41.
71. Glenesk NL, Rahman S, Lopez PP. Anatomy, thorax, intercostal nerves. 2022.
72. Sertcakacilar G, Tire Y, Kelava M, et al. Regional anesthesia for thoracic surgery: a narrative review of indications and clinical considerations. J Thorac Dis. 2022;14(12):5012–28.
73. Guay J, Kopp S. Epidural analgesia for adults undergoing cardiac surgery with or without cardiopulmonary bypass. Cochrane Database Syst Rev. 2019;3(3):CD006715.
74. Landoni G, Isella F, Greco M, Zangrillo A, Royse CF. Benefits and risks of epidural analgesia in cardiac surgery. Br J Anaesth. 2015;115(1):25–32.
75. Ultrasound-Guided Thoracic Paravertebral Block. NYSORA. Available at https://www.nysora.com/pain-management/ultrasound-guided-thoracic-paravertebral-block. Accessed 15 May 2024.
76. Sun L, Li Q, Wang Q, Ma F, Han W, Wang M. Bilateral thoracic paravertebral block combined with general anesthesia vs. general anesthesia for patients undergoing off-pump coronary artery bypass grafting: a feasibility study. BMC Anesthesiol. 2019;19(1):101.
77. Naganuma M, Tokita T, Sato Y, et al. Efficacy of preoperative bilateral thoracic paravertebral block in cardiac surgery requiring full heparinization: a propensity-matched study. J Cardiothorac Vasc Anesth. 2022;36(2):477–82.
78. Cantó M, Sánchez MJ, Casas MA, Bataller ML. Bilateral paravertebral blockade for conventional cardiac surgery. Anaesthesia. 2003;58(4):365–70.
79. Devarajan J, Balasubramanian S, Nazarnia S, Lin C, Subramaniam K. Regional analgesia for cardiac surgery part 1. Current status of neuraxial and paravertebral blocks for adult cardiac surgery. Semin Cardiothorac Vasc Anesth. 2021;25(4):252–64.
80. Olivier JF, Bracco D, Nguyen P, Le N, Noiseux N, Hemmerling T. A novel approach for pain management in cardiac surgery via median sternotomy: bilateral single-shot paravertebral blocks. Heart Surg Forum. 2007;10(5):E357–62.
81. Jiang T, Ting A, Leclerc M, Calkins K, Huang J. Regional anesthesia in cardiac surgery: a review of the literature. Cureus. 2021;13(10):e18808.
82. Battista C, Krishnan S. Pectoralis Nerve Block. In: StatPearls. Treasure Island (FL): StatPearls; 2023.
83. Kumar KN, Kalyane RN, Singh NG, et al. Efficacy of bilateral pectoralis nerve block for ultrafast tracking and postoperative pain management in cardiac surgery. Ann Card Anaesth. 2018;21(3):333–8.
84. Southgate SJ, Herbst MK. Ultrasound guided serratus anterior blocks. In: StatPearls. Treasure Island (FL): StatPearls Publishing; 2022.
85. Berthoud V, Ellouze O, Nguyen M, et al. Serratus anterior plane block for minimal invasive heart surgery. BMC Anesthesiol. 2018;18(1):144.

86. Toscano A, Capuano P, Costamagna A, et al. The serratus anterior plane study: continuous deep serratus anterior plane block for mitral valve surgery performed in right minithoracotomy. J Cardiothorac Vasc Anesth. 2020;34(11):2975–82.
87. Gautam S, Pande S, Agarwal A, Agarwal SK, Rastogi A, Shamshery C, et al. Evaluation of serratus anterior plane block for pain relief in patients undergoing MIDCAB surgery. Innovations (Phila). 2020;15(2):148–54.
88. Krishnan S, Cascella M. Erector spinae plane block. In: StatPearls. Treasure Island (FL): StatPearls; 2023.
89. Krishna SN, Chauhan S, Bhoi D, et al. Bilateral erector spinae plane block for acute post-surgical pain in adult cardiac surgical patients: a randomized controlled trial. J Cardiothorac Vasc Anesth. 2019;33(2):368–75.
90. Macaire P, Ho N, Nguyen T, et al. Ultrasound-guided continuous thoracic erector spinae plane block within an enhanced recovery program is associated with decreased opioid consumption and improved patient postoperative rehabilitation after open cardiac surgery—a patient-matched, controlled before-and-after study. J Cardiothorac Vasc Anesth. 2019;33(6):1659–67.
91. Vaughan BN, Bartone CL, McCarthy CM, Answini GA, Hurford WE. Ultrasound-guided continuous bilateral erector spinae plane blocks are associated with reduced opioid consumption and length of stay for open cardiac surgery: a retrospective cohort study. J Clin Med. 2021;10(21):5022.
92. Nagaraja P, Ragavendran S, Singh N, et al. Comparison of continuous thoracic epidural analgesia with bilateral erector spinae plane block for perioperative pain management in cardiac surgery. Ann Card Anaesth. 2018;21(3):323.
93. Sertcakacilar G, Tire Y, Kelava M, Nair HK, Lawin-O'Brien ROC, Turan A, et al. Regional anesthesia for thoracic surgery: a narrative review of indications and clinical considerations. J Thorac Dis. 2022;14(12):5012–28.
94. Kelava M, Alfirevic A, Bustamante S, Hargrave J, Marciniak D. Regional anesthesia in cardiac surgery: an overview of fascial plane chest wall blocks. Anesth Analg. 2020;131(1):127–35.
95. Kumar AK, Chauhan S, Bhoi D, Kaushal B. Pectointercostal fascial block (PIFB) as a novel technique for postoperative pain management in patients undergoing cardiac surgery. J Cardiothorac Vasc Anesth. 2021;35(1):116–22.
96. Zhang Y, Min J, Chen S. Continuous pecto-intercostal fascial block provides effective analgesia in patients undergoing open cardiac surgery: a randomized controlled trial. Pain Med. 2022;23(3):440–7.
97. Chaudhary V, Chauhan S, Choudhury M, Kiran U, Vasdev S, Talwar S. Parasternal intercostal block with ropivacaine for postoperative analgesia in pediatric patients undergoing cardiac surgery: a double-blind, randomized, controlled study. J Cardiothorac Vasc Anesth. 2021;21:98.
98. Barr AM, Tutungi E, Almeida AA. Parasternal intercostal block with ropivacaine for pain management after cardiac surgery: a double-blind, randomized, controlled trial. J Cardiothorac Vasc Anesth. 2007;21(4):547–53.
99. Zhang Y, Gong H, Zhan B, Chen S. Effects of bilateral pecto-intercostal bascial Block for perioperative pain management in patients undergoing open cardiac surgery: a prospective randomized study. BMC Anesthesiol. 2021;21(1):175.
100. Zhang Y, Li X, Chen S. Bilateral transversus thoracis muscle plane block provides effective analgesia and enhances recovery after open cardiac surgery. J Card Surg. 2021;36(8):2818–23.
101. Aydin ME, Ahiskalioglu A, Ates I, et al. Efficacy of ultrasound-guided transversus thoracic muscle plane block on postoperative opioid consumption after cardiac surgery: a prospective, randomized, double-blind study. J Cardiothorac Vasc Anesth. 2020;34(11):2996–3003.
102. Zhang Y, Chen S, Gong H, Zhan B. Efficacy of bilateral transversus thoracis muscle plane block in pediatric patients undergoing open cardiac surgery. J Cardiothorac Vasc Anesth. 2020;34(9):2430–4.
103. Kaya C, Dost B, Dokmeci O, Yucel SM, Karakaya D. Comparison of ultrasound-guided pecto-intercostal fascial block and transversus thoracic muscle plane block for acute poststernotomy pain management after cardiac surgery: a prospective, randomized, double-blind pilot study. J Cardiothorac Vasc Anesth. 2022;36(8 Pt A):2313–21.

Perioperative Care of the LGBQTA+ Community

Olga C. Nin, Adam H. Fischler, Po-Yi Paul Su, Hamzah Adel Ramawad, Kenneth Higgins Elliott III, and Dane Saksa

1 LGBTQA+ Historical Perspective, Current Status and Future

Those who identify as *lesbian, gay, bisexual,* and *transgender* (LGBT) make up a diverse community of individuals with a large population. The acronym LGBTQ+ is commonly used in place of LGBT; in this instance the "Q" may refer to either *queer* or *questioning*. The acronym is sometimes further expanded to include the *intersex* community ("I") as well as *asexual* individuals or *allies* ("A"). A "+" is commonly included as a marker for those who also identify with this diverse community of individuals. This chapter will introduce the LGBTQ+ community, share some historical perspective, discuss preoperative considerations for transgender care, review types of gender affirmation surgery, and provide an overview of analgesia for this community in the perioperative setting (including regional anesthesia).

O. C. Nin (✉)
Department of Anesthesiology, University of Florida College of Medicine, Gainesville, FL, USA
e-mail: onin@anest.ufl.edu

A. H. Fischler
Department of Anesthesiology, UCONN Health, Farmington, OR, USA

P.-Y. P. Su
Department of Anesthesia, University of California, San Francisco, USA
e-mail: paul.su@ucsf.edu

H. A. Ramawad
Department of Emergency Medicine, NYC Health & Hospital, South Brooklyn Health, Brooklyn, USA

K. H. Elliott III · D. Saksa
UCLA Department of Anesthesiology and Perioperative Medicine, Los Angeles, USA
e-mail: kehiggins@mednet.ucla.edu

D. Saksa
e-mail: dsaksa@mednet.ucla.edu

A. Abd-Elsayed and K. Schroeder (eds.), *Perioperative Pain Management*,
https://doi.org/10.1007/978-3-031-67648-2_23

Vocabulary and definitions are important in helping all patients feel comfortable, safe, and respected by their care team. We therefore begin this chapter with a brief discussion of terminology as it may apply to a patient on the day of surgery. Lesbians, gay men, and bisexual men and women are defined by their sexual orientation, which may be thought of in terms of an overlap of sexual attraction, behavior, and identity. In contrast, transgender individuals identify in accordance with a gender identity and the presentation of that gender identity. The transgender and gender diverse community may also include individuals who reject the traditional male/female gender identity dichotomy outright. The transgender and gender diverse community is diverse in many facets including gender identity, gender expression, and sexual orientation. Female-to-male transgender individuals are sometimes known as FtM, transgender males, and transmen. Male-to-female transgender individuals might be known as MtF, transgender females, and transwomen [1]. It can be helpful to confirm the gender identity with which a patient identifies prior to the day of surgery so that all members of the care team can address them with clarity and respect. While it is difficult to get exact estimates of the size of the diverse LGBTQ+ population, most current data suggests that around 3.5% of the United States population identify as gay, lesbian, or bisexual [2]. Thus, at least 9 million individuals in the United States identify as LGBTQ+ as of 2021 (though some surveys estimate millions more [3]).

Despite growing visibility and awareness of the LGBTQ+ community in the United States, significant health disparities persist as a result of ongoing stigma, prejudice, discrimination, and other critical determinants of health. From a societal perspective, LGBTQ+ individuals are subject to inequitable access to housing, employment, and healthcare, which are well-known pillars of physical and mental health. Due to prior negative experiences with healthcare, members of the LGBTQ+ community are sometimes reluctant to be forthcoming about aspects of their health, further contributing to substandard access to healthcare resources. Furthermore, LGBTQ+ patients have been shown to have increased rates of substance use disorders, mental health disorders, and suicidal ideation. Beyond the realm of mental health, research has also shown a higher burden of chronic disease within the LGBTQ+ community, including increased incidence of cardiovascular risk factors [4, 5]. Additional research has demonstrated that LGBTQ+ youth experience increased rates of adverse health outcomes (physical, mental, and behavioral) and that gender minority youth may be at higher risk for being overweight or obese compared to their cis-gender peers. Specifically, transgender and gender-diverse (TGD) patients seeking gender-affirming care may face difficulty navigating the care system given that perioperative teams may have less experience delivering sensitive, safe, and evidence-based gender-affirming care. Clearly, much remains to be investigated on the disparities experienced by LGBTQ+ patients in the perioperative setting [6].

Importantly, it is not just the patients we must care for in the perioperative arena. We also can help protect the well-being of our LGBTQ+ healthcare professionals. LGBTQ+ status was identified as an independent driver of anesthesiologist burnout, one of four variables identified in a national survey of anesthesiologists [6]. Burnout is correlated with decreased workplace efficacy, increased healthcare costs, and medical errors [7]. Recognizing that burnout among healthcare professionals threatens all aspects of a functional U.S. health system, there have been major investments in finding solutions to help our workforce feel more fulfilled, with a particular focus on systems improvement. As of 2022, burnout has become such an epidemic within medicine that organizations such as the National Academy of Medicine are calling for collective action to address healthcare professional well-being via the National Plan for Health Workforce Well-Being [8]. While more research is needed on the best practices to mitigate LGBTQ+ healthcare professional burnout, energy and attention spent on increasing perceived workplace support may mitigate the burnout of our LGBTQ+ healthcare workforce and help our LGBTQ+ colleagues feel more fulfilled, safe, and engaged. This can translate to a thriving LGBTQ+ workforce and result in better care for our LGBTQ+ patients.

2 Preoperative Considerations

The goal of preoperative assessment is to reduce a patient's perioperative morbidity and mortality by identifying and optimizing risk factors related to the interactions between the patient's medical condition and surgical and anesthetic plans. While the key biology relevant to preoperative assessment of anesthesia is the same across all patients regardless of sexual orientation or gender identity, there are several perioperative nuances specific to the sexual and gender minority (SGM) population that will be discussed in this section. Ever more importantly, SGM patients' health outcomes are disproportionally affected by pervasive socioeconomic structural biases and discrimination; thus, the preoperative assessment requires a non-judgmental, patient-centered, compassionate approach.

Pregnancy Test

The American Society of Anesthesiologists (ASA) suggests "pregnancy testing may be offered to female patients of childbearing age and for whom the results would alter the patient's management" [11]. This is based on reported incidence of 0.3% to 1.2% of positive pregnancy in screening of biological females of childbearing potential. However, in 100% of the cases of pregnancy the scheduled surgery was postponed, cancelled, or had an impact on management. Additionally, these observational studies suggest patient report is an unreliable marker for pregnancy, so further testing should be offered. In retrospect, none of the studies specify SGM patients and are poorly designed with inherent biases such as assuming "sexual activity" of a female is exclusively with a sperm-producing partner [11, 12].

Interruption of hormone therapy in patients may result in ovulation; for example, during the perioperative period. Therefore, it is aligned with the ASA to offer pregnancy tests to individuals capable of ovulation and for whom the results would alter the patient's management. However, no patients should be required to complete a pregnancy test.

HIV+ Infection

The perioperative assessment of patients with positive HIV status is the same regardless of sexual orientation or gender identity. Because HIV and its treatment can have multiorgan implications and HIV disproportionately affects the SGM population, it is prudent to highlight the perioperative considerations for HIV-positive patients by systems (Table 1) [13].

- Undetectable viral loads are optimal for elective surgery. An HIV viral load test can be used to monitor the efficacy of Antiretroviral therapy (ART), and CD4 count is a proxy for immune constitution and function. For patients on stable ART, HIV viral loads are reviewed every 4–6 months and CD4 counts are reviewed every 12 months or optionally in certain circumstances [16]. If results within the appropriate time frame are not available, consider ordering these laboratory tests. Patients on ART therapy with HIV viral loads < 200 copies/ml and CD4 count > 200 cells/mm3 (CDC HIV stages 1 or 2) had similar postsurgical outcomes as HIV-negative patients. In contrast, patients with uncontrolled viral loads and low CD4 counts (CD4 < 200 mm; CDC HIV stage 3) are associated with increased risk of postoperative mortality and complications [17–20].
- These patients could benefit from HIV specialists formulating an individualized plan balancing the HIV treatment and delaying surgery. Additionally, viral suppression minimizes the risk of nosocomial transmission [21, 22].

ARTs and opportunistic infection prophylaxis should be continued throughout the perioperative period [23]. Cessation of ART can result in rapid viral load rebound or immune decompensation [24–26]. Patients should be instructed to bring their ART medications to the hospital in case of formulary discrepancies. Healthcare providers should consult with HIV specialists if ARTs and OI prophylaxis cannot be continued and to consider implications for ART resistance patterns, as well as alternative replacements including liquid formulations, crushing compatible ARTs, or intravenous formulations.

Multiple ARTs are simultaneously used in order to target multiple critical stages of the HIV viral replication. Various ARTs may have anesthetic implications because of potential adverse effects and/or due to potential interactions with anesthetic medications. The commonly prescribed ARTs are summarized in Table 2.

Table 1 Multisystemic manifestations of HIV and associated treatments and considerations for perioperative care [14, 15]

Organ system	Common effects	Notes	Perioperative considerations
Cardiovascular	Myocarditis Pulmonary hypertension Accelerated coronary artery disease/cardiac infarction Pericardial effusion Vasculitis Heart failure/cardiomyopathy	Can be due to HIV infection itself, ARV, and/or as a consequence of infections	Consider ECG and/or further cardiac testing (echocardiogram) in patients with positive cardiac review of systems or physical exam
Pulmonary	Opportunistic upper and lower respiratory infections	High clinical suspicion for opportunistic infection risks with CD4 counts < 200 mm^3	
Gastrointestinal	Dysphagia (due to pharyngitis, esophagitis, gastritis) Esophageal reflux Diarrhea Nausea/vomiting Hepatitis Biliary disease	Severity of upper GI symptoms can impact aspiration risk with general anesthesia Nausea and diarrhea can affect electrolyte and acid/base abnormalities Risk of hepatic dysfunction increased with ARVs and pre-existing hepatic dysfunction	Consider BMP to evaluate for electrolyte abnormalities Consider LFT and coagulation assays for liver dysfunction ARV medications should be continued during the perioperative period ("Perioperative Care in Adults With HIV," n.d.)
Renal	Chronic kidney disease	Nephrotoxicity can be related to ARV or from HIV infection	Consider assessment of renal function Adjust anesthetic for patients with renal disease. May need to renally adjust certain ARVs if renal function changes postoperatively

(continued)

Table 1 (continued)

Organ system	Common effects	Notes	Perioperative considerations
Neurologic	Neurocognitive impairment Opportunistic infections (encephalitis, meningitis) Seizures Demyelinating and degenerative disorders Cranial and peripheral neuropathy		Patients may be more sensitive to opioids and benzodiazepines due to drug-drug interactions from ARV and/or underlying neurologic involvement Intracranial masses or opportunistic infections may increase intracranial pressure Preexisting peripheral neuropathy may impact the risks and benefits of regional anesthesia
Hematologic	Thrombocytopenia Anemia Neutropenia Coagulopathy Lymphadenopathy Malignancies	ARVs can also induce pancytopenia	Consider CBC (with differential)
Endocrine	Lipid dystrophy Metabolic syndrome Lactic acidosis Hypothalamic–pituitary–adrenal axis dysfunction (Cushing's, adrenal insufficiency) Hyper/hypothyroidism SIADH	Common side effects from ARVs	Consider BMP to evaluate for electrolyte disturbances Consider glucose testing (A1C) Consider adrenal and thyroid function tests as needed. Patients with adrenal insufficiency may need glucocorticoids

LFT liver function test, *SIADH* syndrome of inappropriate anti-diuretic hormone secretion, *BMP* basic metabolic panel, *ARV* Antiretroviral medications

Hormone Therapy

Transgender patients may be on hormone therapy for medical management of gender dysphoria (Table 3) [28–30].

Transgender females. Hormone therapy typically consists of estrogen and androgen blockers. Estrogen is available as the naturally occurring 17-beta estradiol (available as transdermal or injection preparations) or the synthetic analog ethinyl estradiol (orally available since it avoids first-pass metabolism). Estrogen increases prothrombotic factors [31]; oral ethinyl estradiol is associated with increased thrombotic risk and is not recommended for transgender patients [32]. Transdermal estrogen may be the least thrombogenic in transgender females [33]. Other risks associated with estrogen therapy include elevated cardiovascular/cerebrovascular risk and impaired lipid and glucose metabolism. The World Professional Association for Transgender

Table 2 Different antiretroviral therapy medications for the treatment of HIV and their possible anesthetic considerations [21, 22, 27]

Drug class	Medications	Common adverse effects	Anesthetic considerations
Nucleosides analog reverse transcriptase inhibitor – Inhibit reverse transcription by binding to viral DNA	Abacavir Adefovir Didanosine Emtricitabine Lamivudine Stavudine Tenofovir Zidovudine	Peripheral neuropathy Pancytopenia GI disturbances (nausea/vomiting)	Consider BMP for electrolyte abnormalities; some medications (lamivudine, tenofovir, etc.) depend on renal clearance and may require dose reduction if kidney function is impaired postoperatively Consider CBC for anemia and thrombocytopenia; risk of bleeding with neuraxial anesthesia (Zidovudine) Implicated in lactic acidosis. Consider avoiding prolonged propofol infusion Does not interact with cytochrome P450 systems. Few significant drug-drug interactions
Nonnucleoside reverse transcriptase inhibitor – Inhibits reverse transcription by inhibiting the reverse transciptase enzyme	Delavirdine Doravirine Efavirenz Nevirapine Rilpivirine	Skin rash/ Stevens-Johnson's Syndrome GI disturbances	Consider BMP for electrolyte abnormalities Induces CYP3A4 (decreases serum levels of midazolam, fentanyl, oxycodone, hydrocodone, tramadol) Consider ECG. May prolong QT interval when administered with other QT-prolonging medications
Protease inhibitors – Inhibit HIV protease	Amprenavir Atazanavir Darunavir Fosamprenavir Indinavir Nelfinavir Ritonavir Saquinavir Tipranavir	GI disturbances Hyperglycemia Peripheral neuropathy Hypertriglyceridemia Elevated liver enzymes	Consider BMP, LFT Consider ECG, drug-drug interactions with calcium channel blockers and beta-blockers to prolong PR interval. Risk of QT prolongation with other QT-prolonging medications (sevofluorane, ondansetron, prochlorperazine, promethazine, droperidol) **Inhibits** CYP3A4 (enhances effects of midazolam and fentanyl, oxycodone, hydrocodone, tramadol.)

(continued)

Table 2 (continued)

Drug class	Medications	Common adverse effects	Anesthetic considerations
Integrase inhibitor – Prevents integration of viral genome into host genome by inhibiting integrase enzyme	Cabotegravir Dolutegravir Elvitegravir Raltegravir	GI disturbances	Consider BMP
CD4 entry inhibitor – Prevents binding of HIV virus to CD4 cells	Enfuvirtide Fostemsavir Maraviroc	GI disturbances	Consider BMP

BMP basic metabolic panel (including creatinine clearance), *CBC* complete blood count, *ECG* electrocardiogram, *LFT* liver function test

Health recommends continuing estrogen hormone therapy through the perioperative period unless specific risk factors such as smoking, family history or previous history of thromboembolic events, or the use of synthetic estrogen preparations are present. Withdrawal symptoms from estrogen include anxiety, depression, autonomic dysfunction, and decreased seizure threshold [28]. Androgen blocking medications function to reduce testosterone levels or activity, thus minimizing masculine characteristics and helping decrease the estrogen dose. Common androgen blocks include spironolactone, cyproterone (not available in the US due to concerns for hepatotoxicity), and finasteride. Spironolactone also is a potent mineralocorticoid receptor blocker and exerts antihypertensive and diuretic functions. Spironolactone may be continued or stopped perioperatively to achieve the desired blood pressure and/or volume status on a case-by-case basis but the anesthesia provider should be aware of the implications on hemodynamics with anesthesia and effects on electrolytes (e.g., the potential for hyperkalemia).

Transgender males. Testosterone is the hormone therapy for transgender males. There is no increased thromboembolic risk as is seen with estrogen and it can be safely continued throughout the perioperative period. Testosterone may lead to an increase in hematocrit and inflammatory markers but otherwise has minimal impact on the delivery of anesthesia [23, 29, 30, 34, 35].

Little is known about the impact of hormone therapy on reference values of laboratory tests [36]. A common approach assumes that laboratory tests reflect the hormone profile; thus, for patients on chronic hormone therapy (> 6 months) the

Table 3 Commonly used gender-affirming hormone therapy and their perioperative implications [28–30]

Medication class	Medications	Notes	Anesthetic considerations
Estrogen		Oral estradiol is associated with increased thromboembolic risk: not recommended Estrogen is associated with coronary artery disease, cerebrovascular disease, and impaired lipid and glucose metabolism	Generally, continue estrogen perioperatively. Joint decision making if other thromboembolic risks such as smoking and/or history of VTE Consider further cardiac and metabolic assessment based on history and physical examination results
Androgen Blocker	Spironolactone Cyproterone acetate Gonadotropin-release hormone receptor 5-alpha reductase inhibitor (finasteride)	Cytoproterone acetate is not available in the US due to concerns of hepatotoxicity	Consider BMP to assess electrolyte abnormalities (potassium specifically) with spironolactone Spironolactone can be safely stopped or continued to target desired volume status/blood pressure perioperatively
Testosterone	Parental (subcutaneous, intramuscular) Transdermal (gel, cream, patch)	Testosterone leads to menstrual cessation but the time to cessation is individually variable Little correlation to testosterone dose (Ahmad and Leinung, 2017)	Safe to continue perioperatively; no increased thromboembolic risk May increase hematocrit count Consider voluntary pregnancy test in childbearing-patients (± those who are sexually active with sperm-producing partners)

VTE Venous Thromboembolism

reference value to interpret laboratory tests should reflect their cisgender counterparts (i.e., transgender male should be referenced to cisgender males). There are tools to help guide health care providers in interpreting some laboratory tests, but ultimately anesthesia providers must exercise clinical judgement when assessing abnormal laboratory values [37].

Gender-Affirming Interventions with Anesthetic Implications

Anesthesia providers need to recognize that gender-affirming interventions may alter the relevant anatomy and mislead conventional physical examination interpretations.

Chest binding. A nonsurgical intervention, chest binding flattens the female breast tissue with garments or other materials around the chest wall. This intervention is associated with negative outcomes including high incidence of pain (back, chest, shoulder), and respiratory symptoms (ranging from shortness of breath to respiratory infections) [38]. In fact, individuals who chronically practice chest binding had abnormal forced spirometry values on pulmonary function testing [39]. The clinical significance in the perioperative setting and interaction with anesthesia is not well described; however, given the known pulmonary effects of general anesthesia (atelectasis, ventilation-perfusion mismatch) anesthesia providers may consider suspending chest binding during the perioperative setting.

Facial feminization. Facial feminization surgeries target the outward sexual characteristics of the feminine face: a heart-shaped jaw, shorter forehead, small narrow nose, arched eyebrows, prominent cheekbones, and fuller lips [40, 41]. Surgeries of the lower face can have significant impacts on the patient's airway. Mandibular osteotomies and genioplasties to reduce chin width and height may create relative-micrognathia and limit movement due to scarring. This may lead to a more challenging mask ventilation and tracheal intubation. Chondrolaryngoplasty to reduce the size of the thyroid cartilage prominence ("Adam's apple") may affect cricothyrotomy in an airway emergency. In addition to cosmetic feminization, various vocal cord feminization procedures have been described with a shared goal of elevating the vocal pitch [40, 42]. This is significant for the anesthesia provider as the previous surgery may increase the difficulty in selecting appropriately sized tracheal tubes and performing endotracheal intubation; reciprocally, this increases the risk of injury to the patient, such as tracheal stenosis and local tissue trauma during intubation [40].

Fascial masculinization. In contrast to facial feminization, facial masculinization seeks to achieve characteristics of the male face: a square-shaped jaw, wider forehead, wider nose and mouth, prominent supraorbital ridge, and facial hair [45]. The anesthetic considerations are similar to facial feminization surgeries, including postoperative scarring limiting movement for mask ventilation and airway instrumentation or distortion of surface landmarks for procedures (such as the cricothyroid membrane for emergent cricothyrotomy). Lowering of the vocal pitch is often achieved with testosterone therapy; laryngeal surgery for voice masculinization is rare but has been described so anesthesia providers should be cognizant of previous laryngeal surgeries as an indicator for possible difficult endotracheal intubation and trauma [46, 47]. More relevantly, anesthesia providers need to be attentive to the anatomically narrower female trachea despite the presence of surgically/hormonally masculinized facial features. Tracheal stenosis may result from impaired regional perfusion due to an oversized endotracheal tube or overinflated cuffs [48].

3 Types of Gender Affirmation Surgery

Gender affirmation surgeries, also known as gender confirmation surgeries or gender reassignment surgeries, have become increasingly recognized as a crucial aspect of medical care for individuals who experience a mismatch between their gender identity and their anatomy. With over 1.3 million adults in the U.S. identifying as transgender, the importance of this type of medical care cannot be overstated. These surgeries can involve a range of procedures, including genital reconstructions, chest surgeries, facial feminization, or masculinization surgeries, in conjunction with hormone replacement therapies. Despite its significant size, the transgender and gender nonconfirming community continues to face significant challenges, including discrimination, insurance exclusions, and lack of transgender health care education by physicians, among others.

Gender affirmation medical care has presented challenging and exciting opportunities for growth since its beginning. The history of gender-affirming surgeries dates to the early twentieth century, when Dr. Magnus Hirschfeld opened the Institute for Sexual Science in Berlin, Germany. It was here that the first vaginoplasty was performed for cisgender women with traumatic, congenital, and oncologic defects. In 1966, Johns Hopkins University in Baltimore, Maryland, unveiled the first Gender Identity Clinic to perform gender-affirming surgeries in the United States. Within its initial 2–3 years, the clinic received nearly 2000 surgery requests [49]. This was a groundbreaking moment in the history of gender affirmation surgeries as it demonstrated the potential for medical intervention to alleviate the suffering of individuals with gender dysphoria, a condition where a person experiences significant distress due to the incongruence between their gender and their physical appearance [50]. Today, these surgeries continue to play a critical role in helping individuals achieve gender congruence and live authentic, fulfilling lives.

For many transgender people, these surgeries are a crucial step in their journey to live as their true selves and can bring immense physical and psychological benefits. Individuals who underwent gender affirmation surgeries reported significant reductions in symptoms of depression, anxiety, and suicidality. In fact, gender affirmation surgeries have been shown to decrease depression and suicidal tendencies compared to those receiving hormone therapy alone [51]. This is further supported by a study that showed that those who underwent one or more gender affirmation surgeries had a 44% reduction of past-year suicidal ideation and psychological distress. Other benefits include improvement in overall quality of life and physical health outcomes [52].

Gender affirmation surgeries come in several forms and are performed by surgical specialists in the fields of gynecology, urology, and plastic surgery. These surgical interventions can be classified into a spectrum of procedures for those who were assigned male at birth (AMAB) and those assigned female at birth (AFAB). As expected, there are potential complications associated with gender-affirming surgery. However, many of these are minor in nature and can be managed with outpatient care. In fact, the incidence of complications is comparable to that of other surgical procedures (i.e., non–gender-affirming surgeries) performed for unrelated diagnoses [53] The complications related to transfeminine and transmasculine procedures are summarized in Tables 4 and 5. Studies conducted on these procedures consistently report a significant increase in overall body image, patient satisfaction, and improvements in depression and anxiety [54].

Gender dysphoria can lead some transgender women to seek "bottom surgery" to remove their penis. This complex surgical procedure typically involves several steps, including penectomy, orchiectomy, vaginoplasty, clitoroplasty, and vulvoplasty. The primary objective is to create a neovagina by inverting the penis. Along with the standard surgical complications such as bleeding and infections, this procedure can lead to complete or partial necrosis of the clitoris, labia, or vagina if blood supply is interrupted. Transwomen who take hormone replacement therapy typically develop

Table 4 Transfeminine procedures

Transfeminine Procedures	LOS	Complications	Complication Rate	Pain Level
Breast augmentation	SD	***Surgical complications***: persistent breast pain, infection, seroma/hematoma, skin necrosis, superficial thrombophlebitis ***Implant based complications***: capsular contracture, rupture of silicone, malposition, breast implant illness. ***Aesthetic concerns***: breast asymmetry, skin rippling	All cause a complication rate of 1.8% [58]	MM + Reg
Thyroid cartilage reduction	SD	***Common***: odynophagia, hoarseness, laryngospasm	20.3, 39.1, and 1.4% respectively [59]	MM
		Rare: infection, hematoma, laryngeal cutaneous fistula, laryngeal edema, numbness of the larynx or superior laryngeal nerve neuralgia	<1%	
Brow reduction	SD	Numbness, eyebrow alopecia, asymmetry, others ***Others***: hematoma, infection, eye-related complication and sinus penetration	***Open:*** alopecia (2.2%), numbness (5.5%), asymmetry (1.5%), others (<1%)	MM
			Endoscopic: alopecia (2.8%), numbness (2%), asymmetry (<1%), others (<1%) [60]	
Facial feminization - Rhinoplasty - Cheek augmentation - Blepharoplasty - Genioplasty - Mandibular angle reduction - Forehead contouring	SD/HS	Dehiscence, infection, hematoma, epistaxis, PE or DVT, ophthalmic injury, CSF leak, nerve injury, and sinus fracture.	5.4, 5.1, 1.3, 2.1, 1.6, 2.5, 0.2, 0, and 0% respectively All cause a complication rate of 5.4% [61, 62]	MM
Thyroplasty ("voice lift")	SD	Intraoperative vocal cord tear, hematoma, laryngeal edema, aspiration pneumonia, bleeding, dysphonia, dysphagia, and infection.	7% rate of wound infection. 29% rate of dysphonia and dysphagia [63]	MM
Orchiectomy	HS	Bleeding, infection, hematoma, and ilioinguinal nerve injury.	All cause complication rate of 2.9% [64]	MM + Reg
Vaginoplasty	SD/HS	***Surgical complication***: bowel injury, vascular injury, urologic injury, strictures, fistula, and infections/bleeds.	1.1, 0.1, 0.2, 3.2, 0.7 and 5.7% respectively.	MM + Reg
		Non-surgical complications: AKI, ileus, bleeding, cardiac event, sepsis, and other infections.	0.3, 5.25, 5.8, 2.5, 1.4, and 1.8% respectively [65]	
Vulvoplasty	SD	Bleeding, infection/abscess, swollen labia, itching, and tissue necrosis.	Bleeding (1.8%), infection (0.3%), and UTI (3.9%) [66]	MM + Reg

● Plastic Surgery, ● Urology, ● Gynecology, *HS* hospital stay, *MM* multimodal, *Reg* regional anesthesia, *SD* same day surgery

Table 5 Transmasculine procedures

Transmasculine Procedures	LOS	Complications	Complication Rate	Pain Level
Mastectomy	HS	Bleeding/hematoma, partial nipple graft loss, full nipple graft loss, seroma, infection, poor aesthetic outcomes (scarring, contour abnormalities)	12, 10, 3, 2, 1, and 13% respectively Up to 10% of patients may need reoperation for acute complications, with bleeding and hematoma being the most common All cause complication rates of 10.4% [53]	MM + Reg
Thyroid cartilage augmentation ("Adam's apple" enhancement)	SD	Sore throat, hoarseness, dysphagia, dysphonia	There is insufficient data	MM
Brow lift	SD	Alopecia, numbness, asymmetry, edema, hematoma/infection/pain	2.8, 2, 0.7, 0.2, and 0.1% respectively [60]	MM
Facial masculinization - Rhinoplasty - Forehead lightening - Cheek augmentation - Chin/jaw contouring	HS	Site infection, dehiscence, seroma	5, 3, and 3% respectively [67]	MM
Thyroplasty ("Voice lift")	SD	Intraoperative vocal cord tear, hematoma, laryngeal edema, aspiration pneumonia, bleeding, dysphonia, dysphagia, and infection	7% rate of wound infection. 29% rate of dysphonia and dysphagia [63]	MM
Phalloplasty - Free flaps - Pedicled flaps The following procedures are typically performed in conjunction with phalloplasty: - *Urethroplasty* - *Glansplasty* - *Scrotoplasty*	HS	***Donor site***: decreased sensory function, decreased motor function, delayed wound healing, lymphedema, intractable pain	14, 11, 10, 1, 1, and 1% respectively [68]	MM + Reg
		Recipient Site (urinary): urethral stricture, uretherocuteneous fistula, delayed wound healing, hematoma, seroma, incontinence, abscess, complete flap loss	32, 36, 12, 13, 12, 1, 1, and 3% respectively. Rate of operative revision as high as 25% [68]	
Metoidioplasty	HS	Urethral stricture, uretherocuteneous fistula, delayed wound healing, hematoma, seroma, incontinence, abscess, decreased sensory function, decreased motor function	21, 41, 10, 22, 0, 0, 3, 6 and 16% respectively [68]	MM + Reg
Penis allotransplantation	HS	Infection, organ rejection, organ failure (loss of sensory and motor function)	Insufficient published data	MM + Reg
Hysterectomy - Abdominal - Vaginal - Laparoscopic	HS	Dehiscence, surgical site infection, bleeding that requires transfusion, PE, DVT, UTI, sepsis	All cause complication of 3.6%	MM + Reg
Vaginectomy		Bleeding, infections, bladder injury, rectal perforation, urethral stricture, fistulas, voiding dysfunction	Insufficient published data	
Oophorectomy	SD/HS	Bleeding, urinary tract injury, nerve injury, infection	All cause complication rates of 3.1% [57]	MM + Reg

● Plastic Surgery, ● Urology, ● Gynecology, *HS* hospital stay, *MM* multimodal, *Reg* regional anesthesia, *SD* same day surgery

breast tissue, and many are content with the outcomes after 12–18 months [55]. However, some choose to undergo breast augmentation to increase their breast size, which carries the standard risk associated with such procedures, such as infections, bleeding, breast pain, and capsular contractures. To achieve a more feminine facial appearance, many transwomen opt for procedures such as eyebrow reduction, thyroid cartilage reduction, rhinoplasty, forehead contouring, and cheek augmentation. The complications related to transfeminine procedures are summarized in Table 4.

Transgender men have different options for gender-affirming surgery such as metoidioplasty, which creates a small phallus for standing urination but not penetrative intercourse. Some patients subsequently undergo phalloplasty. This refers to the creation of a penis with a free flap of skin from the arm or thigh which is then gradated onto the base of the clitoris to retain erotic sensation. Complications can include urinary tract stenosis, fistulas, phallus necrosis, and rectal injuries. Mastectomy or "top surgery" is the most common procedure for transmasculine individuals. It involves removing breast tissue and contouring the chest to create a more masculine appearance. Nipple retention is often possible, and various techniques are used depending on factors such as breast size and skin elasticity. Up to 10% of patients may need reoperation for acute complications, with bleeding and hematoma being the most common [53]. Hysterectomy with bilateral oophorectomy is also a common procedure for many transmen, but some may choose to preserve the option of pregnancy. The incidence of perioperative complications associated with hysterectomy and oophorectomy performed for gender-affirming surgery is the same for cisgender women undergoing the same procedures [56]. The complications related to transmasculine procedures are summarized in Table 5.

Multidisciplinary pain medicine plays a crucial role in these surgeries by helping to manage postoperative pain and discomfort and in some cases chronic pain syndromes. After a gender affirmation procedure, patients may experience pain and discomfort due to the incisions, tissue manipulation, and healing process. Pain management helps patients recover more comfortably and quickly, allowing them to return to their daily activities. Pain medicine can be administered through various methods such as oral medications, topical creams, peripheral nerve blocks, and epidural injections. The choice of pain management methods will depend on the type of procedure, patients' preferences, allergies, and the primary surgeon's recommendation. Physical therapy and rehabilitation programs can also be effective in managing pain after gender-affirming surgery and some patients may benefit from therapy to help them cope with chronic pain and improve their quality of life [57]. Ultimately, the best approach to pain management after gender-affirming surgery will depend on the individual patient's needs, preferences, and underlying health conditions.

4 Anesthesia Care for Sex Reassignment Surgery

Gender-affirming surgeries (GAS) can be divided into cosmetic surgery, "top" or "chest" surgery (mastectomy, breast implants), and "bottom" or "genital" surgery (vaginoplasty, penectomy, orchiectomy, phalloplasty, metoidioplasty, scrotoplasty). Some female-to-male transgender individuals may also wish to have hysterectomies, salpingectomies, and vaginectomies. Sex reassignment surgery (SRS), also referred to as genital affirmation surgery, is a category within the more general umbrella of GAS. SRS encompasses the more complex and irreversible interventions of gender-affirming surgeries and is becoming more common for the transgender community as awareness and acceptance has increased over recent years. While the "top" SRSs for transgender patients require little to no change in the intraoperative anesthetic management from that of cisgender individuals, the "bottom" SRSs are specific to transgender patients and require interesting options for optimal anesthetic and pain management outcomes. Therefore, the focus of the intraoperative material found later in this section will describe the anesthetic management of the transgender patient undergoing "bottom" or "genital" sex reassignment surgery. Collaboration and agreement with surgical colleagues regarding the anesthetic management of these cases is essential.

It is important to understand that there are many recommended safeguards preceding gender-affirming surgeries. The World Professional Association for Transgender Health (WPATH) Standards of Care Version 8 proposes many guidelines, including the necessity for a documented history of gender dysphoria with associated psychological evaluation before starting any component of gender transition [54]. Transgender patients of all ages undergo extensive preoperative evaluation, including mental health screenings, before any proposed surgical procedures and are typically required to be socially transitioned and receiving gender-affirming hormone therapy (GAHT) for at least one year. It is recommended that these patients have one mental health provider referral for chest/breast surgery and two independent referrals before "bottom" surgery. Despite recommendations, final decisions remain with the patient, parents (as applicable), surgeons, mental health providers, and other involved providers.

General Preoperative Considerations for Transgender Patients Presenting for Gender-Affirming Surgery

First things first: it is of the utmost importance that providers understand and are comfortable using preferred pronouns when interacting with transgender patients. Utilizing the transgender patient's preferred name and pronouns is one of the most powerful tools for making the transgender patient feel understood, accepted, respected, and safe. The most common pronouns are he/him/his, she/her/hers/ and they/them/theirs. Providers should introduce themselves with their preferred name and pronouns. The provider can then request the patient to reveal their preferred name and pronouns. For example: "Hello, my name is Dr. Smith; I use he/him pronouns. What are your preferred pronouns and name?" There is no better way to initiate an encounter with a member of the transgender community. Electronic medical records (EMRs) should be designed to identify every patient's assigned sex at birth, legal name, gender identity, and preferred name. This will help providers when caring for transgender patients and prevent unnecessary confusion or mislabeling of gender.

Given the high incidence of mental illness in transgender patients, a complete understanding of the impact of various psychiatric medications is essential in the care of these patients. This is no different than the care of cisgender patients with mental illness. Anxiety, depression, and suicide ideation are frequent psychiatric diagnoses amongst transgender individuals and should be recognized and managed perioperatively. These patients are also more likely to have nicotine and substance use disorders compared to the general population [69]. Anxiety will likely be at its highest level given the significance of the surgery these patients are undertaking. Optimization of psychiatric medications and control of substance use disorders by the patient's mental health provider in conjunction with the provision of a comfortable and low stress preoperative environment is the best approach.

Most if not all transgender patients presenting for GAS will be receiving GAHT. The medications most commonly utilized include testosterone and estrogen. Spironolactone is also commonly used for transgender females for the purpose of blocking the effects of testosterone. While there may be concern regarding a potential increased risk of venous thromboembolism (VTE) in transgender female patients taking estrogen, there is no clear evidence supporting discontinuation of estrogen therapy prior to GAS. WPATH recommends continuation of estrogen therapy before and after surgical procedures in transgender females without additional risk factors such as smoking, family history of venous thromboembolism, or the use of synthetic estrogens such as ethinyl estradiol, which is no longer recommended [28, 70]. Additionally, the use of transdermal estrogen as opposed to oral estrogen seems to have lower risk of VTE and should be considered the best option, especially perioperatively. Regarding transgender male patients, there appears to be no need to routinely discontinue testosterone prior to GAS. A systematic review did not demonstrate any increased association between venous thromboembolism and perioperative testosterone use [34, 35]. Spironolactone has its own intrinsic risks of hyperkalemia and acute kidney injury (AKI) that should be no different in transgender patients versus cisgender patients. A placebo-controlled randomized trial showed no increased risk of kidney injury in the spironolactone group [71]. Intraoperative concerns regarding hypovolemia and hypotension from the diuretic effects of spironolactone are appropriate.

An occasionally pertinent issue that may arise involves risk stratification models for transgender patients. These assessments have the potential to be impacted due to the common inclusion of a binary sex component in the scoring systems. Since the male sex is usually scored higher, there is a chance of underestimating risk in transgender females or overestimating risk in transgender males. Since it remains unclear which sex component is most appropriate to incorporate in various risk stratification models for transgender patients, it may be best to calculate both options and comply with the one indicating higher risk.

Providers should assess for any previous cosmetic gender-affirming surgeries that the transgender patient may have undergone. Facial feminization and masculinization procedures can potentially impact airway anatomy which may create difficulty with intubation or ventilation. Vocal feminization procedures in transgender females may involve anterior (Wendler) glottoplasty, also referred to as anterior commissure web formation, and cricothyroid approximation (CTA). Both of these procedures may affect the glottic opening which could require the need for a smaller endotracheal tube [72]. Also, these procedures may have the additional complications of vocal cord dysfunction, lesions, or paralysis.

When considering preoperative laboratory tests, it is important to consider the appropriateness of a preoperative pregnancy test in transgender males. Given that fertility is inconsistently impacted by testosterone therapy, transgender males with intact female reproductive organs have the potential to become pregnant. Therefore, without absolute knowledge of sexual relations, providers should consider obtaining a pregnancy test on all transgender males of reproductive age.

It is important to recognize that some laboratory tests may seem inconsistent with the transgender patient's affirmed gender. In those cases, the provider must consider the patient's sex at birth. Providers should also be aware that the opposite scenario is possible where typical reference values for various laboratory tests may not apply when considering sex assigned at birth instead of the patient's affirmed gender [73]. Transgender patients on GAHT can have changes in lab values that begin to shift toward the reference values of their affirmed gender by 6 months of therapy [74] Changes include increases in hematocrit, hemoglobin, and creatinine for patients taking testosterone and decreases in these values for those taking estrogen.

Another preoperative consideration specific to transgender males is the practice of chest binding. This process involves using specialized garments to compress breast tissue in order to create a flat chest and therefore appear more male. This behavior helps to reduce the dysphoria related to their physical appearance and allows them to feel more like their affirmed gender [75]. However, the resultant restriction of breathing can produce shortness of breath with associated reduced exercise tolerance and speech difficulties [76]. Skin damage can become an issue as well. Chronic binding has been shown to result in abnormal baseline lung function including an overall reduction in lung volumes, abnormally high FEV1/FVC, lower peak expiratory flow values, and decreases in expiratory vital capacities (both slow vital capacity and forced vital capacity) [76, 77]. Given these findings, patients may be at risk of restrictive lung disease over the long term but very likely will have some degree of atelectasis while engaging in chest binding, which could affect the patient's oxygenation during the perioperative period [77]. Providers should have a plan in place for preoperative discontinuation of chest binding as well as postoperative resumption if desired by the patient. One consideration would be having patients refrain from chest binding for 24 h preoperatively and resume no sooner than 24 h after ambulation. Providers could also require that patients perform incentive spirometry before and after anesthesia [77].

General Logistics Regarding "Bottom" Sex Reassignment Surgery

In general, the "bottom" sex reassignment surgeries take 2 to 6 h depending on which surgeries are undertaken. Most commonly, the postoperative management requires a 3 to 4 day hospitalization. Postoperative ambulation does not usually occur before postoperative day (POD) #2 in many circumstances.

Preoperative Analgesic and Anxiolytic Medications

Sex reassignment surgery, or genital affirmation surgery, is not just generic reconstructive surgery. It also involves the rearrangement of some particularly crucial nerves, some of which are responsible for sexual arousal and pleasure. These sensory nerves are sometimes severed and transported to new locations. Due to this, neuropathic pain is quite common and can be quite uncomfortable and confusing to patients in the postoperative period. Therefore, gabapentinoids should be considered for optimization of pain management. Although most current literature does not indicate a meaningful benefit to using these medications as adjuncts in treating general post-surgical pain, the neuropathic pain and occasional phantom sensations experienced by gender reassignment surgery patients warrant consideration of the use of these medications. Since these patients are typically not elderly, the risks of dizziness and sedation should be low [78]. One important caveat would be to obtain clearance to use these medications from the patient's mental health provider in order to assure that the gabapentinoids will not adversely interact with the patient's other psychiatric medications.

Other preoperative analgesic medications such as acetaminophen and celecoxib can be given orally prior to surgery with a sip of water. Alternatively, the anesthesia provider could administer intravenous acetaminophen and ketorolac along with dexamethasone during the intraoperative phase of care.

Another important preoperative consideration is the management of patient anxiety, as this is a common preexisting condition in transgender patients. Sex reassignment surgery is an enormous undertaking for what are typically young or middle-aged individuals. These patients are having parts of the body that they have known for their entire lives permanently removed or revised. There really is no going back. Midazolam should be effective along with an abundance of compassion and support. When these patients feel safe and respected, anxiety and fear should be greatly reduced.

Intraoperative Anesthetic Plan

The intraoperative phase of care is open to many options, but should be paired with an effective postoperative pain management plan. There is a lack of randomized controlled trials comparing the effectiveness of various anesthetic and pain management approaches to the care of transgender patients undergoing SRS. Therefore, anesthesia providers must rely on their knowledge and experience with similar surgical procedures in order to formulate an appropriate and successful anesthetic plan. While many anesthetic plans could be formulated, the following are three anesthetic plans for sex reassignment surgery that should be considered.

1. **Combined spinal/epidural followed by general anesthesia**

After appropriate sedation is given and monitoring applied, a combined spinal/epidural (CSE) can be performed utilizing bupivacaine and fentanyl in the spinal component of this technique. Following a test dose to rule out an intravascular epidural catheter, the patient can be placed in the supine position for induction of general anesthesia. Total intravenous anesthesia (TIVA) with any combination of preferred anesthetic drugs would be most desirable from a side effect and sustainability standpoint. Low total fresh gas flow general anesthesia with sevoflurane is also a reasonable choice as an adjunct to TIVA or on its own.

Postoperatively, an epidural infusion of bupivacaine/fentanyl or bupivacaine/hydromorphone solutions can be initiated and maintained for analgesia. The local anesthetic component has the additional benefit of producing a sympathectomy to the lower body which may have a beneficial effect by virtue of improving circulation to the newly created tissues and grafts.

Since many of these patients remain on bedrest through the first postoperative day, this epidural infusion can continue. Once ambulation is to proceed , the epidural solution can be switched to opioid only or it can be discontinued if desired by the providers. This technique allows potential elimination of intravenous opioid usage with its multiple associated risks and side effects. Nonopioid multimodal pain medications (acetaminophen, celecoxib, gabapentinoid, dexamethasone) can be continued postoperatively along with oral opioids as needed.

2. **Spinal anesthetic followed by general anesthesia**

This is a similar initial plan to that described above; however, this technique will likely require the use of an opioid patient-controlled analgesia (PCA) pump postoperatively given the typical severity of postoperative pain once the effect of the spinal anesthetic dissipates. If adding preservative-free morphine instead of fentanyl to the bupivacaine spinal anesthetic, caution is advised when starting intravenous opioid PCA in order to avoid delayed respiratory depression. Nonnarcotic multimodal medications (acetaminophen, celecoxib, gabapentinoid, dexamethasone) can be continued postoperatively.

3. **General anesthesia**

This method will require the use of an opioid PCA pump postoperatively. Nonnarcotic multimodal medications (acetaminophen, celecoxib, gabapentinoid, dexamethasone) can be continued postoperatively.

Other intraoperative considerations include providing normotension and proper hydration. It should be noted that the penectomy-orchiectomy-vaginoplasty combination surgery does require a bowel prep. Therefore, these patients are likely to be more dehydrated then the average patient in the preoperative period. Also, if not given preoperatively, anesthesia providers should give the usual multimodal nonnarcotic analgesics and antiemetic medications that are typically given to the vast majority of surgical patients during the intraoperative period.

Postoperative Care

In the postanesthesia care unit (PACU), the patient should be evaluated for anxiety and pain. If an epidural was placed and the effect of the spinal anesthetic has dissipated adequately, a test dose with epinephrine containing local anesthetic can be performed in order to rule out intrathecal and intravascular location of the epidural catheter prior to initiating the infusion. Further pain management actions can proceed as noted in previous sections.

Continuation of the patient's home medication regimen should proceed as tolerated and allowable. Psychiatric medication can be very important in the process of recovery from surgery and should not be taken lightly. Mental health support, physical therapy, and a positive environment provided by staff are all integral to an optimal outcome. Also, a private hospital bed is ideal for patient privacy and comfort.

A very important take-home message regarding SRS is that these gender-affirming surgeries should be considered to be medically-necessary surgeries that can provide potentially life-saving mental health benefits for our transgender patients [17].

References

1. Institute of Medicine (US) Committee on Lesbian, Gay, Bisexual, and Transgender Health Issues and Research Gaps and Opportunities. Introduction. In: The health of lesbian, gay, bisexual, and transgender people: building a foundation for better understanding. Washington, DC: The National Academies Press; 2011. p. 11–24. https://doi.org/10.17226/13128
2. Institute W. LGBT proportion of population: United States. 2021.
3. Newport F. In U.S., estimate of LGBT population rises to 4.5% [Internet]. Gallup. 2018 May 2022 [cited 2023 Apr 24]. Available from: https://news.gallup.com/poll/234863/estimate-lgbt-population-rises.aspx
4. National Academies of Sciences, Engineering, and Medicine. Understanding the well-being of LGBTQI+ populations. Washington, DC: The National Academies Press; 2020. https://doi.org/10.17226/25877
5. Sutter M, Perrin PB. Discrimination, mental health, and suicidal ideation among LGBTQ people of color. J Couns Psychol. 2016;63(1):98–105. https://doi.org/10.1037/cou0000126.
6. Taylor NM, King CK. Sexual health and the LGBTQ+ community. Prim Care. 2021;48(2):271–82. https://doi.org/10.1016/j.pop.2021.02.009.
7. Afonso AM, Cadwell JB, Staffa SJ, Zurakowski D, Vinson AE. Burnout rate and risk factors among anesthesiologists in the United States. Anesthesiology. 2021;134(5):683–96. https://doi.org/10.1097/ALN.0000000000003722.
8. Han S, Shanafelt TD, Sinsky CA, Awad KM, Dyrbye LN, Fiscus LC, et al. Estimating the attributable cost of physician burnout in the United States. Ann Intern Med. 2019;170(11):784–90. https://doi.org/10.7326/M18-1422.
9. National plan for health workforce well being. National Academy of Medicine. 2022 [cited 2023 Apr 24]. Available from: https://nam.edu/initiatives/clinician-resilience-and-well-being/national-plan-for-health-workforce-well-being/
10. Committee on Standards and Practice Parameters; Apfelbaum JL, Connis RT, Nickinovich DG; American Society of Anesthesiologists Task Force on Preanesthesia Evaluation; Pasternak LR, et al. Practice advisory for preanesthesia evaluation: an updated report by the American Society of Anesthesiologists Task Force on Preanesthesia Evaluation. Anesthesiology. 2012;116(3):522–38. doi.org/https://doi.org/10.1097/ALN.0b013e31823c1067

11. Manley S, de Kelaita G, Joseph NJ, Salem MR, Heyman HJ. Preoperative pregnancy testing in ambulatory surgery: incidence and impact of positive results. Anesthesiology. 1995;83(4):690–3. https://doi.org/10.1097/00000542-199510000-00007.
12. Pierre N, Moy LK, Redd S, Emans SJ, Laufer MR. Evaluation of a pregnancy-testing protocol in adolescents undergoing surgery. J Pediatr Adolesc Gynecol. 1998;11(3):139–41. https://doi.org/10.1016/s1083-3188(98)70133-0.
13. Evron S, Glezerman M, Harow E, Sadan O, Ezri T. Human immunodeficiency virus: anesthetic and obstetric considerations. Anesth Analg. 2004;98(2):503–11. https://doi.org/10.1213/01.ANE.0000097193.91244.50
14. Bajwa SJS, Kulshrestha A. The potential anesthetic threats, challenges and intensive care considerations in patients with HIV infection. J Pharm Bioallied Sci. 2013;5(1):10–6. https://doi.org/10.4103/0975-7406.106554.
15. Evron S, Glezerman M, Harow E, Sadan O, Ezri T. Human immunodeficiency virus: anesthetic and obstetric considerations. Anesth Analg. 2004;98(2):503–11. https://doi.org/10.1213/01.ANE.0000097193.91244.50. PMID: 14742395.
16. New York State Department of Health AIDS Institute Clinical Guidelines Program. Virologic and immunologic monitoring in HIV care [Internet]. 2022 June 16 [cited 2023 Apr 24]. Available from: https://www.hivguidelines.org/antiretroviral-therapy/cd4-and-viral-load-monitoring/
17. Horberg MA, Hurley LB, Klein DB, Follansbee SE, Quesenberry C, Flamm JA, et al. Surgical outcomes in human immunodeficiency virus-infected patients in the era of highly active antiretroviral therapy. Arch Surg. 2006;141(12):1238–45. https://doi.org/10.1001/archsurg.141.12.1238.
18. King JT Jr, Perkal MF, Rosenthal RA, Gordon AJ, Crystal S, Rodriguez-Barradas MC, et al. Thirty-day postoperative mortality among individuals with HIV infection receiving antiretroviral therapy and procedure-matched, uninfected comparators. JAMA Surg. 2015;150(4):343–51. https://doi.org/10.1001/jamasurg.2014.2257.
19. Naziri Q, Boylan MR, Issa K, Jones LC, Khanuja HS, Mont MA. Does HIV infection increase the risk of perioperative complications after THA? a nationwide database study. Clin Orthop Relat Res. 2015;473(2):581–6. https://doi.org/10.1007/s11999-014-3855-8.
20. Sandler BJ, Davis KA, Schuster KM. Symptomatic human immunodeficiency virus–infected patients have poorer outcomes following emergency general surgery: a study of the nationwide inpatient sample. J Trauma Acute Care Surg. 2019;86(3):479–88. https://doi.org/10.1097/TA.0000000000002161.
21. Cohen MS, Chen YQ, McCauley M, Gamble T, Hosseinipour MC, Kumarasamy N, et al. Prevention of HIV-1 infection with early antiretroviral therapy. N Engl J Med. 2011;365(6):493–505. https://doi.org/10.1056/NEJMoa1105243.
22. Rodger AJ, Cambiano V, Bruun T, Vernazza P, Collins S, van Lunzen J, et al. Sexual activity without condoms and risk of HIV transmission in serodifferent couples when the HIV-positive partner is using suppressive antiretroviral therapy. JAMA. 2016;316(2):171–81. https://doi.org/10.1001/jama.2016.5148.
23. New York State Department of Health AIDS Institute Clinical Guidelines Program. Perioperative care in adults with HIV [Internet]. 2021 Nov 16 [cited 2023 Apr 24]. Available from: https://www.hivguidelines.org/hiv-care/perioperative-management/
24. Holkmann Olsen C, Mocroft A, Kirk O, Vella S, Blaxhult A, Clumeck N, et al. Interruption of combination antiretroviral therapy and risk of clinical disease progression to AIDS or death. HIV Med. 2007;8(2):96–104. https://doi.org/10.1111/j.1468-1293.2007.00436.x.
25. Li JZ, Etemad B, Ahmed H, Aga E, Bosch RJ, Mellors JW, et al. The size of the expressed HIV reservoir predicts timing of viral rebound after treatment interruption. AIDS. 2016;30(3):343–53. https://doi.org/10.1097/QAD.0000000000000953.
26. Skiest DJ, Su Z, Havlir DV, Robertson KR, Coombs RW, Cain P, et al. Interruption of antiretroviral treatment in HIV-infected patients with preserved immune function is associated with a low rate of clinical progression: a prospective study by AIDS Clinical Trials Group 5170. J Infect Dis. 2007;195(10):1426–36. https://doi.org/10.1086/512681.

27. Russell LA, Craig C, Flores EK, Wainaina JN, Keshock M, Kasten MJ, et al. Preoperative management of medications for rheumatologic and HIV diseases: Society for Perioperative Assessment and Quality Improvement (SPAQI) consensus statement. Mayo Clin Proc. 2022;97(8):1551–71. https://doi.org/10.1016/j.mayocp.2022.05.002.
28. Coleman E, Bockting W, Botzer M, Cohen-Kettenis P, DeCuypere G, Feldman J, et al. Standards of care for the health of transsexual, transgender, and gender-nonconforming people, version 7. Int J Transgend. 2012;13(4):165–232. https://doi.org/10.1080/15532739.2011.700873.
29. Tollinche LE, Rosa WE, van Rooyen CD. Perioperative considerations for person-centered gender-affirming surgery. Adv Anesth. 2021;39:77–96. https://doi.org/10.1016/j.aan.2021.07.005.
30. Tollinche LE, Walters CB, Radix A, Long M, Galante L, Goldstein ZG, et al. The perioperative care of the transgender patient. Anesth Analg. 2018;127(2):359–66. https://doi.org/10.1213/ANE.0000000000003371.
31. Middeldorp S, Meijers JC, van den Ende AE, van Enk A, Bouma BN, Tans G, et al. Effects on coagulation of levonorgestrel- and desogestrel-containing low dose oral contraceptives: a cross-over study. Thromb Haemost. 2000;84(1):4–8.
32. Gomes MPV, Deitcher SR. Risk of venous thromboembolic disease associated with hormonal contraceptives and hormone replacement therapy: a clinical review. Arch Intern Med. 2004;164(18):1965–76. https://doi.org/10.1001/archinte.164.18.1965.
33. Vinogradova Y, Coupland C, Hippisley-Cox J. Use of hormone replacement therapy and risk of venous thromboembolism: nested case-control studies using the QResearch and CPRD databases. BMJ. 2019;364:k4810. https://doi.org/10.1136/bmj.k4810.
34. Argalious MY, Steib J, Daskalakis N, Mao G, Li M, Armanyous S, et al. Association of testosterone replacement therapy and the incidence of a composite of postoperative in-hospital mortality and cardiovascular events in men undergoing cardiac surgery. Anesth Analg. 2020;130(4):890–8. https://doi.org/10.1213/ANE.0000000000004115.
35. Boskey ER, Taghinia AH, Ganor O. Association of surgical risk with exogenous hormone use in transgender patients: a systematic review. JAMA Surg. 2019;154(2):159–69. https://doi.org/10.1001/jamasurg.2018.4598.
36. Goldstein Z, Corneil TA, Greene DN. When gender identity doesn't equal sex recorded at birth: the role of the laboratory in providing effective healthcare to the transgender community. Clin Chem. 2017;63(8):1342–52. doi.org:https://doi.org/10.1373/clinchem.2016.258780
37. UCSF Gender Affirming Health Program, Department of Family and Community Medicine, University of California San Francisco. Guidelines for the primary and gender-affirming care of transgender and gender nonbinary people. 2nd edition [Internet]. Deutsch MB, editor. 2016 June [cited 2023 Apr 24]. Available from: https://transcare.ucsf.edu/guidelines.
38. Peitzmeier S, Gardner I, Weinand J, Corbet A, Acevedo K. Health impact of chest binding among transgender adults: a community-engaged, cross-sectional study. Cult Health Sex. 2017;19(1):64–75. https://doi.org/10.1080/13691058.2016.1191675.
39. Morrison SD, Vyas KS, Motakef S, Gast KM, Chung MT, Rashidi V, et al. Facial feminization: systematic review of the literature. Plast Reconstr Surg. 2016;137(6):1759–70. https://doi.org/10.1097/PRS.0000000000002171.
40. Sayegh F, Ludwig DC, Ascha M, Vyas K, Shakir A, Kwong JW, et al. Facial masculinization surgery and its role in the treatment of gender dysphoria. J Craniofac Surg. 2019;30(5):1339–46. https://doi.org/10.1097/SCS.0000000000005101.
41. Kanagalingam J, Georgalas C, Wood GR, Ahluwalia S, Sandhu G, Cheesman AD. Cricothyroid approximation and subluxation in 21 male-to-female transsexuals. Laryngoscope. 2005;115(4):611–8. https://doi.org/10.1097/01.mlg.0000161357.12826.33.
42. Mastronikolis NS, Remacle M, Biagini M, Kiagiadaki D, Lawson G. Wendler glottoplasty: an effective pitch raising surgery in male-to-female transsexuals. J Voice. 2013;27(4):516–22. https://doi.org/10.1016/j.jvoice.2013.04.004.
43. Thomas JP, Macmillan C. Feminization laryngoplasty: assessment of surgical pitch elevation. Eur Arch Otorhinolaryngol. 2013;270(10):2695–2700. doi.org:https://doi.org/10.1007/s00405-013-2511-3

44. Vowles BJ, Ahmad I, Christodoulides G. Unexpected difficult airway management in a transgender female patient. Anaesth Rep. 2020;8(1):36–9. https://doi.org/10.1002/anr3.12042.
45. McNeill EJM. Management of the transgender voice. J Laryngol Otol. 2006;120(7):521–3. https://doi.org/10.1017/S0022215106001174.
46. Saito Y, Nakamura K, Itani S, Tsukahara K. Type 3 thyroplasty for a patient with female-to-male gender identity disorder. Case Rep Otolaryngol. 2018;2018:4280381. https://doi.org/10.1155/2018/4280381.
47. Lao WP, Crawley BK. Airway considerations in transgender patients: complicated intubation. Ear Nose Throat J. 2021;100(5_suppl):755S–756S. https://doi.org/10.1177/0145561320910680
48. Ahmad S, Leinung M. The response of the menstrual cycle to initiation of hormonal therapy in transgender men. Transgend Health. 2017;2(1):176–9. https://doi.org/10.1089/trgh.2017.0023.
49. Frey JD, Poudrier G, Thomson JE, Hazen A. A historical review of gender-affirming medicine: focus on genital reconstruction surgery. J Sex Med. 2017;14(8):991–1002. https://doi.org/10.1016/j.jsxm.2017.06.007.
50. Weissler JM, Chang BL, Carney MJ, Rengifo D, Messa CA IV, Sarwer DB, et al. Gender-affirming surgery in persons with gender dysphoria. Plast Reconstr Surg. 2018;141(3):388e–96e. https://doi.org/10.1097/PRS.0000000000004123.
51. Tucker RP, Testa RJ, Simpson TL, Shipherd JC, Blosnich JR, Lehavot K. Hormone therapy, gender affirmation surgery, and their association with recent suicidal ideation and depression symptoms in transgender veterans. Psychol Med. 2018;48(14):2329–36. https://doi.org/10.1017/S0033291717003853.
52. Tordoff DM, Wanta JW, Collin A, Stepney C, Inwards-Breland DJ, Ahrens K. Mental health outcomes in transgender and nonbinary youths receiving gender-affirming care. JAMA Netw Open. 2022;5(2):e220978. https://doi.org/10.1001/jamanetworkopen.2022.0978.
53. Cuccolo NG, Kang CO, Boskey ER, Ibrahim AMS, Blankensteijn LL, Taghinia A, et al. Mastectomy in transgender and cisgender patients: a comparative analysis of epidemiology and postoperative outcomes. Plast Reconstr Surg Glob Open. 2019;7(6):e2316. https://doi.org/10.1097/GOX.0000000000002316.
54. Coleman E, Radix A, Bouman WP, Brown GR, de Vries ALC, Deutsch MB, et al. Standards of care for the health of transgender and gender diverse people, version 8. Int J Transgend Health. 2022;23(suppl 1):S1–259. https://doi.org/10.1080/26895269.2022.2100644.
55. Erickson-Schroth L, editor. Trans bodies, trans selves: a resource for the transgender community. New York: Oxford University Press; 2014.
56. Bretschneider CE, Sheyn D, Pollard R, Ferrando CA. Complication rates and outcomes after hysterectomy in transgender men. Obstet Gynecol. 2018;132(5):1265–73. https://doi.org/10.1097/AOG.0000000000002936.
57. Rachlin K, Hansbury G, Pardo ST. Hysterectomy and oophorectomy experiences of female-to-male transgender individuals. Int J Transgend. 2010;12(3):155–66. https://doi.org/10.1080/15532739.2010.514220.
58. Bekeny JC, Zolper EG, Fan KL, Del Corral G. Breast augmentation for transfeminine patients: methods, complications, and outcomes. Gland Surg. 2020;9(3):788–96. https://doi.org/10.21037/gs.2020.03.18.
59. Therattil PJ, Hazim NY, Cohen WA, Keith JD. Esthetic reduction of the thyroid cartilage: a systematic review of chondrolaryngoplasty. JPRAS Open. 2019;22:27–32. https://doi.org/10.1016/j.jpra.2019.07.002.
60. Cho MJ, Carboy JA, Rohrich RJ. Complications in brow lifts: a systemic review of surgical and nonsurgical brow rejuvenations. Plast Reconstr Surg Glob Open. 2018;6(10):e1943. https://doi.org/10.1097/GOX.0000000000001943.
61. Tirrell AR, Abu El Hawa AA, Bekeny JC, Chang BL, Del Corral G. Facial feminization surgery: a systematic review of perioperative surgical planning and outcomes. Plast Reconstr Surg Glob Open. 2022;10(3):e4210. https://doi.org/10.1097/GOX.0000000000004210
62. Namin A, Shokri T, Vincent A, Saman M, Ducic Y. Complications in facial esthetic surgery. Semin Plast Surg. 2020;34(4):272–6. https://doi.org/10.1055/s-0040-1721764.

63. Chang J, Yung K. Gender affirming voice care: a literature review. Int J Head Neck Surg. 2021;12(3):93–7. https://doi.org/10.5005/jp-journals-10001-1448.
64. Russell CB, Hong CX, Fairchild P, Bretschneider CE. Complications after orchiectomy and vaginoplasty for gender affirmation: an analysis of concurrent versus separate procedures using a national database. Urogynecology (Phila). 2023;29(2):202–8. https://doi.org/10.1097/SPV.0000000000001312.
65. Mishra K, Ferrando CA. Postoperative adverse events following gender-affirming vaginoplasty: an American College of Surgeons National Surgical Quality Improvement Program study. Am J Obstet Gynecol. Published online 18 Jan 2023. https://doi.org/10.1016/j.ajog.2023.01.011
66. Melancon DM, Walton AB, Mundinger G, Benson C. Surgical outcomes and complications of genital gender affirmation surgery. Curr Sex Health Rep. 2021;13(4):107–16. https://doi.org/10.1007/s11930-021-00318-3.
67. Salesky M, Zebolsky AL, Benjamin T, Wulu JA, Park A, Knott PD, et al. Gender-affirming facial surgery: experiences and outcomes at an academic center. Facial Plast Surg Aesthet Med. 2022;24(1):54–9. https://doi.org/10.1089/fpsam.2021.0060.
68. Robinson IS, Blasdel G, Cohen O, Zhao LC, Bluebond-Langner R. Surgical outcomes following gender affirming penile reconstruction: patient-reported outcomes from a multi-center, international survey of 129 transmasculine patients. J Sex Med. 2021;18(4):800–11. https://doi.org/10.1016/j.jsxm.2021.01.183.
69. Reece-Nguyen TL, Tollinche L, Van Rooyen C, Roque RA. Current challenges faced by transgender and gender-diverse patients and providers in anesthesiology. Int Anesthesiol Clin. 2023;61(1):26–33. https://doi.org/10.1097/aia.0000000000000384.
70. Kozato A, Fox GWC, Yong PC, Shin SJ, Avanessian BK, Ting J, et al. No venous thromboembolism increase among transgender female patients remaining on estrogen for gender-affirming surgery. J Clin Endocrinol Metab. 2021;106(4):e1586–90. https://doi.org/10.1210/clinem/dgaa966.
71. Barba-Navarro R, Tapia-Silva M, Garza-Garcia C, López-Giacoman S, Melgoza-Toral I, Vázquez-Rangel A, et al. The effect of spironolactone on acute kidney injury after cardiac surgery: a randomized, placebo-controlled trial. Am J Kidney Dis. 2017;69:192–9. https://doi.org/10.1053/j.ajkd.2016.06.013.
72. Kim HT. Vocal feminization for transgender women: current strategies and patient perspectives. Int J Gen Med. 2020;13:43–52. https://doi.org/10.2147/IJGM.S205102.
73. Goldstein Z, Corneil TA, Greene DN. When gender identity doesn't equal sex recorded at birth: the role of the laboratory in providing effective healthcare to the transgender community. Clin Chem. 2017;63(8):1342–52. https://doi.org/10.1373/clinchem.2016.258780.
74. Rosendale N, Goldman S, Ortiz GM, Haber LA. Acute clinical care for transgender patients. JAMA Intern Med. 2018;178(11):1535–43. https://doi.org/10.1001/jamainternmed.2018.4179.
75. Peitzmeier S, Gardner I, Weinand J, Corbet A, Acevedo K. Health impact of chest binding among transgender adults: community-engaged, cross-sectional study. Cult Health Sex. 2017;19(1):64–75. https://doi.org/10.1080/13691058.2016.1191675.
76. Cumming RJM, Sylvester K, Fuld J. P257 Understanding the effects on lung function of chest binder use in the transgender population. Thorax. 2016;71(suppl 3):A227. https://doi.org/10.1136/thoraxjnl-2016-209333.400.
77. Kim E, Mukerji S, Debryn D, Price R, Streed C Jr, Nozari A. Oxygen desaturation in a transgender man: initial concerns and recommendations regarding the practice of chest binding: a case report. J Med Case Rep. 2022;16(1):333. https://doi.org/10.1186/s13256-022-03527-z.
78. Kumar AH, Habib AS. The role of gabapentinoids in acute and chronic pain after surgery. Curr Opin Anaesthesiol. 2019;32(5):629–34. https://doi.org/10.1097/ACO.0000000000000767.
79. Almazan AN, Keuroghlian AS. Association between gender-affirming surgeries and mental health outcomes. JAMA Surg. 2021;156(7):611–8. https://doi.org/10.1001/jamasurg.2021.0952.
80. Aquino NJ, Boskey ER, Staffa SJ, Ganor O, Crest AW, Gemmill KV, et al. A single center case series of gender-affirming surgeries and the evolution of a specialty anesthesia team. J Clin Med. 2022;11(7):1943. https://doi.org/10.3390/jcm11071943.

81. Aquino NJ, Ganor O, Chrisos HA, Oles N, Boskey ER. Perioperative issues with gender-diverse youth. J Pediatr Surg Nurs. 2021;10(1):23–31. https://doi.org/10.1097/jps.0000000000000282.
82. Oles N, Ganor O, Aquino NJ, Boskey ER. Surgical affirmation for gender-diverse youth. J Pediatr Surg Nurs. 2021;10(1):32–9. https://doi.org/10.1097/jps.0000000000000279.
83. Hembree WC, Cohen-Kettenis PT, Gooren L, Hannema SE, Meyer WJ, Murad MH, et al. Endocrine treatment of gender-dysphoric/gender-incongruent persons: an Endocrine Society clinical practice guideline. J Clin Endocrinol Metab. 2017;102(11):3869–903. https://doi.org/10.1210/jc.2017-01658.

Sickle Cell Disease (SCD) and Perioperative Pain Management

Cynthia Iradukunda

Abstract Sickle cell disease is an autosomal recessive disorder that involves the inheritance of a mutant Beta globin gene. The Beta globin gene is encoded at chromosome 11. The defective hemoglobin S (HbS) results from a substitution mutation that occurs at the sixth amino acid where Glutamine is substituted for Valine on chromosome 11 (Kumar et al, Robbins basic pathology, Elsevier, Saint Louis, pp 411–3, 2012 [1]; Lanzkron, Sickle cell anemia straight to the point of care [Internet], 2023 [2]). At least one HbS allele must be present to develop sickle cell disease. In cases where only one HbS allele exists, co-inheritance of defective Beta hemoglobin such as occurs in the setting of Beta thalassemia or Hemoglobin C disease may result in clinical manifestations of sickle cell disease. Inheritance of a hemoglobin S allele from both parents results in the most severe form of sickle cell disease also known as sickle cell anemia (Lanzkron, Sickle cell anemia straight to the point of care [Internet] 2023, [2]). Patients with sickle cell trait have one normal gene (HbA) and another sickle gene and are commonly asymptomatic or have symptoms of diminished magnitude.

Keywords Sickle cell disease (SCD) · Postoperative surgical pain · Acute painful crisis · Chronic pain · And chronic opioid therapy

1 Epidemiology

The Global Prevalence of SCD increased by 41.4%. from 5.46 million people in 2000 to 7.74 million in 2021 [3]. The ancestry of patients with sickle cell disease can be traced back to sub-Saharan Africa, the Caribbean, India, Saudi Arabia, and Mediterranean countries [3, 4]. In the United States of America, approximately 100,000 people suffer from sickle cell disease, and the condition is most prevalent among African Americans. The incidence of sickle cell disease is 1 for every 365 live births

C. Iradukunda (✉)
Department of Anesthesiology, School of Medicine and Public Health, University of Wisconsin, Madison, USA
e-mail: ciradukunda@uwhealth.org

A. Abd-Elsayed and K. Schroeder (eds.), *Perioperative Pain Management*,
https://doi.org/10.1007/978-3-031-67648-2_24

in the African-American population and 1 in every 16,300 Hispanic-American births [5]. Recent advances in medical therapy have made it possible for patients with sickle cell disease to survive into adulthood [5–7]. However, given the pathogenesis of sickle cell disease, there is an increased incidence of surgery in this population compared to the general population [1, 8, 9]. In an earlier cooperative study of surgery and sickle cell disease, 69% of sickle cell patients underwent a single procedure, 21% underwent two procedures and 11% had more than 2 procedures over a10 year study period [9]. Additionally, patients with SCD who underwent surgery were reported to have more complications, increased pain scores, and increased opioid requirements [10–12].

2 Pathogenesis of Sickle Cell Disease

Understanding the pathogenesis of sickle cell disease and sickle cell anemia plays a critical role in optimizing the surgical care of patients with SCD. Normal adult hemoglobin (HbA) is a tetramer with 2 alpha and 2 beta chains encoded at chromosome 16 and chromosome 11 respectively [1]. A substitution mutation of glutamine for valine at chromosome 11 results in a mutated beta Hemoglobin S (HbS). Sickle cell disease follows an inheritance of at least one abnormal beta hemoglobin chain (HbS) from one parent, with varying degrees of severity as dictated by the patient's genotype. With hemoglobin electrophoresis, the most severe forms of sickle cell disease that is HbSS and HbSbeta^0 are found to have more than 80% of the Beta hemoglobin mutant. [13]. Patients with sickle cell anemia (HbSS) can present with severe features as early as 6 months and are bound to endure multiple hospital admissions and blood transfusions [2].

Underlying the unique clinical presentations of sickle cell disease is the process of polymerization of HbS within the red cells in the presence of hypoxia which results in morphological changes of the red blood cell from a normal discoid to a sickle or crescent shape. The rate of HbS polymerization is directly proportional to its concentration within the cell. Once the cells are sickled, they increasingly adhere to endothelium promoting thrombosis, decreased blood flow and a shortened life span of 20 days versus 120 days of life for the normal red cell [1] When sickling occurs in the microvasculature, partial or complete obstruction of blood flow occurs inducing an acute or subacute vaso-occlusive painful crisis, in the affected organs. In organs with increased transit time such as the spleen and bone marrow, the sickled cells are subjected to increased hemolysis resulting in anemia [1, 14]. Tissue and organ infarction usually results from multiple vaso-occlusive episodes following different triggers. Reversing hypoxemia with improved oxygenation has been shown to attenuate further sickling and occasionally reverse sickling. In addition to hypoxemia, dehydration, acidosis, cold temperatures, extreme exertion, inflammation, stress, and infection are the other commonly identified triggers of red blood cell sickling [2].

The two major outcomes of sickled red blood cells are [1]:

1. Recurrent hemolysis resulting in chronic hemolytic anemia.
2. Microvascular obstructions result in thrombosis, vascular congestion, and infarction of multiple organs resulting in sudden vaso-occlusive pain crises including acute chest syndrome, a life-threatening complication.

3 Sickle Cell Disease and Surgery

Beginning in the preoperative period, an Anesthesia professional should work closely with a multidisciplinary team including the patient's primary care physician, Hematologist, and the acute pain service [15–17]. Patients with SCD may require surgical interventions to provide symptomatic relief or to definitively treat the sequalae of infarction. Surgical encounters in SCD start early on in childhood and are generally associated with longer hospital stays secondary to poorly controlled postoperative pain among other factors [8, 18, 19]. Cholecystectomy, splenectomy, and adenotonsillectomy are reported as the most common procedures, however, other procedures may include hip surgery for avascular necrosis of femur, incision and drainage for abscess, surgery for priapism, cardiac surgery, neurosurgery for stroke, arteriovenous malformations, and MoyaMoya disease [9, 20–23].

4 Perioperative Pain Management in Patients with Sickle Cell Disease

Patients with sickle cell disease are most vulnerable in the perioperative period due to the accentuation of multiple triggers for sickling including dehydration, stress, surgery, hypoxia, and increased inflammation following surgical manipulation [16]. Prolonged hours of fasting predispose patients to dehydration, which in turn increases anxiety and stress resulting in a vicious cycle of multiple triggers for polymerization of the defective haemoglobin (HbS) and red cell sickling. Consequentially, vaso-occlusive acute painful crises often occur perioperatively and complicate the management of postoperative surgical pain.

Postoperative pain in patients with SCD remains complex and systematic approaches to analgesia should incorporate the patient and a diverse group of medical professionals.

5 Hematology Consult

Once the patient is scheduled for surgery, the patient should be seen or reviewed by an in-house hematologist to establish and ensure continuity of care. A patient's hemoglobinopathy should be ascertained since some forms of SCD are more severe than others [13]. Ascertaining the genotype of patients from endemic areas of the world [5, 24] is essential in guiding individualized postoperative analgesia plans and appropriating resources as determined by the disease severity [13, 25, 26] Additionally, the expertise of the Hematologist is also crucial to guide the timely initiation of sickle disease-modifying therapies such as hydroxyurea, crizanlizumub, L-glutamine and voxelotor [7].

6 Individualized Pain Plan

Optimizing postoperative pain management in patients with sickle cell disease requires that the provider be familiar with the complex manifestations of the disease in situations of increased stress that may be encountered in the perioperative period. Goal setting is pivotal in managing postoperative pain in SCD patients with a focus on return to baseline functional status which may mean complete pain resolution for some versus baseline chronic pain state in others.

Postoperative pain management in SCD patients begins in the preoperative period with a focused pain history and an assessment of analgesic elements (Table 1) pertinent to SCD patients followed by the drafting of an individualized pain management plan [27, 28]. In general, a multimodal analgesic approach to postoperative pain is suitable for most surgical patients, however, SCD patients present several challenges and may require additional resources. Distinctive in patients with SCD are several factors that impact and compound the presentation of postoperative pain in the perioperative period as outlined in the following paragraphs.

7 Early Recognition and Management of an Acute Painful Crisis

A vaso-occlusive painful crisis in the perioperative period is often multifactorial in etiology [2, 12]. In the postoperative period, an acute painful crisis often presents as a new severe acute pain and may be localized to a non-surgical site often with precipitating factors that should be identified and treated promptly [29, 30]. Maintaining adequate hydration status by allowing clear fluid intake up to 2 h before surgery and careful intravenous fluid maintenance for those who are strict NPO status is advised [31]. Throughout the perioperative period, vigilant monitoring of a patient's input and output should be performed and this can provide valuable information about the patient's hydration status [29]. To prevent hypoxia, supplemental oxygen may be required during the intraoperative and postoperative periods to maintain an oxygen saturation > 95%. Incentive spirometry is encouraged in patients with SCD undergoing surgery to mitigate pulmonary complications and the use of CPAP in patients with Obstructive Sleep Apnea may be necessary [23, 26].

Table 1 Elements for postoperative pain assessmentin SCD

Element	Questions
Triggers for acute pain crisis	Do you often experience painful crises? What triggers your painful crisis? (hypoxia, exercise, infection, dehydration) How often do they occur?
Frequency of ED visits and hospital admission	How many times have you visited the ED due to increased pain, uncontrolled pain or other reasons? Number of times admitted to the hospital in the last (month, 6 months, 1 year)
Location of the chronic pain Location of the any pain including the new pain	1. Where is the pain? Is it localized or generalized 2. Is this pain new or different from the pain you usually experience at home?
Intensity	How severe is this pain? (use a validated pain intensity)
Quality of pain	Is the pain sharp or dull? Is it constant or intermittent?
Aggravating and relieving factors	What makes the pain better or worse?
Current pain regimen	What do you take regularly to remain comfortable? What do you take for breakthrough pain?

[a] Modified from Chou et al. [28]

Avoiding hypothermia throughout the perioperative period can be achieved with the use of Bair huggers, warm blankets, warm intravenous fluids, and prewarming the room for most of the general cases in conjunction with temperature monitoring [29]. In particular, the use of cold ice packs and other cold therapies should be avoided in SCD patients.

Perioperative transfusion of red blood cells increases the proportion of HbA and may alleviate the presentation of a painful crisis. However, this does not represent routine clinical practice and implementation should be considered on a case-by-case basis [12, 23, 29, 32]. Ballas et al. further demonstrated that the use of hydroxyurea among adults experiencing an acute painful crisis resulted in lesser opioid requirements and shorter hospital stays [12]. This modality can be explored with critical input from the Hematologist.

Parenteral opioids are commonly utilized in the severe forms of acute painful crises, and in the setting of acute postoperative pain, this would translate into higher opioid dosing requirements for extended periods. The clinician(s) involved in the postoperative care of SCD patients should be acutely aware of these deviations from the general population to avoid suboptimal pain relief from suboptimal opioid prescription and administration.

Acute chest syndrome is a life-threatening complication [12, 33] and is reported as the most common postoperative cause of morbidity and mortality in sickle cell patients requiring ICU admission. It is defined as a new pulmonary infiltrate on imaging and presents in children with fever, shortness of breath, chest pain, and tachypnea [33]. Risk factors include sickle cell disease genotype, h/o pulmonary disease, and recent surgery [33, 34]. Acute chest syndrome can be triggered by the combination of surgery and other known sickling triggers as noted above. [33, 34]. In cases of acute chest syndrome, multiple interventions including early recognition, prompt hematology consultation coupled with timely institution of mechanical ventilation and transfusion protocols are crucial in preventing fatal outcomes.

8 Management of Persistent Chronic Pain and Chronic Opioid Use

Chronic pain in SCD is considered when painful symptoms are present for most days in the previous 6 months or more [35]. With the high prevalence of chronic pain in SCD adolescents and adults, of more than 50%, most SCD patients will be opioid-tolerant and will require higher than anticipated opioid doses to control postoperative pain [10, 11, 36]. American Pain Society guidelines on the management of postoperative pain strongly recommend early consultation with pain specialists for patients who are at high risk of sub-therapeutic management of postoperative pain such as those on chronic opioid therapy [28, 37]. A multidisciplinary team with a holistic approach to SCD pain presentations encompassing the different aspects of chronic SCD pain compounded by new post-surgical pain is highly recommended [35, 36].

9 Patient-Centered Treatment Plan

Opioids remain the mainstay of management for moderate to severe postoperative pain. Patients with SCD generally require elevated postoperative opioid dosing and it is crucial that frequent patient assessments are performed to establish responses to therapy and monitor for opioid related adverse events [38]. Several guidelines can be referenced to guide pain management in patients on chronic pain therapy. In particular, the American Society of Hematology 2020(ASH 2020) guidelines for sickle cell disease [39] provide recommendations on acute and chronic pain management in SCD patients. It is critical to bear in mind that following surgery, SCD patients will have, in addition to their baseline pain(s), post-surgical pain depending on the extent of the surgical procedure which may also be complicated by an acute painful crisis.

10 Multimodal Analgesia Approach

The American Pain Society and the ASH 2020 guidelines on the management of postoperative pain recommend a multimodal analgesic approach to provide optimal pain relief. While opioids have been routinely prescribed in the immediate postsurgical period, the opioid epidemic has introduced opioid restriction measures that may affect SCD patients negatively [12, 34]. It is therefore important that healthcare professionals find a way to utilize different pain relief modalities bearing in mind the unique pain syndromes and patterns experienced by patients with SCD. [12, 37]. To maximize the efficacy of multimodal analgesic approaches, pain assessment using age-appropriate pain-validated tools is recommended [38, 40]. In adults, visual analog and numerical rating scales are commonly used [40, 41] (Table 2).

Ketamine

SCD patients maintained on chronic opioid therapy may experience refractory pain with minimal responses to escalated opioid doses. Etiologies to blunted analgesic responses following opioid administration may include central sensitization resulting in allodynia, opioid-induced hyperalgesia, and neuropathic pain. Subanesthetic ketamine infusions have demonstrated an ability in patients with SCD to decrease opioid utilization and improve pain control [42].

Table 2 Multimodal analgesia[a]

Reported pain intensity	Recommendedanalgesicmodalities
Mild pain	Acetaminophenand NSAIDs- ibuprofen, ketorolac, naproxen, diclofenac
Moderate	Enteralopioids: codeine, oxycodone, morphine sulphate
Severe pain and acute post-surgical pain	Parenteralopioids IV hydromorphone PCA, IVketamine infusion[42], IV lidocaine [43],fentanyl(nasal, transdermal patches, IV), regional and neuraxialanalgesia[44, 45]
Acute painful crisis	Parenteralopioidsas above Consider transfusion of red blood cells Consider sickle cell modifying therapies such as hydroxyurea [12] Optimal volume status, oxygenation, and temperature regulation (normothermia) [2, 29]

[a]Table 2 constructed from multiple data sources [2, 6, 12, 28, 29, 39, 42–45]

Regional and Peripheral Nerve Blocks

Regional blocks can be performed for anesthesia or analgesia in SCD and may result in less opioid consumption in the immediate postoperative period [44, 45]. In male patients, priapism can develop and if unrecognized, complications of penile infarction, and impotence. Mandatory monitoring in this patient population is highly recommended to facilitate timely surgical decompression and other relevant interventions.

Non-pharmacological Therapies

The American Society of Hematology for Sickle Cell Disease provides no recommendation for or against the use of non-pharmacological therapies for acute pain management in sickle cell disease and these include physical therapy, behavioral therapies, and psychological therapies [39]

11 Compassionate Care

Too frequently, optimal pain management in patients with SCD may be hampered by the prejudices of healthcare professionals responsible for their care [27]. These patients may be labeled as difficult, addicted or drug seeking and may therefore suffer needlessly as their description of pain symptomology is minimized [46]. To combat these potential inherent biases, the development and implementation of specific clinical guidelines may help to ensure that patients receive the essential components of a tailored analgesic regimen. In addition, patients should be empowered as active participants in their healthcare and their descriptions of pain symptomology should be addressed with at least the same attention as any other patient. Finally, staff training in mechanisms to collaborate care and analgesic pathways in patients with SCD may effectively minimize challenges in access to appropriate analgesic care [47].

12 Conclusion

Perioperative pain management in patients with SCD remains a challenging endeavor for healthcare professionals. To optimize pain relief in SCD, a systematic approach that begins in the preoperative period with a focused pain history capturing the baseline chronicity of sickle cell pain, frequency of acute painful crises, and current pattern of opioid consumption together with a multidisciplinary team should be adopted.

Healthcare professionals involved in the perioperative care of patients with SCD should consider the pathogenesis of SCD as this is critical in early diagnosis, differentiation, and management of postoperative surgical pain compounded by acute painful crises, life-threatening acute chest syndrome, and chronic pain. In these circumstances, we recommend frequent patient assessment to quantify the need for escalating opioid dosing for extended periods to achieve the goal of returning to baseline individual functional status.

Key Takeaway Points

1. Starting in the preoperative period, the Anesthesia professional should work closely with other healthcare professionals and draft an individualized pain management plan.
2. Recognize the several facets of pain in patients with Sickle cell disease including the different pain patterns of chronic pain [6, 36], and the challenges associated with chronic or long-term opioid use to avoid the pitfall of subtherapeutic perioperative pain management.
3. Actively prevent and treat the triggers for sickling coupled with timely diagnosis and management of vaso-occlusive painful crises.
4. Return to baseline functional status is the expectant goal of perioperative pain management in patients with SCD and this should be clearly communicated to the patient and the involved healthcare professionals.

References

1. Kumar V, Abbas AK, Aster CJ, Richard M. Hematopoietic and lymphoid systems. In: Robbins basic pathology. Saint Louis: Elsevier. ProQuest Ebook Central, 16 Dec 2023; 2012. p. 411–3.
2. Lanzkron S. Sickle cell anemia Straight to the point of care [Internet]. 2023 [cited 2023 Dec 15]. Available from: https://bestpractice.bmj.com>topics>en-us
3. Thomson AM, McHugh TA, Oron AP, Teply C, Lonberg N, Vilchis Tella V, et al. Global, regional, and national prevalence and mortality burden of sickle cell disease, 2000–2021: a systematic analysis from the Global Burden of Disease Study 2021. Lancet Haematol. 2023;10(8):e585–99.
4. Sickle-Cell Anaemia Report by the Secretariat Prevalence of Sickle-Cell Anaemia. 2006.
5. CDC [Internet] [cited 2023 Dec 15]. Data & Statistics on Sickle Cell Disease. Available from: https://www.cdc.gov/ncbddd/sicklecell/data.html
6. Brandow AM, Liem RI. Advances in the diagnosis and treatment of sickle cell disease. J Hematol Oncol. 2022;15.
7. Higgins T, Menditto MA, Katartzis S, Matson KL. Advances in the management of sickle cell disease: new concepts and future horizons. J Pediatric Pharmacol Therapeut. 2022;27(3):206–13.
8. Hyder O, Yaster M, Bateman BT, Firth PG. Surgical procedures and outcomes among children with sickle cell disease. Anesth Analg. 2013;117(5):1192–6.
9. Koshy M, Weiner SJ, Miller ST, Sleeper LA, Vichinsky E, Brown AK, et al. Surgery and anesthesia in sickle cell disease.
10. Crawford MW, Galton S, Naser B. Postoperative morphine consumption in children with sickle-cell disease. Acute Pain. 2006;8(3).

11. Carroll CP. Opioid treatment for acute and chronic pain in patients with sickle cell disease. Neurosci Lett. 2020;714.
12. Ballas SK, Bauserman RL, McCarthy WF, Castro OL, Smith WR, Waclawiw MA. Hydroxyurea and acute painful crises in sickle cell anemia: Effects on hospital length of stay and opioid utilization during hospitalization, outpatient acute care contacts, and at home. J Pain Symptom Manage. 2010;40(6):870–82.
13. Idowu M, Sridhar A. American of Hematology. 2021. [cited 2023 Dec 16]. Hemoglobin electrophoresis in sickle cell disease: a primer for the clinician. Available from: https://www.hematology.org/education/trainees/fellows/trainee-news/2021/hemoglobin-electrophoresis-in-sickle-cell-disease
14. Sundd P, Gladwin MT, Novelli EM. Pathophysiology of sickle cell disease. In: Annual review of pathology: mechanisms of disease, vol. 14. Annual Reviews Inc.; 2019. p. 263–92.
15. Humphreys José VA. The management of sickle cell disease in a primary care setting. J Family Med Prim Care. 2012;1(1).
16. Oyedeji CI, Welsby IJ. Optimizing management of sickle cell disease in patients undergoing surgery. Hematology (United States). 2021;2021(1).
17. Guyer D, Reagan J, Jennings E, Eskridge P, Cherenzia K. Crisis no more: promoting patient-centered care for patients with sickle cell disease and the integration of palliative care into the multidisciplinary team (SA306). J Pain Symptom Manage. 2022;63(5).
18. Vichinsky EP, Neumayr LD, Haberkern C, Earles AN, Eckman J, Koshy M, et al. The peri-operative complication rate of orthopedic surgery in sickle cell disease: Report of the national sickle cell surgery study group. Am J Hematol. 1999;62(3).
19. Earl J, Neumayr L, Aguilar C, Donthineni R, Quirolo K, Treadwell M, et al. Clinical vignette—avascular necrosis of the femoral head in a 7 year old with sickle cell disease. Am J Hematol. 2011;86.
20. Stephens CG, Scott RB. Cholelithiasis in Sickle Cell Anemia: Surgical or Medical Management. Arch Intern Med. 1980;140(5).
21. Al-Salem AH. Indications and complications of splenectomy for children with sickle cell disease. J Pediatr Surg. 2006;41(11).
22. Adesina O, Brunson A, Keegan THM, Wun T. Osteonecrosis of the femoral head in sickle cell disease: prevalence, comorbidities, and surgical outcomes in California. Blood Adv. 2017;1(16).
23. Walker I, Trompeter S, Howard J, Williams A, Bell R, Bingham R, et al. Guideline on the peri-operative management of patients with sickle cell disease: Guideline from the Association of Anaesthetists. Anaesthesia. 2021;76(6):805–17.
24. Nnodu O, Madu A, Chianumba R, Isa HA, Olanrewaju I, Osagie S, et al. Establishing a database for sickle cell disease patient mapping and survival tracking: The sickle pan-African research consortium Nigeria example. Front Genet. 2022;13.
25. Khurmi N, Gorlin A, Misra L. Perioperative considerations for patients with sickle cell disease: a narrative review. Can J Anesth. 2017;64(8).
26. Brennan-Cook J, Bonnabeau E, Harris-Bloom H, Tanabe P. Improving the care of individuals with sickle cell disease in the emergency department using a quality improvement framework: the emergency department sickle cell assessment of needs and strengths (ed-scans). Adv Emerg Nurs J. 2019;41(3).
27. Masese RV, Bulgin D, Douglas C, Shah N, Tanabe P. Barriers and facilitators to care for individuals with sickle cell disease in central North Carolina: the emergency department providers' perspective. PLoS One. 2019;14(5).
28. Chou R, Gordon DB, De Leon-Casasola OA, Rosenberg JM, Bickler S, Brennan T, et al. Management of postoperative pain: A clinical practice guideline from the American pain society, the American society of regional anesthesia and pain medicine, and the American Society of Anesthesiologists' Committee on regional anesthesia, executive committee, and administrative council. J Pain. 2016;17(2):131–57.
29. Azbell RCG, Lanzkron SM, Desai PC. Current evidence and rationale to guide perioperative management, including transfusion decisions. In: Patients with sickle cell disease. Anesthesia and Analgesia, vol. 136. Lippincott Williams and Wilkins; 2023. p. 1107–14.

30. Ballas SK, Darbari DS. Review/overview of pain in sickle cell disease. In: Complementary therapies in medicine, vol. 49. Churchill Livingstone; 2020.
31. Joshi GP, Abdelmalak BB, Weigel WA, Harbell MW, Kuo CI, Soriano SG, et al. American Society of Anesthesiologists Practice Guidelines for Preoperative Fasting: carbohydrate-containing clear liquids with or without protein, chewing gum, and pediatric fasting duration—a modular update of the 2017 American Society of Anesthesiologists Practice Guidelines for Preoperative Fasting. Anesthesiology. 2023;138(2):132–51.
32. Jaeckel R, Thieme M, Czeslick E, Sablotzki A. The use of partial exchange blood transfusion and anaesthesia in the management of sickle cell disease in a perioperative setting: two case reports. J Med Case Rep. 2010;4.
33. Khalaf Z, Mahmood M. Acute chest syndrome in post-operative sickle cell disease patients: a systematic review of predisposing factors and interventions. Surg Pract Sci. 2022;11:100143.
34. Delatte SJ, Hebra A, Tagge EP, Jackson S, Jacques K, Othersen HB. Acute chest syndrome in the postoperative sickle cell patient. J Pediatr Surg 1999.
35. Dampier C, Palermo TM, Darbari DS, Hassell K, Smith W, Zempsky W. AAPT diagnostic criteria for chronic sickle cell disease pain. J Pain. 2017;18(5):490–8.
36. Osunkwo I, O'Connor HF, Saah E. Optimizing the management of chronic pain in sickle cell disease. Hematology (United States). 2020;20(1).
37. Sinha CB, Bakshi N, Ross D, Krishnamurti L. Management of chronic pain in adults living with sickle cell disease in the era of the opioid epidemic a qualitative study. JAMA Netw Open. 2019;2(5).
38. Smith WR, Penberthy LT, Bovbjerg VE, Mcclish DK, Roberts JD, Dahman B, et al. Daily assessment of pain in adults with sickle cell disease [Internet]. 2008. Available from: https://annals.org
39. Brandow AM, Carroll CP, Creary S, Edwards-Elliott R, Glassberg J, Hurley RW, et al. American Society of Hematology 2020 guidelines for sickle cell disease: Management of acute and chronic pain. Blood advances, vol. 4. American Society of Hematology; 2020. p. 2656–701.
40. Haefeli M, Elfering A. Pain assessment. Eur Spine J 2006;15.
41. Fink R. Pain assessment: the cornerstone to optimal pain management. Baylor Univ Med Center Proc. 2000;13(3):236–9.
42. Tawfic QA, Faris AS, Kausalya R. The role of a low-dose ketamine-midazolam regimen in the management of severe painful crisis in patients with sickle cell disease. J Pain Symptom Manage. 2014;47(2):334–40.
43. Agbakwuru U, AuBuchon JD, Toebe B, LaBarge A, Di Paola J, Hulbert ML. Implementation of an intravenous lidocaine guideline for children and adolescents with sickle cell vaso-occlusive pain. Blood 2021;138(Supplement 1)
44. Karsenty C, Tubman VN, Liu C jy J, Fasipe T, Wyatt KEK. Regional anesthesia for sickle cell disease vaso-occlusive crisis: a single-center case series. Pediatr Blood Cancer. 2022;69(6).
45. Rizvi MB, Kessler DO, Rabiner JE. Role of regional anesthesia in patients with acute sickle cell pain: a scoping review. Pediatric blood and cancer, vol. 70. John Wiley and Sons Inc.; 2023.
46. Labbe E, Hebert D, Haynes J. Labbe-et-al-2005-physicians-attitude-and-practices-in-sickle-cell-disease-pain-management. J Palliat Care. 2005;21(4):246–51.
47. Martinez RM, Osei-Anto HA, McCormick M, editors. Addressing sickle cell disease: a strategic plan and blueprint for action. Washington D.C.: National Academies Press; 2020 [cited 2024 Jan 31]. Available from: https://www.ncbi.nlm.nih.gov/books/NBK566459/

Peripartum Pain Management

Jarna Shah, Kristin Swope, Sudheer Potru, and Sejal Tamakuwala

Abstract In 2021, the US had over 3.6 million deliveries, of which 32% were via Cesarean delivery. Improved monitoring and anesthetic techniques have improved the safety of peripartum care, enabling patients with more complex cardiopulmonary conditions to become pregnant. Each of these factors contribute to an increasing complexity of patients presenting to the labor and delivery ward each day. The accompanying fetal changes of pregnancy complicating these patients' comorbidities makes labor pain management inherently challenging. In this chapter, we present strategies for managing peripartum pain in complex situations.

Keywords Pregnancy · Opioid use disorder · Pain · Obstetric analgesia · Postpartum pain

---

J. Shah
Department of Anesthesiology, University of Arkansas for Medical Sciences, Little Rock, AR, USA
e-mail: jshah2@uams.edu

K. Swope · S. Tamakuwala (✉)
Department of Gynecology and Obstetrics, Emory University School of Medicine, Atlanta, GA, USA
e-mail: sejal.tamakuwala@emory.edu

K. Swope
e-mail: kristin.i.swope@emory.edu

S. Potru
Complex Pain Clinic, Atlanta VA Healthcare System, East Point, GA, USA

Department of Anesthesiology, Emory University School of Medicine, Atlanta, GA, USA

S. Potru
e-mail: sudheer.potru@emory.edu

A. Abd-Elsayed and K. Schroeder (eds.), *Perioperative Pain Management*,
https://doi.org/10.1007/978-3-031-67648-2_25

1 Introduction

In 2021, the US had over 3.6 million deliveries, of which 32% were via Cesarean delivery [1]. In concert, advancing reproductive technologies are allowing for pregnancy at more advanced ages while unplanned pregnancies and obesity rates in pregnancy are rising rapidly. Improved monitoring and anesthetic techniques have improved the safety of peripartum care, enabling patients with more complex cardiopulmonary conditions to become pregnant. Each of these factors contribute to an increasing complexity of patients presenting to the labor and delivery ward each day. The presence of a fetus and accompanying fetal changes of pregnancy complicating these patients' comorbidities makes labor pain management inherently challenging. In these situations, an anesthesiologist must be well-versed in available analgesic modalities to optimize pain control and prevent maternal morbidity and mortality, the latter of which is at an all-time high in the United States [2]. In this chapter, we present strategies for managing peripartum pain in both routine and complex situations.

At baseline, there is a significant female predominance in both episodic and chronic pain syndromes among women of reproductive age, including chronic abdominal and pelvic pain, migraines, fibromyalgia, and several other painful conditions [3]. A study of 1.1 million women found that one in five pregnant patients (21.6%) enrolled in Medicaid filled at least one opioid prescription during pregnancy, although there were pronounced regional and racial variations in dispensation patterns; the majority of these prescriptions were for hydrocodone or codeine [4]. Common indications included abdominal pain, back pain, headaches, or joint pain [4]. Several confounding pain factors during pregnancy and delivery include premature labor pain, contractions, changes in ligamentous laxity, anxiety, stress, depression, and physiologic and hormonal changes. Medication options during pregnancy are few, due to concern for teratogenic effects and limited safety data. Fluoroscopic injections for chronic pain are also contraindicated. These challenges all make treating pain during pregnancy more complex and challenging. Implications of poor acute pain management during labor include the concerns for opioid use and opioid use disorder, development of chronic pain syndromes, and trauma associated with the birthing experience.

2 Intrapartum Pain Management

During labor and delivery, pregnant patients experience significant pain, and it is important to understand the various mechanisms through which pain is caused. Labor is divided in three stages. The first stage consists of uterine cervical dilation caused by rhythmic contractions which can be further categorized into passive (0 to 5 cm dilation) and active stage (6 to 10 cm dilation). Contractions are generally irregular/less frequent during the passive stage and regular/more frequent during the active stage. The second and third stages of labor consist of expulsion of the fetus and placenta respectively. Pain caused during the first stage of labor is visceral and a result of uterine contractions compressing the myometrial blood vessels and causing localized hypoxia. The C-fibers in the myometrial tissue transmit the nociceptive stimuli to the ipsilateral dorsal roots (T10 to L1) during contractions. While in the second stage of labor, pain results from somatic stimulus, caused by stretching of pelvic, perineal, and vaginal tissue, and transmitted to the spinal roots from S2 to S4 [5, 6]. Pain is a subjective experience, and several physical and psychological factors impact its severity and duration. Maternal age, parity, size of the fetus/position of the fetus in relation to the maternal pelvis, maternal medical conditions are some physical factors [6]. Fear, anxiety, apprehension, family member/birthing companion presence are some of the psychological factors that influence pain during childbirth [6].

Non-pharmacologic pain management options most frequently used include childbirth education, emotional support, massage, aroma therapy, and audio analgesia. Non-pharmacologic interventions requiring specialized training or equipment which are not rigorously studied scientifically are acupuncture/acupressure, hypnosis, TENS, biofeedback, hydrotherapy, and intradermal water injections [6].

Childbirth education is practiced worldwide and, over the years, several studies have been conducted to understand its role in use of analgesia, labor duration, and mode of delivery. The results of such studies are inconsistent and are of poor quality [6]. One systematic review and meta-analysis noted that childbirth education antenatally can reduce maternal stress, improve self-efficacy, lower the cesarean birth rate, and decrease the use of epidural anesthesia, but it is unclear what impact these educational efforts have on maternal/fetal outcomes. Education resources are widely different and these materials require standardization before conclusive statements can be made about actual mental and physical effects [7].

Treating pain in obstetric patients is crucial for optimizing patient comfort and satisfaction during labor. Pain management is generally achieved through the administration of neuraxial or non-neuraxial options including parenteral opioids and nitrous oxide. Parenteral opioids that are commonly used include fentanyl, morphine, nalbuphine, butorphanol, and remifentanil. There is no great evidence demonstrating a substantial benefit of one opioid versus others with regard to side effect profiles such as nausea, vomiting and drowsiness. However, a Cochrane review did conclude that there was generally poor pain relief during labor, which could represent a potential impetus for the delivery of some opioid analgesic [8]. Opioids cross the placenta and drug elimination takes longer in newborns than adults. Patients should be counseled that parenteral opioids are not often used near the time of the delivery due to these effects.

Neuraxial anesthesia includes epidural and spinal techniques. The goal of neuraxial techniques is to provide appropriate analgesia with minimal motor block [9]. Epidural analgesia includes a mixture of medications, which typically includes at least a local anesthetic and often an opioid as well. This medication is administered in either a continuous or repeated fashion through a catheter which is placed into the epidural space. Commonly used local anesthetics include bupivacaine and ropivacaine. Commonly used opioids include lipophilic agents, such as fentanyl and sufentanil, or hydrophilic medications such as morphine. Additionally, epinephrine is often added to a local anesthetic to prolong the duration or increase the density of the block. Table 1 lists a series of combinations that could be used for epidural infusions as well as dosing for related adjunct medications.

Other neuraxial options aside from epidural anesthesia include single-injection spinal anesthesia, continuous spinal analgesia, and combined spinal-epidural anesthesia. A single injection spinal anesthesia is often used for patients when delivery is predicted to occur within an hour or for cesarean delivery. Continuous spinal analgesia allows for rapid onset analgesia to be incrementally extended and confirmed to surgical anesthesia. Similar local anesthetic/opioid solutions are utilized, but the rate of infusion is decreased significantly and slowly titrated. This technique is not often intentionally used because of the high incidence of post dural puncture headaches as well as risk for spinal infection secondary to the indwelling catheter. Third, combined spinal-epidural analgesia consists of Tuohy needle placement in the epidural space followed by spinal needle placement through the Tuohy to pierce the dura and access the intrathecal space. A single intrathecal injection provides rapid onset of analgesia and then, after removal of the spinal needle, an epidural catheter is placed and continuous infusions or bolus dosing can be performed to provide sustained labor analgesia. Alternatively, for a dural puncture epidural, the intrathecal space can be accessed to verify midline placement, as noted by the return of cerebrospinal fluid, and then an epidural catheter is placed. This technique is thought to have an increased rate of analgesic onset as compared to a traditional labor epidural.

Table 1 Labor analgesia doses [10]

Standard dilution instructions	• 0.0625% bupivacaine = 35 mL 0.5% bupivacaine + 250 mL normal saline • 0.1% bupivacaine = 60 mL 0.5% bupivacaine + 250 mL normal saline • 0.1255% bupivacaine = 83 mL 0.5% bupivacaine + 250 mL normal saline
Maximum anesthetic doses (with epinephrine)	• Bupivacaine: 3 mg/kg (3 mg/kg) • Lidocaine 5 mg/kg (7 mg/kg • Ropivacaine 2 mg/kg (2 mg/kg) • 2-chloroprocaine 11 mg/kg (14 mg/kg)
Adjuncts	• Epinephrine 2 mcg/mL • Fentanyl 2 mcg/mL • Clonidine 50–100 mcg bolus, then 1–2 mcg/mL

3 Postpartum Pain Management

Multimodal analgesia is critical for postpartum pain management. Common pain sources following vaginal delivery include uterine cramping, perineal pain from lacerations, and discomfort from hemorrhoids. It is important to address all the sources of pain to treat a postpartum patient effectively. Acetaminophen and nonsteroidal anti-inflammatory medications such as ibuprofen should ideally be scheduled as first line agents. If they are ineffective, then opioids can be added on an as-needed basis. Ice packs, ice gels, and local perineal lidocaine spray can be administered for perineal pain. Bowel regimen and topical agents including astringent, steroid, or anesthetic creams can be used for hemorrhoid pain relief [8, 11].

4 ERAS Protocol for Cesarean Section

Enhanced recovery after cesarean delivery (ERAC) was adopted from the enhanced recovery after surgery (ERAS) protocols with the aim of optimizing patient outcomes using evidence-based methods (Table 2 provides an outline of ERAC components). Per the Society of Obstetric Anesthesia and Perinatology (SOAP) guidelines, preoperative goals of an ERAC protocol include patient education, limiting fasting intervals, nonparticulate carbohydrate loading, lactation and breastfeeding education, and hemoglobin optimization.

Active patient participation in the recovery process is paramount to realizing improved outcomes after surgery; this has been demonstrated in studies on ERAS implementation in various surgical specialties [12]. Patients should be instructed on the details of the procedure, postoperative pain management plan, early feeding and mobilization goals, length of stay, and criteria for discharge. Education should also focus on breastfeeding and lactation support services.

The current practice guidelines for obstetric anesthesia from the American Society of Anesthesiologists (ASA) recommend six to eight hour fasting for solids and clear

Table 2 Perioperative components of ERAC [15]

Preoperative	Intraoperative	Postoperative
• Patient education • Limited fasting interval • Carbohydrate loading	• Prevent and treat spinal induced hypotension • Maintain normothermia • Intraoperative and postoperative nausea and vomiting prophylaxis • Optimal uterotonic administration • Multimodal analgesia • Promote breastfeeding	• Early oral intake • Early mobilization • Promote resting periods • Early urinary catheter removal • Venous thromboembolism prophylaxis • Continue multimodal analgesia • Breastfeeding support • Promote return of bowel function

oral fluid intake up to two hours before the initiation of any anesthetic technique [9]. The intake of a high-caloric carbohydrate drink up to two hours before surgery has been shown to reduce preoperative thirst, hunger, and anxiety in patients undergoing abdominal surgery [13]. It has also been associated with a reduction in insulin resistance and a higher anabolic state postoperatively; both of which are likely to promote positive surgical outcomes.

In terms of intraoperative pain management, neuraxial anesthesia (specifically spinal anesthesia) is preferred for elective cesarean deliveries because it facilitates the presence of a support person, skin-to-skin contact with the newborn, and decreases surgical stress responses. Opioids are usually added to regional anesthetic mixtures because they improve intraoperative anesthesia, prolong its duration, decrease local anesthetic requirements, and provide postoperative analgesia. Short-acting opioids such as fentanyl or sufentanil are often considered better for intraoperative pain management, while long-acting intrathecal and epidural opioids such as morphine are effective for postoperative pain control.

For postoperative pain management, adequate analgesia is integral to implementation of ERAC protocols. Suboptimal analgesia after cesarean delivery is associated with delayed functional recovery, delayed mobilization which could increase the risk of thromboembolic complications, poor maternal bonding with the newborn, breastfeeding difficulties, and an increase in the risk of persistent pain and postpartum depression. Using analgesics with different mechanisms of action is emphasized in ERAS protocols to minimize opioid use and improve pain control while minimizing side effects [12]. The combination includes regional anesthesia, neuraxial opioid analgesics, and oral analgesics. Neuraxial morphine is considered the gold standard for pain management after cesarean delivery. Acetaminophen and non-steroidal anti-inflammatory agents such as ibuprofen have additive effects and they should ideally be scheduled; opioids should be administered on an as-needed basis to optimize analgesia.

Other adjuvants for analgesia after cesarean delivery include fascial plane blocks, local anesthetic wound infiltration, and anesthetic/analgesic infusions such as lidocaine, ketamine, dexmedetomidine, and magnesium. Recently, quadratus lumborum (QL) blocks have come into discussion and these may be considered in patients who are not good candidates for neuraxial analgesia [14].

Components of enhanced recovery after cesarean are detailed in Fig. 1 [14].

ERAS, enhanced recovery after surgery; NPO, *nil per os* (nothing by mouth); PONV, postoperative nausea and vomiting.

5 Pregnant Patients with Opioid Use Disorder

Rates of opioid use disorder (OUD) among pregnant women have increased since 1999 [16]. From 1999–2014, the national prevalence of opioid use disorder increased 333%, from 1.5 cases per 1,000 delivery hospitalizations to 6.5 [16]. For pregnant patients who use opioids for pain, it is important to recognize and differentiate

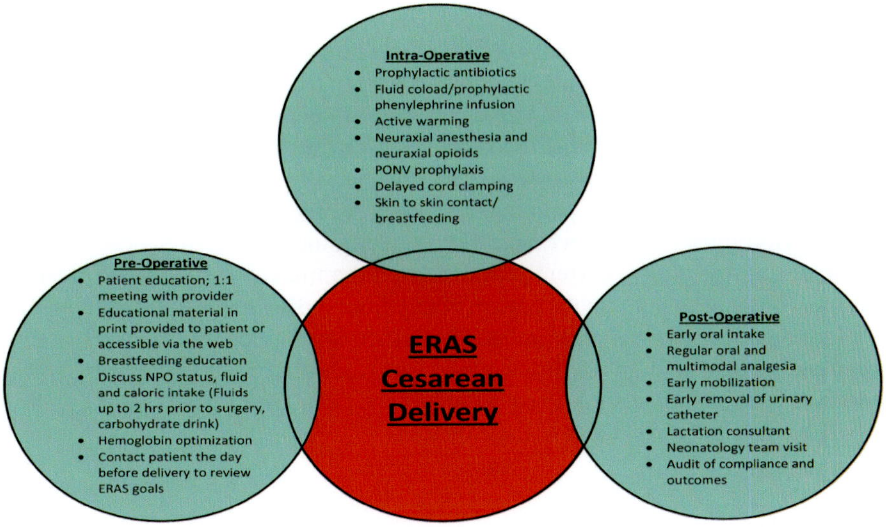

Fig. 1 Enhanced Recovery After Cesarean Delivery

between therapeutic medical opioid use, occasional aberrant behaviors, and untreated opioid use disorder. Pregnant patients with substance use disorders such as OUD face public and political stigma in seeking care, often discouraging them from seeking comprehensive medical care [17].

Treating pain in patients with opioid use disorder requires the consideration of the OUD journey for each individual patient. Patients with long-term sobriety will respond much differently to various anesthetic/analgesic options than those with untreated OUD. In addition, current treatment modalities must be accounted for. Patients with largely untreated OUD may have underlying infections, significant opioid tolerance, and potentially opioid-induced hyperalgesia. These must be considered as they often mandate risk/benefit analysis of catheter placement as well as consideration of non-opioid therapies for pain management.

For vaginal delivery, epidural analgesia should be offered to patients if they have no contraindications. For patients with untreated OUD, long-acting neuraxial opioids such as morphine can be considered in complicated vaginal deliveries or for post-operative pain relief after cesarean sections [18]. Although, evidence does show that patients may need as much as four times the dose required in non-opioid dependent patients [18]. Additionally, withdrawal must be considered in this population of patients, as it can precipitate preterm labor. Neuraxial opioids have not been shown to be as effective in managing opioid withdrawal compared to parenteral or intravenous opioids, although buprenorphine and methadone may be better long-term options for treatment than short-acting, intravenous full opioid agonists [18]. If a pregnant patient is managed with medications for opioid use disorder (MOUD), such as buprenorphine or methadone prior to delivery, those agents should be continued in the intra and postpartum settings.

For planned cesarean delivery in the OUD patient, any neuraxial technique is reasonable, but a combined spinal-epidural may be most optimal for several reasons; the spinal component will quickly provide surgical anesthesia and the epidural catheter placement will allow for treatment of postoperative pain with local anesthetic infusion for a patient whose opioid use may have resulted in substantial receptor upregulation and tolerance to opioids.

The importance of proper pain management for pregnant patients in the perioperative period must be acknowledged. There are limited medications deemed safe for use during pregnancy currently available on the market. Individualized care is necessary to manage pain in this patient population. Individual institutional policies should be evidence based and preferably written with guidance from knowledge experts in the field [19]. In the future, consensus guidelines for management of these patients, in addition to consolidated resources and decreased barriers to access, will be beneficial to the patient and to the care team.

6 Breastfeeding Considerations

Neuraxial opioids for intrapartum pain management have minimal excretion into breast milk and hence are preferred due to minimal effects on the newborn. Parenteral and oral opioids such as morphine, hydromorphone, and fentanyl are excreted into breast milk and thus frequent monitoring of the mother and infant for sedation and respiratory depression is always encouraged. Opioids such as tramadol and codeine are metabolized in the liver by the CYP450 system into morphine to be pharmacologically active. Some patients may be ultrarapid metabolizers, which could lead to supratherapeutic morphine levels. This could lead to sedating levels of morphine in the breast milk and, in extreme cases, respiratory depression and death in the infant. Hence, in 2017, the Food and Drug Administration released a statement recommending against the use of tramadol and codeine in breastfeeding patients [20, 21]. See Table 3 for a non-exhaustive list of agents used in pregnant and postpartum patients and their safety regarding breastfeeding.

Key Takeaways

- Neuraxial anesthesia remains the gold standard for pain management in the laboring patient.
- Multimodal analgesia is critical for postpartum pain management. Most common pain sources after vaginal delivery are uterine cramping, perineal pain from lacerations, and discomfort from hemorrhoids. It is important to address all the sources of pain to effectively treat a postpartum patient. Enhanced Recovery After Cesarean (ERAC) protocols aim to optimize patient outcomes using evidence-based methods.
- Proper pain management for the pregnant person with OUD requires adequate planning, collaboration with all involved parties, and should involve continuation of the patient's prior MOUD.

Table 3 Anesthetic and Analgesic medication safety for breastfeeding mothers [22–25]

Medication	Safe to administer for anesthesia	Safe to breastfeed when awake/alert	Consider pause in breastfeeding
Midazolam	Yes	Yes	Not needed
Propofol	Yes	Yes	Not needed
Etomidate	Yes	Yes	Not needed
Ketamine	Unknown	Unknown	Unknown (so yes)
Volatile anesthetics	Yes	Yes	Not needed
Fentanyl	Yes	Yes	Not needed
Remifentanil	Likely yes	Likely yes	Not needed
Morphine (IV)	Yes	Probably, but need dose discretion	Likely not needed if potency controlled
Hydromorphone (IV)	Yes	Probably, but need dose discretion	Likely not needed if potency controlled
Morphine (epidural)	Yes	Yes	Likely not needed
Meperidine	No	No	Yes
Codeine	N/A	No (due to potential for ultrarapid metabolism)	Yes
Tramadol	N/A	No (due to potential for ultrarapid metabolism)	Yes
NMBAs (depolarizing and non-depolarizing)	Yes	Yes	Not needed
NMBA Reversal Agents	Yes	Yes	Not needed
Lidocaine	Yes	Yes	Not needed
Bupivacaine	Yes	Yes	Not needed
Ondansetron	Yes	Yes	Not needed
Dexamethasone	Yes	Yes	Not needed

- Some pain medications during breastfeeding are minimally excreted into the breastmilk and are therefore safe to use during the postpartum period. Caution should be maintained in attending to the newborn's level of sedation and respiratory depression. Codeine and Tramadol are contraindicated during breastfeeding.

References

1. FastStats [Internet]. Available from: https://www.cdc.gov/nchs/fastats/delivery.htm (2023). Accessed16 Sep 2023.
2. Maternal Mortality Rates in the United States, 2021 [Internet]. Available from: https://www.cdc.gov/nchs/data/hestat/maternal-mortality/2021/maternal-mortality-rates-2021.htm (2023). Accessed16 Sep 2023.
3. Pavlović JM, Derby CA. Pain in midlife women: a growing problem in need of further research. Womens Midlife Health. 2022;8(1):4.
4. Desai RJ, Hernandez-Diaz S, Bateman BT, Huybrechts KF. Increase in prescription opioid use during pregnancy among medicaid-enrolled women. Obstet Gynecol. 2014;123(5):997–1002.
5. Melillo A, Maiorano P, Rachedi S, Caggianese G, Gragnano E, Gallo L, et al. Labor analgesia: a systematic review and meta-analysis of non-pharmacological complementary and alternative approaches to pain during first stage of labor. Crit Rev Eukaryot Gene Expr. 2022;32(2):61–89.
6. Wong CA. Advances in labor analgesia. Int J Womens Health. 2010;1:139–54.
7. Hong K, Hwang H, Han H, Chae J, Choi J, Jeong Y, et al. Perspectives on antenatal education associated with pregnancy outcomes: systematic review and meta-analysis. Women Birth J Aust Coll Midwives. 2021;34(3):219–30.
8. ACOG Practice Bulletin No. 209: Obstetric analgesia and anesthesia. Obstet Gynecol. 2019;133.(3): e208.
9. Practice Guidelines for Obstetric, Anesthesia. An updated report by the american society of anesthesiologists task force on obstetric anesthesia and the society for obstetric anesthesia and perinatology*. Anesthesiol. 2016;124(2):270–300.
10. Schellenberg AG. Anesthesiology pocket guide. Anesth Analg. 1999;88(1):236.
11. Hedayati H, Parsons J, Crowther CA. Topically applied anaesthetics for treating perineal pain after childbirth. Cochrane Database Syst Rev. 2005;(2):CD004223.
12. Kalogera E, Dowdy SC. Enhanced recovery pathway in gynecologic surgery: improving outcomes through evidence-based medicine. Obstet Gynecol Clin North Am. 2016;43(3):551–73.
13. Hausel J, Nygren J, Lagerkranser M, Hellström PM, Hammarqvist F, Almström C, et al. A carbohydrate-rich drink reduces preoperative discomfort in elective surgery patients. Anesth Analg. 2001;93(5):1344–50.
14. Ituk U, Habib AS. Enhanced recovery after cesarean delivery [Internet]. F1000Research. Available from: https://f1000research.com/articles/7-513 (2018). Accessed16 Sep 2023.
15. Patel K, Zakowski M. Enhanced recovery after cesarean: current and emerging trends. Curr Anesthesiol Rep. 2021;11(2):136–44.
16. Haight SC. Opioid Use Disorder Documented at Delivery Hospitalization—United States, 1999–2014. MMWR Morb Mortal Wkly Rep [Internet]. 2018 [cited 2023 Sep 16];67. Available from: https://www.cdc.gov/mmwr/volumes/67/wr/mm6731a1.htm (2018). Accessed16 Sep 2023.
17. Stone R. Pregnant women and substance use: fear, stigma, and barriers to care. Health Just. 2015;3(1):2.
18. Soens MA, He J, Bateman BT. Anesthesia considerations and post-operative pain management in pregnant women with chronic opioid use. Semin Perinatol. 2019;43(3):149–61.
19. Shah JR, Ramseyer A, Coker J. Peripartum management for women with opioid dependence. Curr Opin Anaesthesiol. 2021;34(3):226–32.
20. Koren G, Cairns J, Chitayat D, Gaedigk A, Leeder SJ. Pharmacogenetics of morphine poisoning in a breastfed neonate of a codeine-prescribed mother. The Lancet. 2006;368(9536):704.
21. Research C for DE and. Use of Codeine and Tramadol Products in Breastfeeding Women—Questions and Answers. FDA [Internet]. Available from: https://www.fda.gov/drugs/postmarket-drug-safety-information-patients-and-providers/use-codeine-and-tramadol-products-breastfeeding-women-questions-and-answers (2019). Accessed16 Sep 2023.

22. Cobb B, Liu R, Valentine E, Onuoha O. Breastfeeding after anesthesia: a review for anesthesia providers regarding the transfer of medications into breast Milk. Transl Perioper Pain Med. 2015;1(2):1–7.
23. Lee AI, McCarthy RJ, Toledo P, Jones MJ, White N, Wong CA. Epidural labor analgesia-fentanyl dose and breastfeeding success: a randomized clinical trial. Anesthesiol. 2017;127(4):614–24.
24. Dalal PG, Bosak J, Berlin C. Safety of the breast-feeding infant after maternal anesthesia. Paediatr Anaesth. 2014;24(4):359–71.
25. Drugs and Lactation Database (LactMed®). National Institute of Child Health and Human Development (2006).

Perioperative Pain Management for Chest Wall Procedures

Christopher R. Cowart, Benjamin Hull, Dennis J. Warfield, Shane Barre, and Sanjib Adhikary

Abstract Fascial plane blocks involve injecting local anesthetic between myofascial tissue layers to target multiple nerves or nerve branches. Initially, these blocks were primarily utilized in breast surgery. Recently, they have demonstrated efficacy in both thoracic and cardiac surgery, thus are now being accepted into perioperative analgesic plans. Effective fascial plane blocks for surgeries involving the chest wall include the Pectoralis I and II (PECS I and II), Serratus Anterior Plane (SAP), Erector Spinae Plane (ESP), Transversus Thoracis Plane (TTP), Pectointercostal Fascial Plane (PIF), Retrolaminar Block (RLB), Midpoint Transverse Process to Pleura (MTP), Rhomboid Intercostal Block (RIB), and Rhomboid Intercostal Sub-Serratus (RISS) blocks. Of note, in order to help standardize nomenclature in regional anesthesia, several of these blocks have undergone name changes during the ASRA-ESRA Delphi consensus in 2021 (El-Boghdadly et al. in Reg Anesth Pain Med 46:571–580, 2021 [1]). PECS I blocks are now referred to as Interpectoral Plane blocks and PECS II blocks are now referred to as Pectoserratus Plane blocks. PIF and TTP blocks are now referred to as Superficial and Deep Parasternal Intercostal

C. R. Cowart
Department of Anesthesiology and Perioperative Medicine, Division of Cardiovascular Anesthesiology, Milton S. Hershey Medical Center, Pennsylvania State University College of Medicine, Hershey, PA, USA
e-mail: ccowart@pennstatehealth.psu.edu

B. Hull
Milton S. Hershey Medical Center, Pennsylvania State University College of Medicine, Hershey, PA, USA
e-mail: bhull@pennstatehealth.psu.edu

D. J. Warfield · S. Barre · S. Adhikary (✉)
Department of Anesthesiology and Perioperative Medicine, Division of Regional Anesthesia and Acute Pain Medicine, Milton S. Hershey Medical Center, Pennsylvania State University College of Medicine, 500 University Drive, Hershey, PA 17033, USA
e-mail: sadhikary1@pennstatehealth.psu.edu

D. J. Warfield
e-mail: dwarfield@pennstatehealth.psu.edu

S. Barre
e-mail: sbarre@pennstatehealth.psu.edu

A. Abd-Elsayed and K. Schroeder (eds.), *Perioperative Pain Management*,
https://doi.org/10.1007/978-3-031-67648-2_26

Plane blocks, respectively. The RIP and RISS blocks have since been lumped together as the RIP block while the MTP block has been renamed as one of the Intertransverse Process blocks. The old nomenclature will mostly be referred to in this chapter, as most of the research articles mentioned took place prior to the nomenclature change. These blocks have been shown to reduce postoperative pain scores, intraoperative and postoperative opioid requirements, need for rescue analgesia, and postoperative nausea and vomiting. In some situations, these blocks have not only been shown to improve postoperative lung function and decrease time to extubation, but also improve patient satisfaction. Due to their utility as a component of multimodal analgesia, fascial plane blocks have the potential to be included in enhanced recovery pathways for surgeries involving the chest wall.

Keywords Pectoralis · Serratus anterior · Erector spinae · Transversus thoracis · Retrolaminar · Rhomboid intercostal sub-serratus

1 Introduction

Fascial plane blocks are regional anesthetic techniques that involve the injection of local anesthesia between two myofascial tissue layers. This technique targets nerves found lying within the desired fascial plane, in contrast to locating and targeting a specific nerve or plexus as performed in other regional anesthesia techniques. Originally, these blocks were performed using surface anatomy landmarks and the tactile feeling of the needle tip penetrating through fascial layers, but they are now performed under ultrasound guidance [2]. Chest wall fascial plane blocks were originally employed in breast surgery, but have recently been adopted in both thoracic and cardiac surgery [3, 4].

Classically, neuraxial and paraneuraxial anesthesia, including thoracic epidurals and paravertebral nerve blocks (PVB), have been used in combination with systemic opioids and adjuncts for multimodal analgesia in thoracic surgery. Thoracic epidurals are efficacious; however, they can be contraindicated in some patients and are subject to complications including hypotension, hematoma, infection, and neurologic injury. PVBs have displayed similar analgesic benefits but can share the same major complications and contraindications as thoracic epidurals. As a result, chest wall fascial plane blocks are frequently utilization in thoracic surgery [3]. In cardiac surgery, postoperative analgesia traditionally has been achieved with large doses of intravenous (IV) opioids. However, this convention has changed as practice patterns shifted towards favoring extubating patients either in the operating room or shortly after admission to the intensive care unit (ICU). Neuraxial anesthesia is not widely accepted as an appropriate analgesia option for patients undergoing cardiac surgery due to increased risk associated with intraoperative systemic heparinization and hemodynamic instability [4]. Ultrasound-guided fascial plane blocks have subsequently been adopted as components of multimodal anesthesia in cardiac surgery and have contributed to the practice of earlier extubation in patients undergoing cardiac surgery [4, 5].

In this chapter the techniques, indications, and recent research involving the use of chest wall fascial plane blocks will be reviewed. These blocks include the Pectoralis I and II (PECS I and II), Serratus Anterior Plane (SAP), Erector Spinae Plane (ESP), Transversus Thoracis Plane (TTP), Pectointercostal Fascial Plane (PIF), Retro-laminar Block (RLB), Midpoint Transverse Process to Pleura (MTP), Rhomboid Intercostal Block (RIB), and Rhomboid Intercostal Sub-Serratus (RISS) blocks.

2 Anterior Chest Wall Blocks

Pectoralis I (Renamed to Interpectoral Plane Block) and Pectoralis I (Renamed to Pectoserratus Plane Block)

Technique

The pectoralis I (PECS I) block was originally described by Blanco in 2011 [6]. The PECS I block targets the medial and lateral pectoral nerves by injecting local anesthetic into the interpectoral fascial plane between the pectoralis major and minor muscles [7]. A modified version of the PECS I block, also known as a pectoralis II (PECS II) block, was then later described by Blanco et al. in 2012 [8]. The PECS II block is a PECS I block with a second deep injection in the fascial plane between the pectoralis minor and serratus anterior muscles, further targeting the lateral cutaneous branches of the intercostal nerves, thoracodorsal nerve, and long thoracic nerve (Fig. 1) [7].

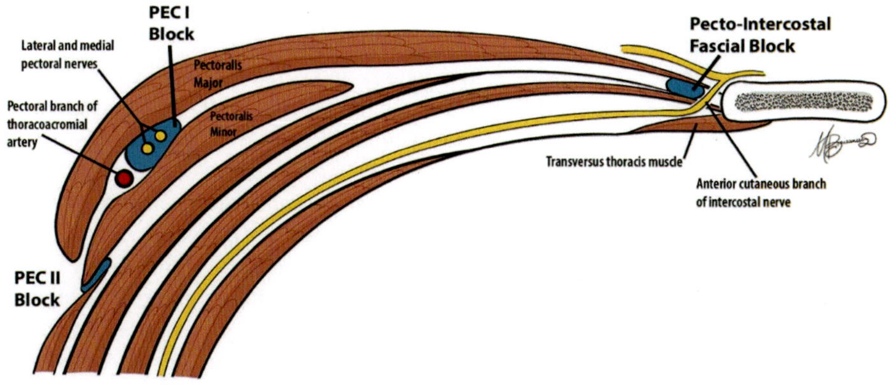

Fig. 1 Image showing relevant anatomy of the anterior chest wall along with injection site locations for PECS I, PECS II, and PIF blocks

To perform the PECS I block, position the patient supine with the ipsilateral arm either at the patient's side or abducted with their head turned to the contralateral side. The plane for this block can be found by placing a straight linear array transducer at the midclavicular parasagittal plane. Identify the pectoralis major and minor muscle, axillary vessels, and pleura. To identify the second and third ribs, slide the transducer inferiorly. The image may be optimized by adjusting the ultrasound probe to be parallel to the deltopectoral groove by rotating the inferior end of the transducer towards the axilla. Insert the needle in-plane or out-of-plane to the ultrasound probe so that the needle tip is within the interpectoral fascia, deep to the pectoralis major and superficial to the pectoralis minor muscle. Inject 1–2 mL of isotonic saline into the interpectoral facia to confirm correct needle placement. After confirming negative aspiration for blood return, inject the desired local anesthetic within the fascial plane [7].

To perform the PECS II block, position the patient and ultrasound transducer as previously described for the PECS I block. The transducer may need to further slide inferiorly towards the mid-axillary line so that the needle tip can be viewed advancing through the pectoralis minor muscle into the fascial plane between the pectoralis minor and serratus anterior muscles. One to two mL of local anesthetic can be injected to confirm the correct plane, followed by the desired dose of local anesthetic after negative aspiration. This block can be performed by either injecting first into the superficial interpectoral fascia then into the deep plane between the pectoralis minor and serratus anterior, or deep-to-superficial. Injecting deep-to-superficial may be preferred, as injecting superficial-to-deep has the potential to result in an unclear ultrasound image of the deep plane by the inadvertent introduction of an air bubble or the downward displacement of the tissue layers from the previous injection [7].

Indications and Recent Research

The PECS I and II blocks have previously been shown to reduce intraoperative and postoperative opioid consumption, the need for postoperative rescue analgesia, postoperative pain scores, and postoperative nausea and vomiting (PONV) in patients undergoing breast surgery [7]. Multiple studies have been conducted that attempt to evaluate the optimal timing and indictions where PECS II block administration optimizes postoperative analgesia.

Ciftci et al. conducted a study in 2021 in which patients undergoing breast augmentation were randomized into a preoperative PECS (pre-group), postoperative PECS (post-group), or control group. They found that the pre-group had significantly lower postoperative opioid consumption at 1, 2, 4, 8, 16, and 24 hours along with significantly lower visual analog scale (VAS) scores at 1, 2, 4, and 8 hours compared to the post-group. Both groups demonstrated significantly lower cumulative opioid and VAS scores at all times compared to the control group [9].

A retrospective cohort study evaluating the PECS II block versus no block on VAS scores and rescue analgesia usage in patients undergoing robot-assisted trans-axillary thyroidectomy showed a PECS II block reduced postoperative pain scores at

10 hours (3.3 ± 2.0 vs. 4.4 ± 2.1; $p = 0.017$) and 25 hours (2.6 ± 1.3 vs. 3.5 ± 1.7, $p = 0.034$); however, there was no statistically significant difference in VAS scores at 4, 20, 35, and 45 hours or in requirements of rescue analgesia [10].

PECS I (Interpectoral Plane) and PECS II (Pectoserratus Plane) Summary

The PECS I and II blocks target the medial and lateral pectoral, lateral intercostal, long thoracic, and thoracodorsal nerves. They are effective fascial plane blocks for analgesia after breast surgery, and reduce intraoperative and postoperative opioid consumption, the need for postoperative rescue analgesia, postoperative pain scores, and PONV. A PECS block administered preoperatively is more effective at reducing postoperative opioid needs and pain scores in breast surgery. PECS I and II blocks have indications beyond breast surgery and may also be utilized in surgical procedures involving the chest wall.

3 Transversus Thoracis Plane Block (Renamed Deep Parasternal Intercostal Plane Block)

Technique

The transversus thoracis plane (TTP) block was originally described by Ueshima and Kitamura in 2015 and has since been renamed to the deep parasternal intercostal plane block [11]. This block targets the anterior cutaneous branches of the second through sixth intercostal nerves in addition to the sympathetic plexus around the internal mammary artery by injecting a local anesthetic into the fascial plane between the internal intercostal and transversus thoracis muscles (Fig. 1) [7].

To perform the deep parasternal intercostal plane block, position the patient either supine or in a semi-inclined position, depending on which is more comfortable for the patient. Use a straight linear array ultrasound transducer and place it on the chest in the parasagittal plane. Use the midclavicular line as a guide and identify the third or fourth rib space and ribs, pleura, pectoralis major, and intercostal muscles. After indentifying ribs, scan in a lateral to medial fashion until the probe is located just lateral to the sternum. Visualize the transversus thoracis muscle deep to the intercostal muscles and superficial to the pleura. Identify the internal thoracic artery running in this plane. Insert the needle in-plane and with a shallow trajectory until the tip is in the fascial plane between the internal intercostal and transversus thoracis muscle. Inject 1–2 mL of normal saline to confirm needle tip placement, and then inject a local anesthetic after negative aspiration for blood [7].

Indications and Recent Research

The TTP block has previously demonstrated usefulness in providing analgesia for surgeries involving the sternum and medial chest, including sternotomy for cardiac surgery and medial breast surgery [7]. Recently, the efficacy of a bilateral TTP block in cardiac surgery has been thoroughly investigated. A systematic review and meta-analysis evaluating ultrasound-guided regional anesthesia in patients undergoing cardiac surgery included patients who received a TTP block. The combination of a TTP block with a SAP block was also evaluated as an option for patients undergoing placement of a subcutaneous implantable cardioverter-defibrillator.

In a double-blinded randomized controlled trial (RCT) in patients undergoing open cardiac surgery, patients who received a bilateral TTP block with 20 mL of 0.4% ropivacaine at the level between the fourth and fifth ribs consumed less intraoperative and postoperative sufentanil when compared to control (74 ± 10mcg vs. 125 ± 30mcg, $p < 0.01$). The block also resulted in lower numeric rating scale (NRS) scores at 1, 2, 4, 6, and 24 hours after extubation, both at rest and with movement ($p < 0.05$) [12].

A systematic review and meta-analysis evaluating the effects of ultrasound-guided regional anesthesia versus placebo in patients undergoing cardiac surgery requiring median sternotomy included five studies investigating the TTP block. Collectively, the TTP block resulted in less opioid consumption compared to no block (MD −10.71 mg, 95% CI −17.08 to −4.33). However, these studies collectively did not show a significant difference in pain scores at 12 and 24 hours after surgery, time to extubation, and ICU length of stay (LOS) when compared to no block [13].

Investigations combining the TTP block with other regional anesthesia techniques have also been conducted. Shariat et al. conducted a small, randomized study with 22 patients comparing the combination of a TTP and SAP block with 0.25% bupivacaine (10 mL and 20 mL, respectively, totaling 30 mL) versus surgical site local anesthetic infiltration with 30 mL of 0.25% bupivacaine in patients undergoing placement of a subcutaneous implantable cardioverter defibrillator (S-ICD). It showed that patients who received a combination TTP-SAP block required less total intraoperative fentanyl compared to surgical site local anesthetic infiltration (45 mcg vs. 90 mcg, $p < 0.026$) [14].

TTP (Deep Parasternal Intercostal Plane) Summary

The TTP block targets the anterior cutaneous branches of the second through sixth intercostal nerves in addition to the sympathetic plexus around the internal mammary artery. It has been shown to provide beneficial analgesia in cardiac and medial breast surgery. A bilateral TTP block may result in less intraoperative and post-operative opioid requirements and lead to lower pain scores in open cardiac surgery. However, a TTP block has not shown reductions in time to extubation or intensive care unit LOS. Combining a TTP block with an SAP block can provide adequate analgesia for patients undergoing S-ICD placement and can reduce total intraoperative fentanyl required compared to those who received only surgical site local anesthetic infiltration.

4 Pectointercostal Fascial Plane Block (Renamed Superficial Parasternal Intercostal Plane Block)

The pectointercostal fascial plane (PIF) block is a potentially safer alternative to the TTP block. The PIF block is performed by injecting local anesthetic in the fascial plane between the pectoralis major and the intercostal muscles directly superficial to the site of injection for a TTP block. Despite being a more superficial block, this technique still manages to anesthetize the anterior branches of the intercostal nerves that are present within the intercostal muscles (Fig. 1) [15]. By utilizing the PIF block, the proceduralist can theoretically decrease overall risk associated with vascular and pericardial puncture, pneumothorax, and local anesthetic systemic toxicity, when compared to TTP.

5 Lateral Chest Wall Blocks

Serratus Anterior Plane Block

Technique

The serratus anterior plane (SAP) block was initially described by Blanco et al. in 2013 [16]. This block targets the long thoracic, thoracodorsal, intercostobrachial, and lateral intercostal nerves by injecting local anesthetic either into the superficial plane created by the latissimus dorsi, teres major, and serratus anterior muscles or into the deep plane created by the serratus anterior and intercostal muscles between the fourth and fifth ribs (Fig. 2) [7].

To perform the SAP block, position the patient supine with their ipsilateral arm abducted. Alternatively, the patient can be placed in the lateral decubitus position with the operative side facing up and the patient's arm flexed forward. Using a straight linear array transducer place the probe in the parasagittal plane inferior to the clavicle. Identify the fourth rib by translating the probe inferiorly. Slide the probe laterally and rotate the inferior end into the midaxillary-to-posterior axillary line to identify the latissimus dorsi and serratus anterior muscles. Insert the needle either in-plane or out-of-plane until the needle tip is within the fascial plane either superficial or deep to the serratus anterior muscle. Inject 1–2 mL of normal saline to confirm the correct placement, followed by local anesthetic after negative aspiration for blood [7].

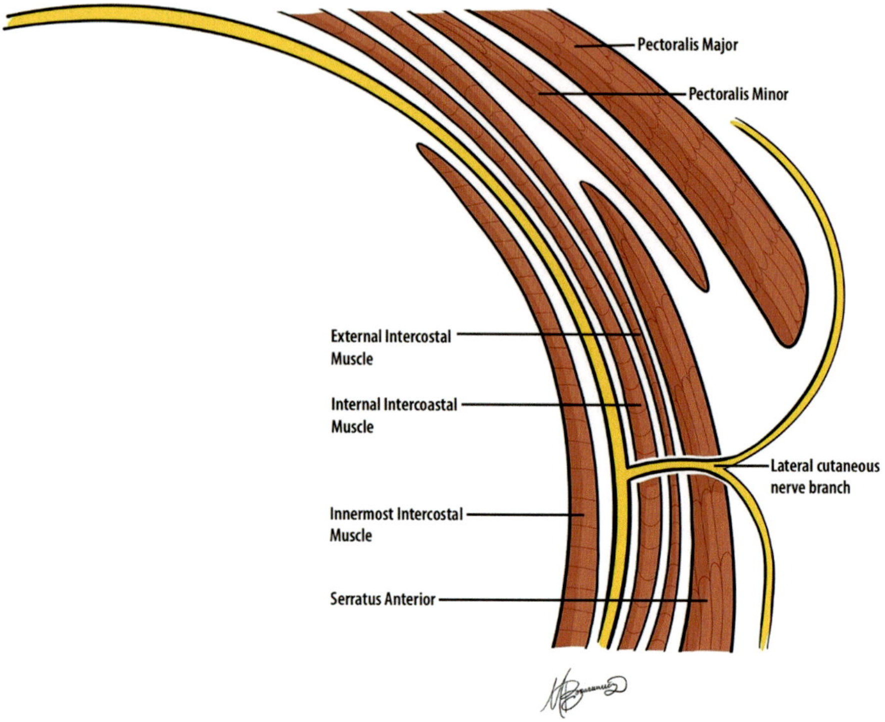

Fig. 2 Image showing relevant anatomy of the lateral chest wall

Indications and Recent Research

The SAP block has displayed efficacy in reducing VAS scores, opioid requirements, and PONV in patients undergoing thoracic surgery [7]. The efficacy and safety profile of the SAP block in pediatric patients undergoing thoracic surgery has been recently studied. The use of a continuous SAP block catheter has also been investigated for patients undergoing video-assisted thoracic surgery (VATS) procedures. In efforts to determine which approach provided more effective analgesia in breast surgery, a comparison study of a superficial versus deep SAP technique was performed. The combination of a SAP with a PECS II block in minimally invasive cardiac surgery and comparisons of the SAP block versus an intercostal nerve block for thoracic surgery also have been evaluated.

A double-blinded RCT performed by Gado et al. investigated the effectiveness and safety of SAP blocks in pediatric patients undergoing thoracotomies. The study demonstrated that pediatric patients undergoing unilateral thoracotomies who received a post-induction SAP block required lower intraoperative (2.1 ± 0.8 mcg/kg vs. 6.9 ± 3.0 mg/kg, $p < 0.001$) and postoperative fentanyl (4.0 ± 1.5mcg.kg vs. 6.3 ± 1.5 mcg/kg, $p < 0.001$) compared to the control, with no significant difference in complication rates. There also was a lengthened time to first rescue analgesia in the SAP block group compared to the control (226.6 ± 73.7 min vs. 64.3 ± 35.8 min, $p < 0.001$) [17].

Gao et al. performed a RCT comparing a continuous SAP block versus an IV sufentanil PCA on the pulmonary function in patients undergoing VATS for lung cancer. Both groups had a substantial decrease in their forced expiratory volume in one second (FEV1), forced vital capacity (FVC), and FEV1/FVC ratio after their procedures ($p < 0.001$). However, patients who received a continuous SAP demonstrated higher postprocedural FEV1, FVC, and FEV1/FVC compared to those with only an opioid PCA ($p < 0.001$). When a subset analysis comparing segmentectomy/lobectomy versus wedge resection was performed, the continuous SAP block group still demonstrated higher postprocedural FEV1, FVC, and FEV1/FVC ($p < 0.05$) [18].

As the SAP block has been described to be performed within both a superficial or deep plane, investigators have set out to examine if there is a superior approach. Edwards et al. conducted a randomized trial with 66 patients comparing a superficial versus a deep SAP block in women undergoing mastectomy. They determined that those who received a deep SAP block required 30% less oral morphine equivalents in the first 24 postoperative hours compared to those who received a superficial block (113.5 mg vs. 147.0 mg, $p = 0.009$) [19].

The SAP block has also been combined with a PECS II block. Torre et al. performed a retrospective cohort study evaluating the combination of a SAP with a PECS II block versus IV opioids alone on postoperative analgesia in patients who underwent mini-thoracotomy for aortic, mitral, or tricuspid valve replacement or atrial myxoma resection. The study revealed critical care pain observation tool (CPOT) scores at 6, 12, and 24 hours after minimally invasive cardiac surgery were lower in the regional group compared to the IV opioids group ($p = 0.0002$; $p = 0.0088$; $p < 0.0001$). The block group also consumed less postoperative sufentanil and morphine ($p < 0.0001$); however, there was not a significant difference in tramadol consumption [20].

When the SAP was compared to an intercostal nerve block in a prospective, double-blinded randomized feasibility trial in patients undergoing VATS there was no statistically significant difference in intraoperative opioid and nonopioid consumption, time to first analgesic request or VAS scores [21].

SAP Summary

The SAP block targets the long thoracic, thoracodorsal, intercostobrachial, and lateral intercostal nerves. It is an effective block in thoracic surgery, as it reduces postoperative pain scores, postoperative opioid needs, and PONV. It can also increase the time until first rescue anesthesia in pediatric patients undergoing unilateral thoracotomies. A continuous SAP block can improve FEV1, FVC, and FEV1/FVC ratios in patients undergoing VATS for lung cancer. Patients who receive a deep SAP block may require less postoperative morphine compared to those who receive a superficial

SAP block. A SAP block can be combined with a PECS II block, and the combination can reduce postoperative pain scores and opioid consumption in patients undergoing minimally invasive cardiac surgery. Patients who receive a SAP block have similar intraoperative opioid needs, time to first analgesic request, and postoperative pain scores as those who receive intercostal nerve blocks for VATS.

6 Posterior Chest Wall Blocks

Erector Spinae Plane Block

Technique

The erector spinae plane (ESP) block was first described by Forero et al. in 2016 [22]. This block targets the dorsal rami of spinal nerves by placing local anesthetic into the posterior chest wall fascial plane between the anterior surface of the erector spinae muscle and the posterior surface of the transverse process of the thoracic vertebrae (Fig. 3) [7]. There has also been shown to be variable and inconsistent anesthetic spread to the ventral rami of spinal nerves via the paravertebral space.

To perform the ESP block, place the patient into the lateral, sitting, or prone position. Use a straight linear or curvilinear array ultrasound transducer dependent on body habitus. Identify the target vertebral level by either counting inferiorly from the C7 spinous process or by using the ultrasound probe to scan inferiorly from the

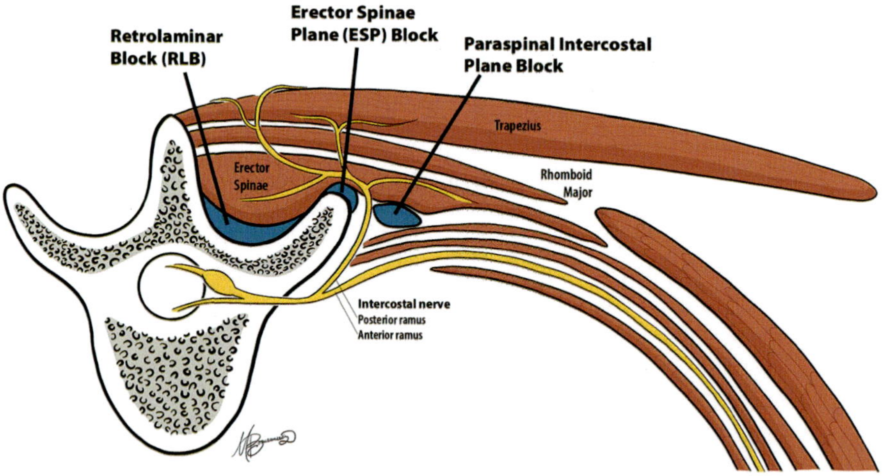

Fig. 3 Image depicting relevant anatomy of the posterior chest wall along with injection site locations of the retrolaminar block (RLB), erector spinae block (ESP) and paraspinal intercostal plane block (PIP)

first rib. Place the transducer in the parasagittal plane approximately 2–3 cm lateral to the spinous process at the desired vertebral level. You can recognize the transverse processes by their "squared-off" appearance versus the "rounded" appearance of the ribs. There will also be a pleural line deep to the ribs. Identify the fascial plane between the anterior surface of the erector spinae muscle and the posterior surface of the transverse processes. Insert the needle either in-plane or out-of-plane to the ultrasound probe. Inserting the needle in-plane and with a shallow trajectory may enhance the ability to effectively open the desired fascial plane or place a catheter. Pass the needle tip into the described fascial plane by skimming off the edge of the desired transverse process and confirm by injecting 1–2 mL of normal saline. Then inject the desired local anesthetic after checking negative aspiration for blood [7].

Indications and Recent Research

The ESP block has been used for analgesia in rib fractures, back surgery, and chest wall procedures including cardiac surgery. The ESP block has previously been shown to reduce VAS scores, intraoperative fentanyl, and postoperative rescue analgesia in epigastric hernia cases. It has demonstrated a reduction in NRS scores as well as opioid rescue analgesia in cardiac surgery and has been associated with improved inspiratory capacity in patients with rib fractures [7]. Further evaluation of the ESP block through systematic reviews and meta-analyses evaluated the effectiveness of the block in cardiac and breast surgery. Additionally, trials comparing the ESP to other techniques, including the PECS II, SAP, thoracic PVB, and intercostal nerve blocks in breast and thoracic surgery have been performed.

Another systematic review and meta-analysis with 861 total patients conducted by Leong et al. compared the ESP to the PECS, PVB, and a control in patients undergoing breast surgery. 147 total patients were in the ESP versus PECS block analysis which revealed that the ESP group required a greater amount of postoperative oral morphine equivalents (MD 14.00 mg, 95% CI 3.91–24.06, $p = 0.007$). 155 total patients were in the ESP versus PVB analysis where there was no significant difference in postoperative oral morphine equivalents consumed (MD −2.15 mg, 95% CI −4.97 to 0.67, $p = 0.14$). Finally, a total of 214 patients were identified in the ESP versus control analysis. There was a significant difference in postoperative oral morphine equivalents consumed in this arm (MD −21.55 mg, 95% CI −23.57 to −10.52, $p = 0.0001$) [23].

Comparisons of ESP blocks to other regional anesthesia techniques have been conducted. A single-blinded RCT compared an ESP block with 0.25% bupivacaine versus PECS II block with 0.25% bupivacaine versus control on postoperative opioid consumption, acute pain, and chronic pain in women undergoing segmental mastectomy with sentinel lymph node biopsy. A total of 95 patients were randomized into the three groups and it was found there was comparable postoperative morphine consumption between the ESP, PECS II and control group, with the control having the highest consumption (4 vs. 3 vs. 5 mg respectively, $p < 0.001$); statistically, yet not clinically significant. Intraoperative remifentanil consumption was also similar between the ESP and PECS II blocks group, but higher in the control group (250 mcg vs. 230 mcg vs. 410 mcg, $p < 0.001$). 23% of patients who received either ESP or PECS II blocks had chronic pain at 3 months compared to 70% of patients who endorsed this in the control group ($p < 0.001$) [24].

Another single-blinded RCT compared the ESP versus SAP versus thoracic epidural in patients undergoing posterolateral thoracotomy for lung cancer. There were no patients in the thoracic epidural group who required postoperative morphine, while 88.2% of patients in the SAP and 47% in the ESP group required post-thoracotomy morphine ($p < 0.001$). There was higher total postoperative morphine consumption in the SAP group compared to the ESP and thoracic epidural groups ($p < 0.001$), while the consumption between the ESP and thoracic epidural groups was similar ($p = 1$). Likewise, the SAP group had significantly higher VAS scores in the post-anesthesia care unit (PACU) and 24 hours postoperatively compared to the thoracic epidural group ($p = 0.002$; $p = 0.017$), while the thoracic epidural and ESP groups were comparable [25].

Turhan et al. also conducted a single-blinded randomized study comparing a 0.5% bupivacaine ESP block versus a 0.5% bupivacaine thoracic PVB versus a 0.5% bupivacaine intercostal nerve block in patients undergoing VATS. Patients who received an ESP block had higher static and dynamic VAS scores at 0, 1, 4, 12, and 24 hours postoperatively ($p < 0.017$) and a higher total amount of morphine compared to the other two groups ($p < 0.017$). There were similar postoperative mobilization times between the ESP, thoracic PVB, and intercostal nerve block groups (4.94 $\pm$ 0.82 hours vs. 5.04 $\pm$ 0.64 vs. 4.98 $\pm$ 0.67 hours, $p > 0.05$). There were also no significant differences in LOS between the groups (4.00 $\pm$ 1.08 days vs. 3.80 $\pm$ 1.15 $\pm$ days vs. 4.05 $\pm$ 1.06 days, $p > 0.05$) [26].

ESP Summary

The ESP block targets the dorsal rami of spinal nerves with variable and inconsistent spread to the ventral rami via the paravertebral space. The block has been shown to reduce pain scores, intraoperative fentanyl requirements, and rescue analgesia requirements in surgeries involving the chest wall and improve inspiratory capacity for rib fractures. An ESP block has not been shown to reduce intensive care LOS or time to extubation in patients undergoing cardiac surgery. When compared to a PECS II block, patients who receive an ESP block may require greater postoperative opioids after breast surgery. An ESP and PVB have displayed similar postoperative opioid requirements in breast surgery. An ESP in thoracic surgery may reduce postoperative morphine requirements and pain scores when compared to an SAP block. An ESP block for VATS may not be as effective at reducing postoperative pain scores and opioid requirements as PVB or intercostal nerve blocks.

7 Retrolaminar Block

Technique

The retrolaminar block (RLB) was first described by Voscopoulous et al. in 2013 [27]. This block is similar to the ESP block as it is still anterior to the erector spinae muscles but is placed more medial to the transverse process and posterior to the lamina of the vertebrae. The same patient positioning and ultrasound scanning technique is used for the RLB as with the ESP block. The lamina of the desired vertebrae is identified on ultrasound by locating the deeper and flatter bony structure between the spinous process and the transverse process. This block targets a similar anesthetic distribution as the ESP (Fig. 3).

Indications and Recent Research

The RLB has demonstrated an ability to provide effective analgesia for rib fractures and breast surgery. The utility of the RLB in thoracic surgery and pediatric patients undergoing cardiac surgery has also been observed.

A double-blinded RCT studying the efficacy of bilateral RLB in pediatric patients undergoing cardiac surgery with median sternotomy revealed that patients who received an RLB required less intraoperative fentanyl (6.9 $\pm$ 2.1 mcg/kg vs. 9.3 $\pm$ 1.2 mcg/kg, $p < 0.001$) and less fentanyl in the first 24 hours after extubation (12.5 $\pm$ 1.4 mcg/kg vs. 16.6 $\pm$ 2.8 mcg/kg, $p < 0.001$). The block group also demonstrated a shorter time to extubation (2. vs. 6 hours, $p < 0.001$), longer time to rescue analgesia after extubation (7 vs. 2 hours, $p < 0.001$), and lower modified objective pain scores at 0, 2, 4, 9, 12, and 16 hours after extubation ($p < 0.05$) [28].

In a randomized study comparing an RLB with a PVB in adult patients undergoing uniport VATS for lung cancer, it was found that NRS scores both at rest and while coughing were lower in patients who received PVB ($p < 0.05$). Total postoperative sufentanil consumption was also lower in the PVB group ($p < 0.001$) while the incidence of postoperative nausea was higher in the RLB group (8 patients vs. 1 patient, $p < 0.05$) [29].

As the RLB is very similar to the ESP block, Sotome et al. conducted a randomized study comparing the two in patients undergoing unilateral mastectomy with sentinel lymph node biopsy. The investigation revealed there was no significant difference in median time to rescue analgesia between patients who received an RLB or ESP block (4.8 hours. [Range 3.0–24 hours] vs. 8.6 h. [Range 2.7—24 hours], $p = 0.8$). There were also no significant differences in intraoperative remifentanil requirements (0.09 mcg/kg/min [SD 0.03] vs. 0.1 mcg/kg/min [SD 0.03], $p = 0.45$) [30].

RLB Summary

The RLB attempts to target the ventral and dorsal rami in addition to the lateral cutaneous and small branches of the intercostal nerves. A continuous RLB has demonstrated effective analgesic effects for rib fractures and breast surgery. It also has been shown to reduce intraoperative and postoperative opioid requirements, shorten time to extubation, and lower pain scores in pediatric patients undergoing cardiac surgery with a medial sternotomy. An RLB may not be as effective as a PVB in reducing pain scores and opioid requirements for patients undergoing VATS. RLB and ESP blocks may be comparable in rescue analgesia and intraoperative opioid needs in patients undergoing breast surgery.

8 Rhomboid Intercostal and Rhomboid Intercostal Sub-Serratus Blocks (Renamed Rhomboid Intercostal Plane Block)

Technique

The rhomboid intercostal block (RIB) and combined rhomboid intercostal and sub-serratus block (RISS) were initially described by Elsharkaway et al. in 2018 and applied in a case study by Kozanhan et al. in 2019 [31, 32]. These blocks target the lateral cutaneous branches of the intercostal nerves with potential spread to the ventral and dorsal rami by performing two injections of local anesthetic into the rhomboid intercostal and sub-serratus spaces. The block is performed by placing the patient in the sitting, lateral, or prone position. A linear array ultrasound is typically used in the parasagittal oblique position and is used to scan in between the spine and scapula at T5-6 to locate the trapezius and rhomboid muscles, deeper ribs, and pleura. To perform the RIB, the needle is then advanced in-plane into the fascial plane between the rhomboid muscle and intercostal muscles. Local anesthetic can then be injected after confirming spread with saline and confirming negative aspiration for blood. In patients receiving a RISS, an additional injection is performed in a more caudal and lateral location between the serratus anterior and external intercostal muscles at T8-9.

Indications and Recent Research

The RIB and RISS blocks have been previously used for analgesia after lung transplants and rib fractures. Multiple studies have evaluated the efficacy of an RIB block in isolation, RIB versus RISS, and the role of these blocks compared to PECS II,

SAP, and ESP blocks. The efficacy of a continuous RISS block for postoperative analgesia in thoracic surgery has also been evaluated.

A randomized trial comparing the effectiveness of a continuous RIB versus PCA with IV sufentanil for postoperative analgesia in patients who underwent unilateral VATS was conducted with 66 patients. Patients who were randomized to the RIB group had a catheter placed in the fascial plane between the rhomboid and intercostal muscles at the level of T5 under ultrasound guidance and 0.2% ropivacaine was administered continuously into the fascial plane. It was found that patients who received the continuous RIB reported higher global quality recovery scores (QoR-40) ($p < 0.001$), lower postoperative NRS scores at rest at 6, 12, and 24 hours ($p < 0.05$), and lower postoperative NRS scores while moving at 3, 6, 12, 18, 24, and 36 hours ($p < 0.05$) compared to patients who received only an opioid PCA [33]. Chen et al. conducted a meta-analysis involving four RCTs, with a total of 216 patients, investigating the analgesia of a RIB in patients undergoing both breast and thoracoscopic surgery. The study revealed that patients who received the RIB versus those who received no block reported lower NRS scores at rest at 0–1 and 6–8 hours after surgery ($p < 0.05$). There was no significant difference in NRS scores at 24 hours ($p = 0.77$). Patients in the RIB groups also required less postoperative opioids (MD −57.52 mcg, 95% CI −106.03 to −9.02, $p < 0.05$) and had a lower incidence of PONV (10.30% vs. 34.60%, OR 0.212, 95% CI 0.100 to 0.447) [34].

Studies have also compared the RIB to other fascial plane blocks, including the PECS II, SAP, and ESP blocks. A prospective RCT compared the analgesic effect of postoperative RIB versus postoperative PECS II versus a control group in patients undergoing breast surgery. The study found there was no significant difference in postoperative fentanyl requirements between patients who received a RIB or a PECS II block, but both block groups required less opioid than the control group (29mcg vs. 20mcg vs. 92.67mcg, $p < 0.001$). There were also no significant differences in VAS scores in patients who received either block [35]. Another RCT compared ultrasound-guided RIB, SAP, and ESP blocks for analgesia status post VATS. The study revealed that patients who had either a RIB or an ESP block required less sufentanil in the first 12 hours after surgery than those who received an SAP block (35.2 ± 2.8 mg vs. 35.4 ± 2.8 mg vs. 43.3 ± 2.7 mg, $p < 0.001$). Similarly, patients who received either a RIB or an ESP block consumed less sufentanil in the first 12–24 hours after surgery than those who received an SAP block ($p < 0.001$), while there were no significant differences between the three groups after 24 hours ($p = 0.192$). The postoperative dynamic NRS scores at 6, 12, 18, and 24 hours were also significantly lower in both the RIB and ESP groups compared to the SAP block group ($p < 0.05$) [36].

While the effectiveness of the RIB has been well documented, additional studies have evaluated the potential differences in efficacy between RIB and RISS blocks. Deng et al. conducted an RCT with 90 patients in 2021 comparing the RIB versus RISS block in patients undergoing VATS. It was found that patients who received a RISS block required less postoperative sufentanil in the first 24 hours compared to patients who received a RIB alone (51.9 ± 2.2 mcg vs. 58.0 ± 3.4 mcg, $p < 0.001$). NRS scores at 12, 18, and 24 hours after surgery were also lower in those who received the RISS block ($p < 0.05$). The time to first postoperative rescue analgesic was longer in the RISS group compared to the RIB group ($p < 0.001$). However, differences in patient satisfaction scores did not show statistical significance between the two blocks [37].

Since more recent studies have demonstrated that a RISS block is more effective than a RIB alone, further investigations have focused on evaluating the RISS block. Kozanhan et al. conducted a randomized trial in 2022 evaluating the analgesic efficacy of a continuous RISS block placed under direct visualization of a thoracic surgeon before surgical site closure and compared it to an IV opioid PCA in patients undergoing VATS. The study demonstrated that NRS scores both at rest and while coughing were lower in patients who received the continuous RISS compared to opioid PCA ($p < 0.001$). Postoperative tramadol consumption in both the first 24 and 48 hours was lower in patients who received the RISS block compared to control (65.0 ± 23.28 mg vs. 174.0 ± 33.78 mg, $p < 0.001$; 178.0 ± 45.38 mg vs. 309.0 ± 67.89 mg. $p < 0.001$). When lung function in each group was compared to each patient's baseline, the RISS group demonstrated higher FEV1 ($p = 0.0047$) and FVC ($p = 0.04$) than those who received an opioid PCA. Patient satisfaction scores were also higher in the RISS group ($p < 0.001$) with similar rates of PONV between both groups [38].

RIB and RISS Summary

The RIB and RISS blocks aim to target both the ventral and dorsal rami of thoracic intercostal nerves. They have been previously used as regional techniques for lung transplants and rib fractures. A RIB alone can reduce postoperative pain scores and opioid requirements in patients undergoing VATS and breast surgery. A RIB compared to a PECS II has shown similar postoperative opioid requirements and pain scores in breast surgery. When compared to an ESP, the RIB has demonstrated similar postoperative opioid requirements and pain scores, while more effective than a SAP block. Regarding a RIB or a RISS for VATS, a RISS can result in fewer postoperative opioid requirements, rescue analgesics, and lower pain scores. A continuous RISS block placed under direct visualization of a surgeon for VATS can reduce pain scores and postoperative opioid requirements while increasing FEV1 and FEVC when compared to an IV opioid PCA.

9 Mid-Point Transverse Process to Pleura Block (Renamed Intertransverse Process Block)

Technique

The mid-point transverse process to pleura (MTP) block was originally described by Costache in 2017 as an alternative to the PVB [39]. It is performed with the patient in the sitting, lateral, or prone position. A linear array or curvilinear ultrasound probe may be used to identify the transverse processes of the vertebrae, using the same scanning technique as with an ESP block. Local anesthetic is injected midway between the transverse process of the vertebrae and the pleura after confirming negative aspiration of blood. By injecting in this exact location, it has been claimed the local anesthetic will penetrate the superior costotransverse ligament and subsequently reach the paravertebral space [40].

Indications and Recent Research

The MTP block has been shown to be of benefit to patients in both the surgical and non-surgical population. The most common indication for an MTP block in a non-surgical setting is in patients presenting with rib fractures [41]. This approach is typically taken when there are contraindications to placing a thoracic epidural or performing a PVB. As such, the MTP block should be considered in patients with rib fractures on anticoagulation or in whom the aforementioned options have proven technically difficult to perform or unsuccessful. In the surgical population, MTP blocks have been proven to provide significant levels of post-operative analgesia in patients undergoing a wide array of chest wall procedures ranging from mastectomies and lymph node dissections [42] to minimally invasive thoracoscopic procedures [40]. In addition to first describing the MTP block in 2017, Costache and colleagues were also the first to describe using the MTP block for complete surgical anesthesia [43]. This ability to provide full surgical anesthesia is one of the benefits of the MTP block that has set it apart from the ESP block in many cases. The ability of the MTP block to provide more reliable and predictable surgical anesthesia is likely due to a more consistent amount of paravertebral spread when compared to the ESP block [43].

Summary

The MTP block has been described as a safe alternative to the PVB in a variety of patients. The MTP block has shown promising results in patients presenting with a wide array of chest wall pain ranging from rib fractures [41] to those experiencing postoperative pain from invasive chest wall surgery [42].

10 Conclusion

Chest wall fascial plane blocks can provide effective analgesia in patients undergoing breast, thoracic, and cardiac surgery. Anesthesiologists have several options, and depending on the surgery, certain blocks may be more efficacious than others. Combinations of these blocks have also been shown to be effective in providing another method for anesthesiologists to plan for patient-specific analgesia. Fascial plane blocks have the potential to be included in several enhanced recovery pathways for surgeries involving the chest wall due to various perioperative benefits.

Key Takeaway Points

1. Fascial plane blocks are a relatively simple, effective means of providing pain control in several types of chest wall surgery.
2. Surgical anesthesia has been demonstrated with some fascial plane blocks, and can be used in patients in which general anesthesia is relatively contraindicated.
3. Many fascial plane blocks can be used in combination with one another to improve their effectiveness and to improve overall block coverage.
4. Fasical plane blocks play a large role in enhanced recovery pathways by broadening the scope of options related to perioperative analgesia.

References

1. El-Boghdadly K, Wolmarans M, Stengel AD, et al. Standardizing nomenclature in regional anesthesia: an ASRA-ESRA Delphi consensus study of abdominal wall, paraspinal, and chest wall blocks. Reg Anesth Pain Med. 2021;46:571–80. https://doi.org/10.1136/rapm-2020-102451.
2. Chin KJ, Versyck B, Elsharkawy H, et al. Anatomical basis of fascial plane blocks. Reg Anesth Pain Med. 2021;46:581–99. https://doi.org/10.1136/rapm-2021-102506.
3. Marciniak D, Kelava M, Hargrave J. Fascial plane blocks in thoracic surgery: a new era or plain painful? Curr Opin Anaesthesiol. 2020;33:1–9. https://doi.org/10.1097/ACO.0000000000000803.
4. Kelava M, Alfirevic A, Bustamante S, et al. Regional anesthesia in cardiac surgery: an overview of fascial plane chest wall blocks. Anesth Analg. 2020;131:127–35. https://doi.org/10.1213/ANE.0000000000004682.
5. Noss C, Prusinkiewicz C, Nelson G, et al. Enhanced recovery for cardiac surgery. J Cardiothorac Vasc Anesth. 2018;32:2760–70. https://doi.org/10.1053/j.jvca.2018.01.045.
6. Blanco R. The "pecs block": a novel technique for providing analgesia after breast surgery. Anaesthesia. 2011;66:847–8. https://doi.org/10.1111/j.1365-2044.2011.06838.x.
7. Warfield DJ, Barre S, Adhikary SD. Current understanding of the fascial plane blocks for analgesia of the chest wall: techniques and indications update for 2020. Curr Opin Anaesthesiol. 2020;33:692–7. https://doi.org/10.1097/ACO.0000000000000909.
8. Blanco R, Fajardo M, Parras Maldonado T. Ultrasound description of Pecs II (modified Pecs I): a novel approach to breast surgery. Rev Esp Anestesiol Reanim. 2012;59:470–5. https://doi.org/10.1016/j.redar.2012.07.003.
9. Ciftci B, Ekinci M, Celik EC, et al. Ultrasound-guided pectoral nerve block for pain control after breast augmentation: a randomized clinical study. Brazil J Anesthesiol (English Edition). 2021;71:44–9. https://doi.org/10.1016/j.bjane.2020.12.004.

10. Chae MS, Park Y, Shim J-W, et al. Clinical application of pectoralis nerve block ii for flap dissection-related pain control after robot-assisted transaxillary thyroidectomy: a preliminary retrospective cohort study. Cancers. 2022;14:4097. https://doi.org/10.3390/cancers14174097.
11. Ueshima H, Kitamura A. Clinical experiences of ultrasound-guided transversus thoracic muscle plane block: a clinical experience. J Clin Anesth. 2015;27:428–9. https://doi.org/10.1016/j.jclinane.2015.03.040.
12. Zhang Y, Li X, Chen S. Bilateral transversus thoracis muscle plane block provides effective analgesia and enhances recovery after open cardiac surgery. J Card Surg. 2021;36:2818–23. https://doi.org/10.1111/jocs.15666.
13. Dost B, De Cassai A, Balzani E, et al. Effects of ultrasound-guided regional anesthesia in cardiac surgery: a systematic review and network meta-analysis. BMC Anesthesiol. 2022;22:409. https://doi.org/10.1186/s12871-022-01952-7.
14. Shariat A, Ghia S, Gui JL, et al. Use of serratus anterior plane and transversus thoracis plane blocks for subcutaneous implantable cardioverter-defibrillator (s-icd) implantation decreases intraoperative opioid requirements. J Cardiothorac Vasc Anesth. 2021;35:3294–8. https://doi.org/10.1053/j.jvca.2021.04.028.
15. Liu V, Mariano ER, Prabhakar C. Pecto-intercostal fascial block for acute poststernotomy pain: a case report. A A Pract. 2018;10:319–22. https://doi.org/10.1213/XAA.0000000000000697.
16. Blanco R, Parras T, McDonnell JG, Prats-Galino A. Serratus plane block: a novel ultrasound-guided thoracic wall nerve block. Anaesthesia. 2013;68:1107–13. https://doi.org/10.1111/anae.12344.
17. Gado AA, Abdalwahab A, Ali H, et al. Serratus anterior plane block in pediatric patients undergoing thoracic surgeries: a randomized controlled trial. J Cardiothorac Vasc Anesth. 2022;36:2271–7. https://doi.org/10.1053/j.jvca.2021.09.014.
18. Gao W, Yang X, Hu J, et al. Continuous serratus anterior plane block improved early pulmonary function after lung cancer surgical procedure. Ann Thorac Surg. 2022;113:436–43. https://doi.org/10.1016/j.athoracsur.2021.02.032.
19. Edwards JT, Langridge XT, Cheng GS, et al. Superficial vs. deep serratus anterior plane block for analgesia in patients undergoing mastectomy: a randomized prospective trial. Journal of Clinical Anesthesia. 2021;75:110470. https://doi.org/10.1016/j.jclinane.2021.110470
20. Torre DE, Pirri C, Contristano M, et al. Ultrasound-guided PECS II + serratus plane fascial blocks are associated with reduced opioid consumption and lengths of stay for minimally invasive cardiac surgery: an observational retrospective study. Life. 2022;12:805. https://doi.org/10.3390/life12060805.
21. Pai P, Hong J, Phillips A, et al. Serratus anterior plane block versus intercostal block with incision infiltration in robotic-assisted thoracoscopic surgery: a randomized controlled pilot trial. J Cardiothorac Vasc Anesth. 2022;36:2287–94. https://doi.org/10.1053/j.jvca.2021.10.022.
22. Forero M, Adhikary SD, Lopez H, et al. The erector spinae plane block: a novel analgesic technique in thoracic neuropathic pain. Reg Anesth Pain Med. 2016;41:621–7. https://doi.org/10.1097/AAP.0000000000000451.
23. Leong RW, Tan ESJ, Wong SN, et al. Efficacy of erector spinae plane block for analgesia in breast surgery: a systematic review and meta-analysis. Anaesthesia. 2021;76:404–13. https://doi.org/10.1111/anae.15164.
24. Genc C, Kaya C, Bilgin S, et al. Pectoserratus plane block versus erector spinae plane block for postoperative opioid consumption and acute and chronic pain after breast cancer surgery: a randomized controlled trial. J Clin Anesth. 2022;79: 110691. https://doi.org/10.1016/j.jclinane.2022.110691.
25. Elsabeeny WY, Ibrahim MA, Shehab NN, et al. Serratus anterior plane block and erector spinae plane block versus thoracic epidural analgesia for perioperative thoracotomy pain control: a randomized controlled study. J Cardiothorac Vasc Anesth. 2021;35:2928–36. https://doi.org/10.1053/j.jvca.2020.12.047.
26. Turhan Ö, Sivrikoz N, Sungur Z, et al. Thoracic paravertebral block achieves better pain control than erector spinae plane block and intercostal nerve block in thoracoscopic surgery: a randomized study. J Cardiothorac Vasc Anesth. 2021;35:2920–7. https://doi.org/10.1053/j.jvca.2020.11.034.

27. Voscopoulos C, Palaniappan D, Zeballos J, et al. The ultrasound-guided retrolaminar block. Can J Anesth/J Can Anesth. 2013;60:888–95. https://doi.org/10.1007/s12630-013-9983-x.
28. Abdelbaser I, Mageed NA, Elfayoumy SI, et al. The effect of ultrasound-guided bilateral thoracic retrolaminar block on analgesia after pediatric open cardiac surgery: a randomized controlled double-blind study. Korean J Anesthesiol. 2022;75:276–82. https://doi.org/10.4097/kja.21466.
29. Wang Q, Wei S, Li S, et al. Comparison of the analgesic effect of ultrasound-guided paravertebral block and ultrasound-guided retrolaminar block in uniportal video-assisted thoracoscopic surgery: a prospective, randomized study. BMC Cancer. 2021;21:1229. https://doi.org/10.1186/s12885-021-08938-7.
30. Sotome S, Sawada A, Wada A, et al. Erector spinae plane block versus retrolaminar block for postoperative analgesia after breast surgery: a randomized controlled trial. J Anesth. 2021;35:27–34. https://doi.org/10.1007/s00540-020-02855-y.
31. Elsharkawy H, Maniker R, Bolash R, et al. Rhomboid intercostal and subserratus plane block: a cadaveric and clinical evaluation. Reg Anesth Pain Med. 2018;43:745–51. https://doi.org/10.1097/AAP.0000000000000824.
32. Kozanhan B, Semerkant T, Esme H, et al. Efficacy of rhomboid intercostal and subserratus plane block performed under direct vision on postoperative pain after thoracotomy. J Clin Anesth. 2019;58:95–7. https://doi.org/10.1016/j.jclinane.2019.05.021.
33. Deng W, Liu F, Jiang C, et al. Continuous rhomboid intercostal block for thoracoscopic postoperative analgesia. Ann Thorac Surg. 2022;114:319–26. https://doi.org/10.1016/j.athoracsur.2021.06.068.
34. Chen R, Su S, Shu H. Efficacy and safety of rhomboid intercostal block for analgesia in breast surgery and thoracoscopic surgery: a meta-analysis. BMC Anesthesiol. 2022;22:71. https://doi.org/10.1186/s12871-022-01599-4.
35. Ciftci B, Ekinci M, Basim P, et al. Comparison of ultrasound-guided type-ii pectoral nerve block and rhomboid intercostal block for pain management following breast cancer surgery: a randomized, controlled trial. Pain Pract. 2021;21:638–45. https://doi.org/10.1111/papr.13004.
36. Zhang J-G, Jiang C-W, Deng W, et al. Comparison of rhomboid intercostal block, erector spinae plane block, and serratus plane block on analgesia for video-assisted thoracic surgery: a prospective, randomized, controlled trial. Int J Clin Pract. 2022;2022:1–9. https://doi.org/10.1155/2022/6924489.
37. Deng W, Hou X, Zhou X, Zhou Q. Rhomboid intercostal block combined with sub-serratus plane block versus rhomboid intercostal block for postoperative analgesia after video-assisted thoracoscopic surgery: a prospective randomized-controlled trial. BMC Pulm Med. 2021;21:68. https://doi.org/10.1186/s12890-021-01432-7.
38. Kozanhan B, Semerkant T, Esme H, et al. Evaluation of rhomboid intercostal and subserratus plane block under direct vision for postoperative analgesia in thoracic surgeries: a prospective, randomized controlled trial. Euro J Cardio-Thoracic Surg. 2022;62:ezac498. https://doi.org/10.1093/ejcts/ezac498
39. Costache I, de Neumann L, Ramnanan CJ, et al. The mid-point transverse process to pleura (MTP) block: a new end-point for thoracic paravertebral block. Anaesthesia. 2017;72:1230–6. https://doi.org/10.1111/anae.14004.
40. Pedoto A, Kalchiem-Dekel O, Baselice S, et al. Ultrasound-guided midpoint transverse process to pleura nerve block for medical thoracoscopy: a case report. A A Pract. 2020;14: e01240. https://doi.org/10.1213/XAA.0000000000001240.
41. Syal R, Kumar R, Kamal M, Bhatia P. Novel block and new indication: ultrasound-guided continuous "mid-point transverse process to pleura" block in a patient with multiple rib fractures. Saudi J Anaesth. 2019;13:365–7. https://doi.org/10.4103/sja.SJA_773_18.
42. Bhoi D, Narasimhan P, Nethaji R, Talawar P. Ultrasound-guided midpoint transverse process to pleura block in breast cancer surgery: a case report. A&A Pract. 2019;12:73. https://doi.org/10.1213/XAA.0000000000000850.
43. Costache I. Mid-point transverse process to pleura block for surgical anaesthesia. Anaesth Rep. 2019;7:1–3. https://doi.org/10.1002/anr3.12003.

Perioperative Considerations in Patients Who Use Cannabis

Ramakrishna Gumidyala, Jacob Loyd, Simrat Kaur, Michael E. Schatman, and Roland Flores

Abstract Cannabis has become the most commonly used illicit substance under federal law, with over 40 million people having used it as of 2019 (1)thirty percent of users potentially having a cannabis use disorder (CUD) (2), and nearly 15% of patients presenting for non-cardiac surgery having reported cannabis use (6). Cannabis use appears to be associated with systemic physiologic effects including the potential for serious cardiopulmonary complications, increased anesthetic and opioid requirements, and postoperative withdrawal. There may be a role for use of cannabis products in the perioperative period to help optimize these patients, though more rigorous studies need to be performed to support its use in this setting. In this chapter, we summarize recently published papers and society guidelines to inform readers on the perioperative management of these patients.

Keywords Cannabis · Marijuana · Perioperative · Pain management

---

R. Gumidyala (✉) · J. Loyd · S. Kaur · R. Flores
Department of Anesthesiology, University of Colorado, Aurora, CO, USA
e-mail: Ramakrishna.Gumidyala@cuanschutz.edu

J. Loyd
e-mail: Jacob.Loyd@cuanschutz.edu

S. Kaur
e-mail: Simrat.Kaur@cuanschutz.edu

R. Flores
e-mail: Roland.Flores@cuanschutz.edu

M. E. Schatman
Department of Anesthesiology, Perioperative Care, and Pain Medicine, NYU Grossman School of Medicine, New York, NY, USA

Department of Population Health—Division of Medical Ethics, NYU Grossman School of Medicine, New York, NY, USA

M. E. Schatman
e-mail: Michael.Schatman@NYULangone.org

A. Abd-Elsayed and K. Schroeder (eds.), *Perioperative Pain Management*,
https://doi.org/10.1007/978-3-031-67648-2_27

1 Introduction

With the legalization and decriminalization of cannabis in many states, it has become the most commonly used illicit substance under federal law, according to the National Survey on Drug Use and Health [1]. The Substance Abuse and Mental Health Services Administration estimates that nearly 43 million people used cannabis at least once as of 2019 [1]. Around 30 percent of cannabis users have a cannabis use disorder (CUD) [2], an established diagnosis in the DSM IV and V, with criteria that include: use for longer periods in larger amounts, inability to cut down use, a strong urge to use, dependence, and withdrawal reactions on cessation, similar to other substance use disorders [3, 4]. Concomitant with the rise in the use of cannabis, more patients are presenting for elective and non-elective surgeries than ever before. It is estimated that approximately 100 million procedures and surgeries are done each year [5], and while the true prevalence of cannabis use is difficult to estimate due to underreporting for a variety of reasons, it is increasingly likely that healthcare providers will care for cannabis-using patients during the perioperative period. According to data from a major healthcare network in the U.S. examining over 200,000 patients undergoing non-cardiac surgery, the prevalence of patients reporting use increased from 4.9% in 2008 to 14.3% in 2020 [6]. Perioperative cannabis use has been associated with higher levels of postoperative healthcare utilization [6] and complications such as myocardial infarction (MI) [7], stroke [8], thromboembolism, neurologic and respiratory complications, sepsis, and poorer disposition at the time of discharge [9]. In addition to these associated complications and a variety of other physiologic impacts, cannabis products are known to modulate pain by both central [10] and peripheral mechanisms [11]. Not surprisingly, there is also an increasing body of literature suggesting that cannabis use may have an impact on pain management and perioperative opioid use among these patients [12–15]. Recommendations for the management of patients who use cannabis have been lacking, likely in part due to its legality, heterogeneity in routes of use, the plurality of types of products, and varying patient physiology. Only recently [16, 17] have guidelines attempted to summarize recommendations for the care of these patients. In this chapter, we will cover the pharmacology of cannabis, the physiologic impacts of cannabis use, and describe the preoperative, intraoperative, and postoperative considerations for the management of patients who use cannabis products.

2 Pharmacology

Cannabis is derived from the cannabis sativa plant and is grown worldwide. The compound consists of two primary cannabinoids, delta-9-tetrahydrocannabinol (THC) and cannabidiol (CBD). THC and CBD generally make up 70% of the plant [18], with minor cannabinoids making up the remainder of the product. THC is the major psychoactive component of cannabis and is the primary constituent driving recreational use. CBD is a weakly psychoactive cannabinoid that is considered safer than THC and is associated with few adverse effects [18].

Pharmacodynamics

Endocannabinoid receptors are found throughout the body including within the nervous system, connective tissue, immune cells, as well as other locations [18, 19]. The predominant receptor types for cannabis are G protein-coupled receptors identified as CB1 and CB2 receptors, with CB1 being the principal receptor type in the central nervous system [19]. CB1 receptors are located in the basal ganglia, hippocampus, cerebellum, association cortices, spinal cord, and peripheral nerves. These receptors are located in the presynaptic membrane and when stimulated, lead to a decrease in the release of acetylcholine and glutamate, thus inducing their inhibitory effects. This leads to a disruption of an individual's psychomotor function, time perception, mood, memory, and learning, all contributing to impaired judgment [18].

Pharmacokinetics

The most common routes of cannabis use are inhalation, either via smoking or vaporization, and ingestion [18]. The mode of use determines the bioavailability, onset, and duration of effects as shown in Table 1.

Cannabis is highly lipophilic which results in its absorption by the liver, kidneys, muscles, and adipose tissue. The result of multi-organ and tissue absorption is a prolonged and unpredictable effect. The half-life of THC in infrequent users ranges from 1.3 days to 5–13 days in frequent users [18]. This lengthy half-life can increase the likelihood of toxicity and other adverse effects. In the perioperative setting, these potential adverse events are dependent to a large extent on the temporal contiguity of the patient's most recent use prior to surgery.

THC is metabolized by the liver, with phase 1 oxidation and phase 2 hydroxylation reactions via the cytochrome p450 system. A small amount undergoes extrahepatic metabolism in the lungs. The inactive metabolites are excreted primarily in the feces

Table 1 Mode of cannabis use, onset time, and time to peak concentration effect [18]

Mode of cannabis use	Onset time	Peak concentration
Inhalation	Fast	22 minutes
Oral	Slow	1–2 hours
Sublingual	Fast	30 minutes
Rectal	Fast	15 minutes
Transcutaneous	Slow	2 hours

(65%) and in the urine (20%), with the majority of the compound excreted within 5 days of consumption [20].

Drug Interactions

THC and CBD inhibit CYP 3A4 and CYP 2C9 and induce CYP 1A2. These resulting processes can lead to altered metabolism of drugs metabolized by the CYP450 system, resulting in prolonged or decreased effect of medications. For example, warfarin is metabolized by the CYP450 system and concomitant cannabis use can lead to bleeding secondary to reduced warfarin metabolism. The durations of action of lithium and tricyclic antidepressants are also prolonged with cannabis use [21]. Furthermore, in patients taking medications that inhibit or induce the CYP450 system, there is an increased risk of experiencing a cannabis overdose versus inadequate effect, respectively. Thus, it is imperative to know all medications that a patient is taking to evaluate potential drug interactions, mitigate deleterious effects, and adjust dosages as necessary.

3 Physiological Impacts and Complications of Cannabis Use

Cannabis is known to adversely affect multiple organ systems in the acute and chronic settings. A summary of potential complications related to prolonged cannabis use is presented in Fig. 1.

Effects on the Autonomic Nervous System

At lower doses, cannabis stimulates the sympathetic nervous system and inhibits the parasympathetic nervous system [20]. This may result in tachycardia and hypertension. The systemic vasodilation associated with cannabis use may also result in reflex tachycardia [20, 21]. The use of propranolol prior to cannabis use is associated with decreased tachycardia, further supporting sympathetic nervous system activation's role in tachycardia [20]. Decreased vagal slowing can occur, as would be expected with Valsalva maneuvers, indicating inhibition of the parasympathetic nervous system [20]. However, with higher doses, cannabis use may result in parasympathetic stimulation, leading to bradycardia and hypotension [20].

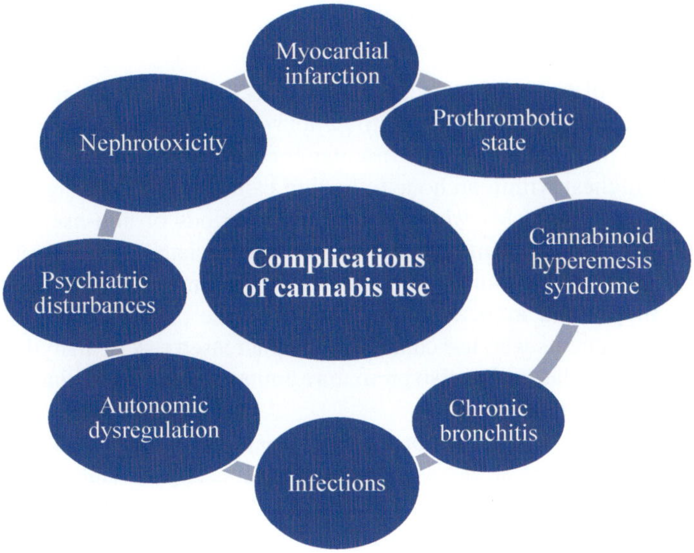

Fig. 1 Complications related to prolonged cannabis use [20, 37, 38, 40, 41]

Psychiatric Effects

Cannabis use has also been associated with either new onset psychiatric disturbances or a worsening of preexisting conditions such as psychosis, anxiety, or depression [21], and may compound elevated anxiety during the perioperative period. Kuepper et al. examined the incidence of psychotic symptoms in individuals with ongoing marijuana use in a 10-year follow-up cohort study. They found a statistically significant increase in the incidence of psychotic symptoms, despite adjusting for confounding variables such as age, other drug use, and environmental stressors [22].

Hines et al. performed a cohort study to assess the relationship between high-potency cannabis use and mental health illnesses. Patients with high-potency cannabis use were four times more likely to use cannabis at least weekly and had a four times higher chance of having generalized anxiety disorder. However, other factors such as environmental stressors may play a role in this, as they can increase the likelihood of substance use disorders or mental health illnesses independently [23].

Effects on the Cardiovascular System

From a cardiovascular standpoint, acute cannabis use leads to a dose-related increase in heart rate and cardiac index lasting up to 72 hours and studies have linked these findings to increased perioperative cardiovascular complications [24, 25]. The increased cardiac risk is highest within an hour following cannabis use, leading to a 4.8-fold higher risk of suffering a MI when compared to periods of non-use, and the risk rapidly decreases after that time [26]. Tachycardia associated with cannabis use can result in increased myocardial oxygen demand which can lead to decreased myocardial oxygen supply and myocardial ischemia in these patients [20]. Tachycardia also predisposes patients who use cannabis to an increased risk of arrhythmias, most commonly atrial fibrillation, but also premature contractions, ventricular tachycardia, and ventricular fibrillation [20].

For patients with CUD who are not actively intoxicated at the time of surgery, there remains an elevated risk of cardiovascular complications. Specifically, a retrospective study identified statistically significant increases in MI and stroke risk among patients undergoing vascular surgery [8] and a 1.88 adjusted odds ratio of perioperative MI in patients with cannabis use disorder undergoing elective surgery [7].

Effects on the Respiratory System

In addition to these cardiovascular risks, cannabis products may contribute to perioperative pulmonary concerns, as these products are most frequently consumed by way of inhalation, notably smoking rolled, unfiltered cigarettes, and vaping either flower or oil concentrates. Use of smoked and vaped products results in the inhalation of several carcinogenic chemicals and irritants such as formaldehyde, tar, benzopyrene, and benzanthracene at much greater levels than during tobacco inhalation [27]. Regular use of smoked cannabis products has not been clearly linked to long-term significant lung dysfunction [28]. While it may provide some bronchodilation in the short-term [27, 29] via interaction with the CB1 receptor [30], there are also negative respiratory effects. Cannabis use is associated with hypersecretion [31], large airway inflammation, increased airway resistance, hyperinflation [32], uvulitis and airway obstruction [33, 34], all of which can impact patients in the perioperative period. Moreover, like with tobacco, cannabis smoking has been associated with lung parenchymal diseases such as chronic bronchitis and emphysema [21]. Cannabis use can also adversely affect the immune system, increasing susceptibility to infections such as pneumonia [35]. There may also exist an association with lung adenocarcinoma with concomitant tobacco smoking [36]. However, the risk of lung cancer from cannabis use alone in not well defined [21], with the high incidence of tobacco use among cannabis users making investigation of the relationship between cannabis use and lung cancer challenging.

Effects on the Renal System

Studies indicate that cannabis, especially synthetic cannabinoids, may cause renal injury and adversely affect renal function, especially in patients who have impaired renal function at baseline. In the multicenter Assessment, Serial Evaluation, and Subsequent Sequelae of Acute Kidney Injury (ASSESS-AKI) study, patients with an estimated glomerular filtration rate (eGFR) of less than 60 ml/min/1.73 m^2 had a more rapid decline in renal function compared to individuals with an eGFR greater than 60 at baseline [37]. One postulated mechanism is that cannabis adversely affects the mitochondrial function of the proximal tubule [37]. These patients are more likely to be diagnosed with acute tubular necrosis through kidney biopsies [37]. Thus, it is important to have a high index of suspicion of cannabis use in individuals with unexplained kidney dysfunction [37]. Cannabis can cause both intrarenal and prerenal injuries, with the latter being due to hypovolemia related to cannabinoid hyperemesis syndrome.

Effects on the Gastrointestinal System

Parikh and colleagues performed a retrospective study comparing gastrointestinal symptomatology in cannabis vs non-cannabis users. This study determined that abdominal pain was the most common presenting symptom among cannabis users, with heartburn being the second most common. They also compared endoscopy findings in cannabis vs non-cannabis users and identified significant inflammatory changes such as gastritis and esophagitis in the cannabis group. With manometry, they found significantly impaired esophageal bolus clearance and greater lower esophageal sphincter pressures in the cannabis group [38].

Cannabinoid hyperemesis syndrome (CHS) is another phenomenon seen in cannabis users. CHS is associated with cyclic nausea, vomiting, and abdominal pain [39]. The syndrome presents in 3 phases: the prodromal phase, hyper-emetic phase, and recovery phase. Patients in the prodromal phase typically present with nausea, anxiety, and autonomic symptoms that can last several months before progressing to the hyper-emetic phase [40]. During the hyper-emetic phase, individuals typically have paroxysms of severe and persistent nausea, vomiting, and abdominal pain, and compulsively begin taking hot showers and baths to alleviate the symptoms [39, 40]. Typical antiemetics are not useful for management of these patients. Rather, they appear to respond better to anxiolytics, sedatives, and antipsychotics. The only definitive treatment is abstinence from cannabis. There is no clear mechanism for this disorder, although one postulated mechanism is prolonged stimulation of the CB1 receptor due to sustained cannabis use leads to dysregulation of the endocannabinoid system, which leads to emesis [40].

Effects on the Hematologic System

Cannabis use is associated with an increased risk of thrombosis due to several different mechanisms. This may be caused by the presence of CB1 and CB2 receptors on the platelet surface leading to enhanced platelet activation. It may also be due to endothelial dysfunction or increased expression of the GP IIb IIIa receptor on the platelet surface [20]. A prothrombotic state coupled with cannabis-induced tachycardia causing increased myocardial demand may further increase the risk of myocardial ischemia. Finally, a prothrombotic state may also increase the risk of peripheral vascular disease and systemic thrombotic events such as stroke [21].

4 Medical Benefits of Cannabinoids

Up to this point, we have focused on several complications or adverse effects of cannabis use. However, there may also be benefits. The most commonly reported indication for medical cannabis is chronic pain [42]. Several studies evaluating the efficacy of cannabis on pain alleviation have been published. In a systematic review, Whiting and colleagues examined 28 trials, with 22 assessing the efficacy of plant-based cannabinoids and 5 examining the effect of synthetic cannabinoids. All of these trials compared cannabis to a control group such as amitriptyline, with the exception of a single trial which compared cannabis to a placebo group. The majority of the trials assessed efficacy for neuropathic pain, while the remaining considered musculoskeletal, rheumatologic, cancer-induced, chemotherapy-induced, or pain due to multiple sclerosis. The results of this review suggested that patients experienced significant improvement in their chronic pain symptoms with the use of cannabis [43]. However, Schatman points out several methodological limitations of this systematic review and meta-analysis of medical cannabinoids. It incorporated studies of a variety of cannabis preparations with differing consumption methods, along with including studies of several pain conditions with varying responses to cannabinoids. Furthermore, the article did not address the wide range of adverse events, dosing issues, and THC/CBD content variance [44], leaving it difficult to make reliable conclusions about the role of cannabinoids in the broad management of chronic pain conditions, without accounting for these limitations. More specifically, cannabis has been shown to be effective in treatment of neuropathic pain [45]. However, it is important to note that these effects are dose-dependent [46] on THC content, and while helpful for neuropathic pain, patients may have significant side effects [45] and impaired neurocognition [46], limiting its use in more functional patients.

Cannabis may also offer benefits as a treatment for nausea and vomiting caused by chemotherapy. While cannabis has been shown to be superior in comparison to a placebo, several studies have failed to demonstrate superiority in comparison to standard antiemetics such as ondansetron or prochlorperazine [43].

Other potential benefits of cannabis use include reduced spasticity associated with multiple sclerosis and reduced insomnia [43] but further evidence may be required before cannabis can be definitively recommended for these indications.

5 Preoperative Considerations

Because of its ubiquity and broad-spanning physiologic impact, recently published guidelines by the Perioperative Pain and Addiction Interdisciplinary Network (PAIN) and the American Society of Regional Anesthesia and Pain Medicine (ASRA Pain Medicine) suggest patients should be screened preoperatively for cannabis use [16, 17]. It has been documented that the potency and dosage of cannabis products have increased over the years [47–49]. In addition, labeled doses may significantly over or underestimate actual cannabinoid content [50, 51], and as a result, accurate quantification of usage amounts may be difficult or impossible. Further, given the likelihood of concomitant use of other substances [42, 52, 53], providers should be aware of the physiologic impacts that these other substances may have and how they present.

Current guidelines recommend that, in order to better understand the effects of cannabis use on our patients, we should ask about the method of consumption (smoking, vaping, ingesting, etc.), how often it is used, the individual's response to cannabis, any withdrawal symptoms experienced, and when the patient last used cannabis or any other substances [16, 17, 54]. This information can help healthcare professionals gain insight into the acute and chronic effects of cannabis or other substances on their patients. The PAIN guidelines recommend quantifying the total dose of cannabis in milligrams or grams per day, given that most products are sold accounting for either percentage of mass in THC or CBD, milligrams of THC/CBD per gram of product, or simply milligrams of cannabis. In terms of defining *significant* use, the PAIN group defined it as 1.5 g/day of inhaled cannabis, 300 mg/day of CBD oil, and 20 mg/day of THC oil, or by frequency of two to three times of usage/day [16]. A validated screening tool [55, 56] can help determine whether a patient has a Cannabis Use Disorder (CUD) and might benefit from a preoperative referral to an addiction medicine specialist. Assays for cannabis and its metabolites exist for determining serum levels of THC [57, 58], though no standardized nomogram or tool exists to correlate use with physiologic impact. Accordingly, toxicology screening is not routinely recommended unless testing for acute intoxication.

Determining whether a patient is experiencing signs and symptoms of acute cannabis use may be challenging, as patients present variably depending on chronicity of use, individual physiologic response and type of cannabis product used. Symptoms of cannabis intoxication can include conjunctivitis, paranoia, anxiety, delirium, hyperkinesis, and hypotension [59, 60]. Both acute and chronic users of cannabis, due to hippocampal effects, are also susceptible to dose-dependent impairment of cognitive function, memory, and ability to process information [35, 61]. An aspect of patient assessment also includes determining whether a patient meets the criteria for consenting to non-emergency surgery. There is evidence that cannabis users may demonstrate susceptibility to false memories [62], so any informed consent process should include thorough documentation of what was discussed and consideration of postponing elective surgery in patients who may not be considered capable of providing consent.

Cannabis use has been associated with tachycardia, arrhythmias [63–65], coronary spasm [66], sudden death [67], and stroke [68]. In discussing anesthetic risk as an element of informed consent, cannabis-using patients should be made aware of their elevated perioperative risk and screened for angina-free functional capacity. Patients with CUDs also are at greater risk of postoperative MI when presenting for elective surgery (adjusted OR 1.88) [7] and greater risk of perioperative MI and stroke when undergoing vascular surgery [8]. In addition to counseling patients that may be at risk for or have coronary artery disease on the potential increase of perioperative MI, the ASRA Pain Medicine guidelines recommend postponing elective surgery for at least 2 hours subsequent to cannabis use due to this elevated risk [17].

As mentioned previously, smoked and vaped cannabis products may be associated with an increased risk of respiratory morbidity. According to one retrospective cohort analysis of over 400,000 patients undergoing elective spine surgery, cannabis users had a twofold increase in the odds of respiratory complications (OR 2.0, 95% CI 1.4–2.9) [9]. Discussing the potential for airway compromise and increased pulmonary complications is recommended by recent guidelines [17]. In addition, providers should consider administration of steroids for treatment of airway edema noted perioperatively [34]. As part of preoperative evaluation and determination of whether to proceed with a given procedure, surgeons and anesthesiologists should weigh the risks and benefits of postponing elective surgery in patients who have recently used cannabis, based on patient comorbidities, surgery-specific pulmonary risk, method and dose of cannabis consumption, and recency of use.

There is conflicting information regarding the relationship between cannabis use before surgery and a higher use of opioids during the perioperative period, as well as how this affects acute pain. However, for patients with chronic pain and opioid use, cannabis use may alleviate pain and reduce chronic opioid consumption [69–72]. Despite the potential benefits of cannabinoids in chronic pain patients perioperatively, these patients demonstrate elevated pain scores postoperatively, lower quality of life, and greater likelihood of using benzodiazepines and opioids for up to 6 months postoperatively [13]. As a result of these potential negative effects, whether patients should taper or discontinue use of cannabis products perioperatively, remains a major concern. The ASRA Pain Medicine guidelines do not recommend for or against a tapering strategy [17]. Further, the Perioperative Pain and Addiction Interdisciplinary Network guideline recommends considering a dose reduction to less than 1.5 g/day of smoked cannabis, 300 mg/day of CBD oil, or 20 mg/day of THC oil within 7 days of surgery, but makes no consensus recommendations regarding tapering between 1 and 6 days preoperatively, and recommends against tapering within 1 day prior to surgery [16]. A U-shaped response to cannabis, with low and elevated THC levels being associated with no reduction in pain [73] suggests a narrow therapeutic window. The narrowness of this window may influence future tapering recommendations, although further research would be necessary to identify the specific duration of this window.

When tapering or discontinuing cannabis preoperatively, one should also consider the risk of cannabis withdrawal syndrome (CWS), discussed in further detail later, among those patients who consume a significant amount of cannabis [16], and determine if this warrants treatment preoperatively.

6 Intraoperative Considerations

Given the broad physiologic and pharmacologic effects of cannabis, one should be diligent when caring for a cannabis user undergoing anesthesia. Unfortunately, there is a paucity of robust clinical research to guide the intraoperative management of these patients. Once a patient's cannabis use has been identified, including the amount, frequency, route, and time of most recent use, the anesthesiologist can better determine how a patient's cannabis history might affect his/her potential intraoperative anesthetic risks. As with other substances, chronic cannabis use and acute intoxication may exert opposing effects and may need to be addressed differently in the perioperative period.

Several clinical studies suggest that chronic cannabis users require higher induction and maintenance doses of anesthesia. A prospective study [69] compared the dose of propofol required to induce general anesthesia and successfully place a laryngeal mask airway in 60 patients, 30 of whom used cannabis more than once a week versus non-using controls and concluded that chronic cannabis use increases the propofol dose required. Similarly, a retrospective study of patients undergoing gastric endoscopies demonstrated that daily or weekly users of cannabis required significantly increased doses of fentanyl, midazolam and propofol, i.e., 14, 19.6 and 220.5% more medication, respectively, when compared to non-users of cannabis.[74] In addition, a retrospective study of patients undergoing open reduction internal fixation of tibial fractures demonstrated a statistically significant increase in sevoflurane dosage for maintenance of anesthesia. However, no significant difference in total dosages of propofol, dexmedetomidine, etomidate, ketamine, desflurane, midazolam, and fentanyl were identified. The definition of cannabis users in this study was broader when compared to the aforementioned studies, with cannabis users defined as any cannabis use within the past month, which may explain why significant differences were not identified with propofol and fentanyl, as had been evidenced in other studies [75].

In contrast to chronic use, acute cannabis intoxication appears to have the opposite effect on tolerance to anesthesia, as evidenced by several animal studies. A reduction in the minimal alveolar concentration (MAC) of sevoflurane in rats [76] and halothane in dogs [77] was identified when the test subjects were treated with THC prior to exposure to inhaled anesthetics. Although animal studies are considered imperfect predictors of human responses, it is logical to conclude that cannabis follows a similar trend with substances such as alcohol, in which it is well documented that acute intoxication leads to decreased MAC anesthesia [78]. In their 2021 consensus recommendations for perioperative management of cannabis users, the PAIN guidelines concluded that acutely intoxicated cannabis users might have lower anesthetic requirements, whereas chronic cannabis users may require higher medication dosages to achieve an adequate depth of anesthesia. In both scenarios, the authors advise considering use of intraoperative EEG monitoring to assist with monitoring [16]. However, recently published consensus guidelines from ASRA Pain Medicine regarding cannabis users concluded that there is still insufficient evidence to support the routine use of intraoperative EEG for depth of anesthesia monitoring in cannabis using patients [17]. The guidelines cite a study comparing bispectral index (BIS) values under general anesthesia between control patients and those who received premedication with cannabis extract Nabiximols. Cannabis premedication was found to increase the BIS value in anesthetized patients, and the authors suggested it was due to a cannabinoid-induced alteration in EEG activity rather than a shallower anesthetic state [79].

7 Postoperative Considerations

The complexity of caring for cannabis users does not end when the patient leaves the operating room. Rather, some of the greatest challenges may lie in the postoperative phase of care. One area of considerable interest is the effect that cannabis use has on achieving effective postoperative analgesia. Studies repeatedly demonstrate that cannabis users experience worse postoperative pain and often require higher doses of opioids as compared to non-users. A study of 3973 patients undergoing major orthopedic surgeries determined that those using recreational or medicinal cannabis had higher pain scores at rest and with movement in the early postoperative period, as well as increased sleep disturbances [14]. Analysis of motor vehicle accident patients across 4 trauma centers determined that habitual cannabis users reported higher pain scores and had increased opioid requirements when compared to non-users and infrequent cannabis users [80]. McAfee and colleagues [13] conducted a prospective study of 1335 patients in which they evaluated clinical characteristics and surgical outcomes of elective surgery patients. The authors determined that not only did cannabis users report higher pain scores both prior to and following surgery, but they also had greater functional impairment, more fatigue, greater sleep disturbances and more symptoms of anxiety and depression versus non-cannabis users. A complicating factor to managing pain in cannabis users is the interaction between cannabinoids and the cytochrome P450 enzymes. Cannabinoids have the potential to increase the effects of medications like warfarin [81], acetaminophen, and benzodiazepines and opioids by inhibition of cytochrome P450 enzymes [82], leading to prolonged half-lives [83]. In vitro and animal studies suggest that cannabinoids can also inhibit cyclooxygenase and may cause a reduced response to non-steroidal anti-inflammatory drugs (NSAIDs) [84]. Despite these interactions, there are no contraindications to common multimodal analgesia medications, including ketamine, dexmedetomidine, NSAIDs, acetaminophen, gabapentinoids, or local anesthetics [16]. A thoughtful approach to pain management is necessary when caring for patients who regularly use cannabis, with multimodal and regional anesthesia techniques being employed as appropriate. Providers should note that higher doses of opioids are often necessary to achieve equianalgesic effects [82, 85].

In addition to postoperative pain management issues, anesthesiologists must be aware of other cannabis-related complications, such as postoperative nausea and vomiting (PONV) as well as cannabis withdrawal syndrome (CWS). A large retrospective analysis of over 27,000 patients indicated that cannabis users had a slightly higher incidence of PONV compared to non-users [86], while another smaller retrospective cohort study found a reduced incidence of PONV in cannabis users [87]. Further contributing to PONV risk may be the association of chronic cannabis use with delayed gastric emptying and decreased intestinal motility [88]. Although it is still premature to make a definitive statement regarding this risk, several studies have demonstrated an association between preoperative cannabis use, elevated postoperative pain scores, and greater opioid use postoperatively [12–14, 85, 89, 90]. This increased opioid use can also contribute to an elevated risk of PONV [91]. As mentioned earlier in this chapter, CHS is a condition where long-term cannabis use can lead to intractable vomiting. While there does not appear to be a link between a history of CHS and anesthesia-related PONV [92], PONV in patients suffering from CHS may be more responsive to butyrophenones (i.e. haloperidol/droperidol) [40, 93] over other anti-emetics. Based on the potential increased risk of PONV in chronic users, practitioners should consider greater PONV prevention and prophylaxis measures.

Cannabis withdrawal syndrome, another potential complication of chronic cannabis use, is related to sudden discontinuation of cannabis after habitual use, which is often a recommendation given to patients by their medical providers prior to surgery. DSM-5 diagnostic criteria state that CWS requires at least 3 of the following: irritability, anger or aggression, nervousness or anxiety, sleep difficulty, decreased appetite or weight loss, restlessness, depressed mood, and one of the following physical discomforts: abdominal pain, shakiness/tremors, sweating, fever, chills and/or headache [4]. Symptoms of CWS can occur 1 to 3 days after cannabis cessation, peaking in the first week, and lasting up to 2 weeks [94] Given that cannabis users are often instructed to stop consuming cannabis prior to surgery, the effects from CWS are more likely to be encountered in the immediate postoperative period. Interestingly, cannabis users who have concurrent opioid dependence rarely present with CWS [95]. Animals experiencing CWS have been shown to have reduced mesolimbic dopamine function [96], while rats with frequent exposure to morphine showed increased dopamine release [97], suggesting a possible mechanism for this reduced CWS symptoms in opioid dependent patients. If CWS is suspected, then symptoms can be attenuated with THC analogs such as dronabinol or nabilone, and gabapentin has exhibited some efficacy, as well [98].

Chronic pain is the leading indication for medical cannabis prescriptions in the United States [99]. Accordingly, it is apparent why researchers have been evaluating the efficacy of cannabis and cannabinoid analogs for treating chronic pain. The results of these studies have been mixed, with some suggesting marked decreases in pain [100, 101], whereas others have identified no reductions in pain as well as side effect profiles that outweigh the potential benefits [45, 102, 103]. The question of whether cannabinoid medications can effectively treat acute postoperative or traumatic pain has recently been garnering more scientific attention. A matched cohort study of dronabinol for treatment of traumatic pain produced a statistically significant reduction in opioid use in the dronabinol cohort, which was more pronounced in patients with a history of cannabis use [104]. Comparably, a THC analog called Cannador was studied for potential postoperative analgesia with dose escalations from 5 to 15 mg, finding an increased analgesic effect with higher doses, yet also more sedation side effects. One study patient experienced a serious vasovagal event at the high dose that ultimately halted the study [105]. A retrospective study of total joint replacement patients determined that the addition of 5 mg dronabinol twice a day resulted in shorter hospital stays and lower daily opioid utilization [106]. These findings are in contrast to two earlier studies of postoperative cannabinoid dosing for analgesia, one of which concluded that there was no difference in pain, and the other determined that pain scores were worse in the patients that received the cannabinoid [107, 108]. The dosing and formulation of cannabinoids varied greatly across these studies, which likely played a large role in their differing outcomes. Further research will need to be done to determine what role, if any, exists for cannabinoid use postoperatively, and if any potential benefits outweigh risks of use.

8 Future Direction

As a growing number of states continue to legalize cannabis and the number of cannabis users continues to rise, the necessity for a better understanding of how cannabis affects anesthesia and pain management needs to grow. To date, the majority of research evaluating the effects of cannabis use on perioperative anesthesia and pain management has been preclinical and observational rather than the high quality randomized controlled trials that are needed [16]. As such, it's difficult to create confident clinical guidelines for managing this patient population. This was evident in the recent consensus guidelines published by ASRA, in which low level of certainty grade C recommendations and insufficient evidence were used to inform the majority of their clinical conclusions [17]. Clearly, this is an area that requires far more scientific attention and higher quality studies. With that said, a 2022 systematic review and meta-analysis of the opioid sparing effects of cannabinoids for analgesia determined that in the five years subsequent to their previous review paper, the number of preclinical (rodent or rhesus monkey) studies published doubled, the number of clinical studies (published and on clinicaltrials.gov) increased fourfold, and the number of study participants increased an impressive sixfold [109]. Irrespective of these substantial increases in published scientific activity, the ubiquitous nature of cannabis use will require dramatic increases in clinical investigation to better inform the perioperative management of both medical and recreational users to evolve from its current status of "medical cannabis neuromysticism".

Key Takeaway Points

1. With the expanding decriminalization and legalization of cannabis, the number of patients presenting with reported cannabis use will increase.
2. Anesthesia providers should be aware of the potential for wide-ranging physiologic impacts of cannabis and how this might influence their anesthetic management.
3. There are limited data to support use of cannabis-related products for clinical applications, but further rescarch may help elucidate what, if any, role there is in this setting. Further research may expand on our understanding of the short and long-term side effects of chronic cannabis use and how it impacts our patients in the perioperative setting.

References

1. Substance Abuse and Mental Health Services Administration. Key Substance Use and Mental Health Indicators in the United States: Results from the 2018 National Survey on Drug Use and Health 2019 Available from: https://www.samhsa.gov/data/report/2018-nsduh-annual-national-report
2. Hasin DS, Saha TD, Kerridge BT, Goldstein RB, Chou SP, Zhang H, et al. Prevalence of Marijuana use disorders in the United States between 2001–2002 and 2012–2013. JAMA Psychiat. 2015;72(12):1235–42.
3. American Psychiatric Association., American Psychiatric Association. Task Force on DSM-IV. Diagnostic and statistical manual of mental disorders : DSM-IV. 4th ed. Washington, DC: American Psychiatric Association; 1994. p. xxvii, 886
4. Battle DE. Diagnostic and statistical manual of mental disorders (DSM). Codas. 2013;25(2):191–2.
5. Wu CL, Raja SN. Treatment of acute postoperative pain. Lancet. 2011;377(9784):2215–25.
6. Ahrens E, Wachtendorf LJ, Chiarella LS, Ashrafian S, Suleiman A, Tartler TM, et al. Prevalence and association of non-medical cannabis use with post-procedural healthcare utilisation in patients undergoing surgery or interventional procedures: a retrospective cohort study. EClinic Med. 2023;57: 101831.
7. Goel A, McGuinness B, Jivraj NK, Wijeysundera DN, Mittleman MA, Bateman BT, et al. Cannabis use disorder and perioperative outcomes in major elective surgeries: a retrospective cohort analysis. Anesthesiology. 2020;132(4):625–35.
8. McGuinness B, Goel A, Elias F, Rapanos T, Mittleman MA, Ladha KS. Cannabis use disorder and perioperative outcomes in vascular surgery. J Vasc Surg. 2021;73(4):1376-87.e3.
9. Chiu RG, Patel S, Siddiqui N, Nunna RS, Mehta AI. Cannabis abuse and perioperative complications following inpatient spine surgery in the United States. Spine (Phila Pa 1976). 2021;46(11):734–43.
10. Hill KP, Palastro MD, Johnson B, Ditre JW. Cannabis and pain: a clinical review. Cannabis Cannabinoid Res. 2017;2(1):96–104.
11. Vučković S, Srebro D, Vujović KS, Vučetić Č, Prostran M. Cannabinoids and pain: new insights from old molecules. Front Pharmacol. 2018;9:1259.

12. Ekrami E, Ozturk SS, Kopac O, Wang D, Mascha EJ, Araujo-Duran J, et al. Association Between cannabis use and postoperative opioid consumption. American Society of Anesthesiologists Annual Meeting; 2022. New Orleans, LA.
13. McAfee J, Boehnke KF, Moser SM, Brummett CM, Waljee JF, Bonar EE. Perioperative cannabis use: a longitudinal study of associated clinical characteristics and surgical outcomes. Reg Anesth Pain Med. 2021;46(2):137–44.
14. Liu CW, Bhatia A, Buzon-Tan A, Walker S, Ilangomaran D, Kara J, et al. Weeding out the problem: the impact of preoperative cannabinoid use on pain in the perioperative period. Anesth Analg. 2019;129(3):874–81.
15. Wallace M, Schulteis G, Atkinson JH, Wolfson T, Lazzaretto D, Bentley H, et al. Dose-dependent effects of smoked cannabis on capsaicin-induced pain and hyperalgesia in healthy volunteers. Anesthesiology. 2007;107(5):785–96.
16. Ladha KS, McLaren-Blades A, Goel A, Buys MJ, Farquhar-Smith P, Haroutounian S, et al. Perioperative Pain and Addiction Interdisciplinary Network (PAIN): consensus recommendations for perioperative management of cannabis and cannabinoid-based medicine users by a modified Delphi process. Br J Anaesth. 2021;126(1):304–18.
17. Shah S, Schwenk ES, Narouze S. ASRA Pain Medicine consensus guidelines on the management of the perioperative patient on cannabis and cannabinoids: an infographic. Reg Anesth Pain Med. 2023;48(3):119.
18. Oberbarnscheidt T, Miller NS. Pharmacology of Marijuana. J Addict Res Therapy. 2016;11(12).
19. Bridgeman MB, Abazia DT. Medicinal Cannabis: history, pharmacology, and implications for the acute care setting. P t. 2017;42(3):180–8.
20. Latif Z, Garg N. The impact of marijuana on the cardiovascular system: a review of the most common cardiovascular events associated with marijuana use. J Clin Med. 2020;9(6):1925.
21. Shah J, Fermo O. Review of systemic and syndromic complications of cannabis use: a review. Medicine (Baltimore). 2022;101(49): e32111.
22. Kuepper R, van Os J, Lieb R, Wittchen HU, Höfler M, Henquet C. Continued cannabis use and risk of incidence and persistence of psychotic symptoms: 10 year follow-up cohort study. BMJ. 2011;342: d738.
23. Hines LA, Freeman TP, Gage SH, Zammit S, Hickman M, Cannon M, et al. Association of high-potency cannabis use with mental health and substance use in adolescence. JAMA Psychiat. 2020;77(10):1044–51.
24. Gregg JM, Campbell RL, Levin KJ, Ghia J, Elliott RA. Cardiovascular effects of cannabinol during oral surgery. Anesth Analg. 1976;55(2):203–13.
25. Malit LA, Johnstone RE, Bourke DI, Kulp RA, Klein V, Smith TC. Intravenous delta9-Tetrahydrocannabinol: effects of ventilatory control and cardiovascular dynamics. Anesthesiology. 1975;42(6):666–73.
26. Mittleman MA, Lewis RA, Maclure M, Sherwood JB, Muller JE. Triggering myocardial infarction by marijuana. Circulation. 2001;103(23):2805–9.
27. Tashkin DP. Effects of marijuana smoking on the lung. Ann Am Thorac Soc. 2013;10(3):239–47.
28. Tan WC, Sin DD. What are the long-term effects of smoked marijuana on lung health? CMAJ. 2018;190(42):E1243–4.
29. Calignano A, Kátona I, Désarnaud F, Giuffrida A, La Rana G, Mackie K, et al. Bidirectional control of airway responsiveness by endogenous cannabinoids. Nature. 2000;408(6808):96–101.
30. Ashton JC, Hancox RJ. The case for cannabinoid cb1 receptors as a target for bronchodilator therapy for β-agonist resistant asthma. Curr Drug Targets. 2018;19(11):1344–9.
31. Gong H Jr, Fligiel S, Tashkin DP, Barbers RG. Tracheobronchial changes in habitual, heavy smokers of marijuana with and without tobacco. Am Rev Respir Dis. 1987;136(1):142–9.
32. Owen KP, Sutter ME, Albertson TE. Marijuana: respiratory tract effects. Clin Rev Allergy Immunol. 2014;46(1):65–81.

33. Boyce SH, Quigley MA. Uvulitis and partial upper airway obstruction following cannabis inhalation. Emerg Med. 2002;14(1):106–8.
34. Mallat A, Roberson J, Brock-Utne JG. Preoperative marijuana inhalation—an airway concern. Can J Anaesth. 1996;43(7):691–3.
35. Abuse NIoD. What are marijuana's long-term effects on the brain? 2021.
36. Zhang LR, Morgenstern H, Greenland S, Chang S-C, Lazarus P, Teare MD, et al. Cannabis smoking and lung cancer risk: pooled analysis in the international lung cancer consortium. Int J Cancer. 2015;136(4):894–903.
37. Rein JL. The nephrologist's guide to cannabis and cannabinoids. Curr Opin Nephrol Hypertens. 2020;29(2):248–57.
38. Parikh M, Sookal S, Ahmad A. Cannabis use in patients presenting to a gastroenterology clinic: associations with symptoms, endoscopy findings, and esophageal manometry. Gastrointestinal Disorders. 2019;1(3):301–7.
39. Chu F, Cascella M. Cannabinoid Hyperemesis Syndrome [Internet]. Treasure Island, FL: StatPearls Publishing. Available from: https://www.ncbi.nlm.nih.gov/books/NBK549915/. (2022). cited 15 Apr 2023
40. DeVuono MV, Parker LA. Cannabinoid hyperemesis syndrome: a review of potential mechanisms. Cannabis Cannabinoid Res. 2020;5(2):132–44.
41. Abuse NIoD. What are marijuana's effects on lung health?; 2021.
42. National Academies of Sciences E, and Medicine; Health and Medicine Division; Board on Population Health and Public Health Practice; Committee on the Health Effects of Marijuana. An Evidence Review and Research Agenda. Cannabis Use and the Abuse of Other Substances. The health effects of cannabis and cannabinoids: the current state of evidence and recommendations for research. Washington, DC: National Academies Press (US); 2017.
43. National Academies of Sciences E, Medicine. The health effects of cannabis and cannabinoids: the current state of evidence and recommendations for research. Washington, DC: The National Academies Press; 2017. p. 486.
44. Schatman ME. Medical use of cannabinoids. JAMA. 2015;314(16):1751.
45. Mücke M, Phillips T, Radbruch L, Petzke F, Häuser W. Cannabis-based medicines for chronic neuropathic pain in adults. Cochrane Database Syst Rev. 2018;3(3):Cd012182.
46. Wallace MS, Marcotte TD, Umlauf A, Gouaux B, Atkinson JH. Efficacy of inhaled cannabis on painful diabetic neuropathy. J Pain. 2015;16(7):616–27.
47. Freeman TP, Groshkova T, Cunningham A, Sedefov R, Griffiths P, Lynskey MT. Increasing potency and price of cannabis in Europe, 2006–16. Addiction. 2019;114(6):1015–23.
48. Freeman TP, Craft S, Wilson J, Stylianou S, ElSohly M, Di Forti M, et al. Changes in delta-9-tetrahydrocannabinol (THC) and cannabidiol (CBD) concentrations in cannabis over time: systematic review and meta-analysis. Addiction. 2021;116(5):1000–10.
49. Kahan M, Srivastava A, Clarke S. Cannabis industry and medical cannabis clinics need regulation. Can Fam Physician. 2019;65(12):864–8.
50. Spindle TR, Sholler DJ, Cone EJ, Murphy TP, ElSohly M, Winecker RE, et al. Cannabinoid content and label accuracy of hemp-derived topical products available online and at national retail stores. JAMA Network Open. 2022;5(7):e2223019.
51. Vandrey R, Raber JC, Raber ME, Douglass B, Miller C, Bonn-Miller MO. Cannabinoid dose and label accuracy in edible medical cannabis products. JAMA. 2015;313(24):2491–3.
52. Lynskey MT, Heath AC, Bucholz KK, Slutske WS, Madden PA, Nelson EC, et al. Escalation of drug use in early-onset cannabis users vs co-twin controls. JAMA. 2003;289(4):427–33.
53. Fergusson DM, Horwood LJ. Does cannabis use encourage other forms of illicit drug use? Addiction. 2000;95(4):505–20.
54. Irvine DMT, Williams J, Huang J. Perioperative considerations of cannabis use on anesthesia administration. Anesthesia Patient Safety Foundation Newsletter. 2022.
55. Schultz NR, Bassett DT, Messina BG, Correia CJ. Evaluation of the psychometric properties of the cannabis use disorders identification test—revised among college students. Addict Behav. 2019;95:11–5.

56. Adamson SJ, Kay-Lambkin FJ, Baker AL, Lewin TJ, Thornton L, Kelly BJ, et al. An improved brief measure of cannabis misuse: the cannabis use disorders identification test-revised (CUDIT-R). Drug Alcohol Depend. 2010;110(1–2):137–43.
57. Connors N, Kosnett MJ, Kulig K, Nelson LS, Stolbach AI. ACMT position statement: interpretation of urine for tetrahydrocannabinol metabolites. J Med Toxicol. 2020;16(2):240–2.
58. Huestis MA, Mitchell JM, Cone EJ. Detection times of marijuana metabolites in urine by immunoassay and GC-MS. J Anal Toxicol. 1995;19(6):443–9.
59. Schep LJ, Slaughter RJ, Glue P, Gee P. The clinical toxicology of cannabis. N Z Med J. 2020;133(1523):96–103.
60. Turner A, Spurling B, Agrawal S. Marijuana Toxicity. Treasure Island, FL: StatPearls Publishing. Available from: https://www.ncbi.nlm.nih.gov/books/NBK430823/. 2023. Cited 10 Apr 2023
61. Shrivastava A, Johnston M, Tsuang M. Cannabis use and cognitive dysfunction. Indian J Psychiatry. 2011;53(3):187–91.
62. Kloft L, Otgaar H, Blokland A, Monds LA, Toennes SW, Loftus EF, et al. Cannabis increases susceptibility to false memory. Proc Natl Acad Sci U S A. 2020;117(9):4585–9.
63. Singh GK. Atrial fibrillation associated with marijuana use. Pediatric Cardiol. 2000;21(3):284.
64. Kosior DA, Filipiak KJ, Stolarz P, Opolski G. Paroxysmal atrial fibrillation following marijuana intoxication: a two-case report of possible association. Int J Cardiol. 2001;78(2):183–4.
65. Desai R, Patel U, Deshmukh A, Sachdeva R, Kumar G. Burden of arrhythmia in recreational marijuana users. Int J Cardiol. 2018;264:91–2.
66. Baskaran J, Anantha Narayanan M, Vakhshoorzadeh J, Ahmad A, Bertog S. Marijuana-induced coronary vasospasm with persistent inter-coronary connection: a case report and review of literature. Cureus. 2019;11(6): e4799.
67. Fischbach P. The role of illicit drug use in sudden death in the young. Cardiol Young. 2017;27(S1):S75–9.
68. Hemachandra D, McKetin R, Cherbuin N, Anstey KJ. Heavy cannabis users at elevated risk of stroke: evidence from a general population survey. Aust N Z J Public Health. 2016;40(3):226–30.
69. Powell D, Pacula RL, Jacobson M. Do medical marijuana laws reduce addictions and deaths related to pain killers? J Health Econ. 2018;58:29–42.
70. Meng H, Hanlon JG, Katznelson R, Ghanekar A, McGilvray I, Clarke H. The prescription of medical cannabis by a transitional pain service to wean a patient with complex pain from opioid use following liver transplantation: a case report. Can J Anaesth. 2016;63(3):307–10.
71. Livingston MD, Barnett TE, Delcher C, Wagenaar AC. Recreational cannabis legalization and opioid-related deaths in Colorado, 2000–2015. Am J Public Health. 2017;107(11):1827–9.
72. Wendelboe AM, Mathew R, Chongsuwat T, Rainwater E, Wendelboe MA, Wickersham E, et al. Is There less opioid abuse in states where marijuana has been decriminalized, either for medicinal or recreational use? a clin-IQ. J Patient Cent Res Rev. 2019;6(4):267–73.
73. Wallace MS, Marcotte TD, Atkinson JH, Padovano HT, Bonn-Miller M. A secondary analysis from a randomized trial on the effect of plasma tetrahydrocannabinol levels on pain reduction in painful diabetic peripheral neuropathy. J Pain. 2020;21(11–12):1175–86.
74. Twardowski MA, Link MM, Twardowski NM. Effects of cannabis use on sedation requirements for endoscopic procedures. J Am Osteopath Assoc. 2019.
75. Holmen IC, Beach JP, Kaizer AM, Gumidyala R. The association between preoperative cannabis use and intraoperative inhaled anesthetic consumption: a retrospective study. J Clin Anesth. 2020;67: 109980.
76. Müller J, Plöchl W, Reiter B, Stimpfl T, Graf A, Baron-Stefaniak J, et al. The effect of oral Δ-9-tetrahydrocannabinol on the minimal alveolar concentration of sevoflurane: a randomised, controlled, observer-blinded experimental study. Eur J Anaesthesiol. 2021;38(1):58–63.
77. Stoelting RK, Martz RC, Gartner J, Creasser C, Brown DJ, Forney RB. Effects of delta-9-tetrahydrocannabinol on halothane MAC in dogs. Anesthesiology. 1973;38(6):521–4.
78. Smith SC. Drug intoxication. Adv Anesthesia Rev. 2023:161.

79. Ibera C, Shalom B, Saifi F, Shruder J, Davidson E. Effects of cannabis extract premedication on anesthetic depth. Harefuah. 2018;157(3):162–6.
80. Salottolo K, Peck L, Tanner Ii A, Carrick MM, Madayag R, McGuire E, et al. The grass is not always greener: a multi-institutional pilot study of marijuana use and acute pain management following traumatic injury. Patient Saf Surg. 2018;12:16.
81. Manini AF, Yiannoulos G, Bergamaschi MM, Hernandez S, Olmedo R, Barnes AJ, et al. Safety and pharmacokinetics of oral cannabidiol when administered concomitantly with intravenous fentanyl in humans. J Addict Med. 2015;9(3):204.
82. Ladha KS, Manoo V, Virji AF, Hanlon JG, McLaren-Blades A, Goel A, et al. The impact of perioperative cannabis use: a narrative scoping review. Cannabis Cannabinoid Res. 2019;4(4):219–30.
83. Yamaori S, Ebisawa J, Okushima Y, Yamamoto I, Watanabe K. Potent inhibition of human cytochrome P450 3A isoforms by cannabidiol: role of phenolic hydroxyl groups in the resorcinol moiety. Life Sci. 2011;88(15–16):730–6.
84. Ruhaak LR, Felth J, Karlsson PC, Rafter JJ, Verpoorte R, Bohlin L. Evaluation of the cyclooxygenase inhibiting effects of six major cannabinoids isolated from cannabis sativa. Biol Pharm Bull. 2011;34(5):774–8.
85. Jefferson DA, Harding HE, Cawich SO, Jackson-Gibson A. Postoperative analgesia in the Jamaican cannabis user. J Psychoactive Drugs. 2013;45(3):227–32.
86. Suhre W, O'Reilly-Shah V, Van Cleve W. Cannabis use is associated with a small increase in the risk of postoperative nausea and vomiting: a retrospective machine-learning causal analysis. BMC Anesthesiol. 2020;20(1):115.
87. Zhang BH, Saud H, Sengupta N, Chen M, Bakshi D, Richardson L, et al. Effect of preoperative cannabis use on perioperative outcomes: a retrospective cohort study. Reg Anesth Pain Med. 2021;46(8):650–5.
88. Bakshi C, Barrett AM. Impact of recreational and medicinal marijuana on surgical patients: a review. Am J Surg. 2019;217(4):783–6.
89. Razzouk J, Chung JH, Lindsey W, Ramos O, Cheng W, Danisa O. Preoperative cannabis use associated with an increased rate of reoperation and postoperative opioid use following anterior cervical decompression and fusion. Cureus. 2022;14(11): e31285.
90. Salottolo K, Peck L, Tanner Ii A, Carrick MM, Madayag R, McGuire E, et al. The grass is not always greener: a multi-institutional pilot study of marijuana use and acute pain management following traumatic injury. Patient Saf Surg. 2018;12(1):16.
91. Gan TJ, Belani KG, Bergese S, Chung F, Diemunsch P, Habib AS, et al. Fourth consensus guidelines for the management of postoperative nausea and vomiting. Anesth Analg. 2020;131(2):411–48.
92. Echeverria-Villalobos M, Todeschini AB, Stoicea N, Fiorda-Diaz J, Weaver T, Bergese SD. Perioperative care of cannabis users: a comprehensive review of pharmacological and anesthetic considerations. J Clin Anesth. 2019;57:41–9.
93. Ruberto AJ, Sivilotti MLA, Forrester S, Hall AK, Crawford FM, Day AG. Intravenous haloperidol versus ondansetron for cannabis hyperemesis syndrome (HaVOC): a randomized. Controll Trial Annal Emerg Med. 2021;77(6):613–9.
94. Hesse M, Thylstrup B. Time-course of the DSM-5 cannabis withdrawal symptoms in poly-substance abusers. BMC Psychiatry. 2013;13:258.
95. Chauchard E, Goncharov O, Krupitsky E, Gorelick DA. Cannabis withdrawal in patients with and without opioid dependence. Subst Abus. 2014;35(3):230–4.
96. Oleson EB, Cheer JF. A brain on cannabinoids: the role of dopamine release in reward seeking. Cold Spring Harb Perspect Med. 2012;2(8): a012229.
97. Nakagawa T, Suzuki Y, Nagayasu K, Kitaichi M, Shirakawa H, Kaneko S. Repeated exposure to methamphetamine, cocaine or morphine induces augmentation of dopamine release in rat mesocorticolimbic slice co-cultures. PLoS ONE. 2011;6(9): e24865.
98. Bonnet U, Preuss UW. The cannabis withdrawal syndrome: current insights. Subst Abuse Rehabil. 2017;8:9–37.

99. Stewart C, Fong Y. Perioperative cannabis as a potential solution for reducing opioid and benzodiazepine dependence. JAMA Surg. 2021;156(2):181–90.
100. Aviram J, Samuelly-Leichtag G. Efficacy of cannabis-based medicines for pain management: a systematic review and meta-analysis of randomized controlled trials. Pain Physician. 2017;20(6):E755–96.
101. Whiting PF, Wolff RF, Deshpande S, Di Nisio M, Duffy S, Hernandez AV, et al. Cannabinoids for medical use: a systematic review and meta-analysis. JAMA. 2015;313(24):2456–73.
102. Martín-Sánchez E, Furukawa TA, Taylor J, Martin JL. Systematic review and meta-analysis of cannabis treatment for chronic pain. Pain Med. 2009;10(8):1353–68.
103. Stockings E, Campbell G, Hall WD, Nielsen S, Zagic D, Rahman R, et al. Cannabis and cannabinoids for the treatment of people with chronic noncancer pain conditions: a systematic review and meta-analysis of controlled and observational studies. Pain. 2018;159(10):1932–54.
104. Schneider-Smith E, Salottolo K, Swartwood C, Melvin C, Madayag RM, Bar-Or D. Matched pilot study examining cannabis-based dronabinol for acute pain following traumatic injury. Trauma Surg Acute Care Open. 2020;5(1): e000391.
105. Holdcroft A, Maze M, Doré C, Tebbs S, Thompson S. A multicenter dose-escalation study of the analgesic and adverse effects of an oral cannabis extract (Cannador) for postoperative pain management. Anesthesiology. 2006;104(5):1040–6.
106. Hickernell TR, Lakra A, Berg A, Cooper HJ, Geller JA, Shah RP. Should cannabinoids be added to multimodal pain regimens after total hip and knee arthroplasty? J Arthroplasty. 2018;33(12):3637–41.
107. Buggy DJ, Toogood L, Maric S, Sharpe P, Lambert DG, Rowbotham DJ. Lack of analgesic efficacy of oral delta-9-tetrahydrocannabinol in postoperative pain. Pain. 2003;106(1–2):169–72.
108. Beaulieu P. Effects of nabilone, a synthetic cannabinoid, on postoperative pain. Can J Anaesth. 2006;53(8):769–75.
109. Nielsen S, Picco L, Murnion B, Winters B, Matheson J, Graham M, et al. Opioid-sparing effect of cannabinoids for analgesia: an updated systematic review and meta-analysis of preclinical and clinical studies. Neuropsychopharmacology. 2022;47(7):1315–30.

Perioperative Analgesic Approach to Patients on Baseline Opioid Antagonist or Mixed Agonist/antagonist Therapy

Ann Heyer, Ashley Shilling, and Brittany Deiling

Abstract Managing patients and optimizing peri-operative outcomes in patients prescribed either opioid antagonists or mixed agonists/antagonists requires strategic planning and specific knowledge of the pharmacokinetics/pharmacodynamics of these agents. Opioid antagonists, including naloxone and naltrexone, block opioid receptors and displace opioid agonists due to their higher affinity for the receptor. Mixed agonist/antagonist therapeutics include buprenorphine, butorphanol, nalbuphine, and pentazocine, with buprenorphine being the most commonly used, currently. Indications for this class of drugs include reversal of respiratory depression caused by opioids, reversal of opioid overdose, reduction in the risk of opioid abuse, and prevention of relapse in those addicted to opioids or alcohol. With addiction and opioid use disorders ascending to become a public health crisis in the United States, the number of patients presenting for surgery prescribed or otherwise self-administering either antagonists or mixed agonist/antagonists has increased. Peri-operative analgesia can be substantially challenging in these patients and therefore instituting appropriate screening and planning management prior to day of surgery is imperative. For patients taking naltrexone, it is important to contact the provider managing the patient's prescription to understand indications and formulate a plan for analgesic strategies. Naltrexone should be stopped before a major surgery in order to provide effective analgesia; this requires either 72 hours prior to procedure for the oral formulation, and 4 weeks for the injectable formulation. Buprenoprhine-naloxone can be continued throughout the perioperative period to reduce the risk of relapse. For isolated buprenorphine preparations, the intrinsic analgesic properties of this agent and altered dosing regimens may be harnessed to provide enhanced analgesia. For any of these partial agonist/antagonist agents, multimodal pain regimens are incredibly

A. Heyer
Department of Anesthesiology, University of Wisconsin, Madison, WI, USA
e-mail: aheyer2@wisc.edu

A. Shilling (✉) · B. Deiling
Department of Anesthesiology, University of Virginia Health System, Charlottesville, VA, USA
e-mail: ABM5F@hscmail.mcc.virginia.edu

B. Deiling
e-mail: bd8hp@uvahealth.org

A. Abd-Elsayed and K. Schroeder (eds.), *Perioperative Pain Management*,
https://doi.org/10.1007/978-3-031-67648-2_28

useful. With naltrexone, it is important to closely monitor patients for signs of overdose, and non-opioid strategies may need to be employed in emergent situations when pre-operative planning is not possible. Follow-up with the patient's regular prescriber for both naltrexone and buprenorphine-naloxone is critical to ensure appropriate continuation of their prescriptions.

Keywords Opioid antagonist · Mixed agonist/antagonist therapy · Naloxone · Naltrexone · Nalbuphine · Suboxone · Buprenorphine · Addiction · Perioperative management

1 Introduction

The most commonly used opioid antagonists include naloxone and naltrexone. With very high affinity for opioid receptors but no activity, their role is to block opioid receptors and displace opioid agonists [1]. Indications for this class of drugs include [1] treatment of opioid overdose and [2] prevention of opioid abuse potential. Antagonists are also used to rapidly reverse opioid-related side effects including respiratory depression and opioid overdose. The use of opioid antagonists can block the effects of other opioids including heroin, morphine, and oxycodone and are therefore used for reducing opioid abuse potential and to prevent relapse [2]. Antagonists can be administered by many routes including intranasal, oral, intramuscular, subcutaneously, or via an endotracheal tube.

Mixed agonist/antagonist therapeutics include suboxone (buprenorphine and naloxone), Embeda (morphine and naltrexone), Targinact (oxycodone and naloxone), and OxyNal (oxycodone and naltrexone). These are oral drug formulations that contain an opioid and an opioid antagonist and are used to reduce the risk of opioid abuse. When given orally, the dose of antagonist is insufficient to antagonize the opioid, but if crushed or injected, the antagonist is released in large enough quantities to perform this function [2]. Additionally, buprenorphine can be used in isolation and acts as a partial agonist.

Although acute use of opioid receptor antagonists in the setting of opioid overdose and respiratory depression are of high concern to anesthesia providers, the long-term use of these agents may complicate perioperative analgesic efforts [3].

2 Patient Population

Substance use disorder (SUD) is a public health crisis in the United States. In 2019, 20.4 million individuals were diagnosed with substance use disorders (SUD). Almost 71,000 people died of drug overdoses in 2019 [4] and the current opioid epidemic is the deadliest in American history [5].

Opioid overdose rates are higher in men than in women, although women aged 40–64 are the demographic showing the fastest growth rates in overdoses and emergency room visits, and death rates are increasing for people of all ages [6]. Non-Hispanic whites represent the racial group associated with the highest overdose risk [7]. Historically, the population hardest hit by the opioid crisis has been white Americans without college degrees from rural areas that have experienced declines in manufacturing and construction jobs [8]. The higher rates in white, non-Hispanic populations has been attributed to bias from providers being less likely to prescribe opioids to non-whites, but the rate of overdose in black populations has been rising as the epidemic shifts from largely prescription opioids to fentanyl and heroin [9].

Additionally, there exists a relationship between mental health disorders and substance abuse. People with anxiety and depression are three times more likely to abuse opioids [10]. In addition to mental health disorders, those with physical ailments are also disproportionately affected by opioid misuse. Examples include those with chronic pain or patients with back or knee pain requiring surgical intervention [11, 12].

Alcoholism is another indication for opioid antagonists and mixed opioid antagonists/agonist treatment. Alcohol abuse is most prevalent in men and whites when compared to blacks, Asians, and Hispanics. It is also more common in those who are unmarried and of lower socioeconomic status [13]. The prevalence of alcohol abuse generally decreases with age, with the highest incidence in those aged 20–29 and generally decreasing with age [14].

Although drug addiction is a large societal problem, only one in six individuals struggling with substance use disorders seeks treatment [15]. The least likely populations to seek treatment for substance use disorders include traditionally underserved groups including the elderly, racial-ethnic minorities, low-income individuals, the un-insured, and people living in rural populations [16]. Therefore, those most likely to be receiving treatment include those with historically better access to healthcare.

3 Implications for the Perioperative Setting

There are many challenges that may be encountered when treating patients prescribed opioid antagonists or mixed agonist/antagonists in the perioperative setting. These include patient concerns and fears of experiencing both pain and bias in the perioperative period as well as the clinical challenges in treating pain. Patients might also be concerned about what analgesic options might be available and how well they will work given the medications they are taking. The following content will discuss preoperative, intraoperative, and postoperative considerations for those patients exposed to baseline opioid antagonists and mixed opioid antagonist/agonist treatment.

4 Preoperative Management

Patients with SUDs often experience significant anxiety surrounding surgery. Fears about stigma and shame about their condition can limit what patients choose to disclose about their medical background, opioid administration history, and struggles with substance use disorders [17]. Patients may also worry about receiving adequate pain relief, experiencing withdrawal symptoms, and relapsing [17]. It is important to keep these worries in mind when treating this population and approach these patients in a non-judgmental fashion.

For preoperative planning, it is important to contact the healthcare professional managing the patient's opioid receptor modulation prescriptions. It is also worth considering a multi-specialty consult that includes the surgical team, acute pain, chronic pain and/or addiction pain medicine services [17]. Involving the patient's baseline opioid receptor modulator prescribers and securing patient buy-in while simultaneously addressing education and patient-specific goals and concerns is an imperative component of successful analgesic planning paradigms. The risks of relapse should be discussed with patients and they should be provided with concerning signs and symptoms that might trigger further evaluation. Table 1 provides an outline of opioid receptor modulators and considerations for use in the perioperative period.

Table 1 Summary of opioid receptor modulators with agonist or partial agonist actions [18–21, 21–31]

	Buprenorphineand buprenorphine-naloxone	Naltrexone
Mechanism of action	Partial agonist at mu receptor, can be combined with naloxonewhich acts as an antagonist at the mu receptor	Full antagonist at mu receptor
Common dosages	2–24 mg with SL or PO daily (for OUD); mcg dosing for chronic pain	PO daily: 50 mg IM depot injection: 380 mg (q 21 days)
Pre-op recommendations	Continue the patient's home dose during the perioperative period	PO: Hold for 72 hours prior to surgery IM: Hold 4 weeks after last injection
Post- op recommendations	Consider splitting daily home dose into BID or TID for improved analgesiafor acute pain	Patients should be monitored carefully for signs and symptoms of inappropriate opioidtherapy

For both buprenorphineand naltrexone, it is important to communicate with the patient's MOUD outpatient prescriber to coordinate preoperative and postoperative discharge planning

Mixed Agonist/Antagonist and Partial Agonist Therapies

The most commonly prescribed agent utilized as an opioid abuse abatement tool is buprenorphine which is a partial mu-opioid receptor agonist and an antagonist at the kappa-opioid receptor. Many healthcare professionals experience trepidation when treating acute postoperative pain in patients prescribed buprenorphine secondary to its long half-life, high affinity for the mu opioid receptor and its ability to displace full mu receptor agonists. Although there are many misconceptions surrounding buprenorphine and its impact on perioperative analgesia, it is important to recall that buprenorphine has potent analgesic properties related to its high affinity for binding to mu opioid receptors. Even with its high binding affinity, at standard dosing of buprenorphine, there remain open receptors available for binding of full mu receptor agonists and therefore it may still be advisable to consider the administration of full opioid receptor agonists. Alternatively, harnessing buprenorphine's analgesic properties through dose escalation or divided dosing may accomplish significant analgesic provision without significantly increasing the risk of respiratory depression or euphoric effects seen with shorter acting mu agonists. [18].

When used for opioid use disorder, buprenorphine can be combined with naloxone (Suboxone) in an abuse deterrent formulation. When left untampered, the naloxone contained within Suboxone is inactive and does not hinder opioid activity at mu receptors. In the event of attempted pharmacologic tampering, the naloxone in suboxone is activated thereby prompting mu receptor antagonism and opioid withdrawal. This class of drugs is indicated in the treatment of both chronic pain and OUD, but the formulations and dosages differ. The indication for OUD is dosed in milligrams, while microgram dosing is used for chronic pain [18].

The perioperative management of patients prescribed buprenorphine has evolved substantially over time as experience with the drug accumulates and further studies have been published. It was previously recommended that buprenorphine be discontinued prior to surgery to increase opioid receptor availability. However, this practice was concerning because of the potential for abuse in patients with a history of substance abuse disorder or medication management challenges in patients who required re-initiation of buprenorphine treatment. Consensus opinion now recommends continuing buprenorphine throughout the perioperative period. According to their 2020 updates on national practice guidelines for the treatment of opioid use disorder, the American Society of Addiction Medicine states that *"discontinuation of methadone or buprenorphine before surgery is not required. Higher potency intravenous full agonist opioids can be used perioperatively for analgesia"* [19].

Furthermore, a clinical practice advisory reports that it is rarely recommended to wean or decrease the patient's home dose [20]. As always, these considerations need to be tailored to the individual patient and the resources available at an individual institution. It is important to have adequate preoperative planning with patients on buprenorphine including communication with their prescriber and discussion with the patient. Utilization of multimodal analgesic and regional anesthesia, when possible, should be considered, in addition to consulting with an acute pain service, depending on location resources.

For patients maintained on buprenorphine-naloxone treatment, the current consensus is to continue treatment; however, discontinuing buprenorphine-naloxone 2–5 days prior to elective surgery has been reported [21, 22]. If a patient has been off buprenorphine-naloxone for greater than 5 days, the patient can be treated with full mu receptor agonist opioids. However, if it was not discontinued, it is important to consider the level of pain associated with the procedure. If there is minimal anticipated postoperative pain, it is appropriate to proceed with the surgery. If moderate to severe pain is anticipated, some protocols suggest canceling the surgery if possible and contacting the patient's buprenorphine-naloxone provider to plan for discontinuing the patient's medication at least 5 days prior to the procedure and transitioning to short acting opioids. However, some protocols suggest holding buprenorphine-naloxone on the day of surgery and others suggest continuing it, so the patient's goals will have to be kept in mind [22–24]. However, the risk of relapse in patients maintained on suboxone is now generally seen as a contraindication to pausing therapy in most patients presenting for surgery.

There are advantages to continuing buprenorphine or buprenorphine-naloxone in the perioperative period that should be considered prior to making medication administration recommendations. Short acting opioids in the absence of opioid receptor antagonism may not the best choice for treating postoperative pain in patients with a history of opioid use disorder as these patients may be susceptible to their euphoria-inducing properties. This property exposes these patients to an elevated risk of relapse during a period when they may already be anxious and vulnerable. Another advantage to continuing preoperative buprenorphine or suboxone regimens is through the maintenance of stable levels of these therapeutics throughout the perioperative period and a diminished need to make outpatient follow-up dosing adjustments [25–27]. Lastly, some case reports have shown that there is no benefit to discontinuing these drugs before surgery and therefore pausing therapy may be exposing patients to an elevated risk profile without an accompanying benefit [28–30]. The risk of relapse with perioperative buprenorphine or suboxone discontinuation is real and one study reported a > 50% chance of recurrence of OUD when buprenorphine was discontinued [32]. Given the evidence that patients' pain can be treated effectively without pausing buprenorphine or buprenorphine-naloxone, it can be advantageous for patients to continue use throughout the perioperative period to reduce their risk of relapse.

Naltrexone

Naltrexone is a full antagonist at the mu-opioid receptor that causes exogenous opioid administration to be ineffective. In addition to the treatment of opioid use disorders, naltrexone is also used in the treatment of alcohol use disorder. Naltrexone is administered as a monthly injectable formulation and an oral formulation. The oral formulation is dosed daily, whereas the longer acting injectable is usually dosed every 21 days. Unlike buprenorphine which is recommended to be continued in the perioperative period, naltrexone will need to be held for surgeries where perioperative opioids will be required. The recommendations on holding naltrexone differ depending on the formulation, but careful planning should include communication with the patient's naltrexone prescriber to ensure adequate analgesia planning. For those maintained on the oral formulation, a wash-out period of at least 72 hours is necessary prior to proceeding with elective surgery. If a patient is maintained on the injectable formulation, elective surgery should be scheduled at least 4 weeks following the last dose. Again, planning should involve the patient's naltrexone prescriber, and concerns for pain management as well as relapse should be discussed. If the patient has any previous experience with surgery and challenging postoperative analgesia, these concerns should be discussed in advance of surgery to allow for the creation of a shared perioperative analgesic management plan [21, 31].

5 Postoperative Management

In all patients with a history of opioid use disorder, it is important to maximize multimodal analgesic therapies. If buprenorphine-naloxone or buprenorphine has been discontinued, a substance abuse or addiction medicine consult is advisable to provide guidance on follow-up and eventual resumption of Suboxone dosing. [21]. Acetaminophen, gabapentin/pregabalin, NSAIDs, ketamine/lidocaine infusions, and alpha-2 agonists (dexmedetomidine) should be considered as agents that might decrease pain in the setting of opioid receptor occupation/antagonism. Non-pharmacologic analgesic approaches including acupuncture, behavioral therapy, massage, etc. may be useful approaches in these patients less likely to respond to opioid analgesics [21]. Long-acting opioids including methadone should be considered as a mechanism for providing consistent opioid receptor action and short acting intravenous opioids, often in the form of a PCA, should be offered for severe breakthrough pain. Regional anesthesia techniques should be maximized to the extent possible and the use of catheter techniques or local anesthetic additives may be more beneficial in these patients less likely to respond to opioid analgesics [21, 33]. The dose of buprenorphine-naloxone or buprenorphine should be divided into 3–4 times per day for better coverage [21]. Finally, patients should be closely monitored after surgery for any signs of cravings or withdrawal, and the patient's emotional state and level of anxiety should be frequently assessed. It is important to ensure that patients feel safe and that their analgesic needs are appropriately addressed. If opioids are needed postoperatively, it is important to ensure that they are stored and administered safely to reduce the risk of misuse, relapse and overdose [21].

With long-term naltrexone use, there is a resulting increase in the density of opioid receptors. If naltrexone is not held prior to a surgical procedure, it is important to keep in mind that higher than expected opioid dosing will be required to accomplish targeted analgesic goals [34]. If naltrexone is held, opioid administration will result in a greater than expected clinical effect secondary to receptor upregulation [35].

This scenario may be challenging because a proportional increase in the patient's sensitivity to opioids may increase the risk of overdose and significant sedation and respiratory depression [36]. It is therefore important to monitor these patients closely for any signs of excessive opioid administration [21]. Multimodal approaches to pain control represents a sound analgesic strategy and regional anesthesia techniques may be of particular benefit in the setting of emergency surgery when there is inadequate time for medication management or optimization [21].

6 Discharge Planning

For patients on both naltrexone, buprenorphine, and buprenorphine-naloxone, it is imperative that good follow-up be arranged with the patient's primary care provider and analgesic prescriber. Any pain medications continued postoperatively and at discharge will need to be accompanied by very clear dosing and monitoring instructions. Coordination with the patient's medication prescriber will help ensure that chronic pain or abuse deterrent medications are continued appropriately or restarted in a timely manner [21]. Finally, patient education that focuses on the risks of overdose and a prescription for naloxone should be strongly considered [21].

Key Points

- Buprenorphine alone or combined with naloxone can be continued throughout the perioperative setting to reduce the risk of relapse.
- If buprenorphine, alone or combined with naloxone, is discontinued prior to surgery, treatment with standard opioid dosing regimens is generally appropriate.
- Regardless of whether buprenorphine or buprenorphine-naloxone is continued into the perioperative period or not, it is important to maximize multimodal pain regimens including acetaminophen, gabapentin, and NSAIDS. Ketamine or alpha-2 agonist infusions/transdermal administration can be considered as analgesic adjuncts or in patients with contraindications to regional anesthetic techniques.
- The dose of buprenorphine and buprenorphine-naloxone should be divided up into 3–4 times per day.
- Naltrexone has a monthly injectable formulation and an oral formulation. For those maintained on the oral formulation, a wash-out period of at least 72 hours is necessary prior to proceeding with elective surgery. If a patient is on the injectable formulation, elective surgery should be scheduled at least 4 weeks after the last dose.
- If naltrexone was not held, it is important to keep in mind that higher than expected amounts of opioids will need to be used.
- If naltrexone was held, any opioids given will cause a greater than expected effect due to the upregulation of receptors. It is therefore very important to monitor these patients closely for any sign of overdose.

- For patients on naltrexone, buprenorphine, and buprenorphine-naloxone, it is imperative that patients be followed closely by their primary care and maintenance regimen prescribers. Excess opioid/overdose monitoring education and a naloxone prescription offer a degree of safety in patients at elevated risk for opioid-related sedation and respiratory depression.

References

1. Choi YS, Billings JA. Opioid antagonists: a review of their role in palliative care, focusing on use in opioid-related constipation. J Pain Symptom Manage. 2002;24:71–90.
2. Barnett V, Twycross R, Mihalyo M, Wilcock A. Opioid antagonists. J Pain Symptom Manage. 2014;47(2):341–52.
3. Matthews S, Dwyer R, Snoek A. Stigma and self-stigma in addiction. J Bioeth Inq. 2017;14:275–86.
4. Substance Abuse and Mental Health Services Administration. 2019 NSDUH detailed tables. National Survey on Drug Use and Health. 2020. Available from: https://www.samhsa.gov/data/report/2019-nsduh-detailed-tables
5. Katz J. Short answers to hard questions about the opioid crisis. The New York Times. 2017
6. Brandeis University Heller School for Social Policy and Management. 2013. Upstream opportunities for reducing the harm of alcohol and drug use.
7. Henry J. Kaiser Family Foundation. 2018. Opioid overdose rates by race and ethnicity.
8. Case A, Deaton A. The media gets the opioid crisis wrong. Here is the truth. The Washington Post. 2017
9. Hansen H, Netherland J. Is the prescription opioid epidemic a White problem? Am J Public Health. 2016;106(12):2127–9.
10. Davis MA, Lin LA, Liu H, Sites BD. Prescription opioid use among adults with mental health disorders in the United States. J Am Board Family Med. 2017;30(4):407–17.
11. Bouckoms AJ, Masand P, Murray GB, Cassem EH, Stern TA, Tesar GE. Chronic nonmalignant pain treated with long-term oral narcotic analgesics. Ann Clin Psychiatry. 1992;4(3):185–92.
12. Brummett CM, Waljee JF, Goesling J, Moser S, Lin P, Englesbe MJ, Nallamothu BK. New persistent opioid use after minor and major surgical procedures in US adults. JAMA Surg. 2017;152(6): e170504.
13. Hasin DS, Stinson FS, Ogburn E, Grant BF. Prevalence, correlates, disability, and comorbidity of DSM–IV alcohol abuse and dependence in the United States: results from the national epidemiologic survey on alcohol and related conditions. Arch Gen Psychiatry. 2007;64(7):830–42.
14. Grant BF, Goldstein RB, Chou SP, et al. Sociodemographic and psychopathologic predictors of first incidence of DSM–IV substance use, mood and anxiety disorders: results from the wave 2 national epidemiologic survey on alcohol and related conditions. Mol Psychiatry. 2009;14(11):1051–66.
15. Brandon T, Irvin VJ, Litvin E. Relapse and relapse prevention. Annu Rev Clin Psychol. 2007;3:257–84.
16. Wang PS, Lane M, Olfson M, Pincus HA, Wells KB, Kessler RC. Twelve-month use of mental health services in the United States: results from the National Comorbidity Survey Replication. Arch Gen Psychiatry. 2005;62(6):629–40.
17. Substance Abuse and Mental Health Services Administration. Behavioral health barometer: United States. Rockville, MD: Substance Abuse and Mental Health Services Administration; 2017.

18. Kohan L, Potru S, Barreveld AM, et al. Buprenorphine management in the perioperative period: educational review and recommendations from a multisociety expert panel. Reg Anesth Pain Med. 2021;46(10):840–59. https://doi.org/10.1136/rapm-2021-103007.
19. American Society of Addiction Medicine. National practice guideline for the treatment of opioid use disorder. Available: https://www.asam.org/docs/defaultsource/quality-science/npg-jam-supplement.pdf?sfvrsn=a00a52c2_2. Accessed 22 Sep 2020. 82 Bentzley BS, Barth K.
20. Goel A, Azargive S, Lamba W. The perioperative patient on buprenorphine: a systematic review of perioperative management strategies and patient outcomes. Le patient en période périopératoire sous buprénorphine: revue systématique des stratégies de gestion périopératoire et de l'évolution des patients. *Can J Anaesth* 2019;66:201–17.
21. Ward EN, Quaye AN, Wilens TE. Opioid use disorders: perioperative management of a special population. Anesth Analg. 2018;127(2):539–47.
22. Wenzel JT, Schwenk ES, Baratta JL, Viscusi ER. Managing opioid-tolerant patients in the perioperative surgical home. Anesthesiol Clin. 2016;34:287–301.
23. Bryson EO. The perioperative management of patients maintained on medications used to manage opioid addiction. Curr Opin Anaesthesiol. 2014;27:359–64.
24. Naloxone Hydrochloride. In: Micromedex solutions. Truven Health Analytics, Inc, Ann Arbor, MI: Available at: http://www.micromedexsolutions.com/micromedex2/librarian. Accessed 12 June 2017.
25. Kampman K, Jarvis M. American Society of Addiction Medicine (ASAM) National Practice Guideline for the use of medications in the treatment of addiction involving opioid use. J Addict Med. 2015;9:358–67.
26. Alford D, Compton P, Samet J. Acute pain management for patients receiving maintenance methadone or buprenorphine therapy. Ann Intern Med. 2007;48:127–34.
27. Anderson TA, Quaye ANA, Ward EN, Wilens TE, Hilliard PE, Brummett CM. To stop or not, that is the question: acute pain management for the patient on chronic buprenorphine. Anesthesiology. 2017;126:1180–6.
28. Chern S, Isserman R, Chen L, Ashburn M, Liu R. Perioperative pain management for patients on chrnoic buprenoprhine: a case report. J Anesth Clin Res. 2013;3:250.
29. Kornfeld H, Manfredi L. Effectiveness of full agonist opioids in patients stabilized on buprenorphine undergoing major surgery: a case series. Am J Ther. 2010;17:523–8.
30. Hansen LE, Stone GL, Matson CA, Tybor DJ, Pevear ME, Smith EL. Total joint arthroplasty in patients taking methadone or buprenorphine/naloxone preoperatively for prior heroin addiction: a prospective matched cohort study. J Arthroplasty. 2016;31:1698–701.
31. Vickers AP, Jolly A. Naltrexone and problems in pain management. BMJ. 2006;332:132–3.
32. Bentzley BS, Barth KS, Back SE, et al. Discontinuation of buprenorphine maintenance therapy: perspectives and outcomes. J Subst Abuse Treat. 2015;52:48–57. https://doi.org/10.1016/j.jsat.2014.12.011. PMID: http://www.ncbi.nlm.nih.gov/pubmed/25601365
33. Anderson TA, Quaye ANA, Ward EN, Wilens TE, Hilliard PE, Brummett CM. To stop or not, that is the question: acute pain management for the patient on chronic buprenorphine. Anesthesiology. 2017;126:1180–6.
34. Yoburn BC, Sierra V, Lutfy K. Simultaneous development of opioid tolerance and opioid antagonist-induced receptor upregulation. Brain Res. 1990;529:143–8.
35. Lesscher HM, Bailey A, Burbach JP, Van Ree JM, Kitchen I, Gerrits MA. Receptor-selective changes in mu-, delta- and kappa-opioid receptors after chronic naltrexone treatment in mice. Eur J Neurosci. 2003;17:1006–12.
36. Dean RL, Todtenkopf MS, Deaver DR, et al. Overriding the blockade of antinociceptive actions of opioids in rats treated with extended-release naltrexone. Pharmacol Biochem Behav. 2008;89:515–22.

Interventions

Chronic Pain Procedures in Anticipation of Surgery/Pain Status Optimization

Loren Shamalov, Yehuda Masturov, and Gary S. Schwartz

Abstract This chapter addresses the issue of chronic pain in anticipation of surgery and the importance of a multidisciplinary approach for pain status optimization. It provides insights into the classification of chronic pain, emphasizing neuropathic and nociceptive pain. Preoperative assessment and evaluation methods, including pain assessment tools and diagnostic tests, are discussed to aid in devising individualized pain management plans. Non-pharmacological interventions, such as physical therapy and rehabilitation, are explored as effective approaches to managing chronic pain. The chapter further discusses the preoperative use of interventional pain procedures, such as peripheral nerve stimulation, epidural steroid injections, and facet joint injections, highlighting their benefits and limitations. Preoperative pain optimization strategies, with a focus on timing interventions and procedures, are also discussed to improve surgical outcomes and reduce postoperative complications.

Keywords Chronic pain · Preoperative pain · Surgical outcomes · Pain management · Interventional pain procedures · Epidural steroid injections · Peripheral nerve stimulation · Facet joint injections · Multidisciplinary approach

---

L. Shamalov · Y. Masturov
CUNY School of Medicine, New York, NY, USA
e-mail: ymastur000@citymail.cuny.edu

G. S. Schwartz (✉)
Maimonides Medical Center, 4802 tenth ave, Brooklyn, NY, USA
e-mail: Gschwartz@maimo.org; Gary.Schwartz@AABPCorp.com

A. Abd-Elsayed and K. Schroeder (eds.), *Perioperative Pain Management*,
https://doi.org/10.1007/978-3-031-67648-2_29

1 Introduction

Background and Significance of Chronic Pain in Anticipation of Surgery

The prevalence of chronic pain prior to surgery is an ever-growing problem with widespread implications. It can complicate the surgical process, which could result in poorer outcomes such as protracted hospital stays and slower recoveries. The increased fear and psychological discomfort that individuals with preoperative pain face only serve to exacerbate these problems. Therefore, it is crucial to control preoperative discomfort in order to optimize surgical outcomes and patient satisfaction. It is imperative to use a multidisciplinary approach combining surgeons, anesthesiologists, pain specialists, and other healthcare professionals to design specialized preoperative pain management regimens. Healthcare practitioners can enhance surgical outcomes and guarantee greater patient satisfaction by managing preoperative discomfort through the use of interventional pain procedures.

2 Understanding Chronic Pain in Anticipation of Surgery

Definition/Classification of Chronic Pain

The general consensus is that chronic pain is persistent or recurrent pain that lasts longer than three months or persists after the anticipated time for tissue healing despite adequate treatment [1]. It is a multifactorial condition that comprises intricate relationships between economic, psychological, and physical elements. The classification of chronic pain can be broken down into neuropathic pain, nociceptive pain, or mixed pain depending on the underlying pathology. Neuropathic pain is a condition that develops as a result of damage or dysfunction to the nervous system. Neuropathic pain is frequently described as an electric, shock-like pain that comes with shooting, burning, or tingling sensations [1]. Since nerve injury is a major cause of neuropathic pain, it can result from disorders such as post-herpetic neuralgia and diabetic neuropathy. In contrast to neuropathic pain, nociceptive pain is induced through the stimulation of nociceptors, specialized nerve endings that detect tissue injury. Nociceptive pain is frequently localized to the area of inflammation or damage and is typically described as dull, achy, or throbbing. It may be triggered by disorders such as osteoarthritis, musculoskeletal trauma, and inflammatory conditions.

3 Preoperative Assessment and Evaluation

In the preoperative phase, a comprehensive assessment that includes the patient's pain history, pain assessment tools, physical examination, and diagnostic tests is crucial for effective management of chronic pain.

Patient History and Pain Assessment Tools

Obtaining a comprehensive patient history helps develop a relationship with the patient and foster an understanding of the nature and impact of chronic pain. Healthcare professionals should inquire about pain duration, location, intensity, and quality, as well as factors that worsen or alleviate pain. Assessing pain's impact on daily activities, sleep, mood, and quality of life aids in developing an individualized pain management plan.

Pain assessment tools, such as visual analog scales (VAS) or numeric rating scales (NRS), provide standardized methods to measure pain intensity and track changes over time [2]. These tools facilitate effective communication between patients and healthcare professionals, enabling accurate pain assessment and monitoring treatment response.

Physical Examination and Diagnostic Tests

A comprehensive physical examination serves as a fundamental component in identifying physical aberrations and manifestations of underlying pathologies that contribute to chronic pain. Thorough evaluation of parameters such as posture, range of motion, muscle strength, and sensory function facilitates the detection of localized tenderness or inflammatory indications.

Diagnostic tests involving imaging modalities (e.g., X-rays, MRI, CT scans), nerve conduction studies, and laboratory assessments are often imperative for further assessment of the root cause of chronic pain. These diagnostic measures provide invaluable insights into structural irregularities, nerve functionality, inflammatory markers, and metabolic factors that exert influence over treatment decisions.

Integrating patient history, pain assessment tools, physical examination findings, and diagnostic test results provides a comprehensive understanding of the patient's pain profile, optimizing preoperative pain control, improving surgical outcomes, and enhancing the patient experience.

4 Multidisciplinary Approach to Pain Management

Collaboration of the Healthcare Team

Managing chronic preoperative pain requires a collaborative, multidisciplinary approach involving surgeons, anesthesiologists, pain specialists, and other healthcare professionals. By integrating patient assessments, developing individualized treatment plans, and fostering communication among team members, this approach ensures comprehensive care and optimal pain control. Patient education and empowerment are vital in promoting active participation and enhancing treatment outcomes. The multidisciplinary approach improves surgical results, minimizes preoperative pain, and increases patient satisfaction.

5 Non-pharmacological Interventions

Physical Therapy and Rehabilitation

Physical therapy and rehabilitation interventions are essential non-pharmacological approaches for managing chronic pain. They aim to reduce pain intensity, improve physical function, and enhance overall well-being. Through the use of techniques, such as manual therapy and therapeutic exercises, physical therapists are able to target specific areas of pain and promote muscle strength, joint flexibility, and mobility. Rehabilitation programs, including occupational therapy, focus on restoring functionality and independence. Physicians widely employ them due to their effectiveness in reducing pain, improving functional outcomes, and enhancing quality of life. Integrating physical therapy and rehabilitation into comprehensive management plans can optimize pain control and improve overall well-being.

6 Pharmacological Interventions

Medications for Chronic Pain Management

Pharmacological interventions play a vital role in managing chronic pain in the preoperative phase. Several medications can be utilized, and careful consideration is needed when selecting and dosing them. Medications commonly used for preoperative chronic pain management include analgesics, nonsteroidal anti-inflammatory drugs (NSAIDs), opioids, and additional medications such as antidepressants or anticonvulsants. The choice of medication depends on the type and severity of pain, individual patient factors, and potential risks and benefits.

Considerations for Medication Selection and Doses

Considerations for medication selection involve assessing the patient's medical history, concurrent medications, allergies, and potential drug interactions. Dosing of medications should be individualized based on the patient's pain intensity, response to treatment, and potential side effects. Starting with the lowest effective dose and titrating as needed is important to achieve optimal pain control while minimizing adverse effects.

7 Interventional Pain Procedures

Overview of Interventional Pain Procedures

Interventional pain procedures aim to specifically target and alleviate the underlying sources of pain, offering an alternative or complementary approach to pharmacological and non-invasive treatments. Interventional pain procedures encompass diverse techniques, including nerve blocks, injections, implantable devices, and minimally invasive surgeries. They serve both diagnostic and therapeutic purposes, allowing for accurate identification of pain origin and tailored treatment interventions.

Peripheral nerve stimulation (PNS) is a common interventional procedure used in the treatment of chronic pain. The procedure begins by implanting a small wire-like electrode next to one of the peripheral nerves [3]. It is then able to modulate the activity of the peripheral nerves by delivering electrical impulses to the nerve, thus providing pain relief and blocking abnormal nerve activity. Although used for chronic pain, recent studies [4, 5] demonstrate the benefits of using percutaneous PNS preoperatively. The peripheral nerve stimulation was shown to decrease pain scores and opioid requirements for at least a week after ambulatory orthopedic surgery, with some studies showing improvement from baseline for 3 months [6]. Interestingly, using percutaneous PNS postoperatively for chronic post amputation pain has demonstrated remarkable improvements of pain, demonstrating its effectiveness in amputees [4, 6]. Percutaneous PNS following amputation reduces chronic pain, permitting for better mobility and quality of life postoperatively. Similarly, the benefits of using PNS postoperatively may change the management of pain in the ambulatory setting.

Epidural steroid injections (ESIs) are a common medical procedure used in the management of chronic pain due to irritation and/or inflammation around the spinal nerves [7]. ESIs involve the injection of an anti-inflammatory corticosteroid medication into the epidural space which surrounds the spinal cord. This provides pain relief to the patient by reducing the inflammation and swelling around the spinal nerves. ESIs are usually given with the assistance of fluoroscopy in order to ensure proper placement of the needle [8]. The real time X-ray allows for the visualization of spinal structures, ensuring accurate needle placement, avoidance of critical structures, and verification of accurate contrast spread [9]. Because needle placement alters the spread of the contrast, and hence the effectiveness of the mit is important to use fluoroscopy to guide ESIs.

ESIs are given to patients with a multitude of conditions, some including herniated discs, degenerative disc disease, spondylosis, and spinal stenosis. ESIs conducted preoperatively in those with radiculopathy have demonstrated immediate improvements in short term radicular pain with no long-term effects [10], thus not having any effect on long term surgery risk. The effectiveness of ESIs in patients with spinal stenosis is considerable, with short-term improvement of radicular pain and no worsening of pain or function [11].

An important consideration is the use of an epidurogram postoperatively following epidural catheter placement. While this technique is generally considered in the setting of chronic pain procedures, the use of an epidurogram postoperatively following epidural catheter placement reliably predicts the clinical functionality of the catheter [12, 13]. The ability of the epidurogram to verify bilateral and appropriate dermatomal coverage supports its use in clinical practice.

Facet joint injections are a widely used interventional pain management technique for relieving pain and inflammation related to facet joint conditions. These injections deliver a combination of local anesthetic and corticosteroid directly to the affected joint, providing both diagnostic and therapeutic benefits. The procedure is guided by imaging techniques to ensure accurate needle placement and maximize the success rate of pain relief [14]. Facet joint injections are most effective for pain originating from the facet joints themselves, but they may not address other underlying causes of pain. The duration of pain relief varies, typically lasting from a few weeks to several months, requiring potential repeat injections. While complications are rare, they can include infection, bleeding, nerve damage, and allergic reactions. Swelling and pain at the injection site are usually temporary, and adverse reactions to the medication used are uncommon and resolve quickly. To achieve optimal long-term outcomes, a comprehensive approach to pain management that considers the patient's overall condition and incorporates other treatment modalities is recommended.

Nerve Blocks and Regional Anesthesia Techniques

Injections involve the targeted delivery of medications, such as corticosteroids or local anesthetics, to specific sites of pain. This can reduce inflammation, numb painful areas, or provide therapeutic benefits. Common injection procedures include epidural steroid injections, trigger point injections, and joint injections.

Implantable devices, such as spinal cord stimulators or intrathecal drug delivery systems, are utilized in certain cases to deliver pain-relieving medications directly to the affected area or to modulate effect of pain. Minimally invasive surgeries, such as radiofrequency ablation or neurolysis, involve precise thermal or chemical destruction of specific pain-causing nerves or tissues to achieve pain relief.

Integrating interventional pain procedures into a comprehensive pain management plan offers personalized and targeted treatment options for individuals with chronic pain. These procedures can significantly alleviate pain, enhance functional outcomes, and improve the overall quality of life. However, careful consideration of potential risks, benefits, and patient-specific factors is essential to achieve optimal outcomes and ensure patient safety.

Limitations of Interventional Pain Procedures

As physicians, considering the limitations to the interventional pain procedures discussed earlier is instrumental in selecting the most appropriate intervention. Peripheral nerve stimulation, despite providing patients with immediate relief and improving function and mobility, can have its efficacy hindered due to inability to place the lead directly near the nerve. This is often due to limitations such as invasiveness, intricacy of lead placement, and risk of nerve damage, infection, pain at the site of pulse generator, lead migration, and hardware/battery failure [15]. In addition, the lead can become dislodged and/or fractured during use or removal [4]. Lastly, other important considerations include the lack of potency of PNS as an analgesic as compared to a peripheral nerve block and the insertion time and technique required for lead placement.

In addition, epidural steroid injections (ESI) are an example of another technique whose limitations must be examined closer for physician consideration. Improper ESI placement, also known as a false ESI, can result in the endangerment of nearby tissue and lack of medication delivery. Staining of paravertebral muscles and ligaments, intravascular injection, inadvertent facet joint injection, dural puncture, subdural injection, nerve injury, and disk injury are examples of possible outcomes of improper ESI placement [8]. Preoperative ESI has also been linked to postoperative infection [10, 16, 17], which has prompted recommendation to wait 1 month after ESI to perform surgery [18]. Other potential risks include hematoma, pain at the site of injection, allergic reaction, and radiation exposure [19].

Facet joint injections have several limitations which physicians must take into consideration. Firstly, accurately diagnosing the exact source of back or neck pain can be challenging, and facet joint injections serve as a diagnostic tool in some cases. Although they can provide temporary pain relief, the facet joint may not always be the primary source of the pain. Additionally, the duration of pain relief varies among individuals, ranging from a few weeks to several months, necessitating potential repeat injections. Moreover, facet joint injections are most effective for pain originating from the facet joints themselves, such as facet joint arthritis or facet joint syndrome, and may not address other underlying causes of pain, such as herniated discs or spinal stenosis. Furthermore, while complications are rare, they can include infection, bleeding, nerve damage, and allergic reactions. It is essential to weigh the benefits and limitations of facet joint injections and develop a comprehensive treatment plan that considers the individual's overall health and medical history for optimal pain management outcomes [14].

8 Preoperative Pain Optimization Strategies

Timing of Interventions and Pain Procedures

Several studies have shown that administering steroids into the knee before knee arthroplasty increases the probability of experiencing postoperative infection [20, 21]. In one meta-analysis, patients who had received an intra-articular corticosteroid injection within 3 months before arthroplasty had a higher risk of postoperative periprosthetic joint infection [20]. Similarly, another meta-analysis revealed that patients who received hyaluronic acid or corticosteroid injections within three months prior to total knee arthroplasty had a significantly higher risk of postoperative infection, whereas no notable difference in infection rates was observed for injections administered between four to six months or seven to twelve months before the procedure [21]. Furthermore, another investigation found that receiving corticosteroid injections within two weeks before total knee arthroplasty significantly raised the risk of postoperative infection, while injections within two to four weeks showed a potential trend towards increased infection risk. However, no significant differences were observed for other injection time frames. The multivariate analysis identified injections within two weeks before total knee arthroplasty as an independent risk factor for postoperative infection. Therefore, several articles suggest that undergoing total knee arthroplasty within four weeks to three months of a corticosteroid injection may be linked to a higher risk of postoperative infection [20–22].

9 Conclusion

Future Directions/Areas for Research

Future research should focus on conducting prospective studies with well-defined time frames to investigate the relationship between preoperative steroid injections and postoperative infection risk in knee arthroplasty. Specifically, studies should evaluate infection rates in patients receiving intra-articular corticosteroid injections within different time intervals before the arthroplasty procedure, such as two weeks, two to four weeks, four to six months, and seven to twelve months. Additionally, exploring the impact of different types and dosages of steroids on infection risk can provide valuable insights into optimizing pain management strategies while minimizing complications. Such evidence-based guidelines can significantly improve patient outcomes in knee arthroplasty procedures.

Key Takeaways and Implications

In conclusion, this chapter has highlighted the significance of addressing chronic pain in anticipation of surgery and the need for a comprehensive, multidisciplinary approach to optimize pain status. Key takeaways from this chapter include the understanding of chronic pain classification, differentiating between neuropathic and nociceptive pain, and the importance of preoperative assessment and evaluation to develop personalized pain management plans.

The role of non-pharmacological interventions, such as physical therapy and rehabilitation, has been emphasized as essential components in reducing pain intensity and improving patient well-being. Similarly, pharmacological interventions, when carefully selected and dosed, play a vital role in managing chronic pain in the preoperative phase.

The chapter delves into various interventional pain procedures, providing insights into their benefits and limitations. Integrating these procedures into a comprehensive pain management plan offers personalized and targeted treatment options for individuals with chronic pain, significantly improving pain relief and overall quality of life. Hence, this chapter serves as a guide to preoperative interventional pain procedures to optimize patient outcomes.

References

1. Kela I, Kakarala CL, Hassan M, Belavadi R, Gudigopuram SVR, Raguthu CC, et al. Chronic pain: a complex condition with a multi-tangential approach. Cureus. 2021.
2. Bielewicz J, Daniluk B, Kamieniak P. VAS and NRS, Same or Different? Are Visual analog scale values and numerical rating scale equally viable tools for assessing patients after microdiscectomy? Pain Res Manag. 2022;2022:e5337483. Available from: https://www.hindawi.com/journals/prm/2022/5337483/#copyright
3. Garcia N. Peripheral nerve stimulation. Neuromodulation.com. 2012. Available from: https://www.neuromodulation.com/PNS
4. Ilfeld BM, Plunkett A, Vijjeswarapu AM, Hackworth R, Dhanjal S, Turan A, et al. Percutaneous peripheral nerve stimulation (neuromodulation) for postoperative pain: a randomized, sham-controlled pilot study. Anesthesiology. 2021.
5. Cohen SP, Gilmore CA, Rauck RL, Lester DD, Trainer RJ, Phan T, et al. Percutaneous peripheral nerve stimulation for the treatment of chronic pain following amputation. Mil Med. 2019;184(7–8):e267–74.
6. Albright-Trainer B, Phan T, Trainer RJ, Crosby ND, Murphy DP, Disalvo P, et al. Peripheral nerve stimulation for the management of acute and subacute post-amputation pain: a randomized, controlled feasibility trial. Pain Management. 2021.
7. Lumbar epidural steroid injections: What it is, benefits, risks and side effects. Cleveland Clinic. Available from: https://my.clevelandclinic.org/health/treatments/22091-lumbar-epidural-steroid-injection
8. Shim E, Lee JW, Lee E, Ahn JM, Kang Y, Kang HS. Fluoroscopically guided epidural injections of the cervical and lumbar spine. Radiographics. 2017;37(2):537–61.
9. Weil L, Frauwirth NH, Kasra Amirdelfan, Grant DS, Rosenberg J. Fluoroscopic analysis of lumbar epidural contrast spread after lumbar interlaminar injection. 2008;89(3):413–6.

10. Chou R, Hashimoto R, Friedly J, Fu R, Bougatsos C, Dana T, et al. Epidural corticosteroid injections for radiculopathy and spinal stenosis. Ann Intern Med. 2015;163(5):373.
11. Wentz K, Chung YC, Patel A. The clinical impact of lumbar epidural steroid injections prior to spine surgery for lumbar spinal stenosis. Intervent Pain Med. 2022;1(2): 100104.
12. Yeager MP, Bae EE, Parra MC, Barr PA, Bonham AK, Sites BD. Fluoroscopy-assisted epidural catheter placement: an exploratory analysis of 303 pre-operative epidurograms. Acta Anaesthesiol Scand. 2015;60(4):513–9.
13. Abdel-Moneem MS, Seam EALH, Eskander FSL, Hamza AH, El-Fawal SM. Fluoroscopy-assisted epidural catheter placement: the effect of dye distribution in preoperative epidurograms on postoperative analgesia. Ain-Shams J Anesthesiology. 2022;14(1).
14. Le DT, Alem N. Facet joint injection. PubMed. Treasure Island (FL): StatPearls Publishing; 2022. Available from: https://www.ncbi.nlm.nih.gov/books/NBK572125/
15. Ranson MT, Pope JE. Reducing risks and complications of interventional pain procedures. Philadelphia, Pa. London: Saunders; 2012.
16. Singla A, Yang S, Werner BC, et al. The impact of preoperative epidural injections on postoperative infection in lumbar fusion surgery. J Neurosurg-Spine. 2017. https://doi.org/10.3171/2016.9.SPINE16484.
17. Yang S, Werner BC, Cancienne JM, Hassanzadeh H, Shimer AL, Shen FH, et al. Preoperative epidural injections are associated with increased risk of infection after single-level lumbar decompression. The Spine J: Official J North Am Spine Soc. 2016 [cited 2023 Jul 25];16(2):191–6. Available from: https://pubmed.ncbi.nlm.nih.gov/26235469/
18. Li P, Hou X, Gao Lifeng, Zheng X. Infection risk of lumbar epidural injection in the operating theatre prior to lumbar fusion surgery. 2020 [cited 2023 Jul 25];13:2181–6. Available from: https://www.ncbi.nlm.nih.gov/pmc/articles/PMC7457848/
19. Goodman BS, Posecion LWF, Mallempati S, Bayazitoglu M. Complications and pitfalls of lumbar interlaminar and transforaminal epidural injections. Curr Rev Musculoskeletal Med. 2008;1(3–4):212–22. Available from: https://www.ncbi.nlm.nih.gov/pmc/articles/PMC2682416/
20. Lai Q, Cai K, Lin T, Zhou C, Chen Z, Zhang Q. Prior intra-articular corticosteroid injection within 3 months may increase the risk of deep infection in subsequent joint arthroplasty: a meta-analysis. Clin Orthop Relat Res. 2021;480(5):971–9.
21. Yang X, Li L, Ren X, Nie L. Do preoperative intra-articular injections of corticosteroids or hyaluronic acid increase the risk of infection after total knee arthroplasty? A meta-analysis. Bone Joint Res. 2022;11(3):171–9.
22. Bhattacharjee S, Wallace S, Luu HH, Shi LL, Lee MJ, Chen AF. Do we need to wait 3 months after corticosteroid injections to reduce the risk of infection after total knee arthroplasty? J Am Acad Orthopaedic Surg. 2021;29(14):e714–21. Available from: https://pubmed.ncbi.nlm.nih.gov/33229905/

Perioperative Management of Pumps and Stimulators

Dylan Lewis, Alexander Bautista, and Alaa Abd-Elsayed

Abstract The number of chronic pain patients with implantable devices presenting for surgery has increased substantially as the indications for these devices has continued to expand. This patient population may present a challenge to health-care professionals and a comprehensive understanding of the devices is necessary to optimize the analgesic and anesthetic care of these patients. Implantable neuromodulation devices include intrathecal pain pumps, spinal cord stimulators, and peripheral nerve stimulators. Specific implications for these devices may vary depending on the type of device, location of the surgical procedure, and whether the implantable device is intended to address analgesic concerns within the realm of the surgical insult.

Keywords Neuromodulation · Intrathecal pain pump · Spinal cord stimulation · Perioperative management · Neuraxial block

1 Introduction

A variety of implantable devices have been utilized to help patients suffering from a diverse scope of chronic pain indications. The use of intrathecal pain pumps has been approved for targeted drug delivery of baclofen in the management of spasticity, and opioids and ziconotide for the management of a wide range of nociceptive, neuropathic, or mixed chronic pain syndromes [1]. Spinal cord and peripheral nerve stimulation has been used in patients with chronic neuropathic pain resulting from failed back surgery, chronic regional pain syndrome types 1 and 2, painful diabetic

D. Lewis · A. Bautista
Department of Anesthesiology and Perioperative Medicine, University of Louisville, Louisville, KY, USA
e-mail: dylan.lewis@louisville.edu

A. Bautista
e-mail: alexander.bautista@louisville.edu

A. Abd-Elsayed (✉)
Anesthesiology, University of Wisconsin-Madison, Madison, WI, USA
e-mail: abdelsayed@wisc.edu

A. Abd-Elsayed and K. Schroeder (eds.), *Perioperative Pain Management*,
https://doi.org/10.1007/978-3-031-67648-2_30

neuropathy, nonsurgical refractory low back pain, visceral, and peripheral nerve pain [2]. There exists a paucity of information in the literature specifically focusing on the perioperative management and essential considerations relevant to patients with implanted pain devices presenting for surgery. In many cases, contacting an individual device manufacturer may represent the optimal method to obtain relevant guideline and labeling information.

2 Mechanism of Action

Spinal cord stimulation functions via the delivery of various waveforms and frequencies to modulate pain signaling and decrease pain symptomology. With this variety in electrical stimulation delivery, there are many theories that attempt to explain how this signaling leads to modulation of pain sensation. The most common form of spinal cord stimulation remains dorsal column stimulation, although other variations such as dorsal root ganglion stimulation, do exist [3]. The original, and still leading, theory describing pain modulation via spinal cord stimulation is the gate control theory. This theory hypothesizes that stimulation of the dorsal column-medial lemniscus pathway results in opening of downstream electrochemical gates and activation of GABA and cholinergic spinal interneurons. Subsequent increased activity in descending analgesic pathways ultimately results in inhibition of pain signal transmission along the lateral spinothalamic tract.

These devices all contain similar componentry: the electrodes or leads, insulated wires connecting the leads to the implantable pulse generator (IPG) or battery, and the charging and reprogramming equipment. Leads that are cylindrical can be placed percutaneously with image guidance, whereas paddle leads require a laminotomy/laminectomy for placement. The type of lead can easily be distinguished with fluoroscopy or x-ray. While older forms of SCS included leads with 4 electrodes, new generations of percutaneous arrays commonly contain 8–16 electrodes with paddle arrays containing 16–32, improving stimulation selectivity and programming options [4, 5].

Notably, it is common for patients to either have a single paddle array or 2 percutaneous leads placed. These electrodes in the form of metal contacts, create an electric field, modulating neurons via the software of the specific device [1]. Prior to permanent implantation, most patients undergo a trial with a percutaneous temporary SCS for 5–7 days and must have significant pain relief before proceeding. During permanent implantation, the wires connected to the electrodes are then tunneled subcutaneously and connected to an implanted pulse generator, commonly in the posterior flank.

Peripheral nerve stimulators work in a similar fashion via both central and peripheral mechanisms. Central mechanisms include inhibition of pain signals via the aforementioned gate control theory, modulation of wide dynamic range neurons on the dorsal horn, and reduction of neural impulses via the medial lemniscal pathway. Peripheral PNS mechanisms include disruption of nociceptive afferent fibers and alteration of the local microenvironmental milieu including downregulation of inflammatory mediators. Combined CNS and PNS mechanisms may improve both central and peripheral sensitization of pain. One specific device has been shown to provide sustained relief at 12 months, following only a 60 day period of peripheral stimulation before the temporary externalized leads were removed. These devices involve percutaneous leads delivered along peripheral nerves, with wires connected to internal pulse generators that are, similar to SCS, implanted in the subcutaneous tissue and anchored to fascia, either directly connected to a power source or connected to an external power source transcutaneously that is worn in a harness overlying the battery [2].

Intrathecal pain pump devices allow for the continuous, with or without bolus, delivery of therapeutic agents directly to the intrathecal space, bypassing first pass metabolism and acting directly on spinal cord ion channels and receptors. This mechanism allows for the utilization of molecules that cannot cross the blood brain barrier, for much smaller doses to be used to achieve therapeutic benefit, and a decreased risk of significant adverse effects [6]. These devices have demonstrated benefit in patients with intractable terminal pain, chronic nonmalignant pain, and an expanding collection of other diagnoses. The only medications FDA-approved for intrathecal administration include morphine and ziconotide for chronic pain and baclofen for spasticity, although many other therapeutic agents are used in an off-label fashion either as monotherapy or combination therapy, including local anesthetics and adrenergic agonists such as clonidine. These devices consist of an integrated battery and implanted pump with a refillable reservoir that is connected to a catheter that delivers medication into the intrathecal space. The most common type of intrathecal pump is the Medtronic SynchroMed® II, introduced in 2004. This device consists of a metal housing that holds a bellow containing the drug, which is surrounded by pressurized gas that exerts pressure on both the bellow and the drug. The drug is then delivered via a battery-powered peristaltic pump which has rollers to compress the catheter tubing and advance the drug forward. Notably, differences in temperature and pressure/altitude will affect pump gas pressures and thus medication dosage delivered. In 2012, the Prometra® Flowonix pump received FDA approval for their device which features a dosing chamber that mitigates, but does not eliminate, the dosing variability caused by changes in pressure and temperature. The dosing is managed by an external programming device. Similar to SCS, the intrathecal catheter is tunneled percutaneously to the pump system which is surgically implanted into a subcutaneous pocket, commonly in the posterior flank or lower lateral abdomen. These systems do require medication withdrawal and refill either before medication runs out or expires. Similar to SCS, most patients undergo a trial period, often a single shot of medication into the intrathecal space with monitored therapeutic response prior to permanent pump placement [7].

3 Perioperative Concerns

Similar to AICD and pacemaker devices, it is advisable for implanted pain devices to be interrogated and reprogrammed to turn the device off or to the lowest possible setting/amplitude prior to a planned surgical procedure. Patients with implanted intrathecal pain pumps will likely have a higher opioid tolerance and may require elevated opioid doses in the perioperative phase of care to maintain hemodynamics and address postoperative pain complaints. It is recommended that devices be interrogated post-operatively to ensure proper functioning or delivery of medication. Regarding SCS or intrathecal pump device removal, dural leak is a known complication and the development of signs and symptoms suggesting postdural puncture headache symptomology should prompt further evaluation. If either type of device must be removed intraoperatively, the SCS leads or intrathecal pump catheter may be done via gentle traction after cutting sutures anchoring to the supraspinous fascia and disconnecting the wires from the IPG or catheter from the pump. Collaboration with the device representative on the day of surgery, either by phone or directly in-person, is recommended [1].

4 Magnetic Resonance Imaging (MRI)

Certain implanted devices have demonstrated safety for use in MRI, however, this is not the case for all. These devices may malfunction during or after MRI, leading to dosing errors. In patients with implanted stimulators, broken devices or circuit disruptions, could generate heat when exposed to the magnetic field and injure the patient [1]. Discussions with the device representative is paramount prior to ordering imaging. Most manufacturers will state if their device is MRI compatible, or more commonly the parameters in which the device is MRI conditional. It is important to consider if the patient's medication can be suspended or delivered via a different route of administration during the MRI. In general, the magnetic field created by the scanner will temporarily suspend the pump, pausing drug delivery, and restarting once MRI exposure has ended. It is recommended to interrogate the device 20–30 minutes after the scan to ensure it has restarted automatically. This is particularly important in patients with intrathecal baclofen pumps as withdrawal can be life-threatening. Notably, if the patient has an older SCS, the battery or IPG may be exchanged for a newer model, making the device MRI compatible/conditional [7].

5 Electrocautery

The use of monopolar electrocautery during surgery may affect electrical conductance posing an increased risk to both the patient and their device. When exposed to monopolar electrocautery, patients have previously described lancinating sensations the location of which is impacted by lead placement. If monopolar electrocautery is deemed necessary, implanted stimulation devices need to be turned off and checked for impedance after the procedure. Intraoperative monopolar cautery utilization should be limited to the lowest effective setting and the grounding pad should be placed as far away from the implanted device as possible.

Bipolar electrocautery is preferrable and may present with less risk to the patient. Bipolar devices do not require a dispersive return electrode pad because both the active and return electrodes are integrated in the energy delivery forceps to a smaller focused area [1].

Care should be taken to not touch any part of the SCS device with active cautery as this could cause thermal damage along the tract of the lead or damage the insulated coat of the wire, making the device nonfunctional and/or stimulating/shocking the patient [3].

6 Device Complications for Spinal Cord Stimulators and Intrathecal Pumps

Following intrathecal pump placement, and less commonly SCS placement, dural leak is a known complication occurring in as many as 20% of cases [8]. To prevent this, some providers place a purse-string suture into the dura at the time of placement. Many of these can be managed conservatively with activity modification, positioning, caffeine, OTC headache medication, and fluid resuscitation. If conservative measures fail, the leak must be sealed with blood patch or primary closure. If an intrathecal pump must be explanted, the decision may be made to leave the tied off catheter in place.

Infections can range from superficial, to pocket infection, to fulminant epidural or intrathecal spread in less than 1% of cases [9]. Management of superficial infections may include culture-guided antibiotic administration alone, whereas deeper infections may require device removal, irrigation, and debridement. Most commonly, pathogens are Staphylococcus or gram-negative bacteria. Notably, approximately 1:4 of infected devices are culture-negative. The site most commonly infected is the pocket containing the pump or IPG. Thorough neurological examination, as well as accompanying imaging, should be performed to evaluate for signs and symptoms of meningitis, epidural abscess, and intrathecal infection [10].

Mechanical device complications are known to occur in up to 20% of patients with implanted pumps [8] and less commonly with spinal cord stimulators [10]. Known mechanical failures include catheter/lead migration, dislocation, breakage, granuloma formation at the catheter tip, and pump failure. These complications should be diagnosed with device interrogation, plain radiographs (with contrast for pumps), and CT imaging (following intracatheter contrast administration for pumps).

Neuraxial injury, including paralysis, has been reported after both SCS and intrathecal pump placement. Thankfully, this has been reported in less than 1% of cases for intrathecal catheter [2] and SCS placement [11]. Injury can be a result of direct needle or hardware trauma, hematoma formation, or infection. If the patient's history or physical examination suggests a spinal cord injury, appropriate imaging is indicated to elucidate reversible causes [12–14].

7 Management

Prior to any procedure in a patient with an implanted pump, the age of device, time of last evaluation, medication dosing, and date of next refill should be determined by the care team. If possible, communication with the healthcare professional responsible for pump-management is encouraged, as well as communication with and ensuring availability of the device representative. It is also important to review the specific device's manufacturer guidelines for perioperative management. As previously mentioned, careful titration of intraoperative and postoperative opiate dosing is required in patients with implanted pumps containing opioids. In these patients, the addition of procedure-related opioids may induce unwanted respiratory depression. In those receiving intrathecal baclofen, addition of opioids may have a greater-than expected response due to the synergistic nature of the drugs. Further complicating the clinical management of these patients is the lack of a reliable method for converting intrathecal opioid dosages to intravenous equivalents. For example, estimates for an equianalgesic dose of oral to intrathecal morphine ranges from 12:1 to 300:1. Careful consideration of patient positioning must account for the location of all device components. Most intrathecal pumps are located in the lower abdomen in a location avoiding contact with the pelvis, ribs, and patient's waist or belt-line. In patients with a larger body habitus, the device may be implanted in the posterior flank. Regarding the catheter, care must be taken to avoid excessive twisting and bending as this may result in catheter damage, kinking, occlusion, or dislodgement. Neuraxial analgesia is not absolutely contraindicated in these patients, but cautious care must be taken to avoid damage to the catheter through needle contact and entry must be made at a level different than that of the catheter. Imaging modalities, such as ultrasound, may be helpful in certain circumstances to identify the location of leads or catheter tubing as they course to either their IPG or reservoir. As previously mentioned, temperature of the patient can affect dosing delivered by older pumps, so the recommendation is to maintain patient body temperature below 39 °C, with a lower limit to be kept within the normal physiologic range. In the event that defibrillation is indicated, the first concern is obviously the termination of aberrant arrhythmias and patient survival. If possible, defibrillation pad placement away from implanted devices is desirable. As for diathermy, it is not absolutely contraindicated. The primary concern with diathermy is device heating, which as previously mentioned may alter infusion rates. Shortwave diathermy is not recommended for use within 30 cm of the pump or catheter for this reason. The use of electroconvulsive therapy has not been established, but there is concern regarding alteration in pump operation and flow rate. There is limited data on lithotripsy, but manufacturers do recommend the focus of the beam be at least 15 cm away from the pump. As for radiation therapy, caution should be used as permanent damage can occur. Manufacturer recommendations are to not direct high radiation sources at the pump, or a shield be placed over the pump if necessary. Notably, there is one study of 39 patients in which 12 received radiation with either the pump or the catheter in the field, and all devices were found to be in working order following completion of treatment. Radiofrequency and microwave ablation in the presence of a pump are not well documented, with the primary concern being overdose due to device heating [7].

A number of the aforementioned complications can occur perioperatively, leading to over- or under-dosing of intrathecal medication. It is imperative to recognize and promptly treat these complications.

Signs of morphine withdrawal include malaise, anxiety, myalgia, insomnia, fever, and worsening pain. Investigation of the catheter with a dye study may be warranted, along with interrogation of the pump. In contrast to withdrawal, morphine overdose can be rapidly life-threatening. Overdose symptoms include confusion, sedation, respiratory arrest, and seizures. The first priority should be to provide airway support and administer naloxone. Notably, intrathecal morphine has a much longer half-life than naloxone and therefore attentive monitoring is required to assess for the need for either repeat naloxone dosing or continuous infusion.

Signs and symptoms of baclofen withdrawal include increased spasticity, pruritis, hypotension, tachycardia, paresthesia, muscle rigidity, fever, hallucinations, delirium, delusions and paranoia. Patients with a spinal cord injury at T6 or higher have an increased risk of autonomic dysreflexia, malignant hyperthermia, and neuroleptic malignant syndrome. Baclofen withdrawal treatment includes expedited pump repair and oral baclofen supplementation. Unfortunately, oral baclofen administration may not effectively replace intrathecal baclofen dosing and drugs with similar properties such as propofol and benzodiazepines may also be required. With insufficient data, dantrolene and cyproheptadine may also address the development of significant withdrawal symptoms. Signs of baclofen overdose include drowsiness, lightheadedness, somnolence, dizziness, respiratory depression, and coma. After necessary breathing and circulatory support are provided, a physician experienced with intrathecal baclofen should be consulted to interrogate the pump and determine potential overdose etiologies. The treatment of baclofen overdose includes a temporary pump interruption for no more than 48 hours to minimize the occurrence of pump damage, CSF aspiration through the pump side port can be considered with careful consideration of the amount of CSF aspirated, and physostigmine administration for symptomatic relief. It is worth mentioning that if a catheter dye study is considered for diagnostic reasons, the pump side port should be aspirated for at least the volume of the catheter to avoid bolusing the patient with more medication [7].

Ziconotide overdose management can include dose reduction if mild symptoms are encountered (nausea, dizziness, weakness, somnolence, vision changes) and termination of drug delivery in the setting of severe symptoms (psychosis, suicidal ideation, deep sedation, confusion) [7].

8 Conclusion

An increasing number of patients with implantable stimulators and intrathecal pumps are presenting for surgery. It is critically important to be familiar with the relevant anatomy, device componentry, mechanism of action, and complications associated with these devices in order to optimize the analgesic and anesthetic care of these patients.

Key Takeaways

1. Prior to any procedure in a patient with an implanted pump, device age, time of last evaluation, medication dosing, and date of next refill should be determined by the care team. It is advisable to turn the device off or to the lowest possible setting prior to a planned surgical procedure.
2. Patients with implanted pain pumps will likely have a higher opioid tolerance and may require elevated opioid doses in the perioperative phase of care to maintain hemodynamics and address postoperative pain complaints.
3. It is important to be familiar with device manufacturer recommendations regarding MRI capability. When in doubt, contact the local device representative.
4. Intraoperative monopolar cautery utilization should be limited to the lowest effective setting and the grounding pad should be placed as far away from the implanted device as possible. Bipolar electrocautery is preferable and may present with less risk to the patient. Care should be taken to not touch any part of an SCS device with active cautery as this could cause thermal damage along the tract of the lead or damage the insulated coat of the wire, making the device nonfunctional and/or stimulating/shocking the patient.
5. It is recommended that devices be interrogated post-operatively to ensure proper functioning or delivery of medication.

References

1. Daniels A, McDonald C, Basques B, Hershman S. Perioperative management of spinal cord stimulators and intrathecal pain pumps. J Am Acad Orthop Surg. 2022;30(17):e1095–105. https://doi.org/10.5435/JAAOS-D-22-00053.
2. Abd-Elsayed A, D'Souza RS. Peripheral nerve stimulation: the evolution in pain medicine. Biomedicines. 2021;10(1):18. https://doi.org/10.3390/biomedicines10010018. PMID: 35052698; PMCID: PMC8773238.

3. Harned ME, Gish B, Zuelzer A, Grider JS. Anesthetic Considerations and perioperative management of spinal cord stimulators: literature review and initial recommendations. Pain Physician. 2017;20(4):319–29. PMID: 28535554.
4. Lempka SF, Patil PG. Innovations in spinal cord stimulation for pain. Curr Opin Biomed Eng. 2018;8:51–60. https://doi.org/10.1016/j.cobme.2018.10.005. Epub 2018 Nov 12. PMID: 30911705; PMCID: PMC6430588.
5. Hasoon J, Berger A, Urits I, Orhurhu V, Viswanath O, Aner M. Spinal cord stimulation for the treatment of chronic pelvic pain after Tarlov cyst surgery in a 66-year-old woman: a case report. Case Rep Women's Health. 2020;25: e00171. https://doi.org/10.1016/j.crwh.2020.e00171.
6. Nelson AM, Jericho BG, Anitescu M. Pump IT up-perioperative care of patients with intrathecal drug delivery systems. Anesth Analg. 2022;134(1):32–4. https://doi.org/10.1213/ANE.0000000000005821. PMID: 34908544.
7. Nadherny W, Anderson B, Abd-Elsayed A. Perioperative and periprocedural care of patients with intrathecal pump therapy. Neuromodulation. 2019;22(7):775–80. https://doi.org/10.1111/ner.12880. Epub 2018 Oct 31. PMID: 30378724.
8. Knight KH, Brand FM, Mchaourab AS, Veneziano G. Implantable intrathecal pumps for chronic pain: highlights and updates. Croat Med J. 2007;48(1):22–34. PMID: 17309136; PMCID: PMC2080496.
9. Esquer Garrigos Z, Farid S, Bendel MA, Sohail MR. Spinal cord stimulator infection: approach to diagnosis, management, and prevention. Clin Infect Dis. 2020;70(12):2727–35. https://doi.org/10.1093/cid/ciz994. PMID: 31598641.
10. Deer T, Stewart D (2008). Complications of spinal cord stimulation: identification, treatment, and prevention. Pain Med. 2008;9(1):S93–S101.
11. Labaran L, Jain N, Puvanesarajah V, Jain A, Buchholz AL, Hassanzadeh H. A retrospective database review of the indications, complications, and incidence of subsequent spine surgery in 12,297 spinal cord stimulator patients. Neuromodulation. 2020;23:634–8.
12. Aprili D, Bandschapp O, Rochlitz C, Urwyler A, Ruppen W. Serious complications associated with external intrathecal catheters used in cancer pain patients. Anesthesiology. 2009;111:1346–55.
13. D'Souza RS, Warner MA, Olatoye OO, et al. Perioperative opioid consumption and clinical outcomes in surgical patients with a pre-existing opioid-based intrathecal drug delivery system. Anesth Analg. 2022;134:35–43.
14. Graham RD, Sankarasubramanian V, Lempka SF. Dorsal root ganglion stimulation for chronic pain: hypothesized mechanisms of action. J Pain. 2022;23(2):196–211. https://doi.org/10.1016/j.jpain.2021.07.008. Epub 2021 Aug 20. PMID: 34425252; PMCID: PMC8943693.

Peripheral Nerve Stimulation for Acute Postoperative Pain

John J. Finneran IV and Brian M. Ilfeld

Abstract The use of electric stimulation for pain control ("neuromodulation") has ancient origins. Although studied more extensively for chronic pain, percutaneous peripheral nerve stimulation, especially when combined with a single injection local anesthetic based peripheral nerve block, has the potential to provide weeks of pain relief following painful orthopedic surgeries. In contrast to nerve blocks with local anesthetic, nerve stimulation produces analgesia with minimal sensory, proprioceptive, or motor deficits. Percutaneous stimulation of the brachial plexus and femoral and sciatic nerves has been utilized for analgesia following orthopedic surgery. This chapter will examine the history and mechanism of action of neuromodulation, its application in acute postoperative pain management, as well as associated contraindications and potential complications.

Keywords Neuromodulation · Peripheral nerve stimulation · Gate control theory · Percutaneous lead · Ultrasound-guidance · Peripheral nerve block · Lead fracture

1 History of Neuromodulation

Electrical stimulation for the treatment of pain, or **neuromodulation**, has been utilized for thousands of years. Ancient Greeks and Romans described using living torpedo fish, which can generate up to 220 V, for the treatment of maladies including gout and headache [1]. During the eighteenth and nineteenth centuries, many descriptions of the physiologic effects of application of electricity to various tissues were published, the first of these by Benjamin Franklin in 1774. The nineteenth century witnessed the development of technology that could create, store, and harness electric current; and the popularization of this knowledge is evident in works such as Mary

J. J. Finneran IV · B. M. Ilfeld (✉)
University of California, San Diego, USA
e-mail: bilfeld@health.ucsd.edu

J. J. Finneran IV
e-mail: jfinneran@health.ucsd.edu

A. Abd-Elsayed and K. Schroeder (eds.), *Perioperative Pain Management*,
https://doi.org/10.1007/978-3-031-67648-2_31

Shelley's *Frankenstein*, published in 1818. In the early twentieth century, many electric devices were marketed for the treatment of pain along with nearly every other conceivable ailment [2]. However, the use and marketing of these devices had little or no scientific support. In 1910, the Carnegie Foundation published the Flexner Report, which called on medical schools to improve standards in admission, graduation, and teaching of scientifically backed clinical practice and recommended the exclusion of electrotherapy from clinical practice [3]. Concomitantly, death by electrocution was becoming a common method for execution in the United States, possibly contributing to a decline in public interest in medical devices employing electric current.

Modern use of **peripheral nerve stimulation** to treat pain can be traced to 1967, when neurosurgeons Sweet and Hall [4] reported successfully treating pain in a series of 8 patients using surgically implanted peripheral nerve stimulators. Unfortunately, the application of such devices required relatively large incisions and extensive surgical dissection, precluding use for acute surgical or traumatic pain. Over subsequent decades, percutaneous leads that could be passed through the skin were developed and transcutaneous neuromuscular stimulation–direct stimulation of large muscles–was described for various chronic pain conditions [5]. The advent of ultrasound-based localization of peripheral nerves and real-time guidance of needles towards those nerves offered the possibility of highly targeted stimulation of peripheral nerves without surgical exposure. Huntoon and Burgher [6] were the first to describe peripheral nerve stimulation for treatment of chronic neuropathic pain using a percutaneously inserted lead placed with ultrasound guidance in 2009. In the following years, various lead placement systems were developed and found to be beneficial for treatment of chronic pain. However, at the time of this writing there is only one percutaneous peripheral nerve stimulator lead system cleared by the United States Food and Drug Administration (USFDA) for treatment of acute pain [7].

2 Mechanism of Analgesia

Many hypotheses about how electric stimulation produces analgesia have been posited. The most commonly accepted explanation is the "**Gate Control Theory**," first described by Melzack and Wall [8]. This theory suggests that the activation of large diameter sensory afferent fibers, those carrying primarily touch and pressure sensation, within peripheral nerves activates a region of the spinal cord, the substantia gelatinosa. Axons from the substantia gelatinosa project to and inhibit signaling via small diameter afferent fibers, those transmitting pain signals. Applying the "Gate Control Theory" to electric neuromodulation, the activation of large diameter fibers (touch) by electrical stimulation closes the "gate" for small diameter fibers (pain). Thus, peripheral nerve stimulation produces a (usually pleasant) touch sensation while inhibiting the transmission of pain signals from the periphery to the brain (Fig. 1).

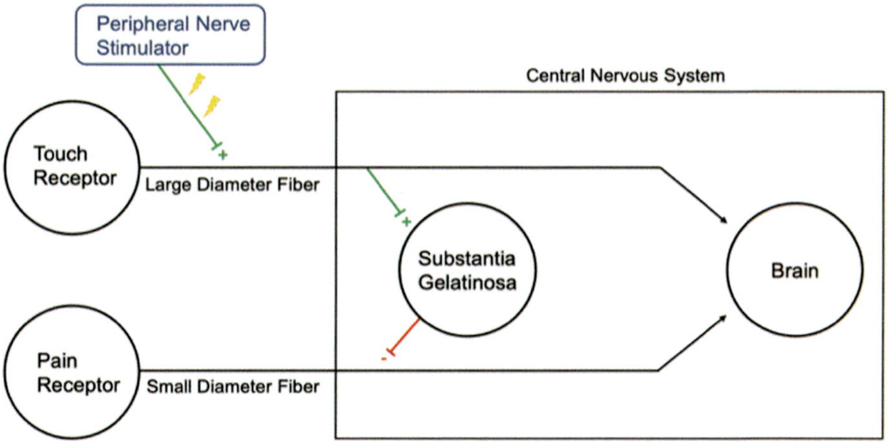

Fig. 1 Schematic representing the "Gate Control Theory" applied to electric neuromodulation of pain

3 Equipment and Insertion Technique for Ultrasound-Guided Percutaneous Peripheral Nerve Stimulation

There is currently one PNS system approved for treatment of acute pain by the USFDA [7]. This system comprises a steel and fluoropolymer **percutaneous lead** connected to a pulse generator/battery pack. The lead itself consists of a 19-strand stainless-steel wire core (160 μm in diameter) insulted with a fluoropolymer. This steel and fluoropolymer wire is wound into an open helical coil (300 μm in diameter) with the distal end bent back at a 75° (approximate) angle to anchor the lead in the tissue adjacent to the target nerve (Fig. 2). As the wire is extremely flexible and thus cannot be threaded through an introducer, the lead is pre-mounted in a 20-Gauge needle to be inserted percutaneously. The needle with its mounted lead is inserted through the skin and guided adjacent to the target nerve using ultrasound or other imaging device. When in the desired position, the needle is withdrawn and the anchor at the end holds the lead in place.

The stimulator lead connects to a pulse generator/battery pack, adherent to the patient via an adhesive mounting pad (Fig. 3). The pulse generator is small (6.2 × 3.7 × 1.4 cm) and light enough (approximately 30 g) to be worn by the patient without interference in activities of daily living. The generator should be secured to the patient's skin in a location that is easily reached by the patient.

The needle with mounted lead may be inserted using in- or out-of-plane **ultrasound guidance** based on the operator's preference (Fig. 4). A small volume of local anesthetic (usually 1% lidocaine) is infiltrated in the skin prior to insertion of the needle/lead. If necessary for patient comfort, the needle tract may be anesthetized as well, however, care should be taken to avoid injecting any local anesthetic adjacent

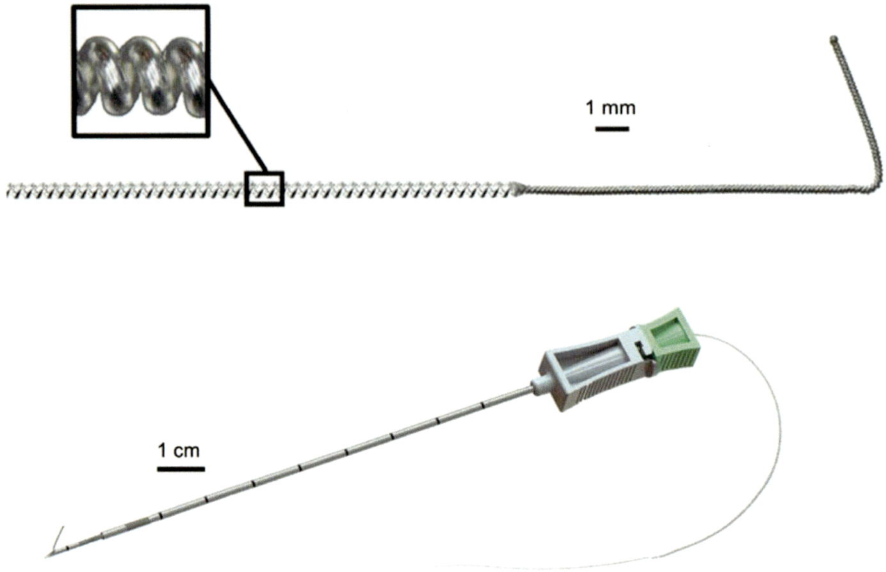

Fig. 2 Percutaneous peripheral nerve stimulation lead and insertion needle. Used with permission from Brian M. Ilfeld, M.D., M.S

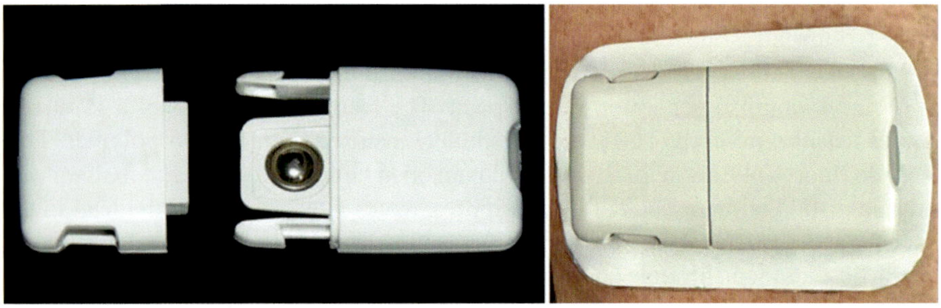

Fig. 3 Pulse generator snaps into place with a rechargeable battery and is attached to a patient's skin by its adhesive mounting pad

to the target nerve/plexus as this will interfere with stimulation. Initial guidance of the needle toward the target nerve or plexus is by ultrasound, with a goal of placing the lead 0.5–1.5 cm from the target.

Following initial advancement of the needle under **ultrasound guidance**, the final location of the lead should be determined by the patient's perceived sensation during testing. Most patients describe a tingling or massage sensation in the region of the expected pain following surgery (i.e., brachial plexus stimulation should elicit a massage sensation in the shoulder for a planned rotator cuff repair). If the patient fails to experience any sensation in the therapeutic window of the device, the lead

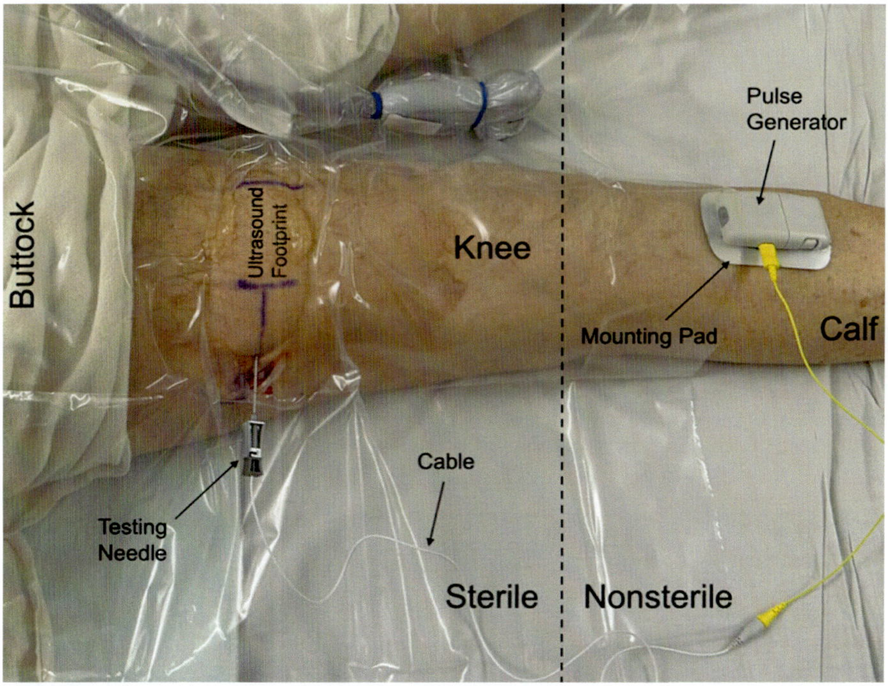

Fig. 4 Set-up for initial test of sciatic nerve stimulation. Used with permission from John J. Finneran IV, M.D.

should be moved closer to the target. If, prior to the patient describing a tingling or massage sensation, pain and/or muscle contraction are experienced, a location further from the nerve or plexus should be trialed as stimulating the nerve from too short a distance may increase activation of small diameter afferent fibers resulting in pain (Fig. 5).

Early PNS lead insertion systems consisted of only a wire lead pre-mounted in a needle. These systems had the significant drawback that the needle could only be advanced when trialing a stimulation location since withdrawing the needle resulted in lead deployment. If suboptimal positioning was found in that initial trajectory and needle repositioning was necessary, an entirely new lead-needle was required. This frequently lead to the need for multiple leads in each patient (the suboptimal leads ultimately removed once the optimal site was determined). Later generation insertion systems employ a testing needle combined with a sleeve that can be advanced and withdrawn to optimize the location prior to placement of the lead. Once the desired location is determined, the testing needle is withdrawn, leaving the sleeve in place. The sleeve then serves as a conduit for insertion of the needle-lead complex (Fig. 6).

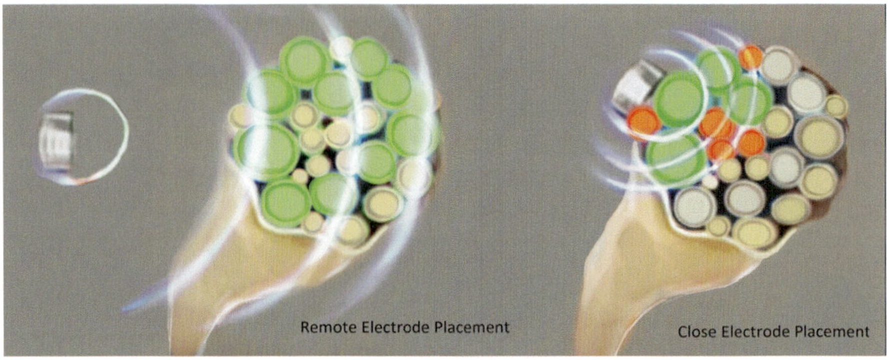

Fig. 5 Remote stimulation of the nerve may allow for more uniform activation of large diameter (touch) afferent fibers, while close stimulation may result in activation of small diameter (pain) afferent fibers. Used with permission from Brian M. Ilfeld, M.D., M.S.

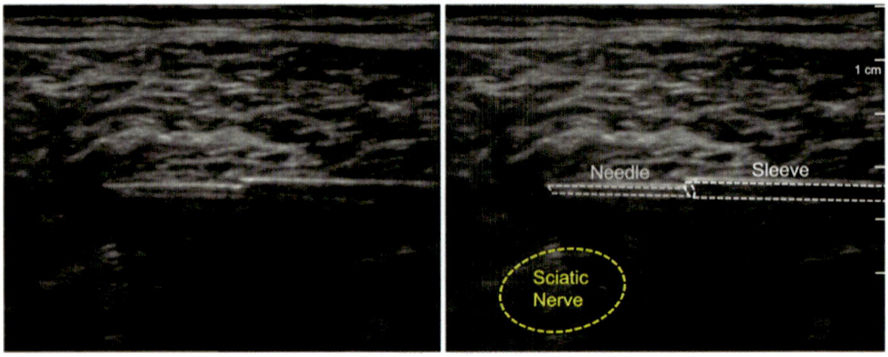

Fig. 6 Ultrasound-guided insertion of the testing needle and percutaneous sleeve to a distance of approximately 1 cm from the sciatic nerve; with and without the needle, sleeve, and nerve labeled

4 Applications for Acute Pain

The United States is currently experiencing an opioid epidemic. Pain following surgery is a common cause of new opioid prescriptions with approximately 80% of patients prescribed either oxycodone or hydrocodone following low risk surgery [9]. **Peripheral nerve blocks** offer a method of potent and targeted analgesia following painful orthopedic surgery; however, both single injection and continuous local anesthetic-based techniques have limitations. Single injection peripheral nerve blocks are limited in duration to hours, while continuous nerve blocks are limited in duration to days due to the size and weight of the external reservoir of local anesthetic as well as infection risk associated with extended duration indwelling catheters [10]. However, pain after orthopedic surgery often lasts for weeks. Further, local anesthetic-based nerve blocks produce weakness of the operative extremity as well as predisposition to falls for lower extremity nerve blocks [12].

In contrast to local anesthetic-based nerve blocks (Table1), PNS offers analgesia without producing weakness or sensory/proprioceptive deficits. Additionally, the device that has been used for most investigations involving PNS for acute postoperative analgesia is cleared by the USFDA for 60 days of continuous use. Thus, PNS may be an analgesic modality better paired with the expected duration of intense pain following major orthopedic surgery. In comparison to local anesthetic nerve blocks, PNS does suffer from substantially increased cost, which may be an order of magnitude more than conventional nerve blocks. In addition, lead placement may be associated with a significant increase in total procedural time. As these leads remain in situ and functioning for a much longer duration than what is expected from a continuous peripheral nerve block, follow-up time requirements are similarly prolonged. In the authors' experience, the intensity of patient interactions and time required for analgesic/complication management is greatly reduced with stimulation techniques.

Percutaneous stimulation of the brachial plexus, femoral nerve, and sciatic nerve has been described [11] for postoperative analgesia (Table 2). Early investigations were aimed at determining if PNS would provide sufficient analgesia in the immediate postoperative period to obviate the need of a local anesthetic-based peripheral nerve block. However, the majority of participants in these studies required a single injection peripheral nerve block prior to discharge. As such, more recent studies on PNS for postoperative analgesia have incorporated a single injection nerve block for all participants, followed by immediate activation of the stimulator in the recovery area.

Table 1 Comparison of single injection and continuous nerve blocks with peripheral nerve stimulation for postoperative analgesia

	Single injection peripheral nerve block	Continuous peripheral nerve block	Peripheral nerve stimulation
Analgesia Duration	Hours	Days	Weeks to Months
Titratability	–	+	++
Administration Time	+	++	+++ to ++++
Sensory deficit	+++	+	–
Motor deficit	++	+	–
Cost	+	++	++++
Follow-up requirements	+	++	++++

Table 2 Sites for peripheral nerve stimulation and corresponding surgical procedures

Stimulation site	Surgical procedure
Upper extremity	
Brachial plexus	Rotator cuff repair
Lower extremity	
Femoral nerve	Anterior cruciate ligament repair
Sciatic nerve	Ankle arthroplasty Hallux valgus surgery
Femoral and sciatic nerves	Total knee arthroplasty

5 Contraindications and Complications

Clinicians will be familiar with most contraindications to PNS as they are similar to other regional anesthetics. The only contraindication specific to PNS is the presence of another electric stimulation device whose current would overlap with that of the nerve stimulator. These include but are not limited to: (1) deep brain stimulator, (2) implanted active cardiac implant (e.g., pacemaker or defibrillator), (3) other implanted neurostimulation device (e.g., spinal cord stimulator). Each of these represents an absolute contraindication to the use of PNS. Other contraindications common to all regional anesthetics include bleeding disorders, infection, pharmacologic anticoagulation, and severe adhesive allergies.

As with its contraindications, complications of PNS are comparable to other regional anesthetic procedures. These include infection, nerve injury, skin irritation, lead dislodgement, and lead fracture. The infection rate for PNS leads is extremely low, with approximately one infection for every 32,000 indwelling days for helically coiled leads [13]. This low rate is likely the result of both the extremely small size of the lead (160 μm) and its helically coiled shape. The small size of the lead correlates to a very small opening in the skin; while the helical coil helps to induce fibrosis around the lead. This fibrosis combined with the helical coil likely prevents pistoning of the lead (microscopic motions in and out of the skin) that can draw potentially pathogenic microbial organisms from the skin subcutaneously while also breaking any bacteriostatic seal at the entry site. When percutaneous brachial plexus stimulation is utilized for shoulder surgery, it is important to keep the lead insertion site high on the neck where it will not be under the strap of the patient's arm sling (Fig. 7). Lead insertion sites under a sling may not fibrose due to the continued motion at the site and therefore not create the same bacteriostatic seal that is normally found at the lead insertion site [14].

Any procedure involving the intentional insertion of a needle or other device adjacent to a peripheral nerve has the potential to produce a nerve injury. However, there has never been a published report of a nerve injury resulting from percutaneous PNS. Compared to conventional nerve blocks with local anesthetic, both single injection and continuous, the theoretical risk of nerve injury should be lower for PNS. Local anesthetic-based nerve blocks require the block needle to be placed within the

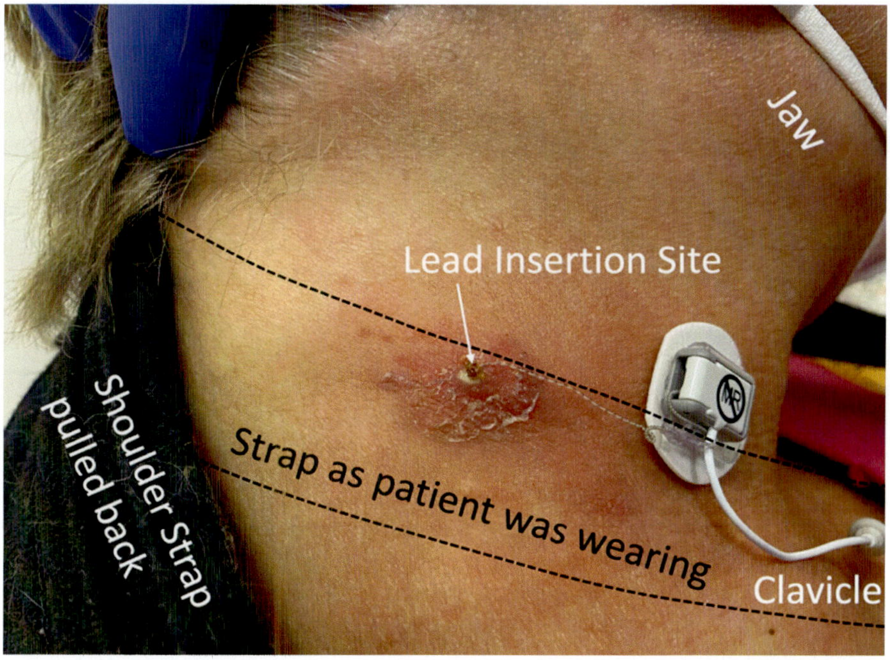

Fig. 7 Infected peripheral nerve stimulation lead insertion site. This infection likely resulted from the lead being inserted under the strap of the patient's sling following rotator cuff repair

connective tissue sheath just surrounding the epineurium; in contrast, PNS leads are placed 0.5–1.5 cm from the epineurium. Thus, there is theoretically less trauma to the nerve associated with placement of a PNS lead than during a conventional nerve block. Additionally, local anesthetic nerve blocks involve the injection of fluid in this perineural space with the potential for unrecognized intraneural injection. As PNS leads may be left in situ far longer than most transcutaneous catheters (USFDA cleared for up to 60 days of use), there is increased risk of skin irritation and breakdown. This risk may be lessened by rotating the site of the adhesive mounting pad and replacing the occlusive dressing covering the lead site regularly. Due to the fibrosis that occurs at the lead insertion site and along its tract as well as the barb shaped distal end, unintentional lead dislodgement is rare and may be further reduced by the use of 2-octyl cyanoacrylate surgical glue at the lead insertion site. When dislodgement does occur, the clinician and patient must weigh the cost and risk of replacement with the patient's pain level following discontinuation of the stimulation therapy.

Reported incidence of lead fracture (breakage at or deep to the insertion site leaving a segment of the wire inside the patient) has varied from 3 to 25% in PNS for acute pain studies. This data is based on the initial lead design, and the manufacturer claims that a newly designed lead is far more durable and associated with a greatly decreased risk of lead fractures. All fractured leads reported in the literature were left in situ with no subsequent negative sequelae reported. This includes infected fractured leads, which have been successfully treated with oral antibiotics and did not require surgical retrieval. Importantly, even if fracture occurs at the insertion site and the entire length of lead is left in situ, patients may still undergo magnetic resonance imaging in machines up to 3.0 Tesla. The risk of fracture may increase when a lead is placed in a highly mobile regional (e.g., sciatic leads placed in the popliteal fossa fracture at a higher rate than those placed in a more proximal thigh position) or when resistance is encountered during removal of the lead. When the latter occurs, slow constant pressure and injection of subcutaneous short acting local anesthetic at the lead insertion site may help to prevent fracture during removal.

6 Summary

Electric stimulation of peripheral nerves is an emerging technology for management of acute postoperative pain. When combined with a single injection peripheral nerve block, PNS offers analgesia for weeks following painful orthopedic surgery of the extremities with no deficits in sensation, strength, or proprioception, and thus may facilitate participation in rehabilitation and return to normal functioning. Ongoing randomized trials will continue to elucidate the role of this novel technology in perioperative care.

References

1. Stillings D. A survey of the history of electrical stimulation for pain to 1900. Med Instrum. 1975;9:255–9.
2. Gildenberg PL. History of electrical neuromodulation for chronic pain. Pain Med. 2006;7:S7-13.
3. Keller T, Krames ES. "On the shoulders of giants": a history of the understandings of pain, leading to the understandings of neuromodulation. Neuromodulation. 2009;12:77–84.
4. Wall PD, Sweet WH. Temporary abolition of pain in man. Science. 1967;155:108–9.
5. Yu DT, Chae J, Walker ME, Hart RL, Petroski GF. Comparing stimulation-induced pain during percutaneous (intramuscular) and transcutaneous neuromuscular electric stimulation for treating shoulder subluxation in hemiplegia. Arch Phys Med Rehabil. 2001;82:756–60.
6. Huntoon MA, Burgher AH. Ultrasound-guided permanent implantation of peripheral nerve stimulation (PNS) system for neuropathic pain of the extremities: original cases and outcomes. Pain Med. 2009;10:1369–77.
7. Ilfeld BM, Finneran JJ. Cryoneurolysis and percutaneous peripheral nerve stimulation to treat acute pain in the time of the opioid crisis: a review. Anesthesiology. 2020;133:1127–49.
8. Melzack R, Wall PD. Pain mechanisms: a new theory. Science. 1965;150:971–9.
9. Wunsch H, Wijeysundera DN, Passarella MA, et al. Opioids prescribed after low-risk surgical procedures in the United States, 2004–2012. JAMA. 2016;315(15):1654–7.
10. Ilfeld BM. Continuous peripheral nerve blocks: an update of the published evidence and comparison with novel, alternative analgesic modalities. Anesth Analg. 2017;124:308–35.
11. Ilfeld BM, Plunkett A, Vijjeswarapu AM, Hackworth R, Dhanjal S, Turan A, Cohen SP, Eisenach JC, Griffith S, Hanling S, Sessler DI, Mascha EJ, Yang D, Boggs JW, Wongsarnpigoon

A, Gelfand H; PAINfRE Investigators. Percutaneous peripheral nerve stimulation (neuromodulation) for postoperative pain: a randomized, Sham-controlled pilot study. Anesthesiology 2021;135 (1):95–110.

12. Ilfeld BM, Duke KB. Donohue: the association between lower extremity continuous peripheral nerve blocks and patient falls after knee and hip arthroplasty. Anesth Analg. 2010;111:1552–4.
13. Ilfeld BM, Gabriel RA, Saulino MF, Chae J, Peckham PH, Grant SA, Gilmore CA, Donohue MC, deBock MG, Wongsarnpigoon A, Boggs JW. Infection rates of electrical leads used for percutaneous neurostimulation of the peripheral nervous system. Pain Pract. 2017;17(6):753–62.
14. Finneran JJ IV, Leek BT, Ilfeld BM, Abdullah B, Said ET. Infection of a retained peripheral nerve stimulation lead: a case report. A A Pract. 2022;16(11): e01626.

Ultrasound-Guided Percutaneous Cryoneurolysis for Acute Pain Management in Surgical and Trauma Patients

Michael Gyorfi, Ian Pillai, and Rodney A. Gabriel

Abstract Ultrasound-guided percutaneous cryoneurolysis is a minimally-invasive procedure that involves the use of extreme cold temperatures to destroy target tissues. Cryoneurolysis has been increasingly used for the treatment of acute pain, particularly in surgical and trauma patients. By applying cold temperatures to target nerves, transmission of pain signals to the brain may be disrupted. This therapeutic modality can provide long-lasting pain relief that persists for weeks to months and diminishes the need for additional opioids. This chapter will cover acute pain indications for cryoneurolysis for surgical (e.g. mastectomy, joint arthroplasty, thoracotomy, limb amputation) and trauma (e.g. acute burns and rib fractures) indications. Several reports have shown that cryoneurolysis can be an effective treatment option with a low risk of complications when provided to the appropriate patient and nerve. As the use of ultrasound-guided percutaneous cryoneurolysis continues to expand, further research is needed to determine the optimal application of this procedure for different pain conditions, as well as to further refine the technique and improve patient outcomes.

Keywords Cryoneurolysis · Cryoangelsia · Cryoablation · Acute pain · Regional anesthesia

M. Gyorfi
Anesthesiology, University of Wisconsin School of Medicine and Public Health, Madison, WI, USA
e-mail: mgyorfi@uwhealth.org

I. Pillai
Midwestern University, Downers Grove, IL, USA
e-mail: ipillai@wisc.edu

R. A. Gabriel (✉)
Anesthesiology, University of California, San Diego, CA, USA
e-mail: ragabriel@health.ucsd.edu

A. Abd-Elsayed and K. Schroeder (eds.), *Perioperative Pain Management*,
https://doi.org/10.1007/978-3-031-67648-2_32

1 Introduction

Despite numerous advancements, acute pain management continues to be a challenging aspect of patient management. Pharmacologic management remains the preferred modality of analgesia in post-surgical and trauma patient populations. With the ongoing opioid epidemic, alternative analgesic modalities are still needed to manage post-intervention pain and prevent pain-related complications. Multimodal analgesic approaches are gaining favor and have demonstrated a reasonable ability to reduce pain even in the setting of heightened pain management complexity. Non-pharmacologic interventions have recently been recognized for their ability to provide adjunctive benefits and facilitate further management and pain reduction in the acute setting. Regional analgesic interventions should be considered broadly, and may offer particular benefits in patient populations with intense and multifaceted acute pain. An important consideration is that adequate analgesia has shown improved rates of recovery and an enhanced ability to modulate the transition of acute to chronic pain symptomology [1]. In this chapter we highlight cryoneurolysis as a developing modality for the treatment and prevention of acute and chronic pain in surgical and trauma settings.

Targeted cryoneurolysis procedures are comparable in many ways to common peripheral nerve blocks using local anesthetics. The major difference between the two interventions is secondary to the mechanism of cryoanalgesia and the destruction of neural tissue that occurs with this technique. The primary mechanism of the cryoneurolysis process is the utilization of isolated and controlled cold temperatures (-20 to -100 °C) that reversibly damage the myelin sheath of the target peripheral nerve. The myelin sheath of the nerve is damaged to such a degree that the resulting edema and neurolysis decrease the targeted nerve's overall ability to transmit sensory information [2]. Afferent and efferent sensory conduction is inhibited in this process, which may markedly reduce pain perception. Furthermore, a degree of neural Wallerian degeneration is observed distal to the site of intervention, further extending analgesic duration until regrowth is achieved over the course of weeks to months at a rate of 1–2 mm per day [3]. Regrowth is possible as neurolysis achieves temperatures incapable of causing damage to the connective tissue of the nerve. The endoneurium, perineurium and epineurium remain completely intact after this procedure [3]. The extent of cryoneurolysis is modulated by the temperature achieved (a process affected by the gaseous medium) and duration of intervention in units of time. The range of targeted temperature application for cryoneurolysis is set between -20 and less than -100 °C and is partially dependent on the gas utilized (e.g., carbon dioxide, nitrous oxide, argon, helium). With this technique, the duration of analgesia may be difficult to predict but may range from weeks to months [4]. Additionally, both motor and sensory nerves may be affected, which makes targeted nerve selection and precise needle tip localization necessary as collateral motor nerve involvement can hinder physical recovery.

The current procedure of cryoneurolysis attempts to optimize the efficiency of targeted analgesia. The localization of the procedure is through focal use of a device called a cryoprobe. The cryoprobe is designed as a hollow tube consisting of both inner and outer chambers that are designed to overlap. This design facilitates travel of a gaseous medium, in many cases nitrous oxide or carbon dioxide. The medium of choice is meant to flow from a high-pressure inner chamber, toward the tip of the probe and double-back through the larger outer chamber [5]. Flow dynamics and thermal equilibrium facilitate the delivery of desired temperatures to neural tissue. The narrowed tip of the cryoprobe allows for targeted therapeutic delivery and rapid heat extraction minimizes collateral tissue destruction. This design creates an effective closed system that maintains a targetted temperature and minimizes gas deposition in patient tissues. The gas is not able to escape the system but the mechanics of this design result in the creation of an ice-ball at the tip of the cryoprobe, through the Joule–Thomson effect. This ice-ball acts as a medium for further delivery of temperature focused treatment [6].

The size and dimensions of the cryoprobe depend on the tissues targeted for cryoneurolysis application. Currently, two divergent systems are available for the application of crynoneurolysis therapy. Cryoprobes may be used by surgeons for the application of cryoneurolysis as a component of a surgical intervention. For example, these probes may be used by surgeons to perform intercostal cryoneurolysis under direct visualization intraoperatively in the setting of thoracic surgery. Cryoneurolysis for pain management often involves the use of smaller gauge needles/probes that may be inserted percutaneously, with the size of these applicators ranging from 18 to 24 gauge. These percutaneous systems often include the ability to perform nerve stimulation [2]. Nerve stimulators facilitate the differentiation between motor and sensory nerves and are therefore utilized for neural target confirmation and improved localization prior to gas delivery. Accurate guidance of the cryoprobe during instrument insertion may be facilitated by the use of an intravenous catheter; termed an introducer. This practice also facilitates the application of local anesthetic to the intended area prior to cryoneurolysis [2]. Careful selection of an introducer of adequate size is necessary as the catheter must be larger than the intended cryoprobe.

Some image-guidance is often included in the procedure, in many cases this includes the initial diagnostic evaluation as well as during the actual cryoneurolytic procedure. Ultrasound, guided fluoroscopy, and computed tomography are all respected and viable options and imaging type is often influenced by the area targeted for intervention. With advances in ultrasound technology, this imaging type has been increasingly utilized secondary to its ability to support accurate needle placement and avoid injury to aberrant anatomic structures [7]. Furthermore, case studies have highlighted the successful use of this imaging modality to support cryoneurolysis application in surgical and trauma settings [8].

Prior to the application of cryoneurolyis, an injection of local anesthetic may be performed to target the presumed loci of pain transmission. This local injection serves to block the afflicted nerve, therefore confirming the target, while also establishing a pain relief baseline for the patient that can be used as a metric during the procedure [2]. The patient can reference this initial nerve block and future procedures can be titrated to the overall level of intervention required to achieve desired relief. Some degree of conscious sedation and local anesthetic is typically used during the cryoneurolysis procedure as well. However, complete sedation is often not needed and negates a thorough intervention as the patient must be conscious enough to express a satisfactory degree of sensation loss [5].

The use of a cryoprobe with nerve stimulator capacity further increases accuracy. Many protocols use 100 Hz as a set frequency to help isolate sensory from motor nerves [2]. While various techniques exist for the use of a cryoprobe, many involve pinning of the targeted nerve to surrounding bone to minimize movement of the nerve and maintain proper contact with the cryoprobe. Repeated cycles of stimulation at sequential decreasing hertz are utilized, with reliable stimulation at a minimal amplitude, often 0.5 V, being the last measure. This is often segued into repeat nerve stimulation at 2 Hz to elicit any nearby motor nerve stimulation as cryoneurolysis of motor nerves may need to be avoided in certain circumstances [6]. From this point, cryoneurolysis is ready to commence. Flow of the selected gas medium should be optimized relative to cryoprobe size. If not already conferred, the patient should be informed that there will be multiple repetitions of cryoneurolysis, with the first being known to elicit pain similar to their initial complaint. Pain should only be appreciated during the first cycle of the process and is generally less than a minute in duration. Ice ball formation is expected with each cycle of cryoneurolysis, often requiring at least one to three minutes of duration for adequate formation and area of effect. Following completion of freezing and thawing cycles, the probe can be withdrawn [5].

Peripheral nerve blocks represent an alternative option to cryoneurolysis for post-surgical and traumatic pain in the acute setting. Peripheral nerve blocks are conducted as a single injection or through continuous infusions, both with the use of local anesthetic. Comparisons between the two options highlight limitations and specific risks of neural blockage versus cryoanalgesia. Both interventions confer a degree of risk for unintended neural damage, circulatory puncture, and local anesthetic systemic toxicity (LAST).

The duration of effect differs between modalities with peripheral nerve blockage generally persisting for a limited number of hours. To warrant analgesia beyond 24 hours, a perineural catheter and continuous infusion is required. With catheter placement, there is an increased risk of infection, hardware migrations, accidental removal, and leakage of local anesthetic. Peripheral nerve blockage has been associated with a degree of muscular weakness, an effect that potentially limits patient ambulation and recovery [9].

2 Applications in Acute Pain Management

Cryoneurolysis is used in a variety of surgical procedures to manage acute pain at an increasing rate. The development of ultrasound-guided cryoneurolysis, which allows for precisely localizing targeted nerves, is largely responsible for the expanded scope of the procedure.

While the cryoneurolysis of the intercostal nerves during thoracotomy surgery was one of the first reported use of cryoanalgesia, it has more recently been investigated for the treatment of postoperative pain following mastectomy surgery, shoulder arthroplasty, and total knee arthroplasty [10].

The remaining chapter summarizes the use of cryoanalgesia in the treatment of acute pain with the expectation that more indications will arise in the near future. The following surgical procedures result in moderate to severe postoperative pain, which, if not properly managed, can become chronic. Thus, the long-term advantages of cryoneurolysis are applicable to these procedures. Recent research has shown that cryoneurolysis is safe, effective, and provides long-lasting pain relief when used in these procedures [10].

Thoracotomy

Thoracotomies are painful operations with significant postoperative pain that is difficult to manage. It has been noted that 22–67% of thoracotomy patients experience chronic postsurgical pain. The gold standard for managing post-thoracotomy pain is typically thoracic epidural analgesia. Epidural anesthesia is not without risk and is not suitable for all patients. Risks and limitations include dural perforation, hematoma, infection, hypotension/bradycardia, and urinary retention. In addition, epidural placement can be technically more challenging to perform, and even the most experienced providers may fail to accurately access the epidural space, leading to unsatisfactory analgesia [11].

When used to treat acute postoperative thoracotomy pain, cryoneurolysis has shown comparable efficacy to epidural analgesia. Numerous studies have demonstrated that intraoperative cryoneurolysis of the intercostal nerve causes significant and enduring postoperative incisional pain relief [12].

In 1974, Nelson et al. [13] demonstrated a decrease in postoperative opioid use without neuritis or neuromas within 24 months of follow-up after cryoneurolysis was performed for thoracic surgery. A similar study performed by Yang et al. [14], combined the use of cryoneurolysis with epidural analgesia and reported that the combination group required less rescue morphine over the first week when compared to epidural analgesia alone. A more recent study performed by Clemence et al. [12] found similar results with an average reduction of 28 morphine milligram equivalents (MME) over the first 10 postoperative days. However, this study did not show a reduction in overall pain scores. Lastly, a study by Chen et al. [15] found a significant reduction in opioid use after thoracotomies in a pediatric oncology population.

Total Knee Arthroplasty

Cryoneurolysis of the infrapatellar branch of the saphenous nerve and anterior femoral cutaneous nerve has been used for postoperative pain management in patients undergoing total knee arthroplasty (TKA) [16].

According to a retrospective study of 100 patients undergoing TKA, preoperative cryoneurolysis of the superficial genicular nerves (SGN) led to an overall improvement in clinical performance when compared to standard multimodal pain regimens. This finding is in line with previous research. The postoperative length of stay was reduced for those who received cryoneurolysis (stayed 2 days, 6% vs. 67%, p 0.0001). The MME opioid consumption in the cryoneurolysis group was 45% lower at the 12 week follow up. Six weeks after the operation, the patients receiving cryoneurolysis also reported lower levels of pain intensity and interference with daily activities, as determined by the Patient-reported Outcomes Measurement Information System (PROMIS) [17].

In 2022, a large retrospective review evaluated total opioid consumption and length of stay following total knee arthroplasties with cryoneurolysis and non cryoneurolysis cases in a similar time frame. They found a small reduction in MME and a reduced length of stay by 1 day [18]. In addition to retrospective data, a recently published randomized control trial of 124 patients compared cryoneurolysis of the superficial genicular nerve to a standard of care control group. This study found a statistically significant reduction in opioid use and overall function improvement in the cryoneurolysis group [19].

Shoulder Arthroplasty

Despite the increased use of brachial plexus blockade, inadequate pain management following shoulder arthroplasty remains a significant concern. Continuous interscalene blocks, which can be used for orthopedic shoulder surgery on moderately painful shoulders, may sometimes have a high failure rate of up to 25% and significant inherent risks (eg, pneumothorax, phrenic nerve injury, and diaphragm paralysis). As a result, patients who have compromised respiratory function might need an alternative method of managing their postoperative pain. For prolonged postoperative analgesia following shoulder procedures, cryoneurolysis of the suprascapular nerve has emerged as a safe and efficious analgesic modality. The suprascapular nerve arises from the upper trunk of the brachial plexus and innervates the supraspinatus, infraspinatus, and the shoulder join [20].

The first report of cryoneurolysis for shoulder arthroplasty analgesia was documented in 2017 after a small case report by Ilfeld et al., which included both shoulder arthroplasty and knee arthroplasty. All 5 patients reported a postoperative pain score of < 2 on a 0–10 numeric rating scale and required less opioids compared to histor controls [8].

Acute Burns

In burn patients, pain management is frequently necessary for both the burn site and the donor sites for autologous split thickness skin grafting (STSG). Since the lower extremity is typically the site of harvesting, the patient's ability to engage in physical therapy is frequently hindered by pain at the graft donor site, which in many patients is worse than the pain from the burn. The lateral femoral cutaneous nerve (LFCN), which innervates the lateral aspect of the thigh, can be seen with ultrasound in the intermuscular space between the tensor fascia latae and sartorius muscles. A case report demonstrated cryoneurolysis as an effective alternative to LFCN blocks performed with bupivacaine. In this report, analgesic duration with cryoneurolysis persisted for weeks and far exceeded what might be expected with local anesthetic-based approaches [21].

Rib Fractures

In trauma patients, rib fractures are a frequent injury that significantly increases morbidity and mortality. There is evidence that local anesthetic-based nerve blocks can significantly reduce pain and prevent complications. However, the duration of this pain frequently lasts for weeks, while the analgesia offered by these blocks is limited to hours for single injection blocks or days for continuous infusions. A study performed evaluated 5 patients with rib fractures and treated their rib fracture pain with ultrasound-guided percutaneous cryoneurolysis and had promising results, which suggests the need for larger studies [22].

Breast Surgery

Post-mastectomy pain is often hard to manage with traditional pain regimens and the incidence of chronic postsurgical pain remains alarmingly high. A case series that consisted of three patients who received preoperative ultrasound-guided percutaneous intercostal nerve cryoneurolysis to treat pain following mastectomy surgery was reported. All three patients reported an average pain score of 0 and received no supplemental opioid analgesics during the measured postoperative period. These findings were a significant improvement over historic cohorts, however appropriately powered randomized controlled clinical trials are necessary to quantify potential risks and benefits [23].

Phantom Limb Pain

It is estimated that 50–85% of people with a lower limb amputation develop chronic pain in the missing limb, termed phantom limb pain. The etiology of phantom limb pain is not fully understood and has few adequately powered and randomized trials to help guide pain management. A randomized trial evaluated 144 patients and randomized them to a singled injection femoral and sciatic nerve block with lidocaine paired with an ultrasound guided percutaneous cryoneurolysis vs sham treatment at the same location. The pain scores were re-evaluated after 4 months without a statistically significant reduction in pain scores, however some benefits are shown in those with below-the-knee amputation (versus above-the-knee amputation). The lack of response to cryoneurolysis in this population was theorized to be a result of the underlying mechanism of phantom limb pain vs non-optimal treatment parameters such as freeze duration and anatomic treatment locations [24].

3 Benefits and Risks of Cryoneurolysis

Cryoneurolysis is a minimally invasive technique that offers several advantages over other treatments for certain medical conditions. One of the main advantages of cryoneurolysis is that it can be performed on an outpatient basis, thus patients can usually go home the same day as the procedure. This can help reduce the cost and inconvenience of hospital stays and allows patients to return to their normal activities more quickly [2].

Another advantage of cryoneurolysis is that it is generally considered to be a safe procedure. The technique uses extreme cold to destroy abnormal tissue or cells with less risk of damage to healthy tissue when compared with other treatments such as radiation therapy or chemotherapy. Additionally, because the procedure is minimally invasive, there is typically less pain and scarring than with traditional surgical procedures [4].

While cryoneurolysis is generally considered a safe and effective procedure, there are still potential risks and complications that patients and clinicians need to consider. One of the most common risks associated with cryoneurolysis is bleeding. Generally, any risk of bruising or bleeding is usually minor and resolves on its own. In rare cases, bleeding can be more significant and require additional treatment or even surgery and the coagulation status of the patient should be considered prior to considering a cryoneurolysis procedure [5].

Another potential complication of cryoneurolysis is damage to nearby organs or tissues. Because the procedure involves freezing tissue, there is a risk that the cold temperature could damage healthy tissue surrounding the area being treated. This can lead to pain, swelling, or even organ dysfunction [5].

In some cases, cryoneurolysis can cause permanent nerve injury. This can lead to numbness, tingling, or weakness in the affected area, and may require additional treatment to manage. The avoidance of nerves with motor innervation should help minimize the risk of any significant and permanent weakness [5]. Finally, like any interventional procedure, there is a risk of infection with cryoneurolysis. The administration of pre-procedure antibiotics may decrease this risk but patients should still be aware of the signs of infection, such as fever, swelling, and redness at the site of probe insertion [5].

4 Contraindications

Cryoneurolysis is relatively safe; however, there are still contraindications. These include Raynaud's syndrome, cryoglobulinemia, cold urticaria, bleeding disorders, localized infection, and anticoagulation. Risks include depigmentation, hyperpigmentation, alopecia in the hairline, and "frostbite" of the skin if the ice ball encompasses the dermis, as well as bruising and bleeding. Three clinical trials involving cryoneurolysis of intercostal nerves through thoracotomy incisions reported an increased risk of postoperative neuropathic pain, while many others found no such association [25].

5 Follow-Up and Recovery After Cryoneurolysis

Following cryoneurolysis, patients are typically monitored for a short duration to ensure that there are no immediate complications associated with the procedure and that any effects associated with conscious sedation have abated.

6 Conclusion

While pain is a constant throughout life, it's management represents an ever-changing sector of medical practice. Today, while a multitude of options exist for the management of acute pain, percutaneous cryoneurolysis represents a potentially effective alternative that extends analgesic efficacy far beyond what is normally experienced with local anesthetic-based regional anesthesia procedures. The high success rate, minimal recovery time, and low complication rate highlight a potential therapeutic niche for cryoneurolysis in the future of acute pain management and prevention of chronic pain. Further research efforts should focus on further optimizing this procedure for various specific pain etiologies.

References

1. Kehlet H, Jensen TS, Woolf CJ. Persistent postsurgical pain: risk factors and prevention. Lancet. 2006;367:1618–25.
2. Filippiadis D, Efthymiou E, Tsochatzis A, Kelekis A, Prologo JD. Percutaneous cryoanalgesia for pain palliation: current status and future trends. Diagn Interv Imaging. 2021;102(5):273–8. https://doi.org/10.1016/j.diii.2020.11.007. Epub 2020 Dec 3. PMID: 33281081.
3. Hsu M, Stevenson FF. Reduction in muscular motility by selective focused cold therapy: a preclinical study. J Neural Transm (Vienna). 2014;121(1):15–20. https://doi.org/10.1007/s00702-013-1077-y. Epub 2013 Aug 6. PMID: 23917804; PMCID: PMC3889817.
4. Ilfeld BM, Preciado J, Trescot AM. Novel cryoneurolysis device for the treatment of sensory and motor peripheral nerves. Expert Rev Med Devices. 2016;13(8):713–25. https://doi.org/10.1080/17434440.2016.1204229. Epub 2016 Jul 13. PMID: 27333989.
5. Law L, Rayi A, Derian A. Cryoanalgesia. 2022. In: StatPearls [Internet]. Treasure Island (FL): StatPearls Publishing; 2023. PMID: 29489178.
6. Trescot AM. Cryoanalgesia in interventional pain management. Pain Phys. 2003;6(3):345–60 PMID: 16880882.
7. Djebbar S, Rossi IM, Adler RS. Ultrasound-guided cryoanalgesia of peripheral nerve lesions. Semin Musculoskelet Radiol. 2016;20(5):461–71. https://doi.org/10.1055/s-0036-1596063. Epub 2016 Dec 21. PMID: 28002868.
8. Ilfeld BM, Gabriel RA, Trescot AM. Ultrasound-guided percutaneous cryoneurolysis providing postoperative analgesia lasting many weeks following a single administration: a replacement for continuous peripheral nerve blocks? A case report. Korean J Anesthesiol. 2017;70(5):567–70. https://doi.org/10.4097/kjae.2017.70.5.567. Epub 2017 Feb 3. PMID: 29046778; PMCID: PMC5645591.
9. Joshi G, Gandhi K, Shah N, Gadsden J, Corman SL. Peripheral nerve blocks in the management of postoperative pain: challenges and opportunities. J Clin Anesth. 2016;35:524–9. https://doi.org/10.1016/j.jclinane.2016.08.041. Epub 2016 Oct 20. PMID: 27871587.
10. Biel E, Aroke EN, Maye J, Zhang SJ. The applications of cryoneurolysis for acute and chronic pain management. Pain Pract. 2023;23(2):204–15. https://doi.org/10.1111/papr.13182. Epub 2022 Dec 4. PMID: 36370129.
11. Ju H, Feng Y, Yang B-X, Wang J. Comparison of epidural analgesia and intercostal nerve cryoanalgesia for post-thoracotomy pain control. Eur J Pain. 2008;12(3):378–84.
12. Clemence J Jr, Malik A, Farhat L, Wu X, Kim KM, Patel H, et al. Cryoneurolysis of intercostal nerves decreased narcotic usage after thoracic or thoracoabdominal aortic aneurysm repair. Semin Thorac Cardiovasc Surg. 2020;32:404–12.
13. Nelson K, Vincent R, Bourke R, Smith D, Blakeley W, Kaplan R, Pollay M. Intraoperative intercostal nerve freezing to prevent post thoracotomy pain. Ann Thorac Surg. 1974;18(3):280–5. https://doi.org/10.1016/S0003-4975(10)64357-3.
14. Yang M, Cho C, Kim Y. The effects of cryoanalgesia combined with thoracic epidural analgesia in patients undergoing thoracotomy. Anaesthesia. 2004;59:1073–7.
15. Chen S, Mack S, Stein J, Kelley-Quon L, Kim E. Intercostal nerve cryoneurolysis is associated with reduced opioid use in pediatric oncology patients. J Surg Res. 2023;283:377–84. https://doi.org/10.1016/j.jss.2022.11.004. Epub 2022 Nov 22. PMID: 36427448.
16. Radnovich R, Scott D, Patel A, et al. Cryoneurolysis to treat the pain and symptoms of knee osteoarthritis: a multicenter, randomized, double-blind, sham-controlled trial. Osteoarthr Cartil. 2017;25(8):1247–56.
17. Dasa V, Lensing G, Parsons M, Harris J, Volaufova J, Bliss R. Percutaneous freezing of sensory nerves prior to total knee arthroplasty. Knee. 2016;23(3):523–8. https://doi.org/10.1016/j.knee.2016.01.011.
18. Lung B, Karasavvidis T, Sharma A, Amirhekmat A, Stepanyan H, McMaster W, Yang S, So D. Cryoneurolysis is a safe, effective modality to improve rehabilitation after total knee arthroplasty. Life. 2022;12:1344. https://doi.org/10.3390/life12091344.

19. Mihalko W, Kerkhof L, Ford M, Crockarell J Jr, Harkess J, Guyton J. Cryoneurolysis before total knee arthroplasty in patients with severe osteoarthritis for reduction of postoperative pain and opioid use in a single-center randomized controlled trial. J Arthroplasty. 2021;36(5):1590–8. https://doi.org/10.1016/j.arth.2020.11.013. Epub 2020 Nov 14. PMID: 33279353.
20. Ilfeld BM, Morey TE, Wright TW, Chidgey LK, Enneking FK. Continuous interscalene brachial plexus block for postoperative pain control at home: a randomized, double-blinded, placebo-controlled study. Anesth Analg. 2003;96(4):1089–95.
21. Finneran JJ, Swisher MW, Gabriel RA, Fiallo A, Hamilton JR, Lee JG, Ilfeld BM. Ultrasound-guided lateral femoral cutaneous nerve cryoneurolysis for analgesia in patients with burns. J Burn Care Res. 2020;41(1):224–7. https://doi.org/10.1093/jbcr/irz192. PMID: 31714578.
22. Finneran IV JJ, Gabriel RA, Swisher MW, Berndtson AE, Godat LN, Costantini TW, Ilfeld BM. Ultrasound-guided percutaneous intercostal nerve cryoneurolysis for analgesia following traumatic rib fracture—a case series. Korean J Anesthesiol. 2020;73(5):455–9. https://doi.org/10.4097/kja.19395. Epub 2019 Nov 5. PMID: 31684715; PMCID: PMC7533180.
23. Gabriel RA, Finneran JJ, Swisher MW, Said ET, Sztain JF, Khatibi B, Wallace AM, Hosseini A, Trescot AM, Ilfeld BM. Ultrasound-guided percutaneous intercostal cryoanalgesia for multiple weeks of analgesia following mastectomy: a case series. Korean J Anesthesiol. 2020;73(2):163–8. https://doi.org/10.4097/kja.19332. Epub 2019 Sep 2. PMID: 31475505; PMCID: PMC7113157.
24. Ilfeld BM, Smith CR, Turan A, Mariano ER, Miller ME, Fisher RL, Trescot AM, Cohen SP, Eisenach JC, Sessler DI, Prologo JD, Mascha EJ, Liu L, Gabriel RA; PAINfRE Investigators. Ultrasound-guided percutaneous cryoneurolysis to treat chronic postamputation phantom limb pain: a multicenter randomized controlled trial. Anesthesiology. 2023;138(1):82–97. https://doi.org/10.1097/ALN.0000000000004429. PMID: 36512721.
25. Khanbhai M, Yap K, Mohamed S, Dunning J. Is cryoanalgesia effective for post-thoracotomy pain? Interact Cardiovasc Thorac Surg. 2014;18:202–9.

Peripheral Nerve Catheters

Jeffrey Grzybowski and Calvin Harberg

Abstract A peripheral nerve catheter (PNC) provides a continuous sensory blockade via either perineural local anesthetic infusion or infusion into a fascial plane or compartment to achieve desired regional analgesic effects. Often used in the perioperative period, PNCs provide sustained analgesia, which can have significant advantages compared to a single shot peripheral nerve block. Their use in the perioperative period has substantially increased with the widespread adoption of ultrasound, and numerous PNC sites have been described in the literature. Like all therapies, PNCs are associated with both benefits and risks, which are further described in this chapter. In addition, some management considerations for different PNC sites and surgical procedures are discussed. This chapter aims to provide an overview of PNC use in perioperative pain management.

Keywords Peripheral nerve catheter · Peripheral nerve blockade · Perineural infusion · Regional anesthesia · Postoperative pain management

1 Introduction

Peripheral nerve catheters (PNCs) were first described in the literature as early as 1946 [1]. With advancements in ultrasound technology/availability, a pressing need to reduce opioid prescriptions, and increasing pressure to limit the duration of hospitalizations, the perioperative use of peripheral nerve blocks and catheter techniques has increased substantially. As new fascial plane and compartment blocks are described and validated, new targets emerge for prolonged analgesia by way of peripheral nerve catheter placement. PNCs have been proven to provide reliable analgesia without

J. Grzybowski (✉) · C. Harberg
Department of Anesthesiology, University of Wisconsin School of Medicine and Public Health, Madison, WI, USA
e-mail: jgrzybowski@wisc.edu

C. Harberg
e-mail: harberg@wisc.edu

A. Abd-Elsayed and K. Schroeder (eds.), *Perioperative Pain Management*,
https://doi.org/10.1007/978-3-031-67648-2_33

the deleterious effects of systemic medications and provide longer duration analgesia than a single-injection regional anesthetic. This chapter will discuss the role of PNCs in perioperative pain management, including indications for placement, placement technique, risks and alternatives, medication infusion strategies, and inpatient/outpatient PNC management considerations.

2 Indications, Benefits, and Alternatives

The primary indication for placement of a PNC is the anticipation of moderate to severe post-operative pain exceeding 24 hours. Patient populations in which it would be beneficial to avoid traditional systemic pain medications either because of pharmacologic side effects or contraindications to those therapies represent additional strong candidates for PNC placement. PNC use at numerous sites has demonstrated improved postoperative analgesia with less opioid use and associated opioid-related side effects [2]. PNCs can be particularly beneficial in patients with pre-existing chronic pain or opioid tolerance, where traditional pain management can be more challenging [2]. Utilization of PNCs for acute trauma is also increasingly common [3, 4]. Placement of catheters for upper/lower extremity trauma, rib fractures, and even chronic or cancer-related pain have been described [5–8]. Utility is further realized in situations where either recent anti-coagulant therapy, positioning constraints, or concern for hemodynamic instability represent contraindications to epidural analgesia (if otherwise indicated). Another advantage of PNCs is the avoidance of pain on block resolution or "rebound pain", which can occur with single shot peripheral nerve blocks (sPNB) at approximately 12–24 hours post-operatively. In the setting of rebound pain, patients experience significantly increased pain compared to patients who did not receive a regional anesthetic technique [9, 10]. Rebound pain can potentially be avoided with early analgesic administration before the local anesthetic has fully lost its therapeutic efficacy [10]. A randomized comparative trial of sPNB vs PNC for ankle surgery showed improved post-operative VAS scores at 12 hours and reduced analgesic consumption in the first 72 hours post-operatively in the PNC group as compared to the sPNB [9]. Additionally, VAS scores were reduced in the PNC group at 2 weeks suggesting a potential long-term benefit [9]. Rebound pain has also been associated with reduced patient satisfaction following a sPNB [10]. Further understanding of rebound pain as a distinct pathology is warranted as it frequently occurs following hospital discharge when there are fewer available analgesic options. The optimal PNC infusion length and/or treatment strategy to prevent rebound pain has yet to be delineated in the literature.

Despite the advantage in duration conveyed by PNCs relative to sPNB, catheters require an additional degree of expertise, are less time-efficient, are associated with an increased risk for complications, while simultaneously burdened with additional equipment, pharmacology, and catheter management expenses and considerations [11, 12]. Alternative competing therapies are emerging including: the use of sPNB with local anesthetic adjuvants, liposomal encapsulated local anesthetic preparations, cryoanalgesia, and percutaneous peripheral nerve stimulation. While a thorough description of these somewhat competing modalities is outside the scope of this chapter, recent reviews have addressed these emerging modalities, including acknowledgement that further investigation is needed to optimize analgesic modalities in the future [13–15].

3 Insertion Techniques

Before the widespread use of ultrasound guidance for catheter placement, PNC placement relied upon identification of anatomic landmarks and/or elicitation of paresthesia with placement. To improve the rate of successful catheter placement, nerve stimulating needles and catheters were then developed where an electrical current is delivered to the target nerve, evoking a specific motor response. However, ultrasound has quickly proven itself to be a superior guidance modality for successful catheter placement, including requiring less time for catheter placement, diminished patient discomfort, and a decreased risk of needle damage to adjacent anatomic structures [16, 17]. Ultrasound guidance has also made PNC placement possible and safer for patients with atypical anatomy, trauma, and coagulopathy. In addition, ultrasound can be advantageous in settings where motor stimulation is not possible or may induce patient discomfort. There is still debate regarding the analgesic efficacy of ultrasound-guided PNC placement versus nerve stimulation-guided PNC placement, but the additional advantages of ultrasound-guidance have quickly made it the most common method used for placement.

Sterile technique should be observed during catheter placement, including sterile gloves, gown and scrub cap to minimize the risk of catheter-associated infections. Sterile towels/drape should be placed around the needle insertion site and a sterile ultrasound probe cover and gel packet further minimize the risk of infectious complications. PNCs can be more difficult and time consuming to place than single shot peripheral nerve blocks and thus familiarity with the procedure, indications, and contraindications is a must to ensure the individual placing the catheter possesses the necessary technical expertise. In addition, appropriate patient selection and monitoring is important to ensure procedural success and safety. If sedation is provided, standard monitors per recommendations of the American Society of Anesthesiologists should be utilized. Resuscitation equipment and emergency medications, including tools for emergency airway management and 20% intravenous lipid emulsion for the treatment of local anesthetic systemic toxicity (LAST), should be readily available.

Commonly, peripheral nerve catheters are inserted through a needle to the target site (Fig. 1). Figure 1 demonstrates an ultrasound-guided catheter through needle technique of a femoral nerve catheter placement. Other techniques include catheter-over-needle (similar to an angiocath) and a needle-over-cannula technique.

If using ultrasound guidance, needle and catheter insertion can be oriented in-plane or out-of-plane with respect to the ultrasound beam; however, most commonly a

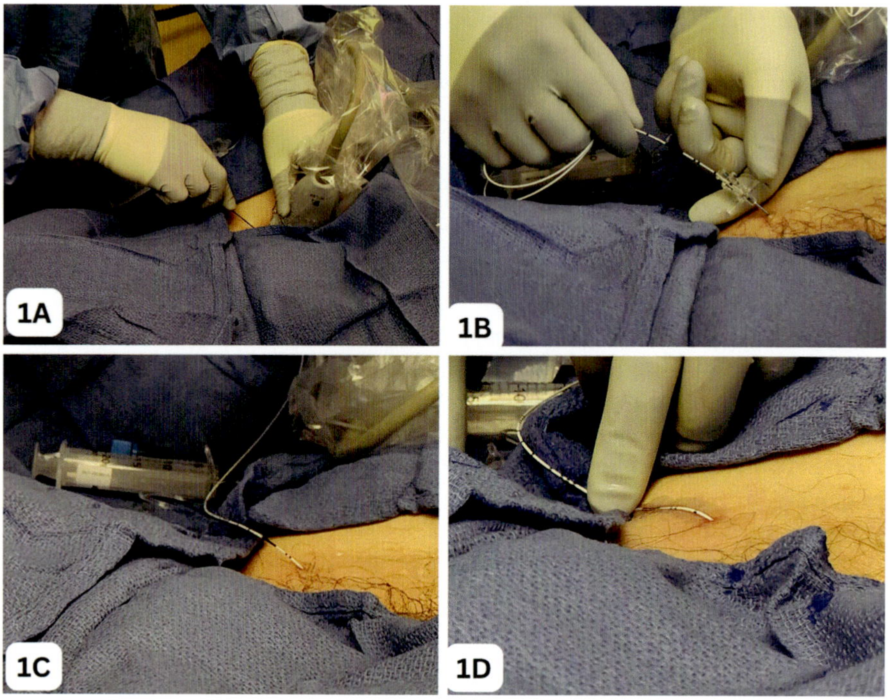

Fig. 1 Demonstration of peripheral nerve catheter insertion. A routine placement of a femoral nerve catheter via a catheter through needle technique is demonstrated. Ultrasound localization of the target nerve/structure is performed, and a Touhy needle with depth markings is inserted, 1A. A wire reinforced peripheral nerve catheter is then over-threaded via the Touhy needle, 1B. The Touhy is then removed along with wire to leave only the nerve catheter in situ, 1C. Lastly, the catheter is secured using a combination of liquid skin adhesive, tunneling, clear adhesive bandages, etc. at the discretion of the provider, 1D

short-axis view of the target nerve (when applicable) and an in-plane needle technique is utilized [18]. This technique allows for visualization of the entire needle path and confirmation of appropriate catheter placement through visualization of perineural spread of the injectate [19–23]. Although optimal distance of threading a PNC past the needle tip is unknown, a maximal distance of 5 cm has been suggested to limit self-coiling of the catheter [24].

If using nerve stimulator and anatomic landmark guidance, a needle with a conducting tip is inserted toward the target nerve with a stimulation current of 1–1.5 mA with a goal of eliciting a specific motor response. Once that response has been achieved, the delivered current is decreased and a sustained motor response at 0.2–0.5 mA is associated with appropriate needle tip proximity to the target nerve for catheter placement. In the case of a sustained motor response at a current < 0.2 mA the needle tip is assumed to be intraneural, and the needle should be withdrawn or repositioned [23, 25]. Once the needle has been appropriately positioned, the catheter is then threaded through the needle for continuous perineural local anesthetic administration. An insulated PNC with a conducting tip could also be inserted with the goal of maintaining the desired motor response with threading of the catheter before local anesthetic administration. The goal of a conducting PNC is to decrease the risk of secondary block failure, which occurs when there is an initially successful block after administration of local anesthetic through the conducting needle, but the catheter then fails to provide adequate analgesia; however, the efficacy of this catheter placement strategy remains questionable [13, 24].

4 Risks and Contraindications

Each anatomic site is associated with unique considerations regarding the risks of PNC placement (Table 1). Amongst the more common risks associated with PNC placement are secondary block failure, catheter dislodgement, and fluid leakage from the catheter site [26]. Although rare, all PNCs share a risk of damage to surrounding anatomic structures, neurologic complications, intravascular injection, systemic local anesthetic toxicity, catheter-associated infection, and bleeding. Nerve injury, when it does occur, is usually transient with only a very small percentage sustaining a long-term injury related to the block [26, 27]; however, patients with preexisting neuropathy are thought to be at higher risk [28, 29]. It is difficult to prove causation, however, since nerve injury is a common risk factor for many surgical procedures as well.

Bacterial colonization of PNCs is common, but infection related to catheter placement is rare [30–33]; PNCs require daily monitoring for signs of active infection and typically are removed 48–72 hours after placement, although infusions of 7–10 days or longer may be indicated in select patients. Risk factors for catheter-associated infections include ICU admission status, axillary and femoral PNC locations, frequent dressing changes, and catheter duration of > 48 hours [32]. In the setting of catheter failure, a risk-benefit assessment should be undertaken regarding replacement of the PNC. While the risk is incredibly low, there also needs to be a high index of suspicion and appropriate monitoring for local anesthetic systemic toxicity given the severity associated with this condition. Relative contraindications to PNC insertion include interference with the surgical site and/or dressings, coagulopathy, infection at the site of catheter placement, and need for close monitoring of motor or sensory function post-operatively. Additionally, for patients at high risk of compartment syndrome, there is concern that regional anesthetic techniques (sPNB and/or PNCs) may mask early clinical symptoms therefore delaying diagnosis and treatment, leading to increased morbidity; however, there is insufficient evidence at this time to either promote or withhold PNCs in these high-risk patients if otherwise indicated. It has been suggested that a high index of suspicion, attention to analgesic consumption and trends, and physical examination are more critical for ensuring timely diagnosis and treatment of compartment syndrome [34].

Table 1 The following table displays numerous commonly utilized PNC sites and refers to specific risks and considerations for each PNC site

PNC site	PNC coverage	Risks	Special considerations
Interscalene	Shoulder, Proximal Humerus, Clavicle	Possibility for respiratory failure secondary to phrenic nerve blockade (~100% incidence) [35, 36] Horner's Syndrome (~20% incidence) [37] Dorsal scapular nerve and long thoracic nerve injury	Injection against a high opening pressure (> 15 psi) is always present with needle-root contact. Multiple needle passes also increase risk for mechanical nerve injury
Supraclavicular	Mid-humerus, elbow, forearm, hand	Phrenic nerve blockade (~50% incidence) [38] Pneumothorax (rare with ultrasound) [39]	Lower risk of phrenic nerve palsy than with interscalene block, but is not reliably avoided. Consider infraclavicular or axillary catheter in patients who cannot tolerate a 27–30% decrease in respiratory function
Infraclavicular	Mid-humerus, elbow, forearm, hand	Pneumothorax (rare)	Needle tip should be visualized posterior to the axillary artery prior to catheter advancement. Confirmation can also by obtained by eliciting a posterior cord motor response (finger or wrist extension)
Axillary	Forearm, hand	Higher risk of catheter-associated infection and dislodgement	A separate injection to target the musculocutaneous nerve is almost always required
Paravertebral	Breast, thorax	Challenging ultrasound placement Hematoma [40] → follow neuraxial guidelines for anticoagulation Pneumothorax (<1%) Epidural/intrathecal spread [40–42]	Unclear benefit of infusion versus single nerve block injection for breast surgery [43], positioning difficulties possible in trauma
Erector Spinae Plane	Posterior thorax, possibly lateral/anterior thorax, abdomen	Correct identification of transverse process results in an injection site distant from pleura and major vessels	Efficacy for pain associated with rib fractures when epidural contraindicated, positioning difficulties possible in trauma

(continued)

Table 1 (continued)

PNC site	PNC coverage	Risks	Special considerations
Serratus Anterior Plane	Anterior and lateral thorax	The pectoral branch of the acromiothoracic artery should be identified-risk for hematoma, intravascular injection	Efficacy for pain associated with rib fractures when epidural contraindicated
Transversus Abdominis Plane (TAP)	Abdomen	Less risk of bleeding than neuraxial analgesia	Provides somatic analgesia below umbilicus when lateral/posterior TAP is chosen
Femoral	Anterior thigh, knee, medial lower leg	Quadriceps weakness → fall risk Bacterial colonization common [31]	Mobility of the inguinal area predisposes femoral PNC to dislodgement. Approach from further lateral may serve to stabilize the catheter
Adductor Canal	Anterior thigh, knee, medial lower leg	Location for catheter placement is in close proximity to femoral artery/vein, increasing the risk for intravascular injection	Less motor weakness than femoral PNC, but high failure rate [14] and no clear advantage over single shot in the first 48 hours after total knee arthroplasty [44]
Fascia Iliaca	Hip, Anterior Thigh, Knee	Lower risk of complications than psoas/lumbar plexus blocks Avoids femoral vessels Quadriceps weakness → fall risk	Similar analgesic efficacy for total hip and knee arthroplasty compared to femoral nerve block [45]. This is a large-volume nerve block requiring 30–40 mL of injectate. Spread should be monitored with ultrasonography
Proximal/ Sub-gluteal Sciatic	Posterior thigh, lower leg with exception of medial portion	Higher risk of bleeding/hematoma than popliteal sciatic (still rare) Insensate extremity → fall risk	Due to the deep nature, consider following neuraxial anticoagulation cessation guidelines
Popliteal Sciatic	Lower leg with exception of medial portion	Insensate extremity → fall risk	Catheter course through the biceps femoris can stabilize the catheter in a lateral approach relative to a posterior approach traversing subcutaneous tissue

This table is not exhaustive and there are numerous other insertion sites that have been reported in the literature [13]

5 Medications and Delivery Strategies

The ideal medication and infusion strategy will provide adequate analgesia, limit side effects, and minimize systemic toxicity. Long-acting dilute local anesthetics remain the primary medication used in peripheral nerve catheter infusions. The most commonly utilized medications include ropivacaine, bupivacaine, and levobupivacaine. Dilute local anesthetics (0.1–0.125% bupivacaine and levobupivacaine and 0.1–0.2% ropivacaine) are preferred to minimize motor blockade and positioning risks associated with an insensate limb.

A variety of adjuncts to local anesthetics have been studied, but there remains a paucity of evidence for their use, and currently local anesthetics are the only FDA approved medications for use in continuous peripheral nerve catheters. Adjuncts that have been studied with variable efficacy include epinephrine, clonidine, dexmedetomidine, dexamethasone, buprenorphine, and opioids [16, 46, 47].

There are three predominant infusion strategies that have been studied for PNCs: continuous infusion, programmed or patient controlled intermittent bolus, and a combination of the two. There is conflicting data on the efficacy of each of these strategies, and currently there is no clear guidance regarding optimal infusion strategies for the different PNC sites [48–50]. This likely reflects overall heterogeneity in practices due to differences in catheters (stimulating versus non-stimulating), insertion techniques (ultrasound-guided versus nerve-stimulator guided), local anesthetics used, anatomic sites of blockade, outcomes measured, and the patient populations.

Proponents of continuous infusion strategy cite improved baseline analgesia, less breakthrough pain, and improved sleep. Intuitively, there remains support that patient-controlled intermittent bolus dosing may be beneficial before potentially painful activities or therapies but that this infusion strategy is accompanied by an increased risk of peaks and valleys in pain control. Programmed intermittent bolus (PIB) dosing has the advantage of continuing to deliver the medication even when the patient is otherwise preoccupied or sleeping and not requesting a dose of medication. Proponents of intermittent bolus dosing cite decreased motor blockade and a diminished risk of an insensate extremity, in addition to improved perineural spread compared to equivalent dosing provided as a basal infusion.

There is some data that PNCs placed in anatomic compartments such as the paravertebral space have better analgesia with a PIB infusion strategy. Two separate RCTs of paravertebral catheters placed for postoperative analgesia following video-assisted thoracic surgery found greater dermatomal spread and improved postoperative analgesia in the programmed intermittent bolus group as compared to the continuous infusion group [51, 52]. Similarly, fascial plane blocks are thought to rely on the spread of local anesthetic in an interfascial plane to provide analgesia; therefore, it's plausible that if a PIB strategy provides superior spread in anatomic compartments, then a PIB strategy may also be superior for fascial plane blocks [53]. A study comparing continuous infusion versus programmed intermittent bolus in popliteal sciatic catheters found improved analgesia and less PCA dose requests in the PIB group [54]. However, another study on popliteal sciatic catheters showed similar analgesic effects between PIB and continuous infusions, but a more profound motor block in the PIB group [55]. An RCT evaluating adductor canal infusion after total knee arthroplasty compared continuous infusion to PIB and found no differences in analgesia, opioid consumption or mobility [56]. Thus, there are currently no clear guidelines regarding the optimal infusion strategy and further studies are needed to delineate the optimal infusion strategy for each specific anatomic site.

6 Inpatient Management

Acute pain management is growing as a perioperative specialty in both academic and non-academic hospitals. Many health systems have established acute pain management services to assist with perioperative pain management. Regional anesthesia and peripheral nerve catheters have demonstrated a recognized ability to contribute in a meaningful way to multimodal pain management. Despite the clear benefits of using peripheral nerve catheters for management of prolonged postoperative pain, there is an increased workload associated with the management of perineural catheters as compared to a single nerve block. This includes education of the healthcare team, including surgical specialties and nursing, as well as patient education on the catheter and associated complications. Ideally, there are systems in place that would allow for daily evaluation and management of the perineural infusion to include medication adjustments, troubleshooting of catheters, catheter replacement, and evaluation for end-of-therapy readiness and transition to an outpatient pain regimen.

7 Outpatient Management

Increasingly, there is interest in providing surgical procedures in outpatient and ambulatory surgical settings. PNCs can help facilitate this transition in care strategy by allowing patients to discharge home sooner with adequate analgesia typically lasting 48–72 hours [57, 58]. There are different outpatient infusion pumps available, primarily electronic and elastomeric pumps, each of which have pros and cons. Elastomeric pumps have a fixed volume reservoir under pressure to deliver the local anesthetic at a programmed hourly rate. Elastomeric pumps have the benefit of being easy to use and program and are disposable, so they do not require pump return, but they have less accurate hourly delivery, a limited ability to adjust dosing regimens, and generally cannot be refilled. Shown in Fig. 2 is an elastomeric pump for home perineural infusion. Benefits of electronic pumps include being very accurate in hourly dosing, accomodating adjustable dosing regimens, and infusate refill capabilities. However, these pumps are more costly and require that equipment be returned either via mail or by having the patient return to the healthcare facility [47].

Appropriate patient selection is important and should include an assessment of the patient and their caregiver's ability to monitor for signs of infection, identify signs of LAST, and the ability to contact their health-care providers if need be. Patients should have 24-h contact information available to them for questions. Ideally, there would be systems in place that allow the anesthesiologist to perform daily follow-up until catheter removal. Increasing familiarity with telehealth by both clinicians and patients may now make this process substantially easier than even a few years prior to COVID. At the therapeutic terminus, PNCs can be removed by the patient at home or possibly in a clinic setting [59, 60]. Caution with outpatient catheter utilization should be exercised in those at higher risk for drug toxicity, including patients with

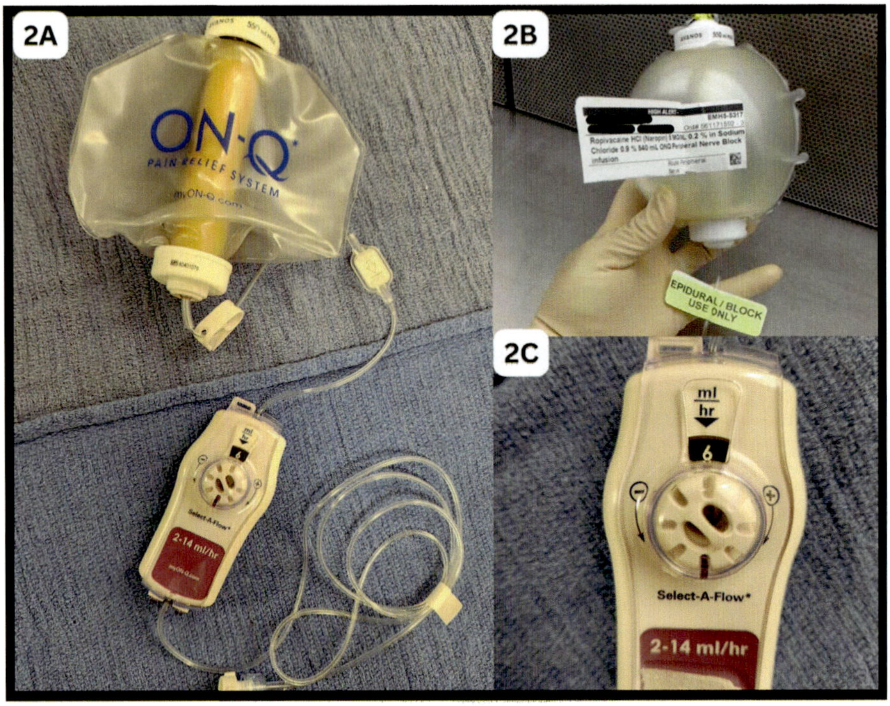

Fig. 2 Shown in Fig. 2A is an empty elastomeric pump that is designed to automatically and continuously deliver a regulated flow of local anesthetic in close proximity to desired nerves to be blocked. This On-Q system (Avanos; Alpharetta, GA) is equipped with a variable rate controller so that flow rate can be selected based on an individual's pain requirements. 2B illustrates the pump "over-filled" with 540 mL of local anesthetic, as recommended by the manufacturer. The variable rate controller (2C) allows for the practitioner to select a flow rate between 2 and 14 mL to run continuously at the catheter site

hepatic and renal dysfunction, and at specific catheter sites where local anesthetic effects could have adverse consequences in the absence of close monitoring. For example, a brachial plexus catheter causing phrenic nerve block in a patient with compromised pulmonary status (ex. obesity, severe COPD) or femoral nerve catheter causing quadriceps weakness and increasing a patient's fall risk [36, 61].

Key Takeaways

- Peripheral nerve catheters require additional expertise and resources for both placement and management; however, they remain an excellent option to treat moderate to severe pain expected to last over 24 h.
- Regional anesthesia via a peripheral nerve catheter has numerous advantages, including avoidance of systemic analgesic medications, but each PNC site also has unique risk factors for both placement and perineural infusion.

- There remains a paucity of data regarding optimal infusion strategies for the majority of PNC sites as well as for specific treatment protocols following various surgical interventions.

References

1. Ansbro FP. A method of continuous brachial plexus block. Am J Surg. 1946;71:716–22.
2. Richman JM, Liu SS, Courpas G, et al. Does continuous peripheral nerve block provide superior pain control to opioids? A meta-analysis. Anesth Analg. 2006;102(1):248–57.
3. Buckenmaier CC, Rupprecht C, McKnight G, et al. Pain following battlefield injury and evacuation: a survey of 110 casualties from the wars in Iraq and Afghanistan. Pain Med. 2009;10:1487–96.
4. Chudinov A, Berkenstadt H, Salai M, et al. Continuous psoas compartment block for anesthesia and perioperative analgesia in patients with hip fractures. Reg Anesth Pain Med. 1999;24:563–8.
5. Dadure C, Motais F, Ricard C, et al. Continuous peripheral nerve blocks at home for treatment of recurrent complex regional pain syndrome I in children. Anesthesiology. 2005;102:387–91.
6. Lierz P, Schroegendorfer K, Choi S, et al. Continuous blockade of both brachial plexus with ropivacaine in phantom pain: a case report. Pain. 1998;78:135–7.
7. Fischer HB, Peters TM, Fleming IM, et al. Peripheral nerve catheterization in the management of terminal cancer pain. Reg Anesth. 1996;21:482–5.
8. Umino M, Kohase H, Ideguchi S, et al. Long-term pain control in trigeminal neuralgia with local anesthetics using an indwelling catheter in the mandibular nerve. Clin J Pain. 2002;18:196–9.
9. Ding DY, Manoli A 3rd, Galos DK, et al. Continuous popliteal sciatic nerve block versus single injection nerve block for ankle fracture surgery: A prospective randomized comparative trial. J Orthop Trauma. 2015;29(9):393–8.
10. Hade AD, Okano S, Pelecanos A, et al. Factors associated with low levels of patient satisfaction following peripheral nerve block. Anaesth Intensive Care. 2021;49(2):125–32.
11. Ahsan ZS, Carvalho B, Yao J. Incidence of failure of continuous peripheral nerve catheters for postoperative analgesia in upper extremity surgery. J Hand Surg Am. 2014;39(2):324–9.
12. Saporito A, Petri GJ, Sturini E, et al. Safety and effectiveness of bilateral continuous sciatic nerve block for bilateral orthopaedic foot surgery: a cohort study. Eur J Anaesthesiol. 2014;31(11):620–5.
13. Ilfeld BM. Continuous peripheral nerve blocks: an update of the published evidence and comparison with novel, alternative analgesic modalities. Anesth Analg. 2017;124(1):308–35.
14. Hauritz RW, Hannig KE, Balocco AL, et al. Peripheral nerve catheters: A critical review of the efficacy. Best Pract Res Clin Anaesthesiol. 2019;33(3):325–39.
15. Ilfeld BM. Continuous peripheral nerve blocks and alternative regional analgesic modalities: clarification regarding relative superiority. Anesth Analg. 2017;124(6):2088.
16. Ilfeld BM. Continuous peripheral nerve blocks: a review of the published evidence. Anesth Analg. 2011;113(4):904–25.
17. Schnabel A, Meyer-Frießem CH, Zahn PK, et al. Ultrasound compared with nerve stimulation guidance for peripheral nerve catheter placement: a meta-analysis of randomized controlled trials. Br J Anaesth. 2013;111(4):564–72.
18. Ilfeld BM, Fredrickson MJ, Mariano ER. Ultrasound-guided perineural catheter insertion: three approaches but few illuminating data. Reg Anesth Pain Med. 2010;35:123–6.
19. Antonakakis JG, Sites BD, Shiffrin J. Ultrasound-guided posterior approach for the placement of a continuous interscalene catheter. Reg Anesth Pain Med. 2009;34:64–8.
20. Dhir S, Ganapathy S. Use of ultrasound guidance and contrast enhancement: a study of continuous infraclavicular brachial plexus approach. Acta Anaesthesiol Scand. 2008;52:338–42.

21. Swenson JD, Davis JJ, DeCou JA. A novel approach for assessing catheter position after ultrasound-guided placement of continuous interscalene block. Anesth Analg. 2008;106:1015–6.
22. Sandhu NS, Capan LM. Ultrasound-guided infraclavicular brachial plexus block. Br J Anaesth. 2002;89:254–9.
23. Merritt CK, Mariano ER, Kaye AD, et al. Peripheral nerve catheters and local anesthetic infiltration in perioperative analgesia. Best Pract Res Clin Anaesthesiol. 2014;28(1):41–57.
24. Enneking K. Close counts. Reg Anesth Pain Med. 2007;32(4):280.
25. Mariano ER (2019) Continuous peripheral nerve blocks. https://www.asra.com/guidelines-articles/original-articles/regional-anesthesia/regional-anesthesia/legacy-b-blog-posts/2019/08/07/continuous-peripheral-nerve-blocks. Accessed 18 Apr 2023.
26. Neuburger M, Breitbarth J, Reisig F, et al. Complications and adverse events in continuous peripheral regional anesthesia: results of investigations on 3491 catheters. Anaesthesist. 2006;55:33–40.
27. Wiegel M, Gottschaldt U, Hennebach R, et al. Complications and adverse effects associated with continuous peripheral nerve blocks in orthopedic patients. Anesth Analg. 2007;104:1578–82.
28. Blumenthal S, Borgeat A, Maurer K, et al. Preexisting subclinical neuropathy as a risk factor for nerve injury after continuous ropivacaine administration through a femoral nerve catheter. Anesthesiology. 2006;105:1053–6.
29. Horlocker TT, O'Driscoll SW, Dinapoli RP. Recurring brachial plexus neuropathy in a diabetic patient after shoulder surgery and continuous interscalene block. Anesth Analg. 2000;91:688–90.
30. Compere V, Legrand JF, Guitard PG, et al. Bacterial colonization after tunneling in 402 perineural catheters: a prospective study. Anesth Analg. 2009;108:1326–30.
31. Cuvillon P, Ripart J, Lalourcey L, et al. The continuous femoral nerve block catheter for postoperative analgesia: bacterial colonization, infectious rate and adverse effects. Anesth Analg. 2001;93:1045–9.
32. Capdevila X, Bringuier S, Borgeat A. Infectious risk of continuous peripheral nerve blocks. Anesthesiology. 2009;110:182–8.
33. Neuburger M, Buttner J, Blumenthal S, et al. Inflammation and infection complications of 2285 perineural catheters: a prospective study. Acta Anaesthesiol Scand. 2007;51:108–14.
34. Walker BJ, Noonan KJ, Bosenberg AT. Evolving compartment syndrome not masked by a continuous peripheral nerve block: evidence-based case management. Reg Anesth Pain Med. 2012;37(4):393–7.
35. Urmey WF, Talts KH, Sharrock NE. One hundred percent incidence of hemidiaphragmatic paresis associated with interscalene brachial plexus anesthesia as diagnosed by ultrasonography. Anesth Analg. 1991;72(4):498.
36. Sanchez M, Malhotra N, Lin L, et al. End-stage pulmonary disease and brachial plexus regional anesthesia: their implications on perioperative pulmonary function. Semin Cardiothoracic Vasc Anesth. 2012;16(1):59–64.
37. Vester-Andersen T, Christiansen C, Hansen A, et al. Interscalene brachial plexus block: area of analgesia, complications, and blood concentrations of local anesthetics. Acta Anaesthesiol Scand. 1981;25(2):81–4.
38. Neal J, Moore J, Kopacz D, et al. Quantitative analysis of respiratory, motor, and sensory function after supraclavicular block. Anesh Analg. 1998;86:1239–44.
39. Brand L, Papper EM. A comparison of supraclavicular and axillary techniques for brachial plexus blocks. Anesthesiology. 1961;22:226.
40. Naja Z, Lönnqvist PA. Somatic paravertebral nerve blockade incidence of failed block and complications. Anaesthesia. 2001;56(12):1181–201.
41. Pace MM, Sharma B, Anderson-Dam J, et al. Ultrasound-guided thoracic paravertebral blockade: a retrospective study of the incidence of complications. Anesth Analg. 2016;122(4):1186–91.

42. Coveney E, Weltz CR, Greengrass R, et al. Use of paravertebral block anesthesia in the surgical management of breast cancer: experience in 156 cases. Ann Surg. 1998;227(4):496.
43. Buckenmaier CC 3rd, Kwon KH, Howard RS, et al. Double-blinded, placebo-controlled, prospective randomized trial evaluating the efficacy of paravertebral block with and without continuous paravertebral block analgesia in outpatient breast cancer surgery. Pain Med. 2010;11(5):790–9.
44. Hussain N, Brull R, Zhou S, et al. Analgesic benefits of single-shot versus continuous adductor canal block for total knee arthroplasty: a systemic review and meta-analysis of randomized trials. Reg Anesth Pain Med. 2023;48:49–60.
45. Fan X, Cao F, Luo A. Femoral nerve block versus fascia iliaca block for pain control in knee and hip arthroplasties: a meta-analysis. Medicine. 2021;100(14): e25450.
46. Ilfeld BM, Morey TE, Enneking FK. Continuous infraclavicular perineural infusion with clonidine and ropivacaine compared with ropivacaine alone: a randomized, double-blinded, controlled study. Anesth Analg. 2003;97:706–12.
47. Ilfeld BM, Enneking FK. Continuous peripheral nerve blocks at home: a review. Anesth Analg. 2005;100:1822–33.
48. Gabriel RA, Ilfeld BM. Continuous peripheral nerve blocks: does automated intermittent bolus administration provide any benefit compared with a continuous infusion? ASRA News. 2019;17(1):22–4.
49. Jagannathan R, Niesen AD, D'Souza R, et al. Intermittent bolus versus continuous infusion techniques for local anesthetic delivery in peripheral and truncal nerve analgesia: the current state of evidence. Reg Anesth Pain Med. 2019;44:447–51.
50. Ilfeld BM, Gabriel RA. Basal infusion versus intermittent boluses for perineural catheters: should we take the 'continuous' out of 'continuous peripheral nerve blocks'? Reg Anesth Pain Med. 2019;44:285–6.
51. Hida K, Murata H, Ichinomiya T, et al. Effects of programmed intermittent thoracic paravertebral bolus of levobupivacaine on the spread of sensory block: a randomized, controlled, double-blind study. Reg Anesth Pain Med. 2019;44:326–32.
52. Chen L, Wu Y, Cai Y, et al. Comparison of programmed intermittent bolus infusion and continuous infusion for postoperative patient-controlled analgesia with thoracic paravertebral block catheter: a randomized, double-blind, controlled trial. Reg Anesth Pain Med. 2019;44:240–5.
53. Finneran Iv JJ, Alexander B, Bechis SK, et al. Continuous erector spinae plane blocks with automated boluses for analgesia following percutaneous nephrolithotomy. Korean J Anesthesiol. 2021;74(2):178–80.
54. Finneran JJ, Said ET, Curran BP, et al. Basal infusion versus automated boluses and a delayed start timer for "continuous" sciatic nerve blocks after ambulatory foot and ankle surgery: a randomized clinical trial. Anesthesiology. 2022;136(6):970–82.
55. Short AJ, Ghosh M, Jin R, et al. Intermittent bolus versus continuous infusion popliteal sciatic nerve block following major foot and ankle surgery: a prospective randomized comparison. Reg Anesth Pain Med. 2019;44:1053–8.
56. Jaeger P, Baggesgaard J, Sørensen JK, et al. Adductor canal block with continuous infusion versus intermittent boluses and morphine consumption: a randomized, blinded, controlled clinical trial. Anesth Analg. 2018;126(6):2069–77.
57. Ilfeld BM, Le LT, Meyer RS, et al. Ambulatory continuous femoral nerve blocks decrease time to discharge readiness after tricompartment total knee arthroplasty: a randomized, triple-masked, placebo-controlled study. Anesthesiology. 2008;108:703–13.
58. Ilfeld BM, Vandenborne K, Duncan PW, et al. Ambulatory continuous interscalene nerve blocks decrease the time to discharge readiness after total shoulder arthroplasty: a randomized, triple-masked, placebo-controlled study. Anesthesiology. 2006;105:999–1007.
59. Swenson JD, Bay N, Loose E, et al. Outpatient management of continuous peripheral nerve catheters placed using ultrasound guidance: an experience in 620 patients. Anesth Analg. 2006;103(6):1436–43.

60. Ilfeld BM, Esener DE, Morey TE, et al. Ambulatory perineural infusion: the patients' perspective. Reg Anesth Pain Med. 2003;28:418–23.
61. Charous MT, Madison SJ, Suresh PJ, et al. Continuous femoral nerve blocks: varying local anesthetic delivery method (bolus versus basal) to minimize quadriceps motor block while maintaining sensory block. Anesthesiology. 2011;115(4):774–81.

Prehabilitation and Rehabilitation as Pathways to Improved Perioperative Analgesia

Sun Mei Liu, Alina Razak, Ashley Wang, Katrina Kerolus, and Genevieve Monanian

Abstract This chapter details a pathway for improved perioperative analgesia when incorporating practices of prehabilitation and rehabilitation. Following a discussion regarding the experience of postoperative pain and the risk factors for the development of chronic pain, the chapter outlines a longitudinal assessment and treatment for patients, including preoperative risk stratification, multimodal analgesic selection, and teams-based approaches for improved care. Prehabilitation and rehabilitation strategies such as physical therapy, water therapy, massage therapy, acupuncture, transcutaneous electrical nerve stimulation, and cryotherapy are explored further.

Keywords Chronic pain · Multimodal analgesia · Postoperative pain · Prehabilitation

1 Introduction

The International Association for the Study of Pain (IASP) defines pain as "an unpleasant sensory and emotional experience associated with, or resembling that associated with, actual or potential tissue damage" [1]. Pain is, by definition, a subjective and highly personal experience shaped by dynamic interactions between

S. M. Liu (✉) · A. Razak · A. Wang · K. Kerolus · G. Monanian
Department of Anesthesiology, Renaissance School of Medicine, Stony Brook University Hospital, Stony Brook, NY, USA
e-mail: sunmei.liu@stonybrookmedicine.edu

A. Razak
e-mail: alina.razak@stonybrookmedicine.edu

A. Wang
e-mail: ashley.wang@stonybrookmedicine.edu

K. Kerolus
e-mail: katrina.kerolus@stonybrookmedicine.edu

G. Monanian
e-mail: Genevieve.Monanian@stonybrookmedicine.edu

A. Abd-Elsayed and K. Schroeder (eds.), *Perioperative Pain Management*,
https://doi.org/10.1007/978-3-031-67648-2_34

a multitude of biological, psychological, and social factors, thus making it especially challenging to assess and treat [2]. The IASP notes that acute pain occurs suddenly, lasting from several minutes to less than six months, and often plays a protective role by warning individuals of an underlying disease or threat to the body, such as the threat that occurs when undergoing a surgery or medical procedure [1]. Chronic pain is often described as maladaptive pain lasting over three months and persisting beyond what is typically expected given the injury. Despite efforts to mitigate acute perioperative pain, surgical interventions have consistently been identified as one of the leading etiologies of chronic pain development [3, 4]. Studies have shown that up to 80–86% of patients reported moderate, severe, or extreme pain shortly after surgery [5, 6]. Inadequate treatment of postoperative pain is often associated with poor recovery outcomes, including impaired rehabilitation, prolonged length of stay in the hospital, increased risk of hospital readmission, and higher overall cost of care [7, 8]. Furthermore, 10–50% of patients may develop persistent postoperative pain more than three to six months following their surgical procedure [9]. Addressing perioperative pain is frequently challenging and the implementation of multi-faceted approaches that optimize several perioperative parameters may be more likely to be associated with analgesic success.

2 Pain Pathways

The experience of pain is unique and influenced by a wide-array of experiential variables; however, three key physiologic pathways have been identified, including nociceptive, inflammatory, and neuropathic pain [9]. Nociceptive pain involves peripheral stimulation of pain receptors (nociceptors) from noxious and intense mechanical, chemical, or thermal stimuli, which are subsequently converted to neural impulses via transduction [10]. These signals are transmitted via nerve fibers to the spinal cord, which then send second-order nerve fibers to the higher central nervous system for perception processing. Inflammatory pain involves increased excitation of nociceptors by inflammatory mediators that are released in response to surgical intervention [9, 11]. Neuropathic pain refers to pathology in the somatosensory system, often from direct injury to peripheral nerves in the perioperative setting, resulting in both positive sensory phenomena, such as spontaneous pain and allodynia, as well as negative sensory phenomena such as numbness and loss of temperature sensation [9, 12].

Despite the termination of ongoing damaging and noxious stimuli, ongoing inflammation and neuropathic changes may cause significant persistent pain following surgical interventions [13]. It has been proposed that complex chronic post-surgical pain results from inflammation, reversible neuroplasticity, and nerve injury [9]. Inflammation at the surgical site causes increased excitability at the nerve terminal and central sensitization via modifications in gene transcription resulting in secondary hyperalgesia involving pain beyond the initial site of injury [14, 15]. Transection of a nerve results in spontaneous firing of action potentials from surrounding neurons resulting in spontaneous pain and hypersensitivity. Further, persistent lack of transmission through the transected nerve fiber results in apoptosis of inhibitory interneurons within the spinal cord itself resulting in potentially permanent changes in the circuitry within the central nervous system [16].

3 Risk Factors for Post-surgical Pain Development

Chronic post-surgical pain has been defined as occurring after a surgical procedure and persisting for at least three months following the exclusion of other causes for the pain [17, 18]. Studies indicate that chronic post-surgical pain develops in 10–30% of patients who are evaluated for ongoing pain symptoms at one year following surgical procedures [18].

Preoperative risk factors for the development of chronic pain include genetic susceptibility to pain, existing preoperative pain, younger age, and psychosocial factors [9, 18]. Gender has been inconsistently associated with increased postoperative pain [19]. Several intraoperative risk factors have been identified including surgical technique (open versus minimally invasive), extensive nerve injury, and inadequate preemptive analgesia [9]. Importantly, the type and extent of the surgical procedure is associated with post-surgical pain development. The German Quality Improvement in Postoperative Pain Treatment study reported that pain intensities were expectedly higher for major orthopedic and spine surgeries. However, pain scores for "minor" procedures such as tonsillectomy and appendectomy were amongst the highest. The authors hypothesized that chronic pain development following "minor" surgical procedures may be secondary to provider underestimation of pain and limited analgesic interventions with such procedures [20]. Despite the increased utilization of minimally invasive surgical techniques, patients can have unmet needs for post-operative analgesic administration [21]. This recognition has facilitated the development of Procedure-Specific Postoperative Pain Management (PROSPECT) strategies that aim to address barriers to effective analgesic management [22].

4 Complex Pain Perception

Complex pain is a composite of the sensation of pain, emotional response, and cognitive interpretation of the current pain [23]. While many individuals experience pain transiently, complex pain occurs when pain perception persistently interferes with daily activities and function.

Individual variability in the experience of pain has been described according to the biopsychosocial model [2]. Biological contributors include genetics, nociceptive thresholds, and inflammation. The sympathetic nervous system, as part of the autonomic nervous system, has been implicated in the development of complex regional pain syndromes [23, 24]. Studies have demonstrated increased pain with intradermal injection of norepinephrine for patients with complex regional pain syndrome compared to those without, which suggests a role for sympathetic blockade in the treatment of these patients [25].

Psychological aspects of pain perception include stress, mood, and catastrophizing. Catastrophizing has been shown to play a significant role in the perioperative setting, where patients may ruminate on the belief that the current lesion will lead to the maximum amount of pain and foster a mindset of helplessness [26, 27]. Preoperative catastrophizing was found to predict complex chronic pain two years following knee arthroplasty [18, 28]. A study performed with individuals who experience pain with walking indicated that the participants perceived pre-marked distances as being further away than did the control group, suggesting a further intersection between cognition, distress, and pain perception [29].

Social aspects of pain perception include environmental stressors and support infrastructure. Many initiatives have sought to understand the association between socioeconomic status and the experience of pain. A study by the Austrian Federal Ministry of Health, Family and Youth determined that those with a lower socioeconomic status had an increase in the prevalence and intensity of pain as well as increased perceived disability due to pain, further highlighting the importance of social factors in the development of complex pain perception [30].

A key tenet to the biopsychosocial model is that each of the three components interact with one another to decode the complexities of pain perception rather than each influencing pain independently. As an example, perceived stress (social) can lead to heightened sympathetic activation (biological), and therefore increased pain perception [2]. The gene coding for catechol-O-methyl-transferase (COMT) has been extensively studied with relation to pain perception [31]. This genetic finding (biological) has been implicated in pain catastrophizing (psychological) and is able to predict pain intensity [32]. The development of complex pain perception is multidimensional, and the biopsychosocial model seeks to create a more comprehensive understanding of how complex pain arises.

5 Barriers to Care

Individuals with chronic pain have historically been underserved due to a variety of factors. The Institute of Medicine's Committee on Advancing Pain Research, Care, and Education underscores chronic pain as a public health concern given the disparities that affect these patients' care [33]. They identify several barriers to adequate pain care, including inadequate education for health care professionals regarding pain assessment, treatment modalities, implicit biases, and stereotypes that further disparities, as well as outdated reimbursement policies that limit time and resources for treatment of chronic pain and need for interdisciplinary research to identify improved treatment modalities. Overall, they call for a cultural transformation to address gaps in care [33].

6 Treatment Approaches to Preoperative Assessment

Given the nuances of postoperative pain management, it is vital to take a multimodal and multidisciplinary approach in preoperative assessment. Patient education and counseling represent essential elements of any successful program that seeks to preemptively address issues related to pain management. A family-centered, individually tailored preoperative education paradigm would cover not only the analgesic options and the risks/benefits of each treatment, but also the methods of pain reporting and possible changes to be made to patients' regular medication regimen around surgery day [34]. Preoperative counseling also allows clinicians to help patients set realistic goals for postoperative pain in order to manage their expectations. Rather than striving for a "zero pain state" after procedures, patients should understand that complete relief from pain may not be attainable [4]. Instead, a shift of focus towards improving postoperative functional status is more productive; these may include resuming regular diet and returning to normal activities of daily living such as toilet hygiene, grooming, and ambulating [35]. In the course of preoperative education administration, healthcare professionals should account for a patient's level of health literacy and be mindful of any cultural or language barriers. Efforts should be made to foster a supportive environment that addresses all questions or concerns [34]. This may also be an appropriate setting to determine a patients' biopsychosocial needs, such as fears or anxieties regarding surgical pain, coping mechanisms, and level of social support [2, 9].

In addition, proper preoperative risk stratification of patients allows better prediction of pain outcomes. Common predictors of poor acute postoperative pain control include: young age, female gender, smoking, history of depressive symptoms, history of anxiety, sleep difficulties, higher BMI, preoperative pain, and preoperative analgesic use [36]. Since higher intensity and longer duration acute postoperative pain are associated with an increased risk of chronic postsurgical pain, understanding a patient's risk factors prior to surgery helps to anticipate potential complications in postoperative pain management [4, 9, 37].

Special considerations must be given to complex surgical patients, namely those with substance use disorders, chronic pain, and/or significant tolerance in the setting of long-term opioid therapy—with careful distinctions made between each. Chronic pain patients may have opioid tolerance, requiring significant opioid dosing escalations to achieve the same level of pain control as someone who is opioid naïve [38]. These patients may be reasonably expected to request additional pain medications until they achieve the desired level of relief. This behavior can be easily, and perhaps erroneously, seen and labeled as "drug-seeking" behavior typically associated with substance use and addiction. In contrast, those with substance use and addiction are more likely to continue seeking opioids even with good pain control and less likely to follow medication plans as prescribed. They may demand specific drugs or claim allergies to non-opioid analgesics [38]. Furthermore, substance use and addiction can include non-opioids (e.g., benzodiazepines, cocaine, alcohol), which could interact differently with traditional analgesics and complicate pain management [34]. Strategies to manage patients with complex pain include conducting a substance use screen, coordinating with other care teams (e.g., pain medicine, behavioral health, addiction medicine), providing education on potential adverse events of postoperative opioid use, and making telehealth available as an alternative to in-person consults [39]. Patients on long-term opioid therapy need coordination with prescribers to continue baseline opioid administration on the day of surgery, whereas those with opioid tolerance require individualized tapering plans for postoperative opioids [39].

Finally, successful multimodal analgesic regimens combine the use of opioid and non-opioid drugs to address pain. This methodology takes advantage of the additive and/or synergistic effects of a variety of analgesic classes to fight pain from different mechanisms of action, thus lowering total drug usage while reducing overall side effects [40]. This strategy is especially beneficial for chronic postoperative pain, as it allows for personalized treatment based on specific factors such as patient profile, surgical procedure, and type of pain [22, 41]. Common agents and techniques for multimodal pain management include acetaminophen, non-steroidal anti-inflammatory drugs (NSAIDs), N-methyl-D-aspartate (NMDA)-receptor antagonists, gabapentinoids, anticonvulsants, antidepressants, and regional anesthesia [8, 37]. Moreover, incorporation of cognitive-behavioral modalities should be considered as part of the multimodal approach to surgical pain management [34]. These include meditation, breathing exercises, guided imagery, hypnosis, and music therapy. These alternative analgesic modalities may be delivered by many different healthcare professionals including psychologists, therapists, nurses, physicians, and social workers. Relatively harmless and non-invasive therapies including cognitive-behavioral modalities should be routinely considered as an adjunct to traditional analgesics.

7 Prehabilitation and Rehabilitation

Prehabilitation and rehabilitation focus on improving functional status and minimizing the stress response of a patient in the perioperative space. As outlined in the literature, a patient's recovery is highly individualized and largely based on a myriad of baseline patient characteristics that includes those patients with complex pain [42]. Pain is a symptom that is closely monitored following surgery and it is an outcome that patients, and providers, care a great deal about. Patients with a history of chronic pain or pain that is difficult to manage present a challenge to both providers and patients in the perioperative period. Multimodal analgesic approaches to prehabilitation and rehabilitation are more likely to be successful in those patients with significant chronic pain or baseline opioid requirements. Including pain specialists in the perioperative management of patients with complex pain further augments opportunities to preemptively address and ultimately recover from surgical insults.

The concept of preoperative evaluation and testing is one that is both well studied, and evidence based. The process of assessing a patient prior to surgery to determine their risks and assess how to intervene and optimize medical conditions has become an important component of the perioperative timeline. When assessing a patient with complex pain prior to surgery, it is key to obtain input from a pain specialist. Designated onsite pain specialists benefit from expertise and specialized training and are uniquely suited to serve patients with complex pain by recognizing their pain states and processes. Pain specialists' intimate knowledge of multimodal anesthesia and the broad range of analgesics available allow them to deliver safe, individualized pain regimens for these patients while avoiding side effects, pain flare-ups and withdrawal symptoms [43, 44].

A risk frequently encountered with surgical pain management is low functional capacity or frailty, a condition known to be associated with a greater chance of death within 30 days after surgery, longer postoperative hospital stays, and a higher rate of surgical complications [45]. Frailty has been conceptualized as syndrome where individuals have a decreased reserve when responding to stressors due to a combination of physical and cognitive decline, medical comorbidities, and nutritional deficits [46]. Numerous frailty assessments have been trialed and utilized to assess preoperative risk such as the Clinical Frailty Scale and the Frailty Index [47, 48]. Frailty has also been associated with increased chronic post-surgical pain [49, 50].

Given what we know about the risks of low preoperative functional capacity, prehabilitation has emerged as a concept that might be widely applicable and beneficial. The term was introduced by Topp et al. [51] to describe a program that incorporated warm-up, aerobic, strength, flexibility, and functional task components to improve the functional status of patients prior to an intensive care unit admission. Surgical prehabilitation is no longer seen as purely physical exercise recommendations that sought to improve functional status. Prehabilitation is now conceptualized as a well-rounded approach that promotes cessation of adverse habits, exercise to address strength, balance, and aerobic fitness, dietary interventions, and practices to alleviate stress and promote resiliency [45]. Research related to prehabilitation is in the earlier stages, however, studies are showing that exercise prior to major surgery is safe and can lead to beneficial outcomes including improved postoperative quality of life, reduced hospital length of stay, and decreased morbidity. Nutritional and psychological interventions have less independently supportive evidence as they are typically included with physical exercise regimens [52]. However, collectively, the multimodal approach is producing results that are encouraging.

Prehabilitation is intended to be a patient-centered pathway that seeks to improve patient outcomes and is intended to be a complement to rehabilitation [42]. The goal of rehabilitation in the postoperative period is to promote recovery from surgery. A well-known and studied representation of this is enhanced recovery after surgery, which spans the preoperative, intraoperative, and postoperative phases of care. Interventions under the enhanced recovery after surgery umbrella attempt to minimize the surgical stress response to bolster early mobilization and improve surgical outcomes [53]. Enhanced recovery after surgery is a well-studied, independent way to improve surgical outcomes. However, there is emerging literature that shows the complementary relationship that it has with prehabilitation efforts.

The discussion to follow will explore various non-pharmacological options that can be utilized in the prehabilitation and rehabilitation period surrounding major surgery for the patient with complex pain. Multiple modalities will be explored, including physical therapy, water therapy, massage therapy, acupuncture, transcutaneous electrical nerve stimulation (TENS), and cryotherapy, as it is important to acknowledge that the pain experience is complex in that it affects each patient differently, making it essential to have multiple options in the healthcare professional's toolbox to allow for dynamic management of pain in the perioperative period.

Physical Therapy

Physical therapy is a familiar therapeutic intervention for rehabilitation from an injury. However, physical therapy has been found to have a role in the perioperative population both in recovering from surgery as well as preparing for surgery. Components of physical therapy can be broken down into several stages [54]. The initial stage of therapy includes education about the healing process, pain management, and what to expect in therapy as well as the initiation of exercises to promote a range of motion, soft tissue massage to decrease inflammation, and joint mobilization. The following stage incorporates strength training and gait and balance training as well as the advancement of a range of motion exercises. In the rehabilitation setting, this stage would also include modalities to reduce scar tissue formation. The final stage of therapy would include further advancement of the exercises that the patient is undergoing with a focus on challenging the patient's proprioception, balance, flexibility, and range of motion with the final goal being an improvement in functional status [54].

The incorporation of physical therapy in the prehabilitation period appears to improve early postoperative pain scores and hasten functional recovery [55]. The purpose of physical therapy in this time frame is similar to the rehabilitation period as the goal is to decrease pain and increase functional status. Unfortunately, studies conducted in setting of lumbar spine surgery have demonstrated that physical therapy is only minimally incorporated in the preoperative period despite outcomes being improved when compared to restricted activity. Given that patients presenting for spine surgery are frequently maintained on opioid prescriptions, there may be ample opportunities to work with these patients, implement prehabilitation pathways, and seek to reduce the need or dosing of opioid prescriptions [56, 57]. Additional research is necessary to further evaluate the content of physical therapy programs offered to patients, however, given the evidence currently available suggesting reductions in pain, decreased complications, and improved functional recovery with the implementation of a multimodal prehabilitation program including a physical therapy or strength training regimen, it seems prudent to expand overall utilization [58, 59].

Physical therapy is well studied in the period of rehabilitation from surgery and as previously discussed the inclusion of therapy in the preoperative period helps decrease pain and prepares patients for the rehabilitation period. There is evidence that preoperative physical therapy and strength training reduces the time to meet milestones in rehabilitation physical therapy and increases readiness for discharge from physical therapy [60]. These milestones specific to inpatient physical therapy included independent transfers in and out of bed as well as on and off commodes, independent ambulation and negotiation of stairs, and independence with an exercise program planned for at home [60]. One study that specifically evaluated the impact of postoperative physical therapy following total knee arthroplasty found that intensive programs focused on functional and strengthening exercises were beneficial and could be conducted in a land- or water-based environment [61]. Early integration of physical therapy serves as a nonpharmacologic treatment for musculoskeletal pain and can serve as an adjunct to oral analgesics [62]. Evidence suggests that outpatient physical therapy may be best suited for addressing long-term outcomes and that progression through exercises is best when guided by both clinical and strength milestones [61].

Water Therapy

Water therapy, also referred to as aquatic therapy, has shown potential as a method of prehabilitation and rehabilitation, particularly in the case of patients dealing with osteoarthritis or a type of degenerative joint condition where symptoms such as chronic pain and loss of function are predominant [63]. The mechanical and thermal properties of the water environment create a beneficial setting for the musculoskeletal system to allow for therapeutic intervention. Therapy conducted in a rehabilitation pool is typically at 34–35 °C and focuses on movement exercises to both strengthen muscles as well as improve mobility through a phased aquatic exercise session with warm up, main phase, and a relaxing phase. The incorporation of aquatic therapy into the prehabilitation and rehabilitation of patients undergoing orthopedic surgery has been shown to allow for an increase in pain threshold, myorelaxation, and re-introduction of movement that was previously painful or pathologic due to an underlying condition [63].

An additional form of hydrotherapy that has been studied is known as Kneipp hydrotherapy where there are alterations of warm and cold-water therapy. The method used in Kneipp hydrotherapy has demonstrated local vasoconstriction followed by vasodilation, hormone modulation, and immunoregulation [64]. This form of hydrotherapy is also shown to be associated with a reduction in pain, increased mobility, and improvement in quality of life. This type of water therapy does not include rehabilitation pool exercise but instead utilizes affusions in combination with traditional physiotherapy. The pathologic area for the patient is targeted for stimulation with alternating cold and warm water affusions followed by a physiotherapy regimen that seeks to promote an increase in function [64]. Studies are presently underway to determine the most beneficial frequency of affusion water therapy with physiotherapy in this patient population and to further examine the impact of this modality on pain reduction and increased functional capacity [64]. Aquatic therapy as a whole has been shown to induce short-term pain reduction and improved mobilization when compared with traditional physiotherapy/physical therapy. Aquatic therapy has also demonstrated efficacy in patients with pain secondary to osteoarthritis and degenerative joint disease not planned to undergo surgery [65]. However, long-term perioperative benefits and support for the inclusion of aquatic therapy in prehabilitation and rehabilitation regimens remains under investigation [63].

Massage Therapy

Massage therapy is a type of non-pharmacological treatment that may be an important component of multimodal perioperative analgesic regimens [66]. The practice of massage therapy involves the manipulation of soft tissue with the therapeutic goal being to prevent or alleviate pain, spasms, tension, and stress [66]. Studies have shown that a single session of massage therapy successfully alleviates postoperative pain and serves as an effective adjuvant therapy for patients in the perioperative phase of care. Massage therapy has also been shown to be safe for adults and children with chronic and cancer-related pain [66]. The frequency of this therapeutic intervention is typically determined by the licensed practitioner conducting the session, however, inpatient studies suggest daily sessions of 20–45 min with outpatient follow-up that is generally conducted in weekly sessions. The number of sessions recommended is not yet well defined in the literature [66].

Studies have been conducted that demonstrate both long- and short-term benefits associated with utilizing massage therapy as an adjunct to traditional pain management in the rehabilitation period [67]. Across a variety of surgical types, massage therapy appears to serve as an effective therapeutic adjunct for pain relief and anxiety reduction in cardiac surgery, labor-related pain, and orthopedic surgery [68–70]. Throughout the literature there is some variation in the efficacy and clinical impact of massage therapy which is likely due to the lack of consensus regarding frequency, duration, practitioner variation, and timing of intervention.[67] However, massage therapy remains a potentially important tool in complex pain cases where flexibility is needed, and diverse therapeutics are needed to improve outcomes.

Acupuncture

Acupuncture has been a common traditional Chinese practice within the eastern world for over 3000 years and it is becoming increasingly popular across the globe as people seek alternative methods to alleviate pain. The National Health Interview Survey (NHIS) from 2007 reports that Americans who participated in acupuncture therapies increased from 4.2 to 6.3% of the population, representing approximately 14.01 million users in 2007 [71]. Acupuncture involves penetrating the skin with thin needles at established sites throughout the body. Additional gentle needle movements or the provision of electric current via the needle may be utilized to enhance the therapeutic efficacy. The theory behind acupuncture involves stimulating energy points referred to as Qi that flow through channels known as meridians. Originally, 365 acupoints were identified over 14 meridians, but now there are over 2000 recognized points that can be activated to alleviate pain [72]. This energy is drawn from two opposite and complementary sources known as Yin and Yang. Yin is described as a passive force associated with cold and darkness, while Yang is seen as an active force associated with heat, light, and assertiveness [73]. Together, Yin and Yang interact between different meridians, which are interconnected between organs, to promote harmony, healing, and overall well-being. Inversely, disruption of the meridians is believed to be the cause of diseases, stress, and pain.

The exact mechanism of acupuncture is not completely understood but multiple theories have been proposed. The process begins with needle insertion at an acupoint, which is a specific point in the body that is believed to control pain. In a study conducted on rats, it was found that acupoints are composed of mast cells, blood cells, and nerve fibers [74]. There are four different nerve fiber types, Aα, Aβ, Aδ, and C fibers. The role of these specialized peripheral nerve endings is to respond to multiple types of stimuli and transmit them to higher brain centers, which then allows for perception of the sensation. Aβ, Aδ, and C fibers are the main nerve endings involved in acupuncture analgesia, with Aδ and C nociceptive fibers found in the highest concentration at acupoints [75]. The Acupuncture/Endoporhin Theory, proposed by Dr. Bruce Pomeranz in 1987, suggests that activation of acupoints via the insertion of a microneedle stimulates Aδ and C afferent nerve fibers to send a message to the brain to release endogenous opiates such as endorphins and encephalins. These neurochemicals are then used to block the transmission of pain messages at two possible sites: the pituitary gland and the midbrain via the periaqueductal grey cells [76]. Therefore, it was proposed as two endorphinergic pathways, where the endorphin is being used as a hormone at the pituitary gland and as a neurotransmitter in the midbrain. This theory has been supported by multiple studies that have seen increased pain thresholds at acupuncture sites [77].

Other forms of acupuncture include electroacupuncture (EA), which uses the same acupoints as acupuncture but pairs the needle with an electrode that introduces electricity to cause vibration at the point. Vibration frequency is dependent on the patient's illness and severity but both low frequencies (2 Hz) and high frequencies (100 Hz) have demonstrated an ability to provide clinically significant pain relief [78]. This works similarly to when the acupuncturist manually causes gentle traction at the point for activation. Electroacupuncture has been found to provide greater pain analgesia than manual acupuncture [78]. Other benefits of electroacupuncture include shorter duration and the ability to affect more flow patterns (meridians) with fewer acupoints.

Transcutaneous Electrical Nerve Stimulation

Transcutaneous Electrical Nerve Stimulation (TENS) is another non-pharmacological modality that can be used for pain control. Similarly, to electroacupuncture, TENS is a small device that utilizes electrical currents to provide pain relief. However, it is applied through patches to variable parts of the skin instead of needles. TENS is proposed to work by activating large-diameter afferent nerve fibers that follow the gate control theory (GCT) developed by Patrick Wall and Ronald Melzack in 1965. This theory suggests that large afferent nerve fibers excite descending inhibitory neurons at the spinal cord, periaqueductal gray, and ventral medulla to close "pain gates" and prevent pain modulation. TENS units are adjustable to frequency, intensity, and pulse control. TENS typically works at two frequency levels, high frequency (50–100 Hz) and low frequency (2–10 Hz), both effective when high intensities are applied. Due to similarities seen in both electroacupuncture and TENS, studies were conducted to compare TENS when applied over acupoints. Interestingly, it has been found that TENS was more effective over acupoints than over non-acupoints when compared to sham TENS [79].

TENS and acupuncture have been used as treatment options for different pain disorders including migraine headaches, chemotherapy-induced nausea, labor pain, and knee and back pain. Low back pain is the leading cause of disability in the United States affecting nearly four out of every five Americans. It is estimated that 200 billion dollars are spent yearly to manage back pain and yet there are no concrete solutions for resolution of back pain. However, though acupuncture and TENS may not alleviate low back pain completely, they do appear to represent reasonable adjuvant therapeutics [80]. In a randomized controlled study that compared acupuncture with sham acupuncture in patients with low back pain, there was no significant difference in pain scores between the two therapies. However, the acupuncture group did show decreased disability associated with low back pain compared to the control group [81]. Similarly in a meta-analysis comparing different intensities of TENS to placebo, it was found that patients' pain levels were lower immediately after in the group that underwent TENS when compared to the placebo group [82]. When comparing TENS and EA in the treatment of knee osteoarthritis, guidelines are conflicting. The American College of Rheumatology conditionally recommends TENS and acupuncture while the National Institute for Health and Care Excellence recommends TENS but does not support the use of acupuncture [83]. However, a recent study comparing TENS and EA to placebo found that EA and TENS provided significant pain relief for patients with knee osteoarthritis with high-intensity TENS providing the most relief [84].

Cryotherapy

Cryotherapy represents a popular non-pharmacological treatment that is frequently utilized by athletes seeking to hasten their recovery and decrease pain. Cryotherapy, also known as cold therapy, is an umbrella term that involves any therapy that utilizes the withdrawal of heat through reductions in core and tissue temperatures to alter blood flow [85]. Within cryotherapeutics, there is whole-body cryotherapy (WBC), partial-body cryotherapy (PBC), cold water immersion (CWI), and ice application. To understand how these therapies are utilized, it is important to first understand the stages of muscle injury or damage to myofilament structures. This occurs in three stages: Initial muscle damage with inflammatory response, regeneration with activation of satellite cells, and remodeling phase. Injury can result from a direct insult or through prolonged training and exercise. This causes muscle necrosis and interrupts homeostasis and can last up to a few days. An inflammatory response will follow the injury with an influx of macrophages, pro-inflammatory cytokines, and growth factors. The repair phase focuses on macrophages that will clear the dead tissues and be regenerated by satellite cells that will become myoblast cells. Together, they will work with fibroblasts to create new muscle fibers and remodel the damaged area. Cryotherapy targets the inflammatory response period. This is done by exposing selective parts of the body to freezing temperatures which cool the skin. This drop in temperature results in localized cutaneous vasoconstriction and limitations in blood flow that subsequently reduce pain and the inflammatory response [86]. This mechanism is supported by studies that found decreased inflammatory markers following WBC suggesting that the dampened inflammatory response caused less secondary tissue damage, augmented the regeneration process, and shortened overall recovery times [86].

Cold-water immersion is commonly utilized by athletes immersing themselves in tubs full of ice for several minutes following periods of intensive and strenuous activities. The best results for CWI are at temperatures between 11 and 15 °C for 11–15 min intervals [87]. In 1963, a study that examined the effect of CWI on muscle strength following exercise fatigue introduced the possibility of cold therapy being used as a therapeutic muscle recovery mechanism [88]. This discovery is believed to be the inspiration of Dr. Gabe Mirkin who introduced the RICE method in 1978 (rest, ice, compression, elevate) to treat acute sports injuries.

Whole-body cryotherapy involves exposing the body or part of the body to cool temperatures as cold as - 110 to - 140 °C (- 166 to 220 °F) for a few minutes. To minimize cold-related injuries, an individual wears minimal clothing, dry socks, shoes, gloves, and a woolen headband during treatment. The first cryochambers were built in Japan in 1978 to treat Rheumatoid Arthritis after Dr. Toshima Yamaguchi discovered that rapidly lowering skin temperatures caused the release of endorphins and improved pain assessment scores [89]. Cryochambers were introduced to Europe shortly after to assist patients with multiple sclerosis and other arthritic conditions. In these patients, cryotherapy achieves therapeutic effects through reductions in nerve conduction velocity along sensory nerve fibers [90]. It is only within the most recent decade that WBC gained popularity among athletes due to its proposed effect of shortening recovery time. PBC also gained popularity as it does not expose the head and neck to extreme temperatures, making it more bearable for individuals. It has gained fame in the beauty industry due to its marketed benefits for skin enhancements, however, the efficacy of PBC compared to WBC has yet to be fully investigated [91].

8 Conclusion

Pain is an experience that is both subjective and personal. As described, the experience of pain depends on a multitude of factors which span from biological to psychological to social [2]. Given the dynamic nature of the pain experience, it is important to be equally dynamic in the assessment and treatment of pain. It is key to acknowledge that pain exists in both the acute and chronic perioperative phases of care with complex pain being a composite of the sensation of pain, emotional response, and perception of pain level [23]. Patients with complex pain are afflicted by pain in a way that interferes with daily activities and function. When approaching pain management in this population it is paramount to engage a pain specialist, especially in the perioperative period. With attention to the preoperative evaluation of a patient, pain specialists' intimate knowledge of multimodal anesthesia and the broad range of analgesics available allow them to deliver individualized pain regimens for these patients. [43, 44] These pain regimens can include various types of analgesics but as previously demonstrated, there is a role for non-pharmacological options to assist with pain management in the patient with complex pain. Multiple modalities have shown evidence to improve pain, including physical therapy, water therapy, massage therapy, acupuncture, transcutaneous electrical nerve stimulation (TENS), and cryotherapy, and their utility has been shown in the prehabilitation and rehabilitation period. Utilization of these modalities will allow for a comprehensive and dynamic approach to the management of pain in the perioperative period for the patient with complex pain.

Key Takeaway Points

1. The biopsychosocial model is used as a framework to better understand the nature of complex pain perception and the need to achieve analgesia holistically. This begins in the preoperative space with setting realistic expectations, involving a pain specialist, and rigorous prehabilitation.
2. Postoperative functional status and quality of life can be improved by early preoperative integration of physical therapy and aquatic therapy by promoting range of motion.
3. A combined approach with multimodal analgesics and prehabilitation modalities such as massage therapy, acupuncture, transcutaneous electrical nerve stimulation, and cryotherapy allows for the targeting of numerous pain pathways including nociceptive, inflammatory, and neuropathic pain.

References

1. Raja SN, Carr DB, Cohen M, Finnerup NB, Flor H, Gibson S, et al. The revised International Association for the Study of Pain definition of pain: concepts, challenges, and compromises. Pain [Internet]. 2020;161(9):1976–82. Available from: https://pubmed.ncbi.nlm.nih.gov/32694387. https://doi.org/10.1097/j.pain.0000000000001939
2. Fillingim RB. Individual differences in pain: understanding the mosaic that makes pain personal. Pain [Internet]. 2017;158(1):S11–S18. Available from: https://pubmed.ncbi.nlm.nih.gov/27902569. https://doi.org/10.1097/j.pain.0000000000000775
3. Yong R, Mullins P, Bhattacharyya N. Prevalence of chronic pain among adults in the United States. Pain [Internet]. 2022;163(2):e328–32. Available from: https://pubmed.ncbi.nlm.nih.gov/33990113. https://doi.org/10.1097/j.pain.0000000000002291
4. Charipova K, Gress KL, Urits I, Viswanath O, Kaye AD. Management of patients with chronic pain in ambulatory surgery centers. Cureus [Internet]. 2020;12(9):e10408. Available from: https://pubmed.ncbi.nlm.nih.gov/33062525. https://doi.org/10.7759/cureus.10408
5. Warfield CA, Kahn CH. Acute pain management: programs in U.S. hospitals and experiences and attitudes among U.S. adults. Anesthesiology [Internet]. 1995;83(5):1090–4. Available from: https://pubmed.ncbi.nlm.nih.gov/7486160. https://doi.org/10.1097/00000542-199511000-00023
6. Apfelbaum JL, Chen C, Mehta SS, Gan TJ. Postoperative pain experience: results from a national survey suggest postoperative pain continues to be undermanaged. Anesthesia Analgesia [Internet]. 2003;97(2):534–40. Available from: https://pubmed.ncbi.nlm.nih.gov/12873949. https://doi.org/10.1213/01.ANE.0000068822.10113.9E
7. Joshi GP, Ogunnaike BO. Consequences of inadequate postoperative pain relief and chronic persistent postoperative pain. Anesthesiol Clin North Am [Internet]. 2005;23(1):21–36. Available from: https://pubmed.ncbi.nlm.nih.gov/15763409. https://doi.org/10.1016/j.atc.2004.11.013
8. Gan TJ. Poorly controlled postoperative pain: prevalence, consequences, and prevention. J Pain Res [Internet]. 2017; 10:2287–98. Available from: https://pubmed.ncbi.nlm.nih.gov/29026331. https://doi.org/10.2147/JPR.S144066
9. Kehlet H, Jensen TS, Woolf CJ. Persistent postsurgical pain: risk factors and prevention. The Lancet [Internet]. 2006;367(9522):1618–25. Available from: https://pubmed.ncbi.nlm.nih.gov/16698416. https://doi.org/10.1016/s0140-6736(06)68700-x
10. Kelly DJ, Ahmad M, Brull SJ. Preemptive analgesia I: physiological pathways and pharmacological modalities. Can J Anaesth [Internet]. 2001 [cited 2023 Jan 14];48(10):1000–10. Available from: https://link.springer.com/article/10.1007/BF03016591
11. Samad TA, Moore KA, Sapirstein A, Billet S, Allchorne A, Poole S, et al. Interleukin-1β-mediated induction of Cox-2 in the CNS contributes to inflammatory pain hypersensitivity. Nature [Internet]. 2001;410(6827):471–5. Available from: https://www.nature.com/articles/35068566. https://doi.org/10.1038/35068566
12. Gilron I, Baron R, Jensen T. Neuropathic pain: principles of diagnosis and treatment. Mayo Clin Proc [Internet]. 2015;90(4):532–45. Available from: https://pubmed.ncbi.nlm.nih.gov/25841257. https://doi.org/10.1016/j.mayocp.2015.01.018
13. Xu Q, Yaksh TL. A brief comparison of the pathophysiology of inflammatory versus neuropathic pain. Curr Opin Anaesthesiol [Internet]. 2011;24(4):400–7. Available from: https://pubmed.ncbi.nlm.nih.gov/21659872. https://doi.org/10.1097/ACO.0b013e32834871df
14. Woolf CJ, King AE. Dynamic alterations in the cutaneous mechanoreceptive fields of dorsal horn neurons in the rat spinal cord. J Neurosci [Internet]. 1990;10(8):2717–26. Available from: https://www.jneurosci.org/content/10/8/2717. https://doi.org/10.1523/JNEUROSCI.10-08-02717.1990
15. Woolf CJ. Pain: moving from symptom control toward mechanism- specific pharmacologic management. Ann Intern Med [Internet]. 2004;140: 441–51. Available from: https://pubmed.ncbi.nlm.nih.gov/15023710. https://doi.org/10.7326/0003-4819-140-8-200404200-00010

16. Woolf CJ, Shortland P, Coggeshall RE. Peripheral nerve injury triggers central sprouting of myelinated afferents. Nature [Internet]. 1992;355:75–8. Available from: https://www.nature.com/articles/355075a0. https://doi.org/10.1038/355075a0
17. Treede RD, Rief W, Barke A, Aziz Q, Bennett MI, Benoliel R, et al. Chronic pain as a symptom or a disease: the IASP Classification of chronic pain for the International Classification of Diseases (ICD-11). Pain [Internet]. 2019;160(1):19–27. Available from: https://pubmed.ncbi.nlm.nih.gov/30586067. https://doi.org/10.1097/j.pain.0000000000001384
18. Bruce J, Quinlan J. Chronic post-surgical pain. Rev Pain [Internet]. 2011;5(3): 23–9. Available from: https://pubmed.ncbi.nlm.nih.gov/26526062. https://doi.org/10.1177/204946371100500306
19. Ip HYV, Abrishami A, Peng P, Wong J, Chung F. Predictors of postoperative pain and analgesic consumption: A qualitative systematic review. Anesthesiology [Internet]. 2009;111:657. Available from: https://pubs.asahq.org/anesthesiology/article/111/3/657/9525/Predictors-of-Postoperative-Pain-and-Analgesic. https://doi.org/10.1097/ALN.0b013e3181aae87a
20. Gerbershagen HJ, Aduckathil S, van Wijck AJ, Peelen LM, Kalkman CJ, Meissner W. Pain intensity on the first day after surgery. Anesthesiology [Internet]. 2013;118(4):934–44. Available from: https://pubmed.ncbi.nlm.nih.gov/23392233 https://doi.org/10.1097/ALN.0b013e31828866b3
21. Aldamluji N, Burgess A, Pogatzki-Zahn E, Raeder J, Beloeil H, PROSPECT Working Group collaborators. PROSPECT guideline for tonsillectomy: systematic review and procedure-specific postoperative pain management recommendations. Anaesthesia [Internet]. 2021;76(7):947–61. Available from: https://pubmed.ncbi.nlm.nih.gov/33201518 https://doi.org/10.1111/anae.15299
22. Joshi GP, Schug SA, Kehlet H. Procedure-specific pain management and outcome strategies. Best Pract Res Clin Anaesthesiol [Internet]. 2014;28(2):191–201. Available from: https://pubmed.ncbi.nlm.nih.gov/24993439. https://doi.org/10.1016/j.bpa.2014.03.005
23. Crofford LJ. Chronic pain: where the body meets the brain. Trans Am Clin Climatol Assoc [Internet]. 2015;126:167–83. Available from: https://www.ncbi.nlm.nih.gov/pmc/articles/PMC4530716
24. Schlereth T, Birklein F. The sympathetic nervous system and pain. Neuromol Med [Internet]. 2008;10(3):141–7. Available from: https://pubmed.ncbi.nlm.nih.gov/17990126. https://doi.org/10.1007/s12017-007-8018-6
25. Ali Z, Raja SN, Wesselmann U, Fuchs PN, Meyer RA, Campbell JN. Intradermal injection of norepinephrine evokes pain in patients with sympathetically maintained pain. Pain [Internet]. 2000;88:161–8. Available from: https://pubmed.ncbi.nlm.nih.gov/11050371. https://doi.org/10.1016/S0304-3959(00)00327-4
26. Katz J, Seltzer Z. Transition from acute to chronic postsurgical pain: risk factors and protective factors. Expert Rev Neurother [Internet]. 2009;9(5):723–44. Available from: https://pubmed.ncbi.nlm.nih.gov/19402781. https://doi.org/10.1586/ern.09.20
27. Hechler T, Endres D, Thorwart A. Why harmless sensations might hurt in individuals with chronic pain: about heightened prediction and perception of pain in the mind. Front Psychol [Internet]. 2016;7:1638. Available from: https://pubmed.ncbi.nlm.nih.gov/27826271. https://doi.org/10.3389/fpsyg.2016.01638
28. Forsythe ME, Dunbar MJ, Hennigar AW, Sullivan MJ, Gross M. Prospective relation between catastrophising and residual pain following knee arthoplasty: two-year follow-up. Pain Res Manage [Internet]. 2008;13(4):335–41. Available from: https://pubmed.ncbi.nlm.nih.gov/18719716. https://doi.org/10.1155/2008/730951
29. Witt JK, Linkenauger SA, Bakdash JZ, Augustyn JS, Cook A, Proffitt DR. The long road of pain: chronic pain increases perceived distance. Exp Brain Res [Internet]. 2009;192(1):145–8. Available from: https://pubmed.ncbi.nlm.nih.gov/18949471 https://doi.org/10.1007/s00221-008-1594-3
30. Dorner TE, Muckenhuber J, Stronegger WJ, Ràsky E, Gustorff B, Freidl W. The impact of socio-economic status on pain and the perception of disability due to pain. Eur J Pain [Internet]. 2011;15(1):103–9. Available from: https://pubmed.ncbi.nlm.nih.gov/20558096. https://doi.org/10.1016/j.ejpain.2010.05.013

31. Zubieta JK, Heitzeg MM, Smith YR, Bueller JA, Xu K, Xu Y, et al. COMT val158met genotype affects mu-opioid neurotransmitter responses to a pain stressor. Science [Internet]. 2003;299(5610):1240–3. Available from: https://pubmed.ncbi.nlm.nih.gov/12595695. https://doi.org/10.1126/science.1078546
32. George SZ, Wallace MR, Wright TW, Moser MW, Greenfield WH III, Sack BK, et al. Evidence for a biopsychosocial influence on shoulder pain: pain catastrophizing and catechol-O-methyltransferase (COMT) diplotype predict clinical pain ratings. Pain [Internet]. 2008 [cited 2023 Jan 20];136(1–2):53–61. Available from: https://pubmed.ncbi.nlm.nih.gov/17686583. https://doi.org/10.1016/j.pain.2007.06.019
33. Institute of Medicine (US) Committee on Advancing Pain Research, Care, and Education. Relieving pain in America: a blueprint for transforming prevention, care, education, and research. Washington (DC): National Academies Press (US); 2011. Available from: https://www.ncbi.nlm.nih.gov/books/NBK92510
34. Chou R, Gordon DB, de Leon-Casasola OA, Rosenberg JM, Bickler S, Brennan T, et al. Management of postoperative pain: A clinical practice guideline from the American Pain Society, the American Society of Regional Anesthesia and Pain Medicine, and the American Society of Anesthesiologists' Committee on Regional Anesthesia, Executive Committee, and Administrative Council. J Pain [Internet]. 2016;17(2):131–57. Available from: https://pubmed.ncbi.nlm.nih.gov/26827847. https://doi.org/10.1016/j.jpain.2015.12.008
35. Levy N, Mills P, Mythen M. Is the pursuit of dreaming (drinking, eating and mobilizing) the ultimate goal of anaesthesia? Anaesthesia [Internet]. 2016;71(9):1008–12. Available from: https://pubmed.ncbi.nlm.nih.gov/27079158. https://doi.org/10.1111/anae.13495
36. Yang MM, Hartley RL, Leung AA, Ronksley PE, Jetté N, Casha S, et al. Preoperative predictors of poor acute postoperative pain control: A systematic review and meta-analysis. BMJ Open [Internet]. 2019;9(4). Available from: https://pubmed.ncbi.nlm.nih.gov/30940757. https://doi.org/10.1136/bmjopen-2018-025091
37. Small C, Laycock H. Acute postoperative pain management. Br J Surg [Internet]. 2020;107(2). Available from: https://pubmed.ncbi.nlm.nih.gov/31903595. https://doi.org/10.1002/bjs.11477
38. Gandhi K, Heitz JW, Viscusi ER. Challenges in acute pain management. Anesthesiol Clin [Internet]. 2011;29(2):291–309. Available from: https://pubmed.ncbi.nlm.nih.gov/21620344. https://doi.org/10.1016/j.anclin.2011.04.009
39. Medical Societies Develop Best Practices to Manage Acute Pain in Complex Surgical Patients. American Society of Anesthesiologists; 2002 [cited 2023 Jan 17]. Available from: https://www.asahq.org/about-asa/newsroom/news-releases/2022/03/15-medical-societies-develop-best-practices-to-manage-acute-pain-in-complex-surgical-patients
40. Kehlet H, Dahl JB. The value of "multimodal" or "balanced analgesia" in postoperative pain treatment. Anesthesia Analgesia [Internet]. 1993;77(5):1048–56. Available from: https://pubmed.ncbi.nlm.nih.gov/8105724. https://doi.org/10.1213/00000539-199311000-00030
41. Lovich-Sapola J, Smith CE, Brandt CP. Postoperative pain control. Surgical Clinics of North America [Internet]. 2015;95(2):301–18. Available from: https://pubmed.ncbi.nlm.nih.gov/25814108. https://doi.org/10.1016/j.suc.2014.10.002
42. Gillis C, Ljungqvist O, Carli F. Prehabilitation, enhanced recovery after surgery, or both? Br J Anaesthesia [Internet]. 2022. Available from: https://pubmed.ncbi.nlm.nih.gov/35012741. https://doi.org/10.1016/j.bja.2021.12.007
43. Thomas D-A, Chang D, Zhu R, Rayaz H, Vadivelu N. Concept of the ambulatory pain physician. Current Pain and Headache Reports [Internet]. 2017;21(1). Available from: https://pubmed.ncbi.nlm.nih.gov/28233267 https://doi.org/10.1007/s11916-017-0611-2
44. Vadivelu N, Kai A, Kodumudi V, Berger J. Challenges of pain control and the role of the Ambulatory Pain Specialist in the outpatient surgery setting. Journal of Pain Research [Internet]. 2016;9:425. Available from: https://pubmed.ncbi.nlm.nih.gov/27382329. https://doi.org/10.2147/jpr.s86579
45. Carli F. Prehabilitation for the Anesthesiologist. Anesthesiology [Internet]. 2020;133(3):645–52. Available from: https://pubmed.ncbi.nlm.nih.gov/32358253. https://doi.org/10.1097/ALN.0000000000003331

46. McIsaac DI, MacDonald DB, Aucoin SD. Frailty for perioperative clinicians: A narrative review. Anesth Analg [Internet]. 2020;130(6):1450–60. Available from: https://pubmed.ncbi.nlm.nih.gov/32384334. https://doi.org/10.1213/ANE.0000000000004602
47. Rockwood K, Song X, MacKnight C, et al. A global clinical measure of fitness and frailty in elderly people. CMAJ [Internet]. 2005;173(5):489–95. Available from: https://pubmed.ncbi.nlm.nih.gov/16129869. https://doi.org/10.1503/cmaj.050051
48. Searle SD, Mitnitski A, Gahbauer EA, Gill TM, Rockwood K. A standard procedure for creating a frailty index. BMC Geriatr [Internet]. 2008;8:24. Available from: https://pubmed.ncbi.nlm.nih.gov/18826625. https://doi.org/10.1186/1471-2318-8-24
49. Esses G, Deiner S, Ko F, Khelemsky Y. Chronic post-surgical pain in the frail older adult. Drugs Aging [Internet]. 2020;37(5):321–9. Available from: https://pubmed.ncbi.nlm.nih.gov/32297246. https://doi.org/10.1007/s40266-020-00761-2
50. Arends BC, Timmerman L, Vernooij LM, et al. Preoperative frailty and chronic pain after cardiac surgery: a prospective observational study. BMC Anesthesiol [Internet]. 2022;22(1):201. Available from: https://pubmed.ncbi.nlm.nih.gov/32297246. https://doi.org/10.1186/s12871-022-01746-x
51. Topp R, Ditmyer M, King K, Doherty K, Hornyak J. The effect of bed rest and potential of prehabilitation on patients in the intensive care unit. AACN Clin Issues [Internet]. 2002;13(2):263–76. Available from: https://pubmed.ncbi.nlm.nih.gov/12011598. https://doi.org/10.1097/00044067-200205000-00011
52. West MA, Jack S, Grocott MPW. Prehabilitation before surgery: is it for all patients? Best Pract Res Clin Anaesthesiol [Internet]. 2021;35(4):507–16. Available from: https://pubmed.ncbi.nlm.nih.gov/34801213. https://doi.org/10.1016/j.bpa.2021.01.001
53. Moningi S, Patki A, Padhy N, Ramachandran G. Enhanced recovery after surgery: an anesthesiologist's perspective. J Anaesthesiol Clin Pharmacol [Internet]. 2019;35(Suppl 1):S5–S13. Available from: https://www.ncbi.nlm.nih.gov/pmc/articles/PMC6515715. https://doi.org/10.4103/joacp.JOACP_238_16
54. Bond TJ, Lundy J. Physical therapy following peripheral nerve surgeries. Clin Podiatr Med Surg [Internet]. 2006;23(3):651–66. Available from: https://pubmed.ncbi.nlm.nih.gov/16958395. https://doi.org/10.1016/j.cpm.2006.04.006
55. Wang L, Lee M, Zhang Z, Moodie J, Cheng D, Martin J. Does preoperative rehabilitation for patients planning to undergo joint replacement surgery improve outcomes? A systematic review and meta-analysis of randomised controlled trials. BMJ Open [Internet]. 2016 [cited 2023 Jan 26];6(2): e009857. Available from: https://pubmed.ncbi.nlm.nih.gov/26839013. https://doi.org/10.1136/bmjopen-2015-009857
56. Carrignan JA, Simmet RT, Coddington M, Gill NW, Greenlee TA, McCafferty R, et al. Are exercise and physical therapy common forms of conservative management in the year before lumbar spine surgery? Arch Phys Med Rehabil [Internet]. 2020;101(8):1389–1395. Available from: https://pubmed.ncbi.nlm.nih.gov/32416147. https://doi.org/10.1016/j.apmr.2020.04.006
57. Sawyer MW. The role of the physical therapist before and after lumbar spine surgery. Orthop Clin North Am [Internet]. 1983;14(3):649–59. Available from: https://pubmed.ncbi.nlm.nih.gov/6866456
58. Jain SR, Kandarpa VL, Yaow CYL, Tan WJ, Ho LML, Sivarajah SS, et al. The role and effect of multimodal prehabilitation before major abdominal surgery: a systemic review and meta-analysis. World J Surg [Internet]. 2023;47(1):86–102. Available from: https://pubmed.ncbi.nlm.nih.gov/36184673. https://doi.org/10.1007/s00268-022-06761-0.
59. Humphrey R, Malone D. Effectiveness of preoperative physical therapy for elective cardiac surgery. Phys Ther [Internet]. 2015;95(2):160–6. Available from: https://pubmed.ncbi.nlm.nih.gov/25343961. https://doi.org/10.2522/ptj.20130323
60. Soeters R, White PB, Murray-Weir M, Koltsov JCB, Alexiades MM, Ranawat AS, et al. Preoperative physical therapy education reduces time to meet functional milestones after total joint arthroplasty. Clin Orthop Relat Res [Internet]. 2018;476(1):40–8. Available from: https://pubmed.ncbi.nlm.nih.gov/29529614. https://doi.org/10.1007/s11999.0000000000000010

61. Pozzi F, Snyder-Mackler L, Zeni J. Physical exercise after knee arthroplasty: a systematic review of controlled trials. Eur J Phys Rehabil Med [Internet]. 2013;49(6):877–92. Available from: https://www.ncbi.nlm.nih.gov/pmc/articles/PMC4131551
62. George SZ, Goode AP. Physical therapy and opioid use for musculoskeletal pain management: competitors or companions? Pain Rep [Internet]. 2020;5(5):e827. Available from: https://pubmed.ncbi.nlm.nih.gov/33490834. https://doi.org/10.1097/PR9.0000000000000827
63. Łyp M, Kaczor R, Cabak A, Tederko P, Włostowska E, Stanisławska I, et al. A water rehabilitation program in patients with hip osteoarthritis before and after total hip replacement. Med Sci Monit [Internet]. 2016;22:2635–42. Available from: https://pubmed.ncbi.nlm.nih.gov/27455419. https://doi.org/10.12659/msm.896203
64. Schencking M, Otto A, Deutsch T, Sandholzer H. A comparison of Kneipp hydrotherapy with conventional physiotherapy in the treatment of osteoarthritis of the hip or knee: protocol of a prospective randomised controlled clinical trial. BMC Musculoskelet Disord [Internet]. 2009;10:104. Available from: https://pubmed.ncbi.nlm.nih.gov/19689824. https://doi.org/10.1186/1471-2474-10-104
65. Lee CH, Kim IH. Aquatic exercise and land exercise treatments after total knee replacement arthroplasty in elderly women: a comparative study. Medicina (Kaunas) [Internet]. 2021;57(6):589. Available from: https://www.ncbi.nlm.nih.gov/pmc/articles/PMC8229167. https://doi.org/10.3390/medicina57060589
66. Tick H, Nielsen A, Pelletier KR, Bonakdar R, Simmons S, Glick R, et al. Evidence-based nonpharmacologic strategies for comprehensive pain care: the Consortium Pain Task Force white paper. Explore (NY) [Internet]. 2018;14(3):177–211. Available from: https://pubmed.ncbi.nlm.nih.gov/29735382. https://doi.org/10.1016/j.explore.2018.02.001
67. Liu C, Chen X, Wu S. The effect of massage therapy on pain after surgery: a comprehensive meta-analysis. Complement Ther Med [Internet]. 2022;71:102892. Available from: https://pubmed.ncbi.nlm.nih.gov/36309174. https://doi.org/10.1016/j.ctim.2022.102892
68. Kukimoto Y, Ooe N, Ideguchi N. The Effects of massage therapy on pain and anxiety after surgery: a systematic review and meta-analysis. Pain Manag Nurs [Internet]. 2017;18(6):378–90. Available from: https://pubmed.ncbi.nlm.nih.gov/29173797. https://doi.org/10.1016/j.pmn.2017.09.001
69. Gönenç IM, Terzioğlu F. Effects of massage and acupressure on relieving labor pain, reducing labor time, and increasing delivery satisfaction. J Nurs Res [Internet]. 2020;28(1):e68. Available from: https://pubmed.ncbi.nlm.nih.gov/31524645. https://doi.org/10.1097/jnr.0000000000000344
70. Braun LA, Stanguts C, Casanelia L, Spitzer O, Paul E, Vardaxis NJ, et al. Massage therapy for cardiac surgery patients—a randomized trial. J Thorac Cardiovasc Surg [Internet]. 2012;144(6):1453–9, 1459.e1. Available from: https://pubmed.ncbi.nlm.nih.gov/22964355. https://doi.org/10.1016/j.jtcvs.2012.04.027
71. Zhang Y, Lao L, Chen H, Ceballos R. Acupuncture use among American adults: What acupuncture practitioners can learn from National Health interview survey 2007? Evid Based Complement Alternat Med [Internet]. 2012;2012:710750. Available from: https://pubmed.ncbi.nlm.nih.gov/22474517. https://doi.org/10.1155/2012/710750
72. Kaptchuk TJ. Acupuncture: theory, efficacy, and practice. Ann Intern Med [Internet]. 2002;136(5):374–83. Available from: https://pubmed.ncbi.nlm.nih.gov/11874310. https://doi.org/10.7326/0003-4819-136-5-200203050-00010
73. Coutaux A. Non-pharmacological treatments for pain relief: TENS and acupuncture. Joint Bone Spine [Internet]. 2017;84(6):657–61. Available from: https://pubmed.ncbi.nlm.nih.gov/28219657. https://doi.org/10.1016/j.jbspin.2017.02.005
74. Mingfu L, Xiaotong D, Xiaojing S, Jin J, Jinling Z, Ying H. Study on the dynamic compound structure composed of mast cells, blood vessels, and nerves in rat acupoint. Evid Based Complement Alternat Med [Internet]. 2013;2013:160651. Available from: https://pubmed.ncbi.nlm.nih.gov/23878591. https://doi.org/10.1155/2013/160651
75. Kagitani F, Uchida S, Hotta H. Afferent nerve fibers and acupuncture. Auton Neurosci [Internet]. 2010;157(1–2):2–8. Available from: https://pubmed.ncbi.nlm.nih.gov/20494626. https://doi.org/10.1016/j.autneu.2010.03.004

76. Vanderploeg K, Yi X. Acupuncture in modern society. J Acupunct Meridian Stud [Internet]. 2009;2(1):26–33. Available from: https://pubmed.ncbi.nlm.nih.gov/20633471. https://doi.org/10.1016/S2005-2901(09)60012-1
77. Pomeranz B. Acupuncture and the endorphins. Ethos [Internet]. 1982;10(4):385–93. Available from: https://psycnet.apa.org/record/1983-28624-001 https://doi.org/10.1525/eth.1982.10.4.02a00070
78. Ulett GA, Han S, Han JS. Electroacupuncture: mechanisms and clinical application. Biol Psychiatry [Internet]. 1998;44(2):129–38. Available from: https://pubmed.ncbi.nlm.nih.gov/9646895. https://doi.org/10.1016/s0006-3223(97)00394-6
79. Vance CG, Dailey DL, Rakel BA, Sluka KA. Using TENS for pain control: the state of the evidence. Pain Manag [Internet]. 2014;4(3):197–209. Available from: https://pubmed.ncbi.nlm.nih.gov/24953072. https://doi.org/10.2217/pmt.14.13
80. Casiano VE, Sarwan G, Dydyk AM, Varacallo M. Back Pain. StatPearls [Internet]. 2022. Available from: https://pubmed.ncbi.nlm.nih.gov/30844200
81. Kong JT, Puetz C, Tian L, Haynes I, Lee E, Stafford RS, et al. Effect of electroacupuncture vs sham treatment on change in pain severity among adults with chronic low back pain: a randomized clinical trial. JAMA Netw Open [Internet]. 2020;3(10):e2022787. Available from: https://pubmed.ncbi.nlm.nih.gov/33107921. https://doi.org/10.1001/jamanetworkopen.2020.22787
82. Johnson MI, Paley CA, Jones G, Mulvey MR, Wittkopf PG. Efficacy and safety of transcutaneous electrical nerve stimulation (TENS) for acute and chronic pain in adults: a systematic review and meta-analysis of 381 studies (the meta-TENS study). BMJ Open [Internet]. 2022;12(2):e051073. Available from: https://pubmed.ncbi.nlm.nih.gov/35144946. https://doi.org/10.1136/bmjopen-2021-051073
83. Birch S, Lee MS, Robinson N, Alraek T. The U.K. NICE 2014 guidelines for osteoarthritis of the knee: lessons learned in a narrative review addressing inadvertent limitations and bias. J Altern Complement Med [Internet]. 2017;23(4):242–6. Available from: https://pubmed.ncbi.nlm.nih.gov/28394671. https://doi.org/10.1089/acm.2016.0385
84. Shi X, Yu W, Zhang W, Wang T, Battulga O, Wang L, et al. A comparison of the effects of electroacupuncture versus transcutaneous electrical nerve stimulation for pain control in knee osteoarthritis: a Bayesian network meta-analysis of randomized controlled trials. Acupunct Med [Internet]. 2021;39(3):163–74. Available from: https://pubmed.ncbi.nlm.nih.gov/32567333. https://doi.org/10.1177/0964528420921193
85. Kwiecien SY, McHugh MP. The cold truth: the role of cryotherapy in the treatment of injury and recovery from exercise. Eur J Appl Physiol [Internet]. 2021;121(8):2125–42. Available from: https://pubmed.ncbi.nlm.nih.gov/33877402. https://doi.org/10.1007/s00421-021-04683-8
86. Rose C, Edwards KM, Siegler J, Graham K, Caillaud C. Whole-body cryotherapy as a recovery technique after exercise: a review of the literature. Int J Sports Med [Internet]. 2017;38(14):1049–60. Available from: https://pubmed.ncbi.nlm.nih.gov/29161748. https://doi.org/10.1055/s-0043-114861
87. Machado AF, Ferreira PH, Micheletti JK, de Almeida AC, Lemes ÍR, Vanderlei FM, et al. Can water temperature and immersion time influence the effect of cold-water immersion on muscle soreness? A systematic review and meta-analysis. Sports Med [Internet]. 2016;46(4):503–14. Available from: https://pubmed.ncbi.nlm.nih.gov/26581833. https://doi.org/10.1007/s40279-015-0431-7
88. Clarke D. Effect of immersion in hot and cold water upon recovery of muscular strength following fatiguing isometric exercise. Arch Phys Med Rehabil [Internet]. 1963;44:565–8. Available from: https://pubmed.ncbi.nlm.nih.gov/14055798
89. Allan R, Malone J, Alexander J, Vorajee S, Ihsan M, Gregson W, et al. Cold for centuries: a brief history of cryotherapies to improve health, injury and post-exercise recovery. Eur J Appl Physiol [Internet]. 2022;122(5):1153–62. Available from: https://pubmed.ncbi.nlm.nih.gov/35195747. https://doi.org/10.1007/s00421-022-04915-5

90. Herrera E, Sandoval MC, Camargo DM, Salvini TF. Motor and sensory nerve conduction are affected differently by ice pack, ice massage, and cold-water immersion. Phys Ther [Internet]. 2010;90(4):581–91. Available from: https://pubmed.ncbi.nlm.nih.gov/20185615. https://doi.org/10.2522/ptj.20090131
91. Malone JJ, Hodges D, Roberts C, Sinclair JK, Page RM, Allan R. Effect of alterations in whole-body cryotherapy (WBC) exposure on post-match recovery markers in elite Premier League soccer players. Biol Sport [Internet]. 2022;39(1):31–36. Available from: https://pubmed.ncbi.nlm.nih.gov/35173360. https://doi.org/10.5114/biolsport.2021.102931

Analgesics

Perioperative Use of Local Anesthetics and Adjuvants

John C. Alexander, James Kim, and Eric Siu

Abstract Local anesthetics have long been a key element in the surgeon and anesthesiologist's perioperative analgesia strategy. The unique pharmacological attributes of this class of medications provides the ability to interrupt the transmission of nociceptive insults at multiple sites in the peripheral and central nervous system. However, this therapeutic class also requires caution to avoid catastrophic toxicity syndromes. Various additives and adjunct therapies can greatly extend local anesthetic duration of action, but their use requires careful consideration to safely and effectively implement into clinical practice. Recent innovations have sought to further extend the duration of local anesthetics through novel formulations, but safety, cost, and efficacy concerns may limit the applicability of these agents.

Keywords Local anesthetic · Adjuvant · Infiltration · Liposomal bupivacaine

1 Pharmacology

Local anesthetics encompass a broad class of medications that are used to provide analgesia in many different settings. The basic structure of a local anesthetic is comprised of an aromatic ring which is the primary lipophilic component, an ester or amide linkage, and a tertiary amine. They act primarily through the interruption of action potential conduction by reversibly inhibiting the ingress of sodium ions through ion channels in the axonal membrane of peripheral nerves [1]. More specifically, local anesthetics display a greater binding affinity for sodium channels during

J. C. Alexander (✉) · J. Kim · E. Siu
Department of Anesthesiology and Pain Management, UT Southwestern, 5323 Harry Hines Blvd, TX 75390-9068, Dallas, TX, USA
e-mail: john.alexander@utsouthwestern.edu

J. Kim
e-mail: james.kim2@utsouthwestern.edu

E. Siu
e-mail: eric.siu@utsouthwestern.edu

A. Abd-Elsayed and K. Schroeder (eds.), *Perioperative Pain Management*,
https://doi.org/10.1007/978-3-031-67648-2_35

their activated and inactivated states, which translates to greater susceptibility of neural fibers that have more rapid firing rates [2]. Additionally, smaller fibers are also typically more susceptible due to a greater blockade of the requisite number of ion channels for a given volume of local anesthetic delivered around a nerve fiber. These factors together account for the difference in susceptibility of different types of fibers in the human body. Small, rapid-firing autonomic nerves are most sensitive, followed by sensory nerves, and then somatic motor nerves [3].

2 Potency

Local anesthetic potency shows a positive correlation with lipid solubility for amide local anesthetics; however, this correlation is not as robust for ester types. At the same time, ester type local anesthetics have greater potency for blockade at the level of the sodium channel than amides. While lipid solubility is commonly viewed as the primary determinant of potency, it more specifically determines the concentration of drug in the axonal membrane. Drug type (amide vs. ester), is also an important determinant of potency because it affects the affinity of the drug for the sodium channel [1].

3 Onset Time

While molecular lipid solubility is associated with an increased potency and quicker onset time in isolated and in vitro studies, a slower onset is generally seen in clinical practice when local anesthetics with higher lipid solubility are utilized. This observed dichotomy is a result of local anesthetics exposure to multiple tissue types and subsequent sequestration in surrounding adipose tissue and systemic vascular uptake [3].

It is important to remember that the active form of local anesthetics is the neutral, or lipophilic, state [1]. The most influential factor in determining onset time for local anesthetics in the clinical setting is the proportion of molecules that exist in an uncharged, lipid-soluble state, allowing them to cross the cell membrane of the nerve fiber where they will then adopt a charged, non-lipid-soluble, configuration to bind at the intracellular portion of the sodium channel. This charge configuration is carried out at the level of the amine group, where the tertiary (uncharged) state provides lipid-solubility, and the quaternary (charged) state promotes water-solubility.

The pKa of the local anesthetic will influence the proportion of molecules that exist in the tertiary vs. quaternary state at the normal physiologic pH of 7.4. All local anesthetics used in clinical practice exist as weak bases and have a pKa greater than 7.4 and thus will show a larger proportion of molecules in the charged state at physiologic pH. However, it follows that the closer the pKa of the local anesthetic to 7.4, the greater the proportion of uncharged, lipid-soluble, molecules and thus the faster the onset.

The clinical relevance of the pKa of local anesthetics is highlighted when these agents are utilized in inflamed tissues or co-administered with additive solutions. Areas of tissue inflammation are relatively acidotic and thus have a local pH less than 7.4. This acidic environment promotes the formation of quaternary, charged, amine groups in local anesthetics injected into inflamed tissues and thus decreases the overall effectiveness of the local anesthetic [3]. In contrast, the co-administration of agents that increase the pH of an injected local anesthetic can elicit an increased availability of local anesthetics in their uncharged and more lipid soluble state.

4 Metabolism

Metabolism of local anesthetics occurs according to their molecular intermediate linkage. Amide-type local anesthetics undergo hepatic transformation and dosing adjustment considerations must be considered in patients based on age and hepatic function [3]. Ester-type local anesthetics are hydrolyzed in the blood stream by plasma esterases and patients exhibiting atypical cholinesterase activity should be treated accordingly with decreased dosages of ester-type local anesthetics or substitution for an amide-type [4].

5 Dosing

Maximum doses for local anesthetics are subject to many factors. Most dosing recommendations aim to reduce the risk of systemic toxicity. In order to avoid toxicity, dosing adjustments should be considered at both ends of the age spectrum. One study showed that when compared to infants aged 3–12 months, those from birth to 3 months displayed higher free plasma concentrations of ropivacaine following caudal injection and have also showed a slower clearance of bupivacaine [5]. A recent multi-society practice advisory notes several factors worthy of consideration in local anesthetic dosing for pediatric patients. Infants have less cytochrome P450 activity to metabolize local anesthetics, a relatively larger volume of distribution, and a relatively high free-fraction of local anesthetic due to lower levels of alpha-1-acid glycoprotein to bind local anesthetic [6]. Given the unique physiology of this population, one reviewer recommends reducing local anesthetic dosing for regional anesthesia by 15% in infants under 4 months old [7].

Elderly patients should also receive lower doses of local anesthetics. Elderly patients display a lower clearance of and increased sensitivity to the blocking action of local anesthetics. This is likely due to direct age-related reductions in blood flow, organ function, and deterioration of axonal structure and conduction. In considering the declining physiology of elderly patients, one reviewer recommends 10–20% dose reductions for patients >70 years old [7].

6 Contraindications/Cautions/Complication Management

Local anesthetics exert their action on all excitable membranes. Channel blocking effects on cardiovascular and central nervous system tissues pose a particular risk with systemic local anesthetic uptake. Toxic blood levels (5–10 ug/ml) interrupt normal cardiac conduction, decrease myocardial contractility and cause peripheral vasodilation. In the central nervous system, toxic levels of local anesthetics lead to depression of inhibitory neurons, which explains the central nervous irritability and convulsions seen clinically [8].

7 Local Anesthetic Infiltration

Infiltration into a surgical wound is likely one of the oldest and original uses of local anesthetics. In modern terminology it is commonly referred to as either wound infiltration (WI) or surgical site infiltration (SSI). This technique is relatively inexpensive, as it does not require the use of expensive technology to perform (e.g.- ultrasound, mechanical or elastomeric pump, etc.), but optimal use of this technique does require a thorough understanding of the innervation of the structures to be anesthetized and the pharmacological properties of the local anesthetic being used (Fig. 1). The use of local anesthetic applied directly adjacent to the surgical site can block afferent nociceptive signals as well as reduce the local inflammatory response due to tissue injury [9].

Infiltration of superficial dermal structures can be utilized as the sole anesthetic for various procedures including laceration repairs [10], hernia surgery [11], and hemorrhoid surgery [12]. In more invasive procedures, infiltration techniques are still commonly used during skin closure to reduce postoperative pain. Procedure-specific postoperative pain management (PROSPECT) guidelines support the use of wound infiltration techniques in multiple surgical procedures including Caesarean section, open colorectal surgery, abdominal hysterectomy, inguinal hernia repair, laparoscopic cholecystectomy, oncologic breast surgery, lumbar laminectomy, hallux valgus surgery, and open radical prostatectomy [10]. Additionally, these techniques can exert analgesic effects through infiltration in and around deeper areas such as intra-articular/peri-articular surfaces [13] or intra-peritoneal sites [14]. In these instances, the use of higher volumes of long-acting local anesthetics in deeper structures is often termed local infiltration analgesia (LIA) and is often a major part of multimodal analgesia and can exert an opioid-sparing benefit [15]. Just as with perineural regional anesthesia techniques, indwelling catheters can be placed

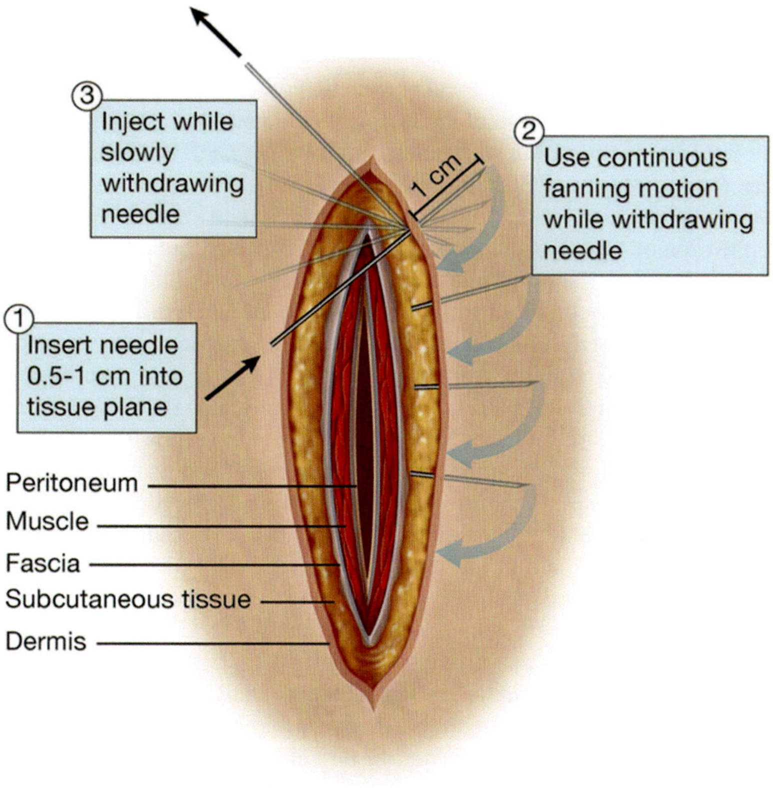

Fig. 1 Local anesthetic infiltration technique (used by permission from Joshi et al. [16])

(usually by surgeons) to extend the duration of analgesia beyond that possible with the one-time infiltration of local anesthetic with additives or extend-release formulations.

Effective SSI or WI requires an understanding of the various types of tissue that are damaged during surgical exposure, which will be unique to each surgical procedure, and then the proper technique to adequately anesthetize each layer. For example, an abdominal surgical incision will induce somatic pain from the disruption of dermal and myofascial structures, while visceral pain will be elicited from disruption of the peritoneum. Thus, effective SSI/WI will require local anesthetic administration within the peritoneal, myofascial, and subdermal layers [16]. For hip/knee arthroplasty, the joint capsule, ligaments, and other soft tissues must be infiltrated [17]. No matter the location of the surgical wound, though, care must be taken to meticulously infiltrate local anesthetic in each layer across the length and the breadth of the wound. The volume injected will thus depend on the size of the wound. Based on the technique described by Joshi, et al., approximately 1–1.5 ml of local anesthetic should be injected via a 22-gauge, 1.5-inch needle for every 1–2 cm of surgical incision per layer, diluted as necessary based on body weight to avoid local anesthetic systemic toxicity. A "moving needle" technique is recommended where the needle is moved in a continuous fanning motion, but infiltration only occurs while withdrawing the needle [16].

Single injection infiltration of local anesthetic confers pain relieving effects that persist for the duration of action of the injected local anesthetic. Continuous wound infiltration (CWI) facilitates the administration of more long-acting analgesia. This technique requires the transcutaneous tunneling of a catheter adjacent to the surgical wound, usually during or prior to wound closure, which then allows the continuous application of local anesthetic at that site. These catheters are simpler to place than advanced regional anesthesia techniques, such as epidural or peripheral nerve catheters, and thus may be more widely utilized if adequately trained anesthesiologists are unavailable or if advanced regional anesthesia procedures are not indicated. Aside from cost and simplicity, another advantage of CWI over epidural or peripheral nerve block is that motor blockade, sympathectomy with resulting hypotension, and urinary retention are unlikely [17]. One systematic review showed improved analgesia, reduced opioid use, higher patient satisfaction, and possible reductions in hospital stay with the use of CWI across multiple surgical procedures [9]. A possible limitation, though, is that subcutaneous CWI catheters are only able to block somatic pain at the surgical site, and not at deeper sites (e.g. visceral pain may be poorly controlled with CWI techniques). A recent meta-analysis showed that preperitoneal CWI catheters provide superior analgesia to subcutaneous CWI catheters and may provide similar analgesia to that provided by an epidural catheter, generally considered the gold-standard technique for perioperative analgesia in major abdominal surgery, but with improved postoperative recovery and patient satisfaction [18].

The push for enhanced recovery and faster return of function has presented a conundrum for certain lower extremity surgical procedures, especially hip and knee arthroplasty. Effective analgesia is paramount in meeting these goals, but the use of peripheral nerve blocks to meet analgesia goals often results in concomitant blockade of motor fibers. This results in transient limb weakness, impaired ability to ambulate, and a higher risk of falls [19]. The need to balance the functional and analgesic requirements necessary to meet enhanced recovery goals has led anesthesiologists to develop motor-sparing nerve blocks such as the adductor canal block rather than femoral nerve block, and the "infiltration between the popliteal artery and capsule of the knee" (iPACK) rather than sciatic nerve block. Additionally, orthopaedic surgeons began to use intra-articular or peri-articular LIA techniques. Literature suggests that both adductor canal block and LIA provide significant analgesia, but the combination appears to provide superior analgesia to either alone [20, 21]. On the other hand, the addition of iPACK to LIA and adductor canal block does not improve analgesia after knee arthroplasty. However, if an adductor canal block is used in isolation, then the addition of iPACK does improve analgesia [22].

While many surgical procedures have been studied, the vast majority of the literature on the use of intraperitoneal local anesthetic instillation are in the setting of laparoscopic cholecystectomy and firm conclusions about its efficacy are limited by significant heterogeneity in study design [14]. Intraperitoneal instillation does appear to be safe, though, with a low risk of local anesthetic toxicity [23]. This has led to the conclusion that this technique may have some short-term benefit in certain laparoscopic procedures, but the effect size is small due to low quality evidence [14, 23].

Potential adverse outcomes related to WI/SSI would include local anesthetic systemic toxicity, hematoma, bruising, technical failure (for CWI), and most concerning, wound infection. Systemic toxicity can usually be avoided through careful calculation of dosing and fastidious technique to avoid intravascular injection. Bruising and hematoma can occur when blood vessels are punctured during infiltration but tend to be mild and self-limited. Studies have not shown a statistically significant increase in wound infections for SSI/WI or CWI techniques [9, 24, 25].

8 Local Anesthetic Adjuvants and Additives

Regional anesthesia has become a key element in the pursuit of opioid-sparing perioperative pain management, but the duration of action of local anesthetics does not always match the duration of postoperative pain. Even intermediate-acting local anesthetics, such as bupivacaine and ropivacaine, have been shown to only provide 8–12 hours of analgesia, resulting in increased pain once the nerve block wears off [26]. Additionally, as more surgical cases are performed in an ambulatory setting, there is a growing need for postoperative analgesic strategies that minimize the adverse effects of analgesics (especially opioids) to help hasten recovery and return to function without compromising analgesia. These potentially confounding goals have led to efforts to find novel means of extending the duration of action for local anesthetics and have led to such innovations as continuous infusions via a perineural catheter and ultra-long-lasting formulations, like liposomal bupivacaine. Prior to the development of these techniques, though, the most common method employed to extend the duration of analgesia after regional anesthesia was to mix various adjuncts and additive agents with local anesthetics. This remains a common technique due to its relative simplicity and low cost when compared to other options. Of note, though, the use of such agents to augment the duration of regional anesthesia, while common and well-described in the literature, is not a Food and Drug Administration approved indication and, as such, is an off-label use. Some authors [27] recommend caution with this technique despite its common use and propose that the unregulated mixture of regulated medications constitute the creation of a new unregistered substance with unknown adverse effects, such as the possibility of precipitation of these mixtures [28, 29]. Given this, care should always be taken when employing the following techniques.

Dexamethasone is a glucocorticoid and one of the most commonly used and well-studied adjuvants. Multiple reviews and meta-analyses have shown consistent prolongation of regional anesthesia across multiple doses, when mixed with a variety of local anesthetics, and when employed in a variety of regional anesthesia techniques [30–32]. Two studies showed equivalency between perineural and intravenous dexamethasone in prolonging the duration of analgesia after block, thus calling into question its utility as an adjuvant agent [33, 34]. A later Cochrane review concluded that while intravenous dexamethasone did prolong sensory block when compared to placebo, the use of perineural dexamethasone provided significantly longer lasting analgesia compared with the intravenous route [31]. Additionally, one in vitro study showed some evidence of neurotoxicity with higher concentrations of perineural dexamethasone [35], but a later *in vivo* study and subsequent review by the same authors [36, 37] concluded that perineural dexamethasone at a dose of 1–2 mg was safe and effective for prolonging block duration.

Another highly studied adjuvant agent is clonidine, an alpha-2-adrenergic agonist. Perineural clonidine administration has been shown to prolong the duration of analgesia provided by local anesthetics through hyperpolarization of cation channels [38]. One review showed significant heterogeneity in the prolongation of the duration of analgesia when clonidine is mixed with both short, intermediate and long-acting local anesthetics across a variety of regional anesthesia procedures, thus the optimal dose and scenario for usage remain unclear [30]. One clear finding, though, is that there is an increased risk of systemic absorption with increasing doses of perineural clonidine, with a coinciding increased risk of hypotension, bradycardia, and fainting. The recommended dose of perineural clonidine is 0.5–1 mcg/kg up to a maximum dose of 150 mcg [39, 40]. Dexmedetomidine is another alpha-2-adrenergic receptor agonist that is more selective than clonidine for the alpha-2 receptor [41]. Thus, the mechanism of action and side effect profile is similar to what is seen with clonidine [30]. One meta-analysis showed that the addition of dexmedetomidine to brachial plexus blocks increased the duration of analgesia by nearly 5 hours. However, this increased duration was not found to be statistically significant [42]. Overall, as with clonidine, there is heterogeneity with the degree of prolongation of analgesia with the addition of dexmedetomidine to local anesthetic solutions, increasing the duration of action by approximately 200-minutes with a dose of 1 mcg/kg [30]. There is some evidence that dexmedetomidine may have a prolonged effect relative to clonidine [43] and may also possess neuroprotective effects [37, 44].

Opioids are another potential adjuvant option and while there is evidence that they could prolong block duration via G-protein receptor-induced hyperpolarization effects on peripheral afferent sensory neurons [45], most of the analgesic benefit seems to be due to systemic absorption, leading to recommendations against their use in the setting of perineural injections [27, 28, 30, 32, 46, 47]. While well established for intrathecal use, extensive review has shown that morphine is not a reliable adjuvant for peripheral blocks [30] due to limited efficacy compared with systemic administration [48]. Another study also noted that patients receiving local anesthetic with a morphine adjunct had significantly more adverse effects (e.g. nausea, sedation), resulting in a stronger patient preference toward blocks with plain local anesthetic [49]. Reviewers have noted similar limitations with the use of fentanyl as a peripheral adjunct, leading to recommendations against the use of both morphine and fentanyl as peripheral adjuvant agents [27, 30, 32]. Tramadol has also been studied for use as an adjuvant due to its diverse effects on both mu-opioid receptors and sodium channels [50, 51]. Although neurotoxicity from perineural administration has not been reported in the literature, tramadol's efficacy in the setting of perineural injection is heterogeneous across multiple studies. One study with 1.5 mg/ml tramadol mixed with levobupivacaine for interscalene brachial plexus block showed significantly increased block duration compared with systemic tramadol and plain levobupivacaine block [52] while another study using lidocaine mixed with 200 mg tramadol for axillary brachial plexus block showed substantially longer duration of block, but delayed time of onset [53]. Robaux, et al. compared 1.5% plain mepivacaine in axillary brachial plexus block to the same agent mixed with increasing doses of tramadol (40, 100, 200 mg) and found no difference in block onset, but prolonged duration of block in a dose-dependent fashion [54]. Another study by Sarsu, et al. using 100 mg tramadol mixed with levobupivacaine and lidocaine showed a slower onset of block, but duration of action was not assessed [55]. Finally, three separate studies found no difference in time of onset or duration of action with a tramadol dose of either 1.5 mg/ml [56, 57] or 100 mg [58]. Given the conflicting evidence of benefit and dearth of safety data, use of tramadol as an adjuvant is not recommended [30, 46, 47]. Buprenorphine is the sole opioid analgesic that still shows promise as a potential adjuvant. Buprenorphine is unique in that while it is primarily a mu-opioid partial agonist, it also displays some degree of blockade of voltage-gated sodium channels [59]. Additionally, it may possess antihyperalgesic effects secondary to reductions in kappa opioid receptor activity and central sensitization [60, 61]. Multiple studies have demonstrated a near doubling of the duration of analgesia with the addition of buprenorphine, mixed with several local anesthetics across multiple types of blocks [62–67]. Buprenorphine's perineural dose ranges from 1–3 mcg/kg up to 300 mcg. One reviewer noted increased postoperative nausea and vomiting (PONV) in buprenorphine patients across several studies leading to a recommendation for the use of PONV prophylaxis and to avoid buprenorphine in patients with a strong history of PONV [30].

Epinephrine is a mixed alpha/beta-adrenergic agonist and is perhaps the oldest adjuvant used to prolong the duration of nerve blocks. It accomplishes this via alpha-1-adrenergic mediated vasoconstriction of the local perineural vasculature leading to reduced systemic absorption and subsequent delayed breakdown of local anesthetics [32, 68]. There has been some consideration of a central analgesic effect, though this appears to be mediated through alpha-2-adrenergic effects in the spinal cord when administered centrally [68, 69]. A dose range of 5–10 mcg/ml is customary [30]. The use of epinephrine has been shown to prolong the duration of a block when used with short to intermediate acting local anesthetics like lidocaine and mepivacaine, but it has not been shown to reliably prolong the duration of analgesia when mixed with bupivacaine or ropivacaine [30]. One additional use of epinephrine as an adjuvant is as a marker for inadvertent intravascular injection, which would result in tachycardia and hypertension immediately following injection. While this may aid in identifying intravascular injection, care must be taken when using epinephrine for this purpose so that the total dose does not cause hemodynamic compromise. The advent of ultrasound-guided regional anesthesia has reduced the utility of epinephrine for this purpose [27]. Furthermore, there is evidence of compromised endoneural blood flow with the use of epinephrine [70] leading to concerns for neurotoxicity and recommendations against its use patient populations at elevated risk of neuropathy, such as those with diabetes mellitus, hypertension, or smokers [47, 71, 72].

Ketamine is an N-Methyl-D-aspartate (NMDA) receptor antagonist with local anesthetic properties [73], but when studied as a perineural adjuvant it was shown to have substantial adverse effects, including hallucinations, sedation, and nausea, leading to recommendations against its use as a local anesthetic adjuvant [74]. Magnesium is another NMDA antagonist that has shown a consistent ability to prolong analgesia in a variety of combinations of nerve blocks and local anesthetics [75–79]. Only in one study [77] did the authors note an increased incidence of adverse effects in the form of nausea during the first 12 hours after the block and this study used a higher dose of magnesium than the other studies (200 mg versus 150 mg). While another study showed histological evidence of neurotoxicity with intrathecal magnesium [80] there are no studies evaluating perineural administration and the development of neurotoxicity. Thus, despite evidence of efficacy in prolonging the duration of nerve blocks, reviewers have consistently recommended against the routine use of magnesium for adjuvant therapy until more robust data are reported to assess for neurotoxicity in perineural use and to elucidate the adverse effect profile [27, 30, 32, 81].

Dextran is a complex branched polysaccharide derived from sucrose that is thought to extend the duration of action of local anesthetics by creating an aqueous solution at the site of injection [82]. Data in human trials have been inconclusive [83, 84] leading to recommendations against its use until safety and efficacy can be established [32].

Midazolam has been proposed as a potential adjuvant agent but has been repeatedly shown to be neurotoxic when administered perineurally and is not recommended for this use [35, 37, 85, 86].

Neostigmine, another potential adjuvant, is thought to prolong analgesia through its effects on acetylcholinesterase inhibitors by increasing endogenous acetylcholine at neural synapses [32]. One small study showed no difference in block onset, block duration, or adverse effects with the addition of neostigmine, but did note lower pain scores and opioid use for 24 hours after block administration [87]. Two other studies showed no analgesic benefit with the addition of neostigmine but did show higher adverse effects in the form of nausea and gastrointestinal distress [88, 89]. Other investigators have noted neurotoxic effects in intrathecal rabbit models [85]. Given the lack of compelling evidence supporting either safety or efficacy, the use of neostigmine as an adjuvant is not recommended.

Adenosine has been shown to have an antinociceptive neuromodulatory effect in the spinal cord that is mediated by A1-subtype adenosine receptors [90]. It has also shown no neurotoxicity in the spinal cord [91]. Given this track record of safety and efficacy, it has been studied as an adjuvant in peripheral nerve blocks but was shown to have no effect in this setting [92] leading to recommendations against its use as an adjuvant in peripheral nerve blocks [32].

9 Local Anesthetic Extended-Release Formulations

Due to the limitations of adjuvant therapy in extending the duration of analgesia with nerve blocks, there have been concerted efforts to find other means of prolonging block duration. Continuous peripheral nerve catheters undoubtedly do this, but they also present distinct potential disadvantages. Compared with single-shot injections, they are more costly and may require additional expertise in placement and maintenance [26]. Additionally, catheters are more susceptible to pump malfunctions, inadvertent catheter migrations, and infection. For instance, a study of 20 volunteers receiving either interscalene or femoral nerve catheters demonstrated catheter dislodgment rates of 5% and 25%, respectively, within 6 hours following regular physical exercises [93].

The search for a safe, long-acting local anesthetic has led to the development of liposomal formulations. Liposomes are microscopic structures that consist of an aqueous core surrounded by at least one phospholipid bilayer. Liposomal bupivacaine (Exparel), created by Pacira Pharmaceuticals, is perhaps the most well-known liposomal local anesthetic and uses multivesicular liposomes (DepoFoam delivery system) containing bupivacaine. DepoFoam has a non-concentric shape that results in slow degradation through internal fusion and division [94]. This slow degradation process has been shown to increase its duration of action to 96 hours and 120 hours for local infiltration and interscalene nerve blocks, respectively.

Liposomal bupivacaine was first approved by the FDA in 2011 for surgical field infiltration after 2 studies demonstrated efficacy in hemorrhoidectomy and bunionectomy surgeries compared with placebo [95]. In 2018, Exparel was approved for interscalene brachial plexus blocks [96]. To date, the interscalene block remains the only peripheral nerve block for which Exparel is approved. Intended as a single shot injection, it is recommended that no greater than 20 mL (266 mg) and 10 mL (133 mg) be used for local surgical field infiltration and interscalene blocks, respectively. The most common side effects include nausea, vomiting, constipation, and pyrexia. Exparel should not be mixed with non-bupivacaine LAs such as lidocaine as this can result in the immediate release of bupivacaine molecules with the potential for life-threatening cardiovascular and central nervous system toxicity. Exparel injection should be delayed at least 20 minutes following lidocaine injection and no additional local anesthetics should be given within 96 hours following the administration of Exparel. Exparel also should not be mixed with hypotonic solutions or water, as this may also disrupt the liposomal structure, and it should not make contact with any antiseptics, such as betadine. Exparel may be mixed with free bupivacaine in a ratio not exceeding 2:1 and may be diluted with normotonic solutions such as normal saline or lactated ringers in a maximum ratio of 1:14 (0.89 mg/mL), usually with the purpose of injecting a greater overall volume [97].

Exparel's indication for interscalene nerve blocks comes from one study involving 155 patients undergoing total shoulder arthroplasty or rotator cuff surgery, which demonstrated improvement in pain scores, opioid consumption, median time to opioid rescue, and percentage of opioid-free patients compared with placebo [98].

It is important to note that the investigators of this study did not compare Exparel to plain bupivacaine. The only specific contraindication is the use of liposomal bupivacaine in obstetric paracervical nerve blocks, which has been shown to result in fetal bradycardia and death [99]. Due to the current lack of pertinent studies regarding safety and efficacy, Exparel is not recommended for epidural, intrathecal, intravascular, and intraarticular injections. Exparel should be avoided in pregnant patients but has recently been approved for weight-based administration (4 mg/kg up to a total dose of 266 mg) for wound infiltration in pediatric patients greater than 6 years old.

While numerous studies have demonstrated Exparel's efficacy compared with placebo in reducing pain and opioid consumption, the studies that led to its FDA approval did not compare its use to plain bupivacaine. Two recently published systematic reviews from February 2021 focused specifically on this topic. A meta-analysis by Hussain et al. compared the efficacy of perineural Exparel to plain bupivacaine or ropivacaine with respect to analgesic outcomes, postsurgical pain, quality of life, and opioid dependence [99]. Nine RCTs involving 619 patients ultimately met the authors' inclusion criteria. The included studies involved patients receiving intercostal, pectoral myofascial plane, fascia iliaca, dorsal penile, interscalene, or adductor canal nerve blocks. Perineural Exparel resulted in a statistically significant reduction in rest pain over 24 through 72 hours versus plain bupivacaine and ropivacaine (the primary outcome); however, the difference in pain scores failed to meet the authors' threshold for clinical significance [99]. Additionally, when the authors excluded one industry sponsored RCT from their analysis, this difference became statistically insignificant. There were no differences in opioid consumption over 72-h, time to first analgesic request, opioid-related side effects, length of hospital stay, functional recovery, or persistent pain at 30 days between patients receiving liposomal versus plain bupivacaine, but patient satisfaction was found to be higher in the liposomal bupivacaine group [99]. One reason why liposomal bupivacaine demonstrated no additional benefits compared with the non-liposomal formulation may be that immediately following bupivacaine injection, local tissue inflammation occurs, resulting in an acidotic medium that prevents further liposomal bupivacaine from penetrating the cellular bilayer and acting on the intracellular voltage-gated sodium channel [99]. A second systematic review by Jin and colleagues yielded similarly negative results. Their study included 13 RCTs comparing the use of liposomal bupivacaine to traditional perineural local anesthetics with respect to opioid use and pain scores. Patients received TAP blocks in 6 of these RCTs, adductor canal blocks in 2 RCTs, brachial plexus blocks in 3 RCTs, fascia iliaca block in 1 RCT, and ankle block in 1 RCT [100]. Although 4 of the 6 RCTs involving TAP blocks reported a longer duration of action with Exparel, the authors were concerned about reliability of these studies given generally small sample sizes, conflicts of interest, and high risk of bias scores [100]. There were conflicting results from the 3 RCTs involving brachial plexus blocks, and all but one of the other RCTs involving alternate types of perineural blocks reported negative findings. Jin and colleagues concluded that "there is currently little evidence that in regional anesthesia, liposomal bupivacaine significantly prolongs the duration of analgesia compared to conventional local anesthetics" [100]. The authors also offered a hypothesis as to why surgical site infiltration with Exparel compared with plain bupivacaine has been shown to be effective whereas regional anesthesia with Exparel has not. Nerves targeted in regional block techniques are larger than those targeted with local infiltration. There must be a high enough concentration and gradient of free bupivacaine surrounding the nerve in order for the local anesthetics to diffuse through the epineurium and perineurium. The authors suggested that after its initial injection and due to the slow-release technology, liposomal bupivacaine may not release enough free bupivacaine molecules at the same time to create a high enough concentration gradient [100]. The authors also noted that factors such as surgical procedure, site of block, and tissue vascularity may influence efficacy as some studies have demonstrated no additional benefit of locally infiltrated Exparel in total knee replacement surgery, laparoscopic urologic surgery, and breast surgery [100–103].

Although Exparel is the most used and clinically relevant long-acting formulation of bupivacaine, others are under development. Heron Therapeutics developed a new drug, HTX-011 (ZYNRELEF), which consists of slow-release bupivacaine as well as meloxicam encapsulated in a bioerodable polymer (Biochronomer) which releases these drugs over 72 hours [94]. ZYNRELEF was FDA approved in May 2021, and has been especially useful in the setting of trauma that may result in the reduction in local anesthetic uptake in the neurons due to lower tissue pH. The low-dose meloxicam functions to normalize the local pH at the incision site, leading to higher efficacy of local anesthetic on the nearby sodium channels. Due to the viscous texture of ZYNRELEF, it must be dripped into the surgical site as opposed to being injected following final irrigation prior to wound closure [104]. Heron Therapeutics is also producing a mepivacaine-containing formulation called APF112 using this Biochronomer technology [94]. HTX-011 has undergone two phase III trials. The first study compared its efficacy to plain bupivacaine and to placebo for local infiltration during bunionectomy surgery, while the second included patients undergoing open inguinal herniorrhaphy with mesh. HTX-011 showed a statistically significant reduction in opioid consumption as well as pain intensity scores in both trials.[105, 106]. Despite these findings, neither HTX-011 nor APF112 is yet FDA-approved.

DURECT Corporation and Sandoz AG are currently developing POSIMIR, which is an extended-release formulation of bupivacaine using SABER-bupivacaine (sucrose acetate isobutyrate extended-release) technology. Sucrose acetate isobutyrate (SAIB) is a biodegradable depot that allows for high concentration bupivacaine storage. Because the drug contains benzyl alcohol, it is not designed for perineural use due to concern for neurotoxicity. After infiltration into the target tissue, POSIMIR releases bupivacaine at a rate of about 10 mg/h over 72 hours. Ekelund et al. compared SABER-bupivacaine versus SABER-placebo in a double-blinded, placebo-controlled trial on 78 patients undergoing shoulder arthroscopy. Compared to placebo, SABER-Bupivacaine reduced pain and opioid analgesic consumption over 72 hours after arthroscopic subacromial decompression and prolonged the time to first use of opioid rescue analgesia [107].

The quest for a safe and effective ultralong-acting local anesthetic remains ongoing. The excitement that came after Exparel's FDA approval may have been tempered by the recent systematic reviews questioning its advantages over traditional local anesthetics in regional anesthesia. Still, liposomal bupivacaine may be a more favorable option for surgical field blocks, and indeed, it remains as a component in intraoperative protocols for hip fracture surgery at many institutions despite this limited evidence.

Key Takeaways

The pharmacokinetics of local anesthetics (LA) involve complex properties of both the LA and its surroundings. LA potency is predominantly determined by lipid solubility, time of onset by the LA's pKa, and duration of action by protein binding.

Surgical site infiltration (SSI) does not require expensive technology or resources, but optimal technique does require an understanding of the innervation of the target structures along with the pharmacological properties of the LA being used. LA adjuvants and additives have been utilized to prolong the duration of action of local anesthetics when used for perineural and fascial plane blocks.

While epinephrine is predominantly used as an intravascular marker, other additives, including dexamethasone, alpha-2 agonists (clonidine, dexmedetomidine), and buprenorphine have been shown to prolong the duration of action with good safety profiles.

With the goal of extending the duration of peripheral nerve blocks, local anesthetic extended-release formulations using liposomal technology are being utilized. Aside from the more commonly used Exparel, other formulations, including HTX-011 and SABER-Bupivacaine are currently being studied as the search for extended-release local anesthetics continues.

References

1. Brau ME, Vogel W, Hempelmann G. Fundamental properties of local anesthetics: half-maximal blocking concentrations for tonic block of Na+ and K+ channels in peripheral nerve. Anesth Analg. 1998;87(4):885–9.
2. Mantegazza M, Catterall WA. Voltage-gated Na+ channels: structure, function, and pathophysiology. In: Noebels JL, Avoli M, Rogawski MA et al (ed) Jasper's basic mechanisms of the epilepsies, 4th ed. Bethesda, MD; 2012. p. 8–9.
3. Becker DE, Reed KL. Local anesthetics: review of pharmacological considerations. Anesth Prog. 2012;59(2):90–101.
4. Kuhnert BR, Philipson EH, et al. A prolonged chloroprocaine epidural block in a postpartum patient with abnormal pseudocholinesterase. Anesthesiology. 1982;56(6):477–8.
5. Hansen TG, Ilett KF, Reid C, et al. Caudal ropivacaine in infants: population pharmacokinetics and plasma concentrations. Anesthesiology. 2001;94(4):579–84.
6. Suresh S, Ecoffey C, Bosenburg A, et al. The European society of regional anaesthesia and pain therapy/American society of regional anesthesia and pain medicine recommendations on local anesthetics and adjuvants dosage in pediatric regional anesthesia. Reg Anesth Pain Med. 2018;43(2):211–6.
7. Rosenberg PH, Veering BT, Urmey WF. Maximum recommended doses of local anesthetics: a multifactorial concept. Reg Anesth Pain Med. 2004;29(6):564–75.

8. Covino BG. Comparative clinical pharmacology of local anesthetic agents. Anesthesiology. 1971;35(2):158–67.
9. Liu SS, Richman JM, Thirlby RC, et al. Efficacy of continuous wound catheters delivering local anesthetic for postoperative analgesia: a quantitative and qualitative systematic review of randomized controlled trials. J Am Coll Surg. 2006;203(6):914–32.
10. Stamenkovic DM, Bezmarevic M, Bojic S, et al. Updates on wound infiltration use for postoperative pain management: a narrative review. J Clin Med. 2021;10(20):4659.
11. HerniaSurge Group. International guidelines for groin hernia management. Hernia. 2018;22(1):1–165.
12. Poskus T, Jakubauskas M, Cekas K, et al. Local perianal anesthetic infiltration is safe and effective for anorectal surgery. Front Surg. 2021. https://doi.org/10.3389/fsurg.2021.730261.
13. Raeder J, Spreng UJ (2023) Intra-articular and periarticular infiltration of local anesthetics. New York School of Regional Anesthesia. Available at https://www.nysora.com/topics/regional-anesthesia-for-specific-surgical-procedures/lower-extremity-regional-anesthesia-for-specific-surgical-procedures/anesthesia-and-analgesia-for-hip-procedures/intra-articular-periarticular-infiltration-local-anesthetics/. Accessed 13 June 2023.
14. Hamill JK, Rahiri JL, Hill AG. Analgesic effect of intraperitoneal local anesthetic in surgery: an overview of systematic reviews. J Surg Res. 2017;212:167–77.
15. Ige O, Kolawole I, Bolaji B. Opioid-sparing effect of bupivacaine wound infiltration after lower abdominal operations. J West Afr Coll Surg. 2011;1(3):62–82.
16. Joshi GP, Janis JE, Haas EM, et al. Surgical site infiltration for abdominal surgery: a novel neuroanatomical-based approach. Plast Reconstr Surg Glob Open. 2016;4(12): e1181.
17. Joshi GP, Machi A. Surgical site infiltration: a neuroanatomical approach. Best Pract Res Clin Anaesthesiol. 2019;33(3):317–24.
18. Mungroop TH, Bond MJ, Lirk P, et al. Preperitoneal or subcutaneous wound catheters as alternative for epidural analgesia in abdominal surgery: a systematic review and meta-analysis. Ann Surg. 2019;269(2):252–60.
19. Ilfeld BM, Duke KB, Donohue MC. The association between lower extremity continuous peripheral nerve blocks and patient falls after knee and hip arthroplasty. Anesth Analg. 2010;111(6):1552–4.
20. Xing Q, Dai W, Zhao D, et al. Adductor canal block with local infiltrative analgesia compared with local infiltrate analgesia for pain control after total knee arthroplasty: a meta-analysis of randomized controlled trials. Medicine (Baltimore). 2017;96(38): e8103.
21. Li Y, Li A, Zhang Y. The efficacy of combined adductor canal block with local infiltration analgesia for pain control after total knee arthroplasty: a meta-analysis. Medicine (Baltimore). 2018;97(49): e13326.
22. Hussain N, Brull R, Sheehy B, et al. Does the addition of iPACK to adductor canal block in the presence of absence of periarticular local anesthetic infiltration improve analgesic and functional outcomes following total knee arthroplasty? A systematic review and meta-analysis. Reg Anesth Pain Med. 2021;46(8):713–21.
23. Gurusamy KS, Nagendran M, Guerrini GP, et al. Intraperitoneal local anaesthetic instillation versus no intraperitoneal local anesthetic instillation for laparoscopic cholecystectomy. Cochrane Database Syst Rev. 2014;13(3):CD007337.
24. Kuan YM, Smith S, Miles C, et al. Effectiveness of intra-operative wound infiltration with long-acting local anaesthetic. ANZ J Surg. 2002;72(1):18–20.
25. Byager N, Hansen MS, Mathiesen O, et al. The analgesic effect of wound infiltration with local anaesthetics after breast surgery: a qualitative systemic review. Acta Anaesthesiol Scan. 2014;58(4):402–10.
26. Chahar P, Cummings KC. Liposomal bupivacaine: a review of new bupivacaine formulation. J Pain Res. 2012;5:257–64.
27. Gasteiger L, Kirchmair L, Hoerner E, et al. Peripheral regional anesthesia using local anesthetics: old wine in new bottles? J Clin Med. 2023;12(4):1541.
28. Nestor CC, Ng C, Sepulveda P, et al. Pharmacological and clinical implications of local anesthetic mixtures: a narrative review. Anaesthesia. 2022;77(3):339–50.

29. Hoerner E, Stundner O, Putz G, et al. Crystallization of ropivacaine and bupivacaine when mixed with different adjuvants: a semiquantitative light microscopy analysis. Reg Anesth Pain Med. 2022;47:625–9.
30. Kirksey MA, Haskins SC, Cheng J, et al. Local anesthetic peripheral nerve block adjuvants for prolongation of analgesia: a systematic qualitative review. PLoS ONE. 2015;10(9): e0137312.
31. Pehora C, Pearson AM, Kaushal A, et al. Dexamethasone as an adjuvant to peripheral nerve block. Cochrane Database Syst Rev. (2017);11(11):CD011770.
32. Emelife PI, Eng MR, Menard BL, et al. Adjunct medications for peripheral and neuraxial anesthesia. Best Pract Res Clin Anaesthesiol. 2018;32(2):83–99.
33. Fanzca MJF, Danesh-Clough TK, White R. Adjuvant dexamethasone for bupivacaine sciatic and ankle blocks: results from 2 randomized placebo-controlled trials. Reg Anesth Pain Med. 2013;38(4):300–7.
34. Desmet M, Braems H, Reynvoet M, et al. I.V. and perineural dexamethasone are equivalent in increasing the analgesic duration of a single-shot interscalene block with ropivacaine for shoulder surgery: a prospective, randomized, placebo-controlled study. Br J Anaesth. 2013;111(3):445–52.
35. Williams BA, Hough KA, Tsui BYK. Neurotoxicity of adjuvants used in perineural anesthesia and analgesia in comparison with ropivacaine. Reg Anesth Pain Med. 2011;36(3):225–30.
36. Williams BA, Ibinson JW, Mangione MP, et al. Research priorities regarding multimodal peripheral nerve blocks for postoperative analgesia and anesthesia based on hospital quality data extracted from over 1,300 cases (2011–2014). Pain Med. 2015;16(1):7–12.
37. Knight JB, Schott NJ, Kentor ML, et al. Neurotoxicity of common peripheral nerve block adjuvants. Curr Opin Anaesthesiol. 2015;28(5):598–604.
38. Kroin JS, Buvanendran A, Beck DR, et al. Clonidine prolongation of lidocaine analgesia after sciatic nerve block in rats is mediated via the hyperpolarization-activated cation current, not by alpha-adrenoreceptors. Anesthesiology. 2004;101(2):488–94.
39. McCartney CJ, Duggan E, Apatu E. Should we add clonidine to local anesthetic for peripheral nerve blockade? A qualitative systematic review of the literature. Reg Anesth Pain Med. 2007;32(4):330–8.
40. Popping DM, Elia N, Marret E, et al. Clonidine as an adjuvant to local anesthetics for peripheral nerve and plexus blocks: a meta-analysis of randomized trials. Anesthesiology. 2009;111(2):406–15.
41. Gertler R, Brown HC, Mitchell DH, et al. Dexmedetomidine: a novel sedative-analgesic agent. Proc (Bayl Univ Med Cent). 2001;14(1):13–21.
42. Abdallah FW, Brull R. Facilitatory effects of perineural dexmedetomidine on neuraxial and peripheral nerve block: a systematic review and meta-analysis. Br J Anaesth. 2013;110(6):915–24.
43. Swami SS, Keniya VM, Ladi SD, et al. Comparison of dexmedetomidine and clonidine (alpha 2 agonist drugs) as an adjuvant to local anaesthesia in supraclavicular brachial plexus block: a randomised double-blind prospective study. Indian J Anaesth. 2012;56(3):243–9.
44. Tufek A, Kaya S, Tokgoz O, et al. The protective effect of dexmedetomidine on bupivacaine-induced sciatic nerve inflammation is mediated by mast cells. Clin Invest Med. 2013;36(2):E95-102.
45. Busch-Dienstfertig M, Stein C. Opioid receptors and opioid peptide-producing leukocytes in inflammatory pain—basic and therapeutic aspects. Brain Behav Immun. 2010;24(5):683–94.
46. Murphy DB, McCartney CJ, Chan VW. Novel analgesic adjuncts for brachial plexus blocks: a systematic review. Anesth Analg. 2000;90(5):1122–8.
47. Brummett CM, Williams BA. Additives to local anesthetics for peripheral nerve blockade. Int Anesthesiol Clin. 2011;49(4):104–16.
48. Racz H, Gunning K, Della Santa D, et al. Evaluation of the effect of perineuronal morphine on the quality of postoperative analgesia after axillary plexus block: a randomized double-blind study. Anesth Analg. 1991;72(6):769–72.
49. Keskinbora K, Aydinli I. Perineural morphine in patients with chronic ischemic lower extremity pain: efficacy and long-term results. J Anesth. 2009;23(1):11–8.

50. Guven M, Mert T, Gunay I. Effects of tramadol on nerve action potentials in rat: comparisons with benzocaine and lidocaine. Int J Neurosci. 2005;115(3):339–49.
51. Sousa AM, Ashmawi HA, Costa LS, et al. Percutaneous sciatic nerve block with tramadol induces analgesia and motor blockade in two animal pain models. Braz J Med Biol Res. 2012;45(2):147–52.
52. Alemanno F, Ghisi D, Fanelli A, et al. Tramadol and 0.5% levobupivacaine for single-shot interscalene block: effects on postoperative analgesia in patients undergoing shoulder arthroplasty. Minerva Anestesiol. 2012;78(3):291–96.
53. Kaabachi O, Ouezini R, Koubaa W, et al. Tramadol as an adjuvant to lidocaine for axillary brachial plexus block. Anesth Analg. 2009;108(1):367–70.
54. Robaux S, Blunt C, Viel E, et al. Tramadol added to 1.5% mepivacaine for axillary brachial plexus block improves postoperative analgesia dose-dependently. Anesth Analg. 2004;98(4):1172–7.
55. Sarsu S, Mizrak A, Karakurum G. Tramadol use for axillary brachial plexus blockade. J Surg Res. 2011;165(1):e23-27.
56. Mannion S, O'Callaghan S, Murphy DB, et al. Tramadol as adjunct to psoas compartment block with levobupivacaine 0.5%: a randomized double-blinded study. Br J Anaesth. 2005;94(3):352–6.
57. Omar AM, Mansour MA, Abdelwahab HH, et al. Role Of ketamine and tramadol as adjuncts to bupivacaine 0.5% in paravertebral block for breast surgery: a randomized double-blind study. Egypt J Anaesth. 2011;27(2):101–5.
58. Kesimci E, Izdes S, Gozdemir M, et al. Tramadol does not prolong the effect of ropivacaine 7.5 mg/ml for axillary brachial plexus block. Acta Anaesthesiol Scand. 2007;51(6):736–41.
59. Leffler A, Frank G, Kistner K, et al. Local anesthetic-like inhibition of voltage-gated Na(+) channels by the partial mu-opioid receptor agonist buprenorphine. Anesthesiology. 2012;116(6):1335–46.
60. Koppert W, Ihmsen H, Korber N, et al. Different profiles of buprenorphine-induced analgesia and antihyperalgesia in a human pain model. Pain. 2005;118(1–2):15–22.
61. Troster A, Ihmsen H, Singler B, et al. Interaction of fentanyl and buprenorphine in an experimental model of pain and central sensitization in human volunteers. Clin J Pain. 2012;28(8):705–11.
62. Viel EJ, Eledjam JJ, De La Coussaye JE, et al. Brachial plexus block with opioids for postoperative pain relief: comparison between buprenorphine and morphine. Reg Anesth. 1989;14(6):274–8.
63. Bazin JE, Massoni C, Bruelle P, et al. The addition of opioids to local anaesthetics in brachial plexus block: the comparative effects of morphine, buprenorphine and sufentanil. Anaesthesia. 1997;52(9):858–62.
64. Candido KD, Franco CD, Khan MA, et al. Buprenorphine added to local anesthetic for brachial plexus block to provide postoperative analgesia in outpatients. Reg Anesth Pain Med. 2001;26(4):352–6.
65. Candido KD, Winnie AP, Ghaleb AH, et al. Buprenorphine added to the local anesthetic for axillary brachial plexus block prolongs postoperative analgesia. Reg Anesth Pain Med. 2002;27(2):162–7.
66. Jadon A, Panigrahi MR, Parida SS, et al. Buprenorphine improves the efficacy of bupivacaine in nerve plexus block: a double blind randomized evaluation in subclavian perivascular brachial block. J Anaesth Clin Pharmacol. 2009;25(2):207–10.
67. Behr A, Freo U, Ori C, et al. Buprenorphine added to levobupivacaine enhances postoperative analgesia of middle interscalene brachial plexus block. J Anesth. 2012;26(5):746–51.
68. Niemi G. Advantages and disadvantages of adrenaline in regional anesthesia. Best Pract Res Clin Anaesthesiol. 2005;19(2):229–45.
69. Reddy SV, Maderdrut JL, Yaksh TL. Spinal cord pharmacology of adrenergic agonist-mediated antinociception. J Pharmacol Exp Ther. 1980;213(3):525–33.
70. Myers RR, Heckman HM. Effects of local anesthesia on nerve blood flow: studies using lidocaine with and without epinephrine. Anesthesiology. 1989;71(5):757–62.

71. Neal JM. Effects of epinephrine in local anesthetics on the central and peripheral nervous systems: neurotoxicity and neural blood flow. Reg Anesth Pain Med. 2003;28(2):124–34.
72. Kroin JS, Buvandendran A, Williams DK, et al. Local anesthetic sciatic nerve block and nerve fiber damage in diabetic rats. Reg Anesth Pain Med. 2010;35(4):343–50.
73. Weber WV, Jawalekar KS, Jawalekar SR. The effect of ketamine on nerve conduction in isolated sciatic nerves of the toad. Neurosci Lett. 1975;1(2):115–20.
74. Lee IO, Kim WK, Kong MH, et al. No enhancement of sensory and motor blockade by ketamine added to ropivacaine interscalene brachial plexus blockade. Acta Anaesthesiol Scand. 2002;46(7):821–6.
75. Gunduz A, Bilir A, Gulec S. Magnesium added to prilocaine prolongs the duration of axillary plexus block. Reg Anesth Pain Med. 2006;31(3):233–6.
76. Dogru K, Yildirim D, Ulgey A, et al. Adding magnesium to levobupivacaine for axillary brachial plexus block in arteriovenous fistule surgery. Bratisl Lek Listy. 2012;113(10):607–9.
77. Lee AR, Yi WH, Chung IS, et al. Magnesium added to bupivacaine prolongs the duration of analgesia after interscalene block. Can J Anaesth. 2012;59(1):21–7.
78. Ekmekci P, Bengisun ZK, Akan B, et al. The effect of magnesium added to levobupivacaine for femoral nerve block on postoperative analgesia in patients undergoing ACL reconstruction. Knee Surg Sports Traumatol Arthrosc. 2013;21(5):1119–24.
79. Elshamaa HA, Ibrahim M, Eldesuky HL. Magnesium sulfate in femoral nerve block, does postoperative analgesia differ? A comparative study. Egypt J Anaesth. 2014;30(2):169–73.
80. Saeki H, Matsumoto M, Kaneko S, et al. Is intrathecal magnesium sulfate safe and protective against ischemic spinal cord injury in rabbits? Anesth Analg. 2004;99(6):1805–12.
81. Bailard NS, Ortiz J, Flores RA. Additives to local anesthetics for peripheral nerve blocks: evidence, limitations, and recommendations. Am J Health Syst Pharm. 2014;71(5):373–85.
82. Aberg G, Friberger P, Sydnes G. Studies on the duration of local anaesthesia: a possible mechanism for the prolonging effect of dextran on the duration of infiltration anaesthesia. Acta Pharmacol Oxical (Copenh). 1978;42(2):88–92.
83. Simpson PJ, Hughes DR, Long DH. Prolonged local analgesia for inguinal herniorrhaphy with bupivacaine and dextran. Ann R Coll Surg Engl. 1982;64(4):243–6.
84. Armstrong DN, Kingsnorth AN. Local anaesthesia in inguinal herniorrhaphy: influence of dextran and saline solutions on duration of action of bupivacaine. Ann R Coll Surg Engl. 1986;68(4):207–8.
85. Demirel E, Ugur HC, Dolgun H, et al. The neurotoxic effects of intrathecal midazolam and neostigmine in rabbits. Anaesth Intensive Care. 2006;34(2):218–23.
86. Yilmaz E, Hough K, Gebhart G, et al. Mechanisms underlying midazolam-induced peripheral nerve block and neurotoxicity. Reg Anesth Pain Med. 2014;39(6):525–33.
87. Bone HG, Van Aken H, Burkle H. Enhancement of axillary brachial plexus block anesthesia by coadministration of neostigmine. Reg Anesth Pain Med. 1999;24(5):405–10.
88. Bouaziz H, Paqueron X, Bur ML, et al. No enhancement of sensory and motor blockade by neostigmine added to mepivacaine axillary plexus block. Anesthesiology. 1999;91(1):78–83.
89. Van Elstraete AC, Pastureau F, Lebrun T, et al. Neostigmine added to lidocaine axillary plexus block for postoperative analgesia. Eur J Anaesthesiol. 2001;18(4):257–60.
90. Sollevi A. Adenosine for pain control. Acta Anaesthesiol Scand Suppl. 1997;110:135–6.
91. Rane K, Karlsten R, Sollevi A, et al. Spinal cord morphology after chronic intrathecal administration of adenosine in the rat. Acta Anesthesiol Scand. 1999;43(10):1035–40.
92. Apan A, Basar H, Ozcan S, et al. Combination of adenosine with prilocaine and lignocaine for brachial plexus block does not prolong postoperative analgesia. Anaesth Intensive Care. 2003;31(6):648–52.
93. Marhofer D, Marhofer P, Triffterer L, et al. Dislocation rates of perineural catheters: a volunteer study. Br J Anaesth. 2013;111(5):800–6.
94. Coppens SJR, Zawodny Z, Dewinter G, et al. In search of the holy grail: poisons and extended release local anesthetics. Best Pract Res Clin Anaesthesiol. 2019;33(1):3–21.
95. Rappaport BA. U.S. Food and drug administration center for drug evaluation and research https://www.accessdata.fda.gov/drugsatfda_docs/nda/2011/022496Orig1s000Approv.pdf (2011). Accessed 13 June 2023.

96. Rabin T. FDA in brief: FDA approves new use of Exparel for nerve block shoulder pain relief following shoulder surgeries. https://www.fda.gov/news-events/fda-brief/fda-brief-fda-approves-new-use-exparel-nerve-block-pain-relief-following-shoulder-surgeries (2018). Accessed 13 June 2023.
97. Food and Drug Administration (FDA) Printed Labeling. https://www.accessdata.fda.gov/drugsatfda_docs/nda/2011/022496Orig1s000Lbl.pdf (2011). Accessed 13 June 2023.
98. Patel MA, Gadsden JC, Nedeljkovic SS. Brachial plexus block with liposomal bupivacaine for shoulder surgery improves analgesia and reduced opioid consumption: results from a multicenter, randomized, double-blind, controlled trial. Pain Med. 2020;21(2):387–400.
99. Hussain N, Brull R, Sheehy B, et al. Perineural liposomal bupivacaine is not superior to nonliposomal bupivacaine for peripheral nerve block analgesia. Anesthesiology. 2021;134(2):147–64.
100. Jin Z, Ding O, Islam A, et al. Comparison of liposomal bupivacaine and conventional local anesthetic agents in regional anesthesia: a systemic review. Anesth Analg. 2021;132(6):1626–34.
101. Knight RB, Walker PW, Keegan KA, et al. A randomized controlled trial for pain control in laparoscopic urologic surgery: 0.25% bupivacaine versus long-acting liposomal bupivacaine. J Endourol. 2015;29(9):1019–24.
102. Schroer WC, Diesfeld PG, LeMarr AR, et al. Does extended-release liposomal bupivacaine better control pain than bupivacaine after total knee arthroplasty (TKA)? A prospective, randomized clinical trial. J Arthroplasty. 2015;30(9 Suppl):64–7.
103. Tan P, Martin MS, Shank N et al (2017) A comparison of 4 analgesic regimens for acute postoperative pain control in breast augmentation patients. Ann Plast Surg. 78(6S Suppl 5):S299–S304.
104. Kang RS, Zhaosheng J, Gan TJ. A novel long-acting local anesthetic—HTX-011 (ZYNRELEF™) for postoperative pain control. Expert Rev Clin Pharmacol. 2022(15:10):1147–53.
105. Viscusi E, Gimbel JS, Pollack RA, et al. HTX-011 reduced pain intensity and opioid consumption versus bupivacaine HCl in bunionectomy: phase III results from the randomized EPOCH 1 study. Reg Anesth Pain Med. 2019;44:700–6.
106. Viscusi E, Minkowitz H, Winkle P, et al. HTX-011 reduced pain intensity and opioid consumption versus bupivacaine HCl in herniorrhaphy: results from the phase 3 EPOCH 2 study. Hernia. 2019;23(6):1071–80.
107. Ekelund A, Peredistijs A, Grohs J, et al. SABER-bupivacaine reduced postoperative pain and opioid consumption after arthroscopic subacromial decompression: a randomized, placebo-controlled trial. J Am Acad Orthop Surg Glob Res Rev. 2022;6(5).

Perioperative Pain Management: Lidocaine

Ryan Ferguson, Alexander Bautista, and Alaa Abd-Elsayed

Abstract The opioid epidemic has fostered a proliferation of strategies aimed at limiting opioid-centric analgesic paradigms in the perioperative phase of care. Effective pain management is a critical component of postoperative care as it affects a myriad of recovery variables and improves patient satisfaction. The use of opioid analgesics has been found to produce untoward side effects and may lead to delayed post-operative recovery. Lidocaine is an amide local anesthetic that has been widely used for local and regional anesthesia while simultaneously possessing antiarrhythmic, anti-nociceptive and anti-bacterial properties. In the management of chronic pain, the intravenous administration of lidocaine has been shown to reduce central pain sensitization. {Chu, 2020 #1} The applicability of intravenous lidocaine for early post-operative pain control has been well studied following laparoscopic and open abdominal surgeries. Intravenous lidocaine has also been shown to be efficacious in the treatment of a variety of acute and chronic pain clinical scenarios.

Keywords Lidocaine · Pain management · Opioid sparing · Analgesia · Anti-inflammatory · Adverse effect

1 Introduction

Lidocaine is a widely used amide-type local anesthetic and antiarrhythmic. It was first synthesized in 1943 by Swedish chemist Nils Lofgren, and its use as a local anesthetic was first described in 1948 by British anesthesiologist L. J. Guedel [1]. Lidocaine is now one of the most used local anesthetics in medical practice after initially gaining widespread popularity due to its superior safety profile when compared to older local anesthetic agents. Lidocaine is a local anesthetic featured on the list of WHO essential

R. Ferguson · A. Bautista
Department of Anesthesiology and Perioperative Medicine, University of Louisville, Louisville, KY, USA

A. Abd-Elsayed (✉)
Anesthesiology, University of Wisconsin-Madison, Madison, WI, USA
e-mail: abdelsayed@wisc.edu

A. Abd-Elsayed and K. Schroeder (eds.), *Perioperative Pain Management*,
https://doi.org/10.1007/978-3-031-67648-2_36

medications given its evidence of efficacy, safety and comparative cost-effectiveness [2]. Lidocaine is available in a variety of formulations, including injectable solutions, topical creams and gels, and transdermal patches. Its dosage and administration depend on the intended use, the patient's age and weight, and other factors that may affect its pharmacokinetics and pharmacodynamics. As a local anesthetic, lidocaine can be used for surface anesthesia, infiltration anesthesia, intravenous regional analgesia and nerve block and dental anesthesia. Moreover, research has recently come to light suggesting intravenous lidocaine may have potential benefits in the perioperative setting. It may have a role in reducing both pain and postoperative nausea and vomiting, which are two of the most common complaints after surgery and anesthesia. In this chapter we discuss lidocaine's use in the perioperative window. Its use in this context can provide a range of benefits, including reduced pain and inflammation, and improved postoperative recovery.

2 Pharmacology

Structure

Lidocaine is a synthesized amide–type local anesthetic that was preceded by amino esters such as cocaine. Ester and amide anesthetics share a similar structure, consisting of an aromatic (lipophilic) portion, an intermediate chain (ester or amide), and an amine (hydrophilic) portion [3]. The protein binding, potency, duration of action, and other clinical aspects of use are influenced by structural variations in the aromatic and amine portions. The intrinsic potency of the anesthetic is often correlated with its lipophilicity. For instance, bupivacaine, which is more lipophilic than lidocaine, has a higher potency and a longer duration of action. Chiral modifications of local anesthetics have their own pharmacodynamic, pharmacokinetic, and toxicity profiles. Generally, the S-enantiomer is more potent and longer-lasting than the R-enantiomer or the racemic mixture of both forms. Additionally, the S-enantiomer is typically less toxic [4]. For example, ropivacaine and levobupivacaine are pure S-enantiomers, offering less neurotoxicity and cardiotoxicity.

Pharmacokinetic—Pharmacokinetics refers to the way a drug is absorbed, distributed, metabolized, and eliminated from the body. Here are the pharmacokinetic properties of lidocaine.

Absorption

The absorption of Lidocaine depends on the site of administration and the dosage form. It can be absorbed through the skin, mucous membranes, and gastrointestinal tract. Topical formulations are absorbed slowly, resulting in lower bioavailability compared to injection solutions. The rate and extent of absorption of injected anesthetics into the bloodstream are influenced by several factors, including the properties of the agent, the presence of a vasoconstrictor in the solution, the site and quantity of drug injection, and the injection technique. Local anesthetics, except for cocaine, have varying degrees of vasodilatory effects. Therefore, epinephrine is commonly added to local anesthetics to induce vasoconstriction and extend the duration of the anesthetic effect. In the absence of epinephrine, lidocaine's effect lasts for approximately 30–60 minutes. However, with epinephrine, the duration of lidocaine's effect can be prolonged to approximately 120–360 minutes [5].

Distribution

As discussed above, the relative lipophilicity of local anesthetics determines their potency and protein binding impacts local anesthetic duration. Lidocaine, which is 60–80% protein bound, has an elimination half-life of 1.5–2.0 hours. Animal studies suggest that lidocaine is widely distributed in all body tissues [6]. However, each local anesthetic varies in the rate and degree of penetration in different tissues and organs. Lidocaine has a volume of distribution of approximately 1–2 L/kg, [7] indicating its widespread distribution throughout the body. The use of lipid nanoparticles as delivery systems for infiltrative and topical local anesthetics has enabled the modification of drug release rates and increased bioavailability, resulting in prolonged duration of action, reduced toxicity, and improved therapeutic potency.

Metabolism

Lidocaine is primarily metabolized in the liver into two active compounds: monoethylglycinexylidide (MEGX) and glycinexylidide (GX) [8]. MEGX possesses 80–90% of the potency of lidocaine, while GX possesses 25% [9]. Lidocaine has an initial half-life of 7–30 minutes, followed by a terminal half-life of 1.5–2 hours, while MEGX has a half-life of 0.5–3.3 hours. Despite having a longer half-life than lidocaine, MEGX exhibits lower potency as a sodium channel blocker, leading to diminished anesthetic effects. The metabolic pathway primarily involves the CYP1A2 enzyme, with CYP3A4 playing a minor role. Following intravenous administration, serum concentrations of MEGX and GX range between 11–36% and 5–11%, respectively, compared to lidocaine concentrations [10, 11]. Lidocaine and its metabolites are excreted by the kidneys, with more than 98% of an absorbed dose recoverable in the urine as metabolites or parent drug, and less than 10% excreted unchanged in adults [12]. Impaired metabolism due to significant hepatic dysfunction increases the risk of systemic toxicity when relatively high volumes of an amide local anesthetic are used. The CYP3A4 system, which specifically metabolizes lidocaine, has significant implications regarding drug interactions.

3 Pharmacodynamics

The pharmacodynamics of lidocaine refer to how the drug produces its effects on the body, particularly in terms of its mechanism of action, potency, and efficacy. Here are the key pharmacodynamic properties of lidocaine.

Mechanism of Action

An understanding of normal nerve conduction physiology provides a framework for considering the mechanism of action of lidocaine. A normal nerve impulse, also known as an action potential, is a brief electrical signal that travels along the axon of a neuron. When a nerve axon is at rest, its membrane maintains a transmembrane electric potential between 290 and 260 mV due to the action of an active transport sodium–potassium pump that transports sodium ions into the extracellular space. During this resting state, the sodium ion channels are closed, resulting in a negatively charged axonal cytoplasm. However, when the nerve is stimulated, the sodium channels open and allow a massive influx of sodium ions, depolarizing the membrane towards the sodium equilibrium potential of 140 mV, which changes the internal negative charge to a positive charge. Following this, the sodium channels inactivate while potassium channels open, allowing potassium ions to leave. The transmembrane potential is then restored to its baseline level by the sodium–potassium pump, allowing nerve impulses to be transmitted down axons and between cells [13].

Lidocaine works by blocking voltage-gated sodium channels in nerve fibers. This prevents the influx of sodium ions that is required for depolarization of the cell membrane and the initiation of a nerve impulse. As a result, lidocaine can prevent or reduce the transmission of pain signals from the nerve fibers to the brain. Specifically, lidocaine binds to the intracellular portion of the sodium channel, blocking the channel from opening and thus preventing sodium from entering the cell. By blocking these channels, lidocaine reduces the number of action potentials that can be generated in the affected nerve fibers, leading to a decrease in pain perception [14, 15].

As an anti-inflammatory agent, the exact mechanism of lidocaine is not fully understood. However, there is evidence to suggest that lidocaine may have several different effects on the immune system that could contribute to its anti-inflammatory properties. Here are some of the proposed mechanisms of action for lidocaine as an anti-inflammatory.

Inhibition of cytokine production: Lidocaine has been shown to inhibit the production of pro-inflammatory cytokines, such as tumor necrosis factor-alpha (TNF-alpha) and interleukin-6 (IL-6), by immune cells such as macrophages and monocytes. This reduction in cytokine activity may help to reduce inflammation and prevent tissue damage [16].

Modulation of immune cell function: Lidocaine has been shown to modulate the function of various immune cells, including T cells, B cells, and natural killer (NK) cells. For example, lidocaine can inhibit T cell proliferation and activation, which may help to reduce inflammation [17].

Lidocaine has also been shown to inhibit leukocyte adhesion and migration [18].

Stabilization of cell membranes: Lidocaine has been shown to stabilize cell membranes, which can prevent the release of pro-inflammatory mediators such as histamine and prostaglandins from damaged cells. This may help to reduce inflammation and prevent tissue damage [19].

Overall, while the precise mechanism of action for lidocaine as an anti-inflammatory medication is not fully understood, it is thought to involve multiple pathways and effects on the immune system, neuronal activity, and cell membranes.

Potency, Dosing, and Efficacy

The potency of intravenous lidocaine used in the perioperative setting is determined by several factors. The dosage administered, the patient's age, weight, and overall health, and the specific surgical procedure are important determinants of the potency of intravenous lidocaine.

In general, lidocaine is considered a potent analgesic when used in appropriate doses. Studies have shown that intravenous lidocaine reduces the incidence of chronic pain following surgery, suggesting that it has a potent analgesic effect. The recommended perioperative dosing of intravenous lidocaine is first initiated with a loading dose of no more than 1.5 mg/kg that is given as an infusion over 10 min. After the loading dose has been administered, an infusion of no more than 1.5 mg/kg/h is continued for no longer than 24 hours [20]. Ideal body weight should be used for dose calculation to prevent toxicity. This can be calculated using the simple formula: ideal body weight = (height in cm − 100) for men; and (height in cm − 105) for women.

Intravenous lidocaine is a potent analgesic with a multifaceted mechanism of action. It has been shown to have anti-inflammatory properties, which may be responsible for its ability to reduce postoperative pain and opioid consumption. Intravenous lidocaine also acts on several neurotransmitter systems, including glutamate and GABA, which may contribute to its analgesic effects [21].

Studies have shown that intravenous lidocaine is effective in reducing postoperative pain scores and opioid consumption in a variety of surgical procedures. For example, a meta-analysis of 29 randomized controlled trials found that intravenous lidocaine reduced postoperative pain and opioid requirement, ileus recovery time, and hospital length of stay. The effect was particularly pronounced in abdominal surgeries [22]. See Table 1 for details on lidocaine infusion protocols.

Intravenous lidocaine has also been shown to have a beneficial effect on postoperative nausea and vomiting (PONV). A meta-analysis of 5 randomized controlled trials found that intravenous lidocaine reduced the incidence of PONV by 20% [26].

Table 1 Lidocaine infusion protocols utilized in the setting of open abdominal procedures [23–25]

Type of surgery	References	Bolus	Infusion	Duration	Results
Open abdominal colorectal	Kuo et al. [23]	2 mg/kg	3 mg/kg/h	30 min before to end surgery	Decreased pain scores and opioid consumption; decreased nausea, duration of ileus, and length of hospitalization
	Herroeder et al. [24]	1.5 mg/kg	2 mg/min	Before induction to 4 h postoperatively	
	Swenson et al. [25]	No bolus	1–3 mg/min	Before induction to return of bowel function	

Although this effect could be partially attributed to the reduction of opioids required for adequate analgesia.

Within the framework of Enhanced Recovery After Surgery (ERAS) protocols, intravenous lidocaine infusions are frequently incorporated into multimodal pain management strategies. ERAS encompasses a comprehensive approach to perioperative care that aims to optimize patient outcomes and expedite recovery following surgery. By integrating intravenous lidocaine, which possesses both analgesic and anti-inflammatory attributes, ERAS protocols can effectively manage postoperative pain, diminish opioid usage, and facilitate a swifter recovery.

Overall, intravenous lidocaine is a potent analgesic that is effective in reducing postoperative pain scores and opioid consumption. Its anti-inflammatory properties and ability to modulate neurotransmitter systems may contribute to its analgesic effects. Intravenous lidocaine may also have a beneficial effect on PONV. The efficacy of intravenous lidocaine should be carefully considered in the context of the specific patient and surgical procedure, as factors such as the patient's age, weight, and overall health may affect its potency and efficacy.

4 Side Effects and Toxicity

Side effects of lidocaine can vary depending on the dose, route of administration, and individual patient factors. In patients considered for lidocaine administration, in particular intravenous infusions, baseline ECG, electrolytes and liver function tests may be helpful to avoid potential complications. Use of lidocaine should be carefully monitored especially in patients with liver disease as lidocaine undergoes hepatic metabolism through the cytochrome P450 (CYP) system, primarily via the CYP1A2 and CYP3A4 enzymes as discussed above. In patients with liver failure, there may be a decreased clearance of lidocaine leading to an increased risk of toxicity.

5 Local Anesthetic Systemic Toxicity (LAST)

LAST is a rare but potentially life-threatening complication that can occur when local anesthetic reaches the systemic circulation resulting in supratherapeutic blood and tissue levels resulting in systemic toxicity. This can result in central nervous system excitation, central nervous system (CNS) inhibition, cardiovascular excitation and cardiovascular inhibition resulting in symptoms such as seizures, confusion, cardiac arrest, and respiratory depression. These findings can be severe and require immediate medical attention [27].

Effective LAST management involves several key considerations. To prevent toxicity, dosing should be carefully controlled, considering factors such as administered dosage, patient age, weight, health status, and the specific surgical procedure. Adherence to recommended dosing guidelines and vigilant monitoring are imperative.

Additionally, it's crucial to recognize that local anesthetic sources extend beyond intravenous lidocaine. Comprehensive assessment must encompass various routes of administration, including local anesthetic infiltration and regional nerve blocks, which collectively contribute to systemic levels.

Furthermore, caution is advised when dealing with liposomal local anesthetic preparations. Avoid mixing lidocaine with these agents, as the interaction can impact pharmacokinetics and potentially lead to unforeseen effects.

Continuous monitoring is paramount for patients receiving intravenous lidocaine. Vigilant observation of vital signs, CNS status, cardiovascular function, and respiratory effort is essential. It is important for healthcare providers to keep in mind the potential for toxicity, even if there are alternative explanations for a patient's symptoms. To ensure prompt treatment in case of toxicity, a 20% lipid emulsion should be easily accessible in any setting where intravenous lidocaine is administered.

6 Methemoglobinemia

Although rare, the use of lidocaine has been associated with the development of methemoglobinemia, particularly when it is administered in high doses or for prolonged periods of time. Lidocaine-induced methemoglobinemia occurs when lidocaine is metabolized in the body to produce a compound called 2,6-xylidine, which can cause oxidation of hemoglobin and the subsequent formation of methemoglobin [28, 29].

Symptoms of methemoglobinemia can vary, but commonly include cyanosis (a blue discoloration of the skin), shortness of breath, headache, dizziness, and confusion. Treatment typically involves stopping the use of lidocaine and administering medication to reduce the levels of methemoglobin in the blood, such as methylene blue or ascorbic acid.

In addition to these two rare complications of lidocaine toxicity, other adverse effects are divided into organ systems and listed below.

7 Nervous System

When high levels of lidocaine (more than 6 mcg/mL free base) are achieved, it can cross the blood–brain barrier and cause significant central nervous system (CNS) toxicity. CNS toxicity can manifest as excitatory or depressive symptoms, including lightheadedness, anxiety, restlessness, confusion, drowsiness, tinnitus, blurred or double vision, vomiting, metallic taste, dysgeusia, sensations of heat or cold, numbness, hyperesthesia, hypoesthesia, asthenia, twitching, tremor, convulsions, unconsciousness, respiratory depression, and respiratory arrest. CNS toxicity can also lead to agitation, dysarthria, oral hypoesthesia, and disorientation. Drowsiness is often an early sign of a high blood concentration of the drug and may occur because of rapid absorption. Some patients experience only minor and transient symptoms of CNS toxicity.

8 Cardiovascular System

Lidocaine is a Class Ib antiarrhythmic that suppresses both the initiation and conduction of nerve impulses by decreasing the neuronal membrane's permeability to sodium ions resulting in inhibition of depolarization with resultant blockade of conduction. As such it is contraindicated in individuals with cardiac abnormalities such as Adam-Stokes syndrome, Wolff-Parkinson-White syndrome, severe degrees of SA, AV, or intraventricular heart block. Even in healthy individuals, lidocaine can also cause adverse cardiovascular effects such as myocardial depression, sinus bradycardia, hypotension, cardiovascular collapse, and cardiac arrest. These effects typically occur with high plasma drug concentrations but have occurred with smaller doses in rare cases. Lidocaine administration should be closely monitored, and if cardiovascular or CNS side effects occur, general supportive physiologic measures such as oxygen therapy, assisted ventilation, and IV fluids should be initiated. Blood pressure and electrocardiogram should also be monitored during intravenous administration. If cardiovascular side effects occur, lidocaine administration should be discontinued, and treatment options should be re-evaluated. Combining lidocaine with a vasoconstrictor increases the likelihood of producing various side effects such as anxiety, palpitations, dizziness, headache, restlessness, tremor, angina, and hypertension.

Respiratory System

Lidocaine can cause respiratory depression, especially when administered intravenously. This side effect is more commonly seen in patients with compromised respiratory function.

Gastrointestinal System

Lidocaine has been associated with nausea and vomiting, especially when administered intravenously.

Renal System

Lidocaine and its metabolites are excreted by the kidneys. High doses or prolonged administration of lidocaine can lead to renal dysfunction and impaired clearance of the drug, leading to an increased risk of toxicity.

Local Tissue Reaction

When lidocaine is applied topically or transdermal, systemic adverse reactions are unlikely to occur due to the small amount of lidocaine that is absorbed. However, the skin at the site of treatment may experience abnormal sensations such as erythema, swelling, or dysesthesia. Additionally, application site reactions may occur during or immediately after treatment with the lidocaine transdermal patch. These reactions can include mild and transient symptoms such as blisters, ecchymosis, depigmentation, skin erosion, exfoliation, flushing, skin irritation, papules, petechiae, pruritus, or vesicles, and usually resolve within a few minutes to hours.

Allergic Reactions

Lidocaine can cause allergic reactions, including anaphylaxis, which is a severe and potentially life-threatening reaction. These reactions are rare but can occur in patients who are hypersensitive to lidocaine or any of its components.

9 Perioperative Use

Lidocaine is commonly used in various forms during the perioperative period to provide anesthesia and analgesia.

Intravenous Lidocaine

Intravenous (IV) lidocaine is used perioperatively for its analgesic and anti-inflammatory properties. It has been shown to reduce postoperative pain, decrease the need for opioid medications, and decrease the incidence of postoperative nausea and vomiting. IV lidocaine works by blocking sodium channels in nerve fibers, inhibiting the transmission of painful stimuli. It also modulates the inflammatory response by reducing the production of pro-inflammatory cytokines.

Lidocaine infiltration: Lidocaine can be injected directly into tissues to provide local anesthesia. It has been used for various procedures, including dental procedures, joint injections, and nerve blocks. Lidocaine injection can also be used for postoperative pain management.

Topical lidocaine: Topical lidocaine is applied directly to the skin or mucous membranes to provide local anesthesia. It has been used during procedures such as endoscopy, bronchoscopy, and urologic procedures. Topical lidocaine is also used for wound care, including debridement and dressing changes.

Transdermal lidocaine patches: Transdermal lidocaine patches provide continuous delivery of lidocaine through the skin. They have been used to manage chronic pain conditions, such as neuropathic pain and postherpetic neuralgia. Some patches are intended for 12-hour wear, while others are designed for 24-hour wear. The instructions provided by the manufacturer should be followed regarding the appropriate duration of patch wear. Common concentrations of lidocaine in patches are 5 and 4%. The typical recommended daily dose of lidocaine from patches can vary, but it often falls within the range of 200–700 mg per day, depending on the concentration and the patient's individual factors.

10 Conclusion

The use of lidocaine perioperatively has been studied extensively and has shown promising results in reducing postoperative pain, nausea and vomiting, and opioid consumption. Lidocaine can be administered in various forms, including intravenous infusion, nerve blocks, and topical application.

Intravenous lidocaine has been shown to have a systemic analgesic effect and can be used as an adjunct to general anesthesia or as a standalone technique in certain surgeries. However, the optimal dosing and timing of administration are still debated, and further studies are needed to determine its effectiveness in reducing chronic postoperative pain.

Local anesthetic nerve blocks using lidocaine have also been shown to provide effective perioperative analgesia, particularly for regional surgeries such as orthopedic and plastic surgery. These blocks can be performed using various techniques, such as single injection, continuous infusion, or intermittent boluses, and can be guided by ultrasound or nerve stimulation. However, the efficacy of nerve blocks depends on proper technique and patient selection, and potential complications such as nerve injury and systemic toxicity should be considered.

Overall, the use of lidocaine perioperatively is a promising approach to reducing postoperative pain and opioid consumption. However, more research is needed to determine the optimal dosing, timing, and administration techniques to maximize its benefits and minimize potential risks.

Key Points

1. IV Lidocaine's Potential: IV lidocaine shows advantages for surgical patients, yet its benefits must be weighed against potential risks.
2. Varied Impact: The effects of risks and benefits differ based on patient characteristics and surgery type.
3. Risk Management: Cautious administration of IV lidocaine can help mitigate potential dangers associated with its use.

References

1. Löfgren N. Studies on local Anaesthetics: xylocaine, a new synthetic drug. Ph.D. Thesis, Stockholm University, Stockholm, Sweden; 1948.
2. World Health Organisation. Lidocaine. WHO model lists of essential medicine. Available online: https://list.essentialmeds.org/medicines/8. Accessed 18 Oct 2021.
3. Covino BG. Local anesthesia. 1. N Engl J Med. 1972;286(18):975–83.
4. McClure JH. Ropivacaine. Br J Anaesth. 1996;76(2):300–7.
5. Berde CB, Strichartz GR. Local anesthetics. In: Miller R, editor. Anesthesia. Philadelphia: Saunders; 2015. p. 1028–54.
6. Katz J. The distribution of 14-C-labelled lidocaine injected intravenously in the rat. Anesthesiology. 1968;29(2):249–53.
7. Rang HP. Pharmacology. Edinburgh: Churchill Livingstone; 2003. p. 103. ISBN 0-443-07145-4.
8. Bennett PN, Aarons LJ, Bending MR, et al. Pharmacokinetics of lidocaine and its deethylated metabolite: dose and time dependency studies in man. J Pharmacokinet Biopharm. 1982;10:265–81.
9. Thomson AH, Elliott HL, Kelman AW, Meredith PA, Whiting B. The pharmacokinetics and pharmacodynamics of lignocaine and MEGX in healthy subjects. J Pharmacokinet Biopharm. 1987;15:101–15.
10. Kenkel JM, Lipschitz AH, Shepherd G, Armstrong VW, Streit F, Oellerich M, Luby M, Rohrich RJ, Brown SA. Pharmacokinetics and safety of lidocaine and monoethylglycinexylidide in liposuction: a microdialysis study. Plast Reconstr Surg. 2004;114(2):516–24; discussion 525–6. https://doi.org/10.1097/01.prs.0000128423.84607.61. PMID: 15277825.

11. Halkin H, Meffin P, Melmon KL, et al. Influence of congestive heart failure on blood vessels of lidocaine and its active monodeethylated metabolite. Clin Pharmacol Ther. 1975;17:669–76.
12. Beckett AH, Boyes RN, Appleton PJ. The metabolism and excretion of lignocaine in man. J Pharm Pharmacol. 1966;18:76S-81S.
13. Strichartz GR, Ritchie JM. The action of local anesthetics on ion channels of excitable tissues. In: Strichartz G, editor. Local Anesthetics, vol. 81. Berlin: Springer-Verlag; 1987. p. 21–53.
14. Omoigui S. The pain drugs handbook. St. Louis, MO: Mosby Year Book; 1995.
15. Butterworth JF 4th, Strichartz GR. Molecular mechanism of local anesthesia: a review. Anesthesiology. 1990;72(4):711–34.
16. Ortiz MP, Godoy MC, Schlosser RS. Effect of endovenous lidocaine on analgesia and serum cytokines: double-blinded and randomized trial. J Clin Anesth. 2016;35:70–7. https://doi.org/10.1016/j.jclinane.2016.07.021.
17. Ramirez MF, Tran P, Cata JP. The effect of clinically therapeutic plasma concentrations of lidocaine on natural killer cell cytotoxicity. Reg Anesth Pain Med. 2015;40(1):43–8. https://doi.org/10.1097/AAP.0000000000000191. PMID: 25469757.
18. Fischer LG, Bremer M, Coleman EJ, Conrad B, Krumm B, Gross A, Hollmann MW, Mandell G, Durieux ME. Local Anesthetics attenuate lysophosphatidic acid-induced priming in human neutrophils. Anesth Analg. 2001;92:1041–7.
19. Yanagi H, Sankawa H, Saito H, Iikura Y. Effect of lidocaine on histamine release and Ca2+ mobilization from mast cells and basophils. Acta Anaesthesiol Scand. 1996;40:1138–44.
20. Foo I, Macfarlane AJR, Srivastava D, Bhaskar A, Barker H, Knaggs R, Eipe N, Smith AF. The use of intravenous lidocaine for postoperative pain and recovery: international consensus statement on efficacy and safety. Anaesthesia. 2021;76:238–50.
21. Werdehausen R, Mittnacht S, Bee LA, Minett MS, Armbruster A, Bauer I, Wood JN, Hermanns H, Eulenburg V. The lidocaine metabolite N-ethylglycine has antinociceptive effects in experimental inflammatory and neuropathic pain. Pain. 2015;156(9):1647–59. https://doi.org/10.1097/j.pain.0000000000000206. PMID: 25932687; PMCID: PMC4617288.
22. Vigneault L, Turgeon AF, Côté D, Lauzier F, Zarychanski R, Moore L, McIntyre LA, Nicole PC, Fergusson DA. Perioperative intravenous lidocaine infusion for postoperative pain control: a meta-analysis of randomized controlled trials. Can J Anaesth. 2011;58(1):22–37. https://doi.org/10.1007/s12630-010-9407-0. PMID: 21061107.
23. Kuo CP, Jao SW, Chen KM, Wong CS, Yeh CC, Sheen MJ, Wu CT: Comparison of the effects of thoracic epidural analgesia and I.V. infusion with lidocaine on cytokine response, postoperative pain and bowel function in patients undergoing colonic surgery. Br J Anaesth. 2006;97:640–6.
24. Herroeder S, Pecher S, Schönherr ME, Kaulitz G, Hahnenkamp K, Friess H, Böttiger BW, Bauer H, Dijkgraaf MG, Durieux ME, Hollmann MW. Systemic lidocaine shortens length of hospital stay after colorectal surgery: a double-blinded, randomized, placebo-controlled trial. Ann Surg. 2007;246:192–200.
25. Koppert W, Weigand M, Neumann F, Sittl R, Schuettler J, Schmelz M, Hering W: Perioperative intravenous lidocaine has preventive effects on postoperative pain and morphine consumption after major abdominal surgery. Anesth Analg. 2004;98:1050–5, table of contents.
26. Marret E, Rolin M, Beaussier M, Bonnet F. Meta-analysis of intravenous lidocaine and postoperative recovery after abdominal surgery. Br J Surg. 2008;95(11):1331–8. https://doi.org/10.1002/bjs.6375. PMID: 18844267.
27. Weinberg GL. Lipid emulsion infusion: resuscitation for local anesthetic and other drug overdose. Anesthesiology. 2012;117(1):180–7. https://doi.org/10.1097/ALN.0b013e31825ad8de. PMID: 22627464; PMCID: PMC4609208.
28. Mansouri A, Lurie AA. Concise review: methemoglobinemia. Am J Hematol. 1993;42(1):7–12. https://doi.org/10.1002/ajh.2830420104. PMID: 8416301.
29. Higuchi R, Fukami T, Nakajima M, Yokoi T. Drug Metab Dispos. 2013;41(6):1220–1230. https://doi.org/10.1124/dmd.113.051714.

The Role of Antiepileptics for Postoperative Pain Management

Junyong In, Kevin Huynh, Jennifer Luong, Dillon Sooknanan, and Sakura Kinjo

Abstract Antiepileptic drugs provide an analgesic effect and have been used to treat chronic pain for decades. During the past twenty years, some of these medications have been used in perioperative settings, as part of a multimodal pain regimen. In this context, the most commonly used and studied drugs are gabapentinoids, such as gabapentin and pregabalin. In contrast to the results of multiple RCTs in the past, a recent well-regarded systematic review and meta-analysis including 281 trials ($N = 24{,}682$), published in 2020, reported that gabapentin and pregabalin provided no clinically meaningful analgesic efficacy in treating acute postoperative pain. This study also reported that they did not significantly reduce postoperative chronic pain but did contribute to a greater risk of adverse events such as dizziness and visual disturbance. Therefore, these authors concluded that routine use of gabapentin or pregabalin is not recommended for postoperative pain management. This study aggregated results across different types of surgeries. Other studies however have studied the risks and benefits of using gabapentinoids as part of a pain regimen for specific types of surgeries. Results from these studies indicate a reduction in postoperative pain for certain types of surgeries but not others. Results of pain studies for specific surgeries will be summarized in this chapter. Other Antiepileptic drugs

J. In
Department of Anesthesiology and Pain Medicine, Dongguk University Ilsan Hospital, Goyang, Republic of Korea
e-mail: dragona1@dumc.or.kr

K. Huynh · J. Luong · D. Sooknanan · S. Kinjo (✉)
Department of Anesthesia and Perioperative Care, University of California, San Francisco, CA, U.S.A.
e-mail: Sakura.Kinjo@ucsf.edu

K. Huynh
e-mail: Kevin.Huynh@ucsf.edu

J. Luong
e-mail: Jennifer.Luong@ucsf.edu

D. Sooknanan
e-mail: Dillon.Sooknanan@ucsf.edu

A. Abd-Elsayed and K. Schroeder (eds.), *Perioperative Pain Management*,
https://doi.org/10.1007/978-3-031-67648-2_37

such as carbamazepine, phenytoin, lamotrigine, lacosamide, zonisamide, and GABA-acting anticonvulsants (tiagabine, vigabatrin, felbamate) have not been commonly used for acute postoperative pain. Due to limited data, it is difficult to make any definitive conclusions regarding their effectiveness in perioperative settings.

Keywords Antiepileptic drug · Gabapentinoids · Carbamazepine · Phenytoin · Lamotrigine · Lacosamide · Zonisamide · GABA-acting anticonvulsants

1 Introduction

For decades, antiepileptic drugs (AEDs) have been used for various chronic pain conditions such as trigeminal neuralgia, diabetic neuropathy, and postherpetic neuralgia (PHN). Each AED has its unique mechanisms of action, and most of the AEDs exert multiple pharmacologic effects. For example, phenytoin and carbamazepine work as sodium channel blockers and also decrease glutamate transmission. Gabapentin, despite the name of this agent, exerts its effect on voltage-gated calcium channels (Table 1). The mechanisms of action are often complex, not all of which are well understood. All AEDs have different side effect profiles which may limit their use in perioperative settings. In the last decade, gabapentinoids (gabapentin and pregabalin) were introduced to treat acute pain. It was hoped that this class of drugs would decrease pain and reduce opioid use. In this context, these medications have been rigorously studied, and more data exists for them compared with than other types of AEDs.

In this chapter, in addition to gabapentin and pregabalin, we will discuss clinical data for different types of AEDs, including a newer gabapentinoid (mirogabalin), carbamazepine, phenytoin, lacosamide, zonisamide, and GABA-acting drugs (tiagabine, vigabatrin, and felbamate).

Table 1 Commonly used antiepileptic drugs: mechanisms of action

Na channel blockade	Ca channel blockade	GABA potentiation	Decreased glutamate transmission
Carbamazepine Felbamate Lamotrigine Oxycarbazepine Phenytoin Topiramate Zonisamide	Carbamazepine Ethosuximide Felbamate Gabapentin Lamotrigine Levetiracetam Oxycarbazepine Pregabalin Topiramate Valproic acid Zonisamide	Barbiturates Benzodiazepines Felbamate Levetiracetam Topiramate	Carbamazepine Felbamate Gabapentin Lamotrigine Oxcarbazepine Pregabalin Phenytoin Valproic acid

GABA = gamma-amino butyric acid

2 Specific Antiepileptic Drugs

Gabapentinoids

Background

Gabapentinoids, including gabapentin and pregabalin were introduced in the 1990s as anticonvulsant medications and subsequently approved to treat chronic neuropathic pain or fibromyalgia. As a part of enhanced recovery after surgery (ERAS) protocols and multimodal analgesia, the use of gabapentinoids have increased significantly for postoperative pain management over the past decade in order to reduce opioid consumption and opioid-related adverse effects [1, 2].

Gabapentin

1. **Pharmacodynamics and Pharmacokinetics**

Gabapentin is an amino acid derived from γ-aminobutyric acid (GABA). It shows strong and specific binding for the $\alpha_2\delta$ subunits of presynaptic P/Q-type voltage-gated calcium channels in the central nervous system. By modulating these calcium channels, the calcium influx necessary for neurotransmitter release from activated nociceptors is mediated [3] (Fig. 1). This, in turn, modulates the subsequent release of glutamate from activated pain-transmitting neurons. The effects of gabapentin are affected by the presence, structure, and biochemical state of the $\alpha_2\delta$ subunit [4–6].

Gabapentin is absorbed from the small part of the duodenum through an active transport system of amino acid carriers. The active transport system becomes saturated within the clinical dose range [7–9]. Once the system is saturated, blood levels of gabapentin do not rise proportionately with higher levels of gabapentin ingestion [10]. Gidal et al. [11] reported wide inter-subject variability in gabapentin absorption and bioavailability. This means that the same dose will likely result in different plasma concentrations in individual patients and therefore, a variable therapeutic effect. Gabapentin exhibits minimal or no binding to plasma proteins and is nearly eliminated entirely via the kidneys without biotransformation [12]. Therefore, the dose of gabapentin must be adjusted for patients with renal dysfunction or those on dialysis [13]. (Table 2) Concomitant use of magnesium oxide affects the absorption of gabapentin and reduces the bioavailability of gabapentin even though pharmacokinetic interactions of gabapentin are minimal [14]. The elimination half-life of gabapentin is 4.8–8.7 hours [3].

2. **Dosing and Route of Administration**

The oral dose of gabapentin is generally 300–1200, mg 1–2 hours before surgery. Administration may also be continued in the postoperative period [15] (Table 3). When continued into the postoperative period, gabapentin is generally administered three times a day (TID). As a strategy to limit the development of sedation and

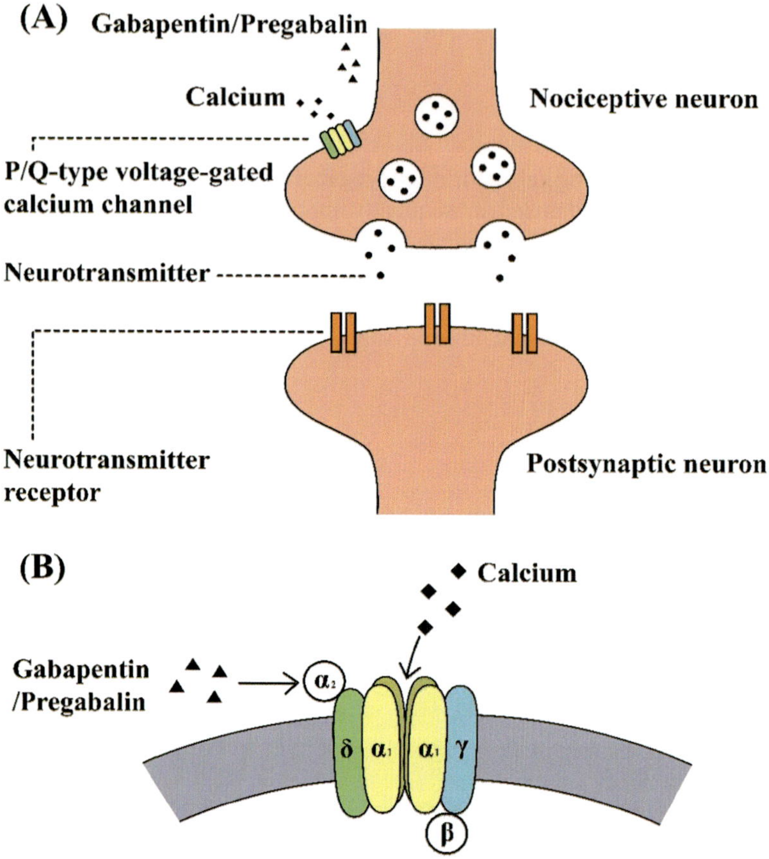

Fig. 1 Schematic action mechanisms of gabapentin/pregabalin. (A) Gabapentin/pregabalin binds to the $\alpha_2\delta$ subunit of P/Q-type voltage-gated calcium channels and modulates calcium influx through these channels. (B) Subunit architecture of P/Q-type voltage-gated calcium channel with gabapentin/pregabalin

Table 2 Example of gabapentin dosage adjustments for renal impairment [13]

Renal function creatinine clearance (ml/min)	Total daily dose range (mg/day)
≥60	900–3600
30–59	400–1400
15–29	200–700
<15	100–300

nausea, dosing of gabapentin is generally started low (i.e., 300 mg TID) and titrated to higher doses as tolerated. As noted above, dosing adjustments are necessary for patients with significant renal disease. Additional dosing reductions/considerations are discussed in more detail below and should be made in the elderly and others at elevated risk for excessive sedation.

3. **Perioperative Uses**

While several randomized controlled trials (RCTs) and meta-analyses reported a modest decrease in postoperative opioid consumption [16–18], other studies have failed to confirm this benefit [19–21]. Here are examples of the use of gabapentinoids for different types of surgery.

A. Mastectomy: Premedication with oral gabapentin significantly reduces postoperative morphine consumption without an increase in adverse effects after radical mastectomy compared to a placebo [22, 23].
B. Spine surgery: Three meta-analyses for spine surgeries reported that preemptive gabapentinoids reduced morphine consumption, lowered pain scores, and decreased the incidence of morphine-related adverse effects such as postoperative nausea/vomiting, pruritus, and urinary retention, while gabapentinoid-related sedation or dizziness was not different between the gabapentinoid and placebo groups [24–26].
C. Cardiac surgery: 600 mg of gabapentin before cardiac surgery lowered opioid requirements, pain scores, and postoperative nausea/vomiting [27]. Gabapentinoids are recommended with acetaminophen, tramadol, and dexmedetomidine as part of the multimodal analgesia regimen after cardiac surgery [28].
D. Gynecologic/oncologic surgery: Routine preoperative administration of oral gabapentin with acetaminophen and celecoxib is recommended to reduce pain and opioid requirements in gynecologic/oncologic surgery [29, 30].
E. Joint surgery: There is a lack of evidence on whether gabapentinoids reduce postoperative pain in total hip and knee replacement surgery, so gabapentinoids are not included in routine premedication even though gabapentinoids reduce postoperative opioid consumption [31].

Table 3 Example of analgesic doses of gabapentin [150–153]

Phase	Dose	Comments
Preoperative	300 mg if < 65 years old 100–300 mg if 65 ≥ years or if any renal impairment	1–2 hours before surgery May consider avoiding in patients at high risk of respiratory depression, delirium, or dizziness, if risks outweigh opioid-sparing benefits
Intraoperative	None	None
Postoperative	600 mg, two or three times per day	As a single dose or in multiple doses

F. Cesarean surgery: Preoperative gabapentin of 300 mg [32] or 600 mg [33] has been reported to reduce pain in cesarean delivery under spinal anesthesia in some studies but not all [34]. Therefore, gabapentin is not listed as a recommended medication for enhanced recovery after cesarean section [35].
G. Liver surgery: The Enhanced Recovery After Surgery (ERAS) Society does not recommend gabapentinoids as pre-anesthetic medication for liver surgery [36]. This recommendation is based on a meta-analysis of perioperative use of gabapentinoids for postoperative acute pain management in liver and major surgeries [18].
H. Thoracic surgery: There is no evidence that gabapentin reduces acute or chronic pain following thoracic surgery [37]. Furthermore, Huot et al. [38] reported that it also does not mitigate post-thoracotomy shoulder pain.

Systematic Reviews

Several meta-analysis studies concluded that gabapentinoids reduce postoperative pain and opioid consumption for pain management [15, 19, 39–42]. Based on these results, multimodal analgesia regimens often include gabapentin to mitigate and treat perioperative pain and decrease opioid requirements [15, 43].

A recent larger meta-analysis from 2020 included a total of 281 trials (24,682 patients) [18]. In this study, compared with controls, gabapentinoids were associated with lower postoperative pain but this effect was not clinically significant. In addition, the opioid-sparing effect was small, and they had no effect on preventing postoperative chronic pain. Although it was associated with a lower risk in postoperative nausea and vomiting, they seemed to contribute to a higher incidence of side effects such as dizziness and visual disturbance. Therefore, the authors concluded that routine use of these medications is not recommended for postoperative pain management. However, clinical heterogeneity of included studies and statistical heterogeneity have been pointed out [44], therefore, one should cautiously adapt the applicability of the results of this meta-analysis to clinical practice for specific types of surgery.

4. **Adverse Effects**

Even though gabapentinoids are generally well tolerated, the dose is initiated at a low level to avoid adverse effects such as sedation, dizziness or headache, visual disturbances, and peripheral edema [45, 46]. In populations that already have an elevated risk of periprocedural sedation, the dose of gabapentin should be used with caution and initiated at a lower dose. For example, some studies suggest using a dose of 100 mg of gabapentin, then titrating to a target range. As with all sedatives, patients should be instructed not to drive until the sedative effect of gabapentin has dropped to a safe level. There is also a concern that gabapentinoids may cause significant respiratory depression in patients with coexisting respiratory illnesses such as: chronic obstructive pulmonary disease; patients undergoing opioid therapy; and in elderly patients [47–50]. These adverse effects should be evaluated and managed with proper dose reduction.

Pregabalin

1. **Pharmacodynamics and Pharmacokinetics**

Pregabalin is a GABA analog that is a potent ligand for the $\alpha_2\delta$ subunit of voltage-gated calcium channels. Although a GABA analog, it is pharmacologically inactive at GABA receptors and therefore does not act through the GABAergic system [51]. Similar to gabapentin, pregabalin demonstrates anticonvulsant and anti-hyperalgesic properties [52]. It has 90% oral bioavailability and a dose-independent absorption profile with rapid absorption. Peak plasma levels are seen 1 hour after administration, and pregabalin has an elimination half-life of 5–6 hours [53]. Pregabalin is minimally metabolized and eliminated primarily by the kidneys [53].

2. **Dosing and Route of Administration**

Pregabalin can be prescribed up to 600 mg per day for epilepsy or neuropathic pain. The commonly used regimen for perioperative settings are: for single dose 75–300 mg 1–2 h before surgery, and some studies continued to administer 50–75 mg twice a day after surgery [54]. Because of predominately renal elimination, dose adjustment is recommended for patients with renal insufficiency [55].

3. **Perioperative Uses**

Perioperative use of pregabalin has been studied in numerous surgical settings.

A. Orthopedic surgery: Pregabalin before and after total knee arthroplasty has been associated with a significant decrease in the need for epidural or oral opioids, compared to placebo [56]. In an RCT of 40 patients undergoing lumbar discectomy, pregabalin at 300 mg before surgery and 150 mg at 12 and 24 hours postoperatively was associated with decreased pain intensity scores at 3 months [57]. Pain scores were also significantly reduced in an RCT of patients undergoing single-level microdiscectomy [58].
B. Cardiac surgery: Elderly patients who received pregabalin before and after surgery reduced their total oxycodone consumption by 48% compared to placebo [59]. Another RCT of 40 patients undergoing off-pump coronary artery bypass randomized to pregabalin 150 mg preoperatively and 75 mg two times a day for two days postoperatively versus placebo had significantly decreased pain scores at 6, 12, 24, and 36 hours from extubation [60].
C. Gynecologic surgery: RCTs investigating the role of pregabalin in hysterectomy showed decreased opiate consumption and higher satisfaction scores [61, 62].
D. Abdominal Surgery: A study examining pregabalin for postoperative pain control for laparoscopic cholecystectomies showed improved pain scores and reduced postoperative fentanyl consumption [63]. Similar findings were seen in an RCT of patients undergoing laparoscopic sleeve gastrectomy [64].

Systematic Reviews

A meta-analysis in 2015 [41] has suggested that pregabalin has opioid-sparing effects and reduces pain scores in the postsurgical setting. Another meta-analysis [54] assessing analgesic efficacy and adverse events of pregabalin in various surgical procedures showed that pregabalin was associated with reduced pain at 2 hours after surgery in all surgical categories, and all surgical categories at 24 hours with the exception of cardiothoracic and spine procedures. Total morphine consumption at 24 hours post-surgery was significantly reduced in all surgical categories with the exception of cardiothoracic and ENT procedures. As stated in the Gabapentin section, the recent larger meta-analysis in 2020 [18] showed that the use of gabapentinoids had no clinically significant benefit for postoperative pain.

4. **Adverse Effects**

The most common adverse effects of pregabalin seen in these RCTs include an increased incidence of sedation, blurry vision, and dizziness [65, 66]. However, some RCTs reported no significant adverse events [64, 67]. A Cochrane review in 2019 which evaluated pregabalin use for acute and chronic neuropathic pain, found that serious adverse events occurred at the same rate as placebo with "high-quality evidence" [68]. In contrast, some studies have shown that pregabalin resulted in significant adverse effects such as sedation and visual disturbances [41, 54]. The recent meta-analysis [18] referenced earlier also showed that gabapentinoids were associated with a greater risk of adverse events (dizziness and visual disturbances) in the perioperative period.

Conclusions for the Use of Gabapentin/Pregabalin for Postoperative Pain

Overall, gabapentinoids may induce a slight decrease in postoperative pain and opioid consumption. However, the results from the meta-analysis studies are conflicting. These studies included different types of surgery, timing of administration, and dose, which makes any general conclusions difficult.

Considering the adverse effects of gabapentinoids and unclear effects on post-operative pain, one should be cautious applying the results to clinical practice. Further studies for a more evident conclusion on the type of surgery and different patient population (e.g., patient's co-morbidities and presence of neuropathic pain) are warranted.

Mirogabalin

1. **Introduction**

Mirogabalin besylate (hereafter mirogabalin) is an orally administered gabapentinoid developed initially by Daiichi Sankyo for the treatment of peripheral neuropathic pain (PNP) [69]. It is a novel ligand for the $\alpha_2\delta$ subunit of voltage-gated calcium channels. Initial approval was granted in Japan based on trials demonstrating efficacy for the treatment of diabetic peripheral neuropathic pain (DPNP) or PHN. Compared to its counterparts (gabapentin and pregabalin), mirogabalin offers more sustained analgesia and a wider safety margin leading to less adverse events [70]. While not currently FDA-approved, the drug is relatively new and has the potential for wider adoption based on recent trials demonstrating possible superiority over pregabalin [71].

2. **Pharmacodynamics/Pharmacokinetics**

Like conventional gabapentinoids, mirogabalin acts on the α2δ subunit of voltage-gated calcium channels (VGCCs) and does not act through the GABAergic system. VGCCs are usually made up of the main pore-forming α1 subunit and auxiliary subunits, including the β and α2δ, or sometimes γ subunits. Four α2δ (α2δ-1, α2δ-2, α2δ-3, and α2δ-4) subunit genes have been cloned. Neuropathic pain pharmacokinetics involve the α2δ-1 subunit, which is distributed in the skeletal, smooth, and cardiac muscles, as well as the central and peripheral nervous systems and endocrine tissues. However, the α2δ-2 subunit has been associated with adverse side effects such as ataxia and dizziness, possibly due to its concentration in the Purkinje cells of the cerebellum [72]. Mirogabalin binds to both α2δ-1 and α2δ-2 subtypes but has a higher binding affinity to them and a longer dissociation half-life from the $\alpha_2\delta$-1 subunit compared to other gabapentinoids [73]. It has a mean terminal half-life of 2–3 hours after a single dose and 2–5 hours after multiple doses [74]. It is excreted primarily through the kidneys and the dose may have to be adjusted based on renal function [75].

3. **Dosing and Route of Administration**

Oral formulations are available in 2.5, 5, 10, and 15 mg tablets with a recommended starting dose of 5 mg twice daily (BID), then increasing weekly by 5 mg up to a maximum dose of 15 mg BID [75, 76]. The median time to maximum plasma concentration (Tmax) after oral administration was 0.5–1.5 hours (possibly increased by 0.5 hours if taken in a fed state) with an oral bioavailability of >85%.

4. **Adverse Effects**

The most common adverse drug reactions are similar to conventional gabapentinoids (e.g., dizziness, somnolence, and headache). Others include gastrointestinal (e.g., constipation, nausea, diarrhea), generalized reactions (e.g., peripheral edema, fatigue, weight gain, and urinary tract infection). The risk of abuse at recommended dosing has been studied and shown to be limited to patients with a history of recreational polydrug abuse. There is an increased risk of abuse if given at doses 4–7× the recommended dose (e.g., 60 and 105 mg), though this risk is similar to pregabalin at therapeutic doses [77].

5. **Conclusions**

Overall, mirogabalin is a relatively new drug that appears to offer a new, effective and safe alternative for treatment in patients with DPNP and PHN and is currently approved in Japan. However, the number of published studies and trials is limited, and the drug is not yet approved by the FDA.

Carbamazepine

1. **Introduction**

Carbamazepine was discovered in the 1950s and became marketed and used in the 1960s for trigeminal neuralgia and epilepsy [78]. Carbamazepine exerts its effects by binding to the extracellular aspect of voltage-gated sodium channels resulting in channel inhibition [79]. It is given orally as there are no intravenous formulations available. Since the 1960s, carbamazepine has effectively treated chronic pain conditions such as PHN, trigeminal neuralgia, and central post-stroke pain [80–82].

2. **Pharmacodynamics and Pharmacokinetics**

It is primarily metabolized by hepatic CYP3A4 and CYP2C8 pathways into the inactive metabolite carbamazepine-10,11-trans dihydrodiol, which is then excreted via the kidneys [83]. Carbamazepine causes upregulation of hepatic enzymes, including CYP3A4 and CYP2C8, resulting in increased hepatic clearance with chronic use necessitating a dosage increase over time [78]. The increased expression of hepatic enzymes can also result in significant drug-drug interaction resulting in decreased effectiveness of other medications (e.g., warfarin, antipsychotics, and other antiepileptics).

3. **Dosing and Route of Administration**

RCTs of carbamazepine had large dose ranges between 100 to 2400 mg per day. Bioavailability has been estimated to be 75–80% [78]. [84]. There are no recommendations for dose adjustment in patients with renal insufficiency or hepatic impairment.

4. **Perioperative Uses**

To date, there is only one RCT that has evaluated carbamazepine in the setting of acute pain. An RCT of 40 patients compared carbamazepine 400 mg daily versus prednisolone 40 mg daily for 10 days to manage acute herpes zoster. At two months, 13 out of 20 (65%) who were treated with carbamazepine developed significant PHN compared to 3 out of 20 (15%) patients who were treated with prednisolone. No studies have evaluated the use of carbamazepine in the perioperative setting.

5. **Adverse Effects**

There is often wide inter-patient variability in terms of clinical response to carbamazepine. Patients with HLA-B*15:02 allele are at high risk of developing Stevens-Johnson syndrome (SJS) and/or toxic epidermal necrolysis (TEN) [85]. Because of these potentially serious adverse reactions to carbamazepine, it is recommended that patients from demographics of higher risk (e.g., Asian ancestry) undergo genetic testing [86, 87]. Patients may still develop SJS or TEN even if they test negative for the HLA-B*15:02 allele. Common adverse effects include nausea, vomiting, ataxia, dizziness, and drowsiness [88]. Carbamazepine also carries a black box warning for the possible development of aplastic anemia and agranulocytosis [89]. In addition, there have been case reports suggesting an association between carbamazepine and the development of hyponatremia and urinary retention [90, 91].

6. **Conclusions**

Carbamazepine has been shown to be effective for specific chronic pain conditions such as PHN and trigeminal neuralgia. However, no existing trials examine the use of carbamazepine in the acute pain setting. Because of variable inter-patient response, significant drug-drug interaction, and potential for serious adverse reactions, its role in the acute pain setting remains limited.

Phenytoin

1. **Introduction**

Phenytoin is an antiepileptic primarily used for tonic–clonic and partial seizures [92]. Additionally, it has anxiolytic and mood-stabilizing properties that allow its use for bipolar disorder and has also been repurposed for use in wound healing and trigeminal neuralgia [93]. While phenytoin has been used for chronic pain, including neuropathic pain, rheumatoid arthritis pain, and fibromyalgia, meta-analyses have not demonstrated significant efficacy [94, 95]. Limited studies exist regarding its perioperative use, though one study compared gabapentin to phenytoin as an analgesic regimen prior to craniotomy. The study administered either drug for 1 week prior to surgery and found that while gabapentin had a small but significant reduction in pain, patients who had phenytoin were significantly less sedated in the initial hours postoperatively [96, 97].

2. **Pharmacodynamics and Pharmacokinetics**

Phenytoin's antiepileptic effects come from its action on voltage-gated sodium channels [98]. It is a hydantoin derivative that stabilizes the sodium channel's inactive state, prolonging the neuronal refractory period [92]. This allows it to reduce the influx of Na^+ and Ca^{2+} into nerve cells to promote the release of GABA and prevent abnormal neuronal discharges. Phenytoin is metabolized by the liver and excreted by the kidneys. It has a large volume of distribution and is about 90% plasma protein bound [99]. The hepatic enzyme CYP2C9 is also involved in its metabolism and must be noted in patients who are poor or intermediate CYP2C9 metabolizers [100].

3. **Dosing and Route of Administration**

Given the lack of evidence in the perioperative use of phenytoin for pain, the doses for refractory trigeminal neuralgia and neuropathic pain seen in case reports will be described. Phenytoin can be administered orally, intravenously, or intramuscularly for seizure prophylaxis. Oral doses of phenytoin range from 100 to 300 mg per day (100 mg three times a day) for diabetic neuropathy, rheumatoid arthritis, cancer pain, and irritable bowel syndrome [99, 101, 102]. Studies and case reports have used the IV formulation for acute flareups of neuropathic pain, trigeminal neuralgia crisis, and refractory trigeminal neuralgia. One-time doses of 250 to 1000 mg or 15 mg/kg of phenytoin were given over 20–120 minutes or no more than 50 mg/minute. This dosing regimen approximates a fosphenytoin dose of 1 phenytoin gram equivalent (PE) or mean 14 mg/kg over 150 mg phenytoin equivalents [PE]/minute [103–105]. Fosphenytoin, a prodrug of phenytoin, is often preferred over phenytoin when administered intravenously for seizures, given its better tolerability at the injection site and lower risk of cardiac dysrhythmias [106]. However, given the many potential side effects of phenytoin, discussed below, the starting dose should be lower, especially for patients with hepatic impairment.

4. **Adverse Effects**

Phenytoin is known for its many side effects and narrow therapeutic index. Dose-related side effects include sedation, ataxia, dizziness, nystagmus, nausea, cognitive impairment, and rash. Phenytoin has been associated with life-threatening hypersensitivity reactions, including phenytoin-induced SJS and TEN. The genetic variations in cytochrome P450 (CYP)2C9 (CYP2C9) cause variability in drug-related phenotypes. The US Food and Drug Administration recommends considering avoiding phenytoin in patients who are positive for the HLA-B*15:02 allele, given the increased risk of SJS and TEN [100, 107]. Additional side effects include gingival hyperplasia, teratogenic effects, and hematologic toxicity, including leukopenia or pancytopenia [108].

5. **Conclusion**

Phenytoin has been used to treat neuropathic pain and trigeminal neuralgia, but its perioperative use is not well studied. Further studies are necessary to elucidate its validity but are limited by its broad range of negative side effects and narrow therapeutic range.

Lacosamide

1. **Introduction**

Lacosamide was first approved in 2008 as an adjunct for partial onset seizures and is being increasingly studied for treating neuropathic pain [109]. A multicenter randomized, double-blinded study showed that lacosamide had better pain relief than placebo in patients with peripheral diabetic neuropathy [110]. Another lab successfully generated a novel chimeric compound, (R)-7 r, derived from lacosamide that showed positive effects for treating neuropathic pain. A rat tibial nerve model was designed in which a single injection of the chimeric compound demonstrated a significant reversal of tactile hypersensitivity [111]. Lacosamide is a promising medication for pain, given its high bioavailability and favorable and predictable side effect profile.

2. **Pharmacodynamics and Pharmacokinetics**

Lacosamide is a functionalized amino acid. Unlike most antiepileptics that block voltage-dependent sodium channels to affect fast inactivation, lacosamide selectively binds to inactivated channels to enhance sodium channel slow inactivation. This stabilizes the hyperexcitable neuronal membranes and then inhibits neuronal firing and sodium channel availability [109, 112]. Lacosamide is metabolically degraded in the liver, with 40% excreted through the kidneys. It is effectively removed by hemodialysis in patients with end-stage renal impairment [109].

3. **Dosing and Administration**

Dosing for seizures ranges from 100 to 600 mg/day. Short and long-term phase 2 clinical trials have attenuated diabetic neuropathic pain with dosing between 100 and 400 mg/day [110, 113].

Lacosamide reaches peak plasma concentrations 0.5–4 hours after intake. It is rapidly absorbed irrespective of food intake due to its amphiphilic properties. It is water-soluble and lipophilic, allowing fast absorption, with the ability to cross the blood–brain barrier [114]. It has a high bioavailability (100%) with doses up to 800 mg. Therefore, no dosing adjustments are needed for mild-to-moderate renal impairment. However, the maximum dose for patients with severe renal impairment is 300 mg/day in the U.S. and 250 mg/day in Europe. For hepatic impairment, the maximum dose is 300 mg/day [115, 116]. Given its predictable pharmacokinetics, drug monitoring is not routine for lacosamide.

4. **Perioperative Uses**

To the best of our knowledge, no studies have been conducted applying lacosamide in a perioperative setting.

5. **Adverse Effects and Safety**

Lacosamide has minimal drug-drug interactions and has not been shown to clinically affect the CYP isoenzymes, except for inhibition of CYP2C19 in *vitro* studies [109, 117]. The most prominent side effects for doses of 200–400 mg/day are dizziness, headache, nausea, diplopia, vomiting, dyspepsia, somnolence, nasopharyngitis, and fatigue [118]. Given the few reports of cardiac dysrhythmias, care should also be taken in patients with cardiac disorders and conduction problems [119]. A small study showed that side effects could be minimized by increasing the frequency of oral dosing from two times daily to three times daily [120]. Another study demonstrated the safety of IV lacosamide infusions of 200–800 mg/day for. A multicenter, open-label inpatient trial enrolled 160 patients and showed that adverse events were similar but more frequent, though not severe, with doses >400 mg/day. Additionally, there was no significant increase in adverse events when administered in equivalent IV dosing over 10, 15, or 30 minutes [121].

6. **Conclusions**

While lacosamide has been a promising medication for neuropathic pain, no studies have demonstrated the utility of lacosamide in the perioperative setting. A retrospective analysis of patients with trigeminal neuralgia showed pain relief during a hospital stay in 77.8% of 63 patients receiving lacosamide infusions [122]. A case report also demonstrated immediate pain relief from chemotherapy-induced peripheral neuropathy with oral lacosamide [123]. These findings support the further study of lacosamide in the acute setting. Given its tolerable pharmacokinetic profile, lacosamide is an antiepileptic that is an attractive candidate for further studies for perioperative pain management.

Zonisamide

1. **Introduction**

Zonisamide is a sulphonamide drug first approved for use in the U.S. in 2000 as an adjunctive treatment of partial seizures [124]. Like other antiepileptics, it blocks sodium channels to inhibit the propagation of action potentials and is postulated to have analgesic benefits.

2. **Pharmacodynamics and Pharmacokinetics**

Zonisamide exerts its effects through various mechanisms. It prolongs the inactive phase of voltage-dependent sodium channels and reduces T-type calcium currents to prevent seizure discharges between cells [125, 126]. It also has been thought to alter the metabolism of dopamine, 5-hydroxytryptamine (5-HT), and acetylcholine [125, 127–129]. Other modes of action are its modulatory effect on GABA-mediated neuronal inhibition, weak inhibition of carbonic anhydrase, and inhibition of glutamate release [130–134].

Studies of oral zonisamide have demonstrated 100% bioavailability irrespective of food intake [135]. It is primarily metabolized in the liver with CYP3A4-mediated reduction and renally excreted [136].

3. **Dosage and Route of Administration**

Oral zonisamide doses usually range between 200 to 600 mg daily for seizure prophylaxis. Literature suggests dosing between 100 to 600 mg/day to treat diabetic neuropathy [137] and 200 mg for migraines [138].

4. **Perioperative Uses**

No studies have investigated the use of zonisamide in the perioperative setting.

5. **Adverse Effects**

Data pooling 848 patients from four placebo-controlled trials have demonstrated that zonisamide is well tolerated for treating epilepsy at doses of 200–600 mg/day [139].

Zonisamide's most prominent side effects are somnolence, dizziness, and anorexia. A long-term open-label extension study of 317 patients with a 3-year follow-up period demonstrated a good safety profile [140].

6. **Conclusion**

Zonisamide is unique from other antiepileptics due to its various modes of action. This provides a broad spectrum of activity, including the potential for treating perioperative pain. Given its safety and tolerability, zonisamide may be another antiepileptic with possible benefits that requires further study to determine its applicability in the perioperative setting.

GABA-Acting Drugs

1. **Introduction**

Drugs that enhance γ-aminobutyric acid (GABA) activity by interacting with postsynaptic GABAA receptors have long been used as hypnotics, sedatives, tranquillizers, and anticonvulsants. There has been a shift to a new group of drugs with GABAergic actions mediated through various mechanisms not directly involving the GABAA receptor, also for use as hypnotics, sedatives, tranquillizers, and anticonvulsants. Here we discuss the utility as an analgesic of some of these GABAergic drugs: Tiagabine, vigabatrin, and felbamate.

2. **Pharmacodynamics and Pharmacokinetics**

Tiagabine potently and specifically inhibits uptake of the inhibitory neurotransmitter GABA into astrocytes and neurons, ultimately classifying it as a re-uptake inhibitor [141]. Vigabatrin was designed to have a specific effect on brain chemistry by inhibiting the GABA-degrading enzyme, GABA transaminase, resulting in a widespread increase in GABA concentrations in the brain [142]. Felbamate's mechanism of action is more uncertain, but it is thought to act both as an NMDA inhibitor and potentiator of GABA (possibly via inhibition of GABA antagonist or enhanced GABA-elicited Cl^- currents). Overall, all three drugs have GABAergic effects with the exception of felbamate, which has NMDA antagonistic effects.

3. **Dosing and Administration**

Tiagabine has been shown to be an effective treatment for painful sensory neuropathy at low doses of 4–8 mg, though it did not have any impact on dull and deep pain [143]. One study compared tiagabine (max dose 24 mg/day) to gabapentin (max dose 2400 mg/day) for the management of chronic pain [144]. They found a significant reduction in pain with both drugs but a more remarkable improvement in sleep quality with tiagabine [145]. Vigabatrin has been used for infantile spasms and refractory complex partial seizures, but currently, data is limited for treating pain in humans (though previous studies have indicated possible utility for neuropathic pain or attenuating morphine tolerance in mice) [146–148]. Felbamate has been shown to act as an antihyperalgesic and antiallodynic (rather than analgesic) in rats- but there is limited data suggesting dosing for pain relief in humans [149].

4. **Perioperative Uses**

There is limited data on the use of vigabatrin, tiagabine, and felbamate for postoperative pain management. Clinical studies in humans are scarce, and more research is needed to determine their effectiveness and safety in perioperative pain management.

5. **Adverse Effects**

While all three drugs carry some degree of CNS side effect risk (e.g., drowsiness, dizziness, behavioral changes), some also have other notable risks. The use of Felbamate for example, significantly declined due to the risk of life-threatening adverse events (aplastic anemia, hepatic failure) not seen in pre-approval studies [144]. Vigabatrin carries a risk of peripheral visual field deficit and requires monitoring of vision along with signs of anemia [148]. These drugs also require close attention to hepatic and renal function to titrate dosing.

6. **Conclusions**

Currently, the mentioned GABA-acting drugs (tiagabine, vigabatrin, felbamate) have possible utility in seizure and spasm-related disorders, but there are limited human data regarding their utility to treat pain. These drugs' complex side effect profile also warrants caution when prescribing.

Key Takeaway Points

1. As a part of a multimodal analgesia regimen, gabapentin and pregabalin have been commonly used for perioperative pain management. Recent literature has shown that they offer minimal clinical benefits and potential adverse effects, thus more tailored use of these medications is recommended.
2. Traditional AEDs such as carbamazepine and phenytoin have been used for chronic pain conditions, however the data is limited for perioperative use due to their potential severe side effects.
3. Lacosamide, zonisamide, and GABA-acting drugs (tiagabine, vigabatrin, felbamate) have limited data regarding their utility in the management of acute pain, and more research is needed to determine their effectiveness and safety in this context.

References

1. Martinez V, Carles M, Marret E, Beloeil H, Regional A, Pain Committee of the French Society of A, et al. Perioperative use of gabapentinoids in France. Mismatch between clinical practice and scientific evidence. Anaesth Crit Care Pain Med. 2018;37(1):43–7.
2. Johansen ME. Gabapentinoid use in the United States 2002 through 2015. JAMA Intern Med. 2018;178(2):292–4.

3. Weinbroum AA. Non-opioid IV adjuvants in the perioperative period: pharmacological and clinical aspects of ketamine and gabapentinoids. Pharmacol Res. 2012;65(4):411–29.
4. Sills GJ. The mechanisms of action of gabapentin and pregabalin. Curr Opin Pharmacol. 2006;6(1):108–13.
5. Brown JT, Randall A. Gabapentin fails to alter P/Q-type Ca2+ channel-mediated synaptic transmission in the hippocampus in vitro. Synapse. 2005;55(4):262–9.
6. Bauer CS, Nieto-Rostro M, Rahman W, Tran-Van-Minh A, Ferron L, Douglas L, et al. The increased trafficking of the calcium channel subunit alpha2delta-1 to presynaptic terminals in neuropathic pain is inhibited by the alpha2delta ligand pregabalin. J Neurosci. 2009;29(13):4076–88.
7. Stewart BH, Kugler AR, Thompson PR, Bockbrader HN. A saturable transport mechanism in the intestinal absorption of gabapentin is the underlying cause of the lack of proportionality between increasing dose and drug levels in plasma. Pharm Res. 1993;10(2):276–81.
8. Su TZ, Lunney E, Campbell G, Oxender DL. Transport of gabapentin, a gamma-amino acid drug, by system l alpha-amino acid transporters: a comparative study in astrocytes, synaptosomes, and CHO cells. J Neurochem. 1995;64(5):2125–31.
9. Taylor CP, Angelotti T, Fauman E. Pharmacology and mechanism of action of pregabalin: the calcium channel alpha2-delta (alpha2-delta) subunit as a target for antiepileptic drug discovery. Epilepsy Res. 2007;73(2):137–50.
10. Piyapolrungroj N, Li C, Bockbrader H, Liu G, Fleisher D. Mucosal uptake of gabapentin (neurontin) versus pregabalin in the small intestine. Pharm Res. 2001;18(8):1126–30.
11. Gidal BE, Radulovic LL, Kruger S, Rutecki P, Pitterle M, Bockbrader HN. Inter- and intra-subject variability in gabapentin absorption and absolute bioavailability. Epilepsy Res. 2000;40(2–3):123–7.
12. Vollmer KO, von Hodenberg A, Kolle EU. Pharmacokinetics and metabolism of gabapentin in rat, dog and man. Arzneimittelforschung. 1986;36(5):830–9.
13. Highlights of prescribing information 2021 [Available from: https://labeling.pfizer.com/showlabeling.aspx?id=630. Accessed 11 June 2023
14. Yagi T, Naito T, Mino Y, Umemura K, Kawakami J. Impact of concomitant antacid administration on gabapentin plasma exposure and oral bioavailability in healthy adult subjects. Drug Metab Pharmacokinet. 2012;27(2):248–54.
15. Hurley RW, Cohen SP, Williams KA, Rowlingson AJ, Wu CL. The analgesic effects of perioperative gabapentin on postoperative pain: a meta-analysis. Reg Anesth Pain Med. 2006;31(3):237–47.
16. Hah J, Mackey SC, Schmidt P, McCue R, Humphreys K, Trafton J, et al. Effect of perioperative gabapentin on postoperative pain resolution and opioid cessation in a mixed surgical cohort: a randomized clinical trial. JAMA Surg. 2018;153(4):303–11.
17. Rupniewska-Ladyko A, Malec-Milewska M, Kraszewska E, Pirozynski M. Gabapentin before laparoscopic sleeve gastrectomy reduces postoperative oxycodone consumption in obese patients: a randomized double-blind placebo-controlled trial. Minerva Anestesiol. 2018;84(5):565–71.
18. Verret M, Lauzier F, Zarychanski R, Perron C, Savard X, Pinard AM, et al. Perioperative use of gabapentinoids for the management of postoperative acute pain: a systematic review and meta-analysis. Anesthesiology. 2020;133(2):265–79.
19. Seib RK, Paul JE. Preoperative gabapentin for postoperative analgesia: a meta-analysis. Can J Anaesth. 2006;53(5):461–9.
20. Wright R, Wright J, Perry K, Wright D. Preoperative pain measures ineffective in outpatient abdominal surgeries. Am J Surg. 2018;215(5):958–62.
21. Fabritius ML, Geisler A, Petersen PL, Nikolajsen L, Hansen MS, Kontinen V, et al. Gabapentin for post-operative pain management - a systematic review with meta-analyses and trial sequential analyses. Acta Anaesthesiol Scand. 2016;60(9):1188–208.
22. Dirks J, Fredensborg BB, Christensen D, Fomsgaard JS, Flyger H, Dahl JB. A randomized study of the effects of single-dose gabapentin versus placebo on postoperative pain and morphine consumption after mastectomy. Anesthesiology. 2002;97(3):560–4.

23. Grover VK, Mathew PJ, Yaddanapudi S, Sehgal S. A single dose of preoperative gabapentin for pain reduction and requirement of morphine after total mastectomy and axillary dissection: randomized placebo-controlled double-blind trial. J Postgrad Med. 2009;55(4):257–60.
24. Han C, Kuang MJ, Ma JX, Ma XL. The efficacy of preoperative gabapentin in spinal surgery: a meta-analysis of randomized controlled trials. Pain Physician. 2017;20(7):649–61.
25. Liu B, Liu R, Wang L. A meta-analysis of the preoperative use of gabapentinoids for the treatment of acute postoperative pain following spinal surgery. Medicine (Baltimore). 2017;96(37): e8031.
26. Yu L, Ran B, Li M, Shi Z. Gabapentin and pregabalin in the management of postoperative pain after lumbar spinal surgery: a systematic review and meta-analysis. Spine (Phila Pa 1976). 2013;38(22):1947–52.
27. Menda F, Koner O, Sayin M, Ergenoglu M, Kucukaksu S, Aykac B. Effects of single-dose gabapentin on postoperative pain and morphine consumption after cardiac surgery. J Cardiothorac Vasc Anesth. 2010;24(5):808–13.
28. Engelman DT, Ben Ali W, Williams JB, Perrault LP, Reddy VS, Arora RC, et al. Guidelines for perioperative care in cardiac surgery: enhanced recovery after surgery society recommendations. JAMA Surg. 2019;154(8):755–66.
29. Ong CK, Seymour RA, Lirk P, Merry AF. Combining paracetamol (acetaminophen) with nonsteroidal antiinflammatory drugs: a qualitative systematic review of analgesic efficacy for acute postoperative pain. Anesth Analg. 2010;110(4):1170–9.
30. Nelson G, Bakkum-Gamez J, Kalogera E, Glaser G, Altman A, Meyer LA, et al. Guidelines for perioperative care in gynecologic/oncology: Enhanced Recovery After Surgery (ERAS) society recommendations-2019 update. Int J Gynecol Cancer. 2019;29(4):651–68.
31. Wainwright TW, Gill M, McDonald DA, Middleton RG, Reed M, Sahota O, et al. Consensus statement for perioperative care in total hip replacement and total knee replacement surgery: Enhanced Recovery After Surgery (ERAS((R))) Society recommendations. Acta Orthop. 2020;91(1):3–19.
32. Najafi Anaraki A, Mirzaei K. The effect of gabapentin versus intrathecal fentanyl on post-operative pain and morphine consumption in cesarean delivery: a prospective, randomized, double-blind study. Arch Gynecol Obstet. 2014;290(1):47–52.
33. Moore A, Costello J, Wieczorek P, Shah V, Taddio A, Carvalho JC. Gabapentin improves postcesarean delivery pain management: a randomized, placebo-controlled trial. Anesth Analg. 2011;112(1):167–73.
34. Short J, Downey K, Bernstein P, Shah V, Carvalho JC. A single preoperative dose of gabapentin does not improve postcesarean delivery pain management: a randomized, double-blind, placebo-controlled dose-finding trial. Anesth Analg. 2012;115(6):1336–42.
35. Wilson RD, Caughey AB, Wood SL, Macones GA, Wrench IJ, Huang J, et al. Guidelines for antenatal and preoperative care in cesarean delivery: enhanced recovery after surgery society recommendations (Part 1). Am J Obstet Gynecol. 2018;219(6):523 e1–e15.
36. Joliat GR, Kobayashi K, Hasegawa K, Thomson JE, Padbury R, Scott M, et al. Guidelines for perioperative care for liver surgery: enhanced recovery after surgery (ERAS) society recommendations 2022. World J Surg. 2023;47(1):11–34.
37. Batchelor TJP, Rasburn NJ, Abdelnour-Berchtold E, Brunelli A, Cerfolio RJ, Gonzalez M, et al. Guidelines for enhanced recovery after lung surgery: recommendations of the Enhanced Recovery After Surgery (ERAS(R)) Society and the European Society of Thoracic Surgeons (ESTS). Eur J Cardiothorac Surg. 2019;55(1):91–115.
38. Huot MP, Chouinard P, Girard F, Ruel M, Lafontaine ER, Ferraro P. Gabapentin does not reduce post-thoracotomy shoulder pain: a randomized, double-blind placebo-controlled study. Can J Anaesth. 2008;55(6):337–43.
39. Doleman B, Heinink TP, Read DJ, Faleiro RJ, Lund JN, Williams JP. A systematic review and meta-regression analysis of prophylactic gabapentin for postoperative pain. Anaesthesia. 2015;70(10):1186–204.
40. Eipe N, Penning J, Yazdi F, Mallick R, Turner L, Ahmadzai N, et al. Perioperative use of pregabalin for acute pain-a systematic review and meta-analysis. Pain. 2015;156(7):1284–300.

41. Mishriky BM, Waldron NH, Habib AS. Impact of pregabalin on acute and persistent postoperative pain: a systematic review and meta-analysis. Br J Anaesth. 2015;114(1):10–31.
42. Peng PW, Wijeysundera DN, Li CC. Use of gabapentin for perioperative pain control—a meta-analysis. Pain Res Manag. 2007;12(2):85–92.
43. Debono B, Wainwright TW, Wang MY, Sigmundsson FG, Yang MMH, Smid-Nanninga H, et al. Consensus statement for perioperative care in lumbar spinal fusion: Enhanced Recovery After Surgery (ERAS(R)) Society recommendations. Spine J. 2021;21(5):729–52.
44. Araujo BLC. Perioperative use of gabapentinoids: comment. Anesthesiology. 2021;134(4):664.
45. Zhang J, Ho KY, Wang Y. Efficacy of pregabalin in acute postoperative pain: a meta-analysis. Br J Anaesth. 2011;106(4):454–62.
46. Parsons B, Tive L, Huang S. Gabapentin: a pooled analysis of adverse events from three clinical trials in patients with postherpetic neuralgia. Am J Geriatr Pharmacother. 2004;2(3):157–62.
47. Cavalcante AN, Sprung J, Schroeder DR, Weingarten TN. Multimodal analgesic therapy with gabapentin and its association with postoperative respiratory depression. Anesth Analg. 2017;125(1):141–6.
48. Deljou A, Hedrick SJ, Portner ER, Schroeder DR, Hooten WM, Sprung J, et al. Pattern of perioperative gabapentinoid use and risk for postoperative naloxone administration. Br J Anaesth. 2018;120(4):798–806.
49. Weingarten TN, Jacob AK, Njathi CW, Wilson GA, Sprung J. Multimodal analgesic protocol and postanesthesia respiratory depression during phase i recovery after total joint arthroplasty. Reg Anesth Pain Med. 2015;40(4):330–6.
50. Myhre M, Diep LM, Stubhaug A. Pregabalin has analgesic, ventilatory, and cognitive effects in combination with remifentanil. Anesthesiology. 2016;124(1):141–9.
51. Baidya DK, Agarwal A, Khanna P, Arora MK. Pregabalin in acute and chronic pain. J Anaesthesiol Clin Pharmacol. 2011;27(3):307–14.
52. Ben-Menachem E. Pregabalin pharmacology and its relevance to clinical practice. Epilepsia. 2004;45(Suppl 6):13–8.
53. Bockbrader HN, Radulovic LL, Posvar EL, Strand JC, Alvey CW, Busch JA, et al. Clinical pharmacokinetics of pregabalin in healthy volunteers. J Clin Pharmacol. 2010;50(8):941–50.
54. Lam DMH, Choi SW, Wong SSC, Irwin MG, Cheung CW. Efficacy of pregabalin in acute postoperative pain under different surgical categories: a meta-analysis. Medicine (Baltimore). 2015;94(46): e1944.
55. Randinitis EJ, Posvar EL, Alvey CW, Sedman AJ, Cook JA, Bockbrader HN. Pharmacokinetics of pregabalin in subjects with various degrees of renal function. J Clin Pharmacol. 2003;43(3):277–83.
56. Buvanendran A, Kroin JS, Della Valle CJ, Kari M, Moric M, Tuman KJ. Perioperative oral pregabalin reduces chronic pain after total knee arthroplasty: a prospective, randomized, controlled trial. Anesth Analg. 2010;110(1):199–207.
57. Burke SM, Shorten GD. Perioperative pregabalin improves pain and functional outcomes 3 months after lumbar discectomy. Anesth Analg. 2010;110(4):1180–5.
58. Baloch SR, Hashmi IA, Rafi MS, Wasim A, Mazar S, Malick N, et al. Role of pregabalin to decrease postoperative pain in microdiscectomy: a randomized clinical trial. Cureus. 2021;13(1): e12870.
59. Pesonen A, Suojaranta-Ylinen R, Hammaren E, Kontinen VK, Raivio P, Tarkkila P, et al. Pregabalin has an opioid-sparing effect in elderly patients after cardiac surgery: a randomized placebo-controlled trial. Br J Anaesth. 2011;106(6):873–81.
60. Joshi SS, Jagadeesh AM. Efficacy of perioperative pregabalin in acute and chronic postoperative pain after off-pump coronary artery bypass surgery: a randomized, double-blind placebo controlled trial. Ann Card Anaesth. 2013;16(3):180–5.
61. Fassoulaki A, Melemeni A, Tsaroucha A, Paraskeva A. Perioperative pregabalin for acute and chronic pain after abdominal hysterectomy or myomectomy: a randomised controlled trial. Eur J Anaesthesiol. 2012;29(11):531–6.

62. Ittichaikulthol W, Virankabutra T, Kunopart M, Khamhom W, Putarawuthichai P, Rungphet S. Effects of pregabalin on post operative morphine consumption and pain after abdominal hysterectomy with/without salphingo-oophorectomy: a randomized, double-blind trial. J Med Assoc Thai. 2009;92(10):1318–23.
63. Balaban F, Yagar S, Ozgok A, Koc M, Gullapoglu H. A randomized, placebo-controlled study of pregabalin for postoperative pain intensity after laparoscopic cholecystectomy. J Clin Anesth. 2012;24(3):175–8.
64. Cabrera Schulmeyer MC, de la Maza J, Ovalle C, Farias C, Vives I. Analgesic effects of a single preoperative dose of pregabalin after laparoscopic sleeve gastrectomy. Obes Surg. 2010;20(12):1678–81.
65. Jokela R, Ahonen J, Tallgren M, Haanpaa M, Korttila K. A randomized controlled trial of perioperative administration of pregabalin for pain after laparoscopic hysterectomy. Pain. 2008;134(1–2):106–12.
66. Chang SH, Lee HW, Kim HK, Kim SH, Kim DK. An evaluation of perioperative pregabalin for prevention and attenuation of postoperative shoulder pain after laparoscopic cholecystectomy. Anesth Analg. 2009;109(4):1284–6.
67. Bornemann-Cimenti H, Lederer AJ, Wejbora M, Michaeli K, Kern-Pirsch C, Archan S, et al. Preoperative pregabalin administration significantly reduces postoperative opioid consumption and mechanical hyperalgesia after transperitoneal nephrectomy. Br J Anaesth. 2012;108(5):845–9.
68. Derry S, Bell RF, Straube S, Wiffen PJ, Aldington D, Moore RA. Pregabalin for neuropathic pain in adults. Cochrane Database Syst Rev. 2019;1(1):CD007076.
69. Burgess J, Javed S, Frank B, Malik RA, Alam U. Mirogabalin besylate in the treatment of neuropathic pain. Drugs Today (Barc). 2020;56(2):135–49.
70. Chen EY, Beutler SS, Kaye AD, Edinoff AN, Khademi SH, Stoltz AE, et al. Mirogabalin as a novel gabapentinoid for the treatment of chronic pain conditions: an analysis of current evidence. Anesth Pain Med. 2021;11(6): e121402.
71. Tetsunaga T, Tetsunaga T, Nishida K, Misawa H, Takigawa T, Yamane K, et al. Short-term outcomes of mirogabalin in patients with peripheral neuropathic pain: a retrospective study. J Orthop Surg Res. 2020;15(1):191.
72. Dolphin AC. The alpha2delta subunits of voltage-gated calcium channels. Biochim Biophys Acta. 2013;1828(7):1541–9.
73. Domon Y, Arakawa N, Inoue T, Matsuda F, Takahashi M, Yamamura N, et al. Binding characteristics and analgesic effects of mirogabalin, a novel ligand for the alpha(2)delta subunit of voltage-gated calcium channels. J Pharmacol Exp Ther. 2018;365(3):573–82.
74. Brown K, Mendell J, Ohwada S, Hsu C, He L, Warren V, et al. Tolerability, pharmacokinetics, and pharmacodynamics of mirogabalin in healthy subjects: results from phase 1 studies. Pharmacol Res Perspect. 2018;6(5): e00418.
75. Kim JY, Abdi S, Huh B, Kim KH. Mirogabalin: could it be the next generation gabapentin or pregabalin? Korean J Pain. 2021;34(1):4–18.
76. Deeks ED. Mirogabalin: first global approval. Drugs. 2019;79(4):463–8.
77. Mendell J, Levy-Cooperman N, Sellers E, Vince B, Kelsh D, Lee J, et al. Abuse potential of mirogabalin in recreational polydrug users. Ther Adv Drug Saf. 2019;10:2042098619836032.
78. Tolou-Ghamari Z, Zare M, Habibabadi JM, Najafi MR. A quick review of carbamazepine pharmacokinetics in epilepsy from 1953–2012. J Res Med Sci. 2013;18(Suppl 1):S81–5.
79. Alrashood ST. Carbamazepine. Profiles Drug Subst Excip Relat Methodol. 2016;41:133–321.
80. Keczkes K, Basheer AM. Do corticosteroids prevent post-herpetic neuralgia? Br J Dermatol. 1980;102(5):551–5.
81. Killian JM, Fromm GH. Carbamazepine in the treatment of neuralgia. Use of side effects. Arch Neurol. 1968;19(2):129–36.
82. Leijon G, Boivie J. Central post-stroke pain–a controlled trial of amitriptyline and carbamazepine. Pain. 1989;36(1):27–36.
83. Puranik YG, Birnbaum AK, Marino SE, Ahmed G, Cloyd JC, Remmel RP, et al. Association of carbamazepine major metabolism and transport pathway gene polymorphisms and pharmacokinetics in patients with epilepsy. Pharmacogenomics. 2013;14(1):35–45.

84. Spina E, Pisani F, Perucca E. Clinically significant pharmacokinetic drug interactions with carbamazepine. An update. Clin Pharmacokinet. 1996;31(3):198–214.
85. Cheung YK, Cheng SH, Chan EJ, Lo SV, Ng MH, Kwan P. HLA-B alleles associated with severe cutaneous reactions to antiepileptic drugs in Han Chinese. Epilepsia. 2013;54(7):1307–14.
86. Adler NR, Aung AK, Ergen EN, Trubiano J, Goh MSY, Phillips EJ. Recent advances in the understanding of severe cutaneous adverse reactions. Br J Dermatol. 2017;177(5):1234–47.
87. Chung WH, Hung SI, Hong HS, Hsih MS, Yang LC, Ho HC, et al. Medical genetics: a marker for Stevens-Johnson syndrome. Nature. 2004;428(6982):486.
88. Koliqi R, Polidori C, Islami H. Prevalence of side effects treatment with carbamazepine and other antiepileptics in patients with epilepsy. Mater Sociomed. 2015;27(3):167–71.
89. Peselow ED, Clevenger S, IsHak WW. Prophylactic efficacy of lithium, valproic acid, and carbamazepine in the maintenance phase of bipolar disorder: a naturalistic study. Int Clin Psychopharmacol. 2016;31(4):218–23.
90. Hmouda H, Ben Salem C, Grira M, Slim R, Bouraoui K. Carbamazepine-induced urinary retention. Br J Clin Pharmacol. 2007;64(6):833–4.
91. Kaeley N, Kabi A, Bhatia R, Mohanty A. Carbamazepine-induced hyponatremia—a wakeup call. J Family Med Prim Care. 2019;8(5):1786–8.
92. Patocka J, Wu Q, Nepovimova E, Kuca K. Phenytoin—an anti-seizure drug: overview of its chemistry, pharmacology and toxicology. Food Chem Toxicol. 2020;142: 111393.
93. Keppel Hesselink JM. Phenytoin repositioned in wound healing: clinical experience spanning 60 years. Drug Discov Today. 2018;23(2):402–8.
94. McQuay H, Carroll D, Jadad AR, Wiffen P, Moore A. Anticonvulsant drugs for management of pain: a systematic review. BMJ. 1995;311(7012):1047–52.
95. Birse F, Derry S, Moore RA. Phenytoin for neuropathic pain and fibromyalgia in adults. Cochrane Database Syst Rev. 2012;2012(5):CD009485.
96. Türe H, Sayin M, Karlikaya G, Bingol CA, Aykac B, Türe U. The analgesic effect of gabapentin as a prophylactic anticonvulsant drug on postcraniotomy pain: a prospective randomized study. Anesth Analg. 2009;109(5):1625–31.
97. Vadivelu N, Kai AM, Tran D, Kodumudi G, Legler A, Ayrian E. Options for perioperative pain management in neurosurgery. J Pain Res. 2016;9:37–47.
98. Yaari Y, Selzer ME, Pincus JH. Phenytoin: mechanisms of its anticonvulsant action. Ann Neurol. 1986;20(2):171–84.
99. Richens A. Clinical pharmacokinetics of phenytoin. Clin Pharmacokinet. 1979;4(3):153–69.
100. Caudle KE, Rettie AE, Whirl-Carrillo M, Smith LH, Mintzer S, Lee MT, et al. Clinical pharmacogenetics implementation consortium guidelines for CYP2C9 and HLA-B genotypes and phenytoin dosing. Clin Pharmacol Ther. 2014;96(5):542–8.
101. Chadda VS, Mathur MS. Double blind study of the effects of diphenylhydantoin sodium on diabetic neuropathy. J Assoc Physicians India. 1978;26(5):403–6.
102. Vinik A. Clinical Review: use of antiepileptic drugs in the treatment of chronic painful diabetic neuropathy. J Clin Endocrinol Metab. 2005;90(8):4936–45.
103. Cheshire WP. Fosphenytoin: an intravenous option for the management of acute trigeminal neuralgia crisis. J Pain Symptom Manage. 2001;21(6):506–10.
104. McCleane GJ. Intravenous infusion of phenytoin relieves neuropathic pain: a randomized, double-blinded, placebo-controlled, crossover study. Anesth Analg. 1999;89(4):985–8.
105. Tate R, Rubin LM, Krajewski KC. Treatment of refractory trigeminal neuralgia with intravenous phenytoin. Am J Health Syst Pharm. 2011;68(21):2059–61.
106. DeToledo JC, Ramsay RE. Fosphenytoin and phenytoin in patients with status epilepticus: improved tolerability versus increased costs. Drug Saf. 2000;22(6):459–66.
107. Karnes JH, Rettie AE, Somogyi AA, Huddart R, Fohner AE, Formea CM, et al. Clinical Pharmacogenetics Implementation Consortium (CPIC) Guideline for CYP2C9 and HLA-B genotypes and phenytoin dosing: 2020 update. Clin Pharmacol Ther. 2021;109(2):302–9.

108. Kaplan YC, Demir O. Use of phenytoin, phenobarbital carbamazepine, levetiracetam lamotrigine and valproate in pregnancy and breastfeeding: risk of major malformations, dose-dependency, monotherapy versus polytherapy Pharmacokinetics and clinical implications. Curr Neuropharmacol. 2021;19(11):1805–24.
109. Cawello W. Clinical pharmacokinetic and pharmacodynamic profile of lacosamide. Clin Pharmacokinet. 2015;54(9):901–14.
110. Rauck RL, Shaibani A, Biton V, Simpson J, Koch B. Lacosamide in painful diabetic peripheral neuropathy: a phase 2 double-blind placebo-controlled study. Clin J Pain. 2007;23(2):150–8.
111. Park KD, Yang XF, Dustrude ET, Wang Y, Ripsch MS, White FA, et al. Chimeric agents derived from the functionalized amino acid, lacosamide, and the α-aminoamide, safinamide: evaluation of their inhibitory actions on voltage-gated sodium channels, and antiseizure and antinociception activities and comparison with lacosamide and safinamide. ACS Chem Neurosci. 2015;6(2):316–30.
112. Jo S, Bean BP. Lacosamide inhibition of Nav1.7 voltage-gated sodium channels: slow binding to fast-inactivated states. Mol Pharmacol. 2017;91(4):277–86.
113. Wymer JP, Simpson J, Sen D, Bongardt S, Group LSS. Efficacy and safety of lacosamide in diabetic neuropathic pain: an 18-week double-blind placebo-controlled trial of fixed-dose regimens. Clin J Pain. 2009;25(5):376–85.
114. Hovinga CA. SPM-927 (Schwarz Pharma). IDrugs. 2003;6(5):479–85.
115. EMA summary of product characteristics http://www.ema.europa.eu/docs/en_GB/document_library/EPAR__Product_Information/human/000863/WC500050338.pdf. Accessed 11 June 2023.
116. Highlights of prescribing information 2022 [updated 9.2022. Available from: https://www.ucb-usa.com/sites/default/files/2022-10/VIMPAT%20current%20COL-%20rev.%2009-2022_0.pdf. Accessed 11 June 2023
117. de Biase S, Valente M, Gigli GL, Merlino G. Pharmacokinetic drug evaluation of lacosamide for the treatment of partial-onset seizures. Expert Opin Drug Metab Toxicol. 2017;13(9):997–1005.
118. Beydoun A, D'Souza J, Hebert D, Doty P. Lacosamide: pharmacology, mechanisms of action and pooled efficacy and safety data in partial-onset seizures. Expert Rev Neurother. 2009;9(1):33–42.
119. Yadav R, Schrem E, Yadav V, Jayarangaiah A, Das S, Theetha KP. Lacosamide-related arrhythmias: a systematic analysis and review of the literature. Cureus. 2021;13(12): e20736.
120. Sattler A, Schaefer M, May TW, Rambeck B, Brandt C. Fluctuation of lacosamide serum concentrations during the day and occurrence of adverse drug reactions–first clinical experience. Epilepsy Res. 2011;95(3):207–12.
121. Krauss G, Ben-Menachem E, Mameniskiene R, Vaiciene-Magistris N, Brock M, Whitesides JG, et al. Intravenous lacosamide as short-term replacement for oral lacosamide in partial-onset seizures. Epilepsia. 2010;51(6):951–7.
122. Muñoz-Vendrell A, Teixidor S, Sala-Padró J, Campoy S, Huerta-Villanueva M. Intravenous lacosamide and phenytoin for the treatment of acute exacerbations of trigeminal neuralgia: a retrospective analysis of 144 cases. Cephalalgia. 2022;42(10):1031–8.
123. Ibrahim SA, Albany Z, Albany C. Significant response to lacosamide in a patient with severe chemotherapy-induced peripheral neuropathy. J Community Support Oncol. 2015;13(5):202–4.
124. Brodie MJ. Zonisamide as adjunctive therapy for refractory partial seizures. Epilepsy Res. 2006;68(Suppl 2):S11–6.
125. Okada M, Kaneko S, Hirano T, Ishida M, Kondo T, Otani K, et al. Effects of zonisamide on extracellular levels of monoamine and its metabolite, and on Ca2+ dependent dopamine release. Epilepsy Res. 1992;13(2):113–9.
126. Rock DM, Macdonald RL, Taylor CP. Blockade of sustained repetitive action potentials in cultured spinal cord neurons by zonisamide (AD 810, CI 912), a novel anticonvulsant. Epilepsy Res. 1989;3(2):138–43.

127. Kaneko S, Okada M, Hirano T, Kondo T, Otani K, Fukushima Y. Carbamazepine and zonisamide increase extracellular dopamine and serotonin levels in vivo, and carbamazepine does not antagonize adenosine effect in vitro: mechanisms of blockade of seizure spread. Jpn J Psychiatry Neurol. 1993;47(2):371–3.
128. Okada M, Hirano T, Kawata Y, Murakami T, Wada K, Mizuno K, et al. Biphasic effects of zonisamide on serotonergic system in rat hippocampus. Epilepsy Res. 1999;34(2–3):187–97.
129. Mizuno K. Effects of carbamazepine and zonisamide on acetylcholine levels in rat striatum. Nihon Shinkei Seishin Yakurigaku Zasshi. 1997;17(1):17–23.
130. Biton V. Clinical pharmacology and mechanism of action of zonisamide. Clin Neuropharmacol. 2007;30(4):230–40.
131. Masuda Y, Karasawa T. Inhibitory effect of zonisamide on human carbonic anhydrase in vitro. Arzneimittelforschung. 1993;43(4):416–8.
132. Masuda Y, Noguchi H, Karasawa T. Evidence against a significant implication of carbonic anhydrase inhibitory activity of zonisamide in its anticonvulsive effects. Arzneimittelforschung. 1994;44(3):267–9.
133. Mimaki T, Suzuki Y, Tagawa T, Karasawa T, Yabuuchi H. Interaction of zonisamide with benzodiazepine and GABA receptors in rat brain. Med J Osaka Univ. 1990;39(1–4):13–7.
134. Ueda Y, Doi T, Tokumaru J, Willmore LJ. Effect of zonisamide on molecular regulation of glutamate and GABA transporter proteins during epileptogenesis in rats with hippocampal seizures. Brain Res Mol Brain Res. 2003;116(1–2):1–6.
135. Kochak GM, Page JG, Buchanan RA, Peters R, Padgett CS. Steady-state pharmacokinetics of zonisamide, an antiepileptic agent for treatment of refractory complex partial seizures. J Clin Pharmacol. 1998;38(2):166–71.
136. Shah J, Shellenberger K, Canafax D. Zonisamide. Chemistry, biotransformation, and pharmacokinetics. In: Levy R, Mattson R, Meldrum B, EP, editors. Antiepileptic drugs. 5th ed. Philadelphia: Lippincott, Williams and Wilkins; 2002. p. 873–9.
137. Atli A, Dogra S. Zonisamide in the treatment of painful diabetic neuropathy: a randomized, double-blind, placebo-controlled pilot study. Pain Med. 2005;6(3):225–34.
138. Mohammadianinejad SE, Abbasi V, Sajedi SA, Majdinasab N, Abdollahi F, Hajmanouchehri R, et al. Zonisamide versus topiramate in migraine prophylaxis: a double-blind randomized clinical trial. Clin Neuropharmacol. 2011;34(4):174–7.
139. Brodie MJ, Ben-Menachem E, Chouette I, Giorgi L. Zonisamide: its pharmacology, efficacy and safety in clinical trials. Acta Neurol Scand Suppl. 2012;194:19–28.
140. Wroe SJ, Yeates AB, Marshall A. Long-term safety and efficacy of zonisamide in patients with refractory partial-onset epilepsy. Acta Neurol Scand. 2008;118(2):87–93.
141. Brodie MJ. Tiagabine pharmacology in profile. Epilepsia. 1995;36(Suppl 6):S7–9.
142. Ben-Menachem E. Mechanism of action of vigabatrin: correcting misperceptions. Acta Neurol Scand Suppl. 2011;192:5–15.
143. Novak V, Kanard R, Kissel JT, Mendell JR. Treatment of painful sensory neuropathy with tiagabine: a pilot study. Clin Auton Res. 2001;11(6):357–61.
144. Hanrahan B, Carson RP. Felbamate. StatPearls. Treasure Island (FL) 2023.
145. Todorov AA, Kolchev CB, Todorov AB. Tiagabine and gabapentin for the management of chronic pain. Clin J Pain. 2005;21(4):358–61.
146. Alves ND, de Castro-Costa CM, de Carvalho AM, Santos FJ, Silveira DG. Possible analgesic effect of vigabatrin in animal experimental chronic neuropathic pain. Arq Neuropsiquiatr. 1999;57(4):916–20.
147. Chavooshi B, Saberi M, Pournaghash Tehrani S, Bakhtiarian A, Ahmadiani A, Haghparast A. Vigabatrin attenuates the development and expression of tolerance to morphine-induced antinociception in mice. Pharmacol Biochem Behav. 2009;93(2):155–9.
148. Singh R, Carson RP. Vigabatrin. StatPearls. Treasure Island (FL) 2023.
149. Imamura Y, Bennett GJ. Felbamate relieves several abnormal pain sensations in rats with an experimental peripheral neuropathy. J Pharmacol Exp Ther. 1995;275(1):177–82.
150. Chou R, Gordon DB, de Leon-Casasola OA, Rosenberg JM, Bickler S, Brennan T, et al. Management of postoperative pain: a clinical practice guideline from the american pain

society, the american society of regional anesthesia and pain medicine, and the american society of anesthesiologists' committee on regional anesthesia, executive committee, and administrative council. J Pain. 2016;17(2):131–57.

151. Kim MP, Godoy C, Nguyen DT, Meisenbach LM, Chihara R, Chan EY, et al. Preemptive pain-management program is associated with reduction of opioid prescriptions after benign minimally invasive foregut surgery. J Thorac Cardiovasc Surg. 2020;159(2):734–44 e4.
152. Kurd MF, Kreitz T, Schroeder G, Vaccaro AR. The role of multimodal analgesia in spine surgery. J Am Acad Orthop Surg. 2017;25(4):260–8.
153. Yang HH, Wu TJ, Suh JD, Wang MB, Holliday MA, Beswick DM, et al. Postoperative gabapentin's effect on opioid consumption and pain control following sinonasal surgery. Laryngoscope. 2022.

Antidepressants in Perioperative Pain Management

Alexis M. Hanson, Ryan M. Rossos, Brittany Walker, Joseph Parks, and Nalini Sehgal

Abstract Opioids are the cornerstone therapy in perioperative pain management. Although opioids are strong analgesics, they are less effective in controlling neuropathic pain and are associated with multiple adverse effects such as delirium, sedation, respiratory depression, postoperative nausea and vomiting (PONV), constipation, and opioid induced hyperalgesia. Furthermore, opioids prescribed for postoperative pain control are associated with an increased risk of opioid use disorder (OUD). In order to limit opioid use and associated adverse effects, and optimize pain management, non-opioid analgesics have been studied as adjunctive therapies in perioperative pain management. The role of antidepressants is well established in chronic pain management. Recent studies have evaluated the efficacy of antidepressants in acute pain settings. This chapter will review antidepressants as adjunctive therapies in perioperative scenarios. We will discuss the pharmacology of tricyclic antidepressants (TCA), serotonin norepinephrine receptor inhibitors (SNRI), and serotonin selective reuptake inhibitors (SSRI) and then review salient studies on the use of antidepressants in a variety of surgical settings.

Keywords Perioperative pain · Postoperative pain · Antidepressants · SNRI · Duloxetine · TCA

A. M. Hanson · B. Walker
University of Wisconsin School of Medicine and Public Health, UW Madison, Madison, WI, USA
e-mail: almhanson@salud.unm.edu

B. Walker
e-mail: bcwalker4@wisc.edu

R. M. Rossos · J. Parks · N. Sehgal (✉)
Department of Orthopedics and Rehabilitation, University of Wisconsin School of Medicine and Public Health, UW Madison, Madison, WI, USA
e-mail: sehgal@rehab.wisc.edu

R. M. Rossos
e-mail: RRossos@uwhealth.org

J. Parks
e-mail: JParks@uwhealth.org

A. Abd-Elsayed and K. Schroeder (eds.), *Perioperative Pain Management*,
https://doi.org/10.1007/978-3-031-67648-2_38

1 Introduction

Current approaches to perioperative pain management predominantly rely on the administration of opioid analgesics. In surgical settings, opioids are often started preoperatively, continued postoperatively, and prescribed at discharge [1]. Although opioids are strong analgesics, perioperative use is associated with several adverse effects: one in ten patients experience nausea, vomiting, ileus, urinary retention, delirium, or respiratory depression postoperatively. In addition, a significant number of these patients continue with opioid use far beyond the anticipated duration required for return to a baseline pain level. In fact, it is estimated that 7.7% of previously opioid naïve patients continue to use opioids 1 year after surgery [2, 3]. Chronic opioid use is associated with frequent dose escalations, opioid dependence, opioid use disorder and decreased quality of life [4]. Furthermore, less than half of the patients administered opioids postoperatively report satisfactory pain relief. Over 75% of patients consuming opioids postoperatively continue to experience moderate, severe, or extreme pain [5]. The intensity of acute postoperative pain is a predictor for developing chronic postoperative pain and highlights the need for optimizing perioperative pain management [6].

The perception of pain and pain intensity can be reduced pharmacologically by various drugs that act on peripheral and central pain pathways. Nociceptive pain during surgery results from disruption and surgical trauma in soft tissues, bones, or internal organs. Neuropathic pain develops after direct nerve damage, during select surgeries, such as thoracotomy or inguinal hernia repair and is poorly controlled with routine perioperative opioid therapy [7]. Multimodal analgesia is advocated for the control of perioperative pain in an effort to simultaneously reduce the use of opioid analgesics and improve pain relief. Studies have demonstrated the efficacy of acetaminophen, NSAIDs, gabapentinoids in perioperative pain management. Several studies have investigated use of antidepressants in acute pain and perioperative pain. Serotonin noradrenaline reuptake inhibitors (SNRI) and tricyclic antidepressants (TCA), are first line therapy for neuropathic and chronic pain [7]. Antidepressants may improve patient satisfaction and quality of life following surgery, and reduce postoperative pain and risk of delirium. The preoperative treatment of preexisting psychiatric diseases, such as anxiety and depression, can improve outcomes. This chapter discusses role of antidepressants in perioperative settings.

2 Pharmacology of Antidepressant Drugs

Tricyclic Antidepressants

Tricyclic antidepressants (TCAs) provide therapeutic benefits by increasing the presynaptic concentration of monoamine neurotransmitters, serotonin and norepinephrine. Both serotonin and norepinephrine modulate endogenous analgesic mechanisms via descending inhibitory pain pathways in the brain and spinal cord. An increase in serotonin and norepinephrine increases descending inhibition of nociceptive input and improves pain relief.

TCAs are absorbed in the small intestine and undergo first pass metabolism in the liver. On entry into the systemic circulation, the drug is highly protein bound. TCA's are lipophilic and widely distributed throughout the body. The peak plasma concentration of TCA's is about 2–6 hours, with an elimination half-life of around 24 hours. TCA's are metabolized by cytochrome p450 oxidative enzymes in the liver.

TCAs are competitive antagonists on post synaptic histaminergic, muscarinic and alpha cholinergic receptors. Their ability to act on these different receptors leads to a wide variety of side effects. TCA's action on histamine receptors results in sedation. Dry mouth, constipation, blurred vision, urinary retention, represent common side effects of TCAs and are due to antagonistic effects on muscarinic and cholinergic receptors. Other anticholinergic effects of TCAs include tachycardia, altered mental status and ocular crisis in patients with narrow angle glaucoma. Sexual dysfunction, diaphoresis and tremor can occur with TCA's at therapeutic doses. At higher doses, TCAs lower seizure thresholds and should be avoided or used cautiously in patients with a history of seizure disorder.

A serious adverse effect of TCAs is their propensity to cause QT prolongation. QT prolongation increases the risk of arrhythmias, specifically ventricular tachycardia, which can potentially lead to cardiac arrest. TCA's should not be prescribed with other QT prolonging drugs. TCAs block alpha adrenergic receptors and can cause orthostatic hypotension. Individuals with preexisting postural hypotension or those prescribed antihypertensive medications are at elevated risk for hypotension. TCAs may also increase the risk of sudden death in patients with ischemic heart disease. In the absence of an underlying heart disease, patients on high doses (300 mg or more) may be at increased risk of sudden cardiac death.

Before initiating treatment with TCAs, a thorough history, review of systems, and family history should be obtained. Baseline screening laboratory tests include serum potassium to evaluate for hypokalemia. An EKG should be performed on individuals over the age of 40 with cardiac symptoms, and also in those taking other drugs with known QT prolonging action. TCAs should be avoided in individuals with a QT interval greater than 500 ms. Other relative contraindications to TCA administration are ischemic heart disease, heart failure, conduction disorder, and arrhythmias.

Due to multiple adverse effects, and risk of significant cardiac side effects TCA's are not suitable in perioperative settings and there is no study describing TCA use in perioperative settings.

Serotonin Norepinephrine Receptor Inhibitors

Serotonin Norepinephrine Reuptake Inhibitors (SNRIs) inhibit the reuptake of serotonin and/or norepinephrine by binding serotonin and norepinephrine transporters in CNS. This results in increased synaptic availability of 5-HT and norepinephrine and enhanced action of descending inhibitory pain pathways. SNRIs vary in their affinity for the serotonin receptor or norepinephrine receptor, for example duloxetine and venlafaxine have a greater effect on inhibiting serotonin reuptake whereas levomilnacipran and milnacipran are potent blockers of norepinephrine reuptake.

The pharmacokinetics of each SNRI vary depending on the specific drug. Duloxetine is well absorbed, has a half-life of 12–15 hours, and can be dosed once daily. It is tightly bound to proteins and undergoes extensive oxidative metabolism via CYP2D6 and CYP1A2. Hepatic impairment significantly alters duloxetine levels. Other SNRIs are less protein bound and renal excretion plays a larger role.

Duloxetine is a moderate inhibitor of hepatic cytochrome p450 enzyme CYP2D6 and can cause drug-drug interactions. Duloxetine should not be given with codeine, hydrocodone and oxycodone because duloxetine interferes with their metabolism and conversion to active metabolites. Duloxetine should not be taken with monoamine oxidase inhibitors or SSRI due to the potential for an increased risk of serotonin toxicity and hypertensive crisis. It is important to allow 14 days between discontinuation of one before starting the other. Duloxetine should not be prescribed to patients with hepatic insufficiency, liver disease or alcohol use disorder. Duloxetine, in addition to other SNRI drugs, requires dose adjustment in the setting of renal impairment.

The most common side effects of SNRIs include nausea, dizziness and diaphoresis. SNRIs and SSRIs enhance serotonergic tone, not just in the brain but throughout the body. Increased serotonergic activity in the gut is commonly associated with nausea, gastrointestinal upset, and diarrhea. GI adverse effects usually emerge early and tend to improve after 1 week. Increased serotonergic tone in the spinal cord and above is associated with decreased sexual function and interest. In addition, SNRIs may also have noradrenergic effects, including increased blood pressure and heart rate, and CNS activation such as insomnia, anxiety and agitation. Duloxetine is rarely associated with hepatic toxicity in patients with a history of liver damage. Discontinuation syndrome characterized by dizziness, paresthesia's, beginning 1 or 2 days after stopping the drug and persisting for 1 week or longer has been reported.

The effectiveness of SNRIs in various neuropathic pain syndromes varies, duloxetine is more effective in the treatment of neuropathic pain caused by root compression, venlafaxine is more appropriate for patients with spinal cord injury presenting with depression and/or nociceptive pain [8].

Serotonin Selective Reuptake Inhibitors

Serotonin Selective Reuptake Inhibitors are a class of antidepressants that exert their action by increasing serotonin levels in the nervous system.

SSRIs are well absorbed in the gastrointestinal tract and are primarily metabolized and eliminated in the liver. Their peak plasma levels are reached within one to eight hours. They bind to plasma proteins and their lipophilic characteristics allow them to be widely distributed throughout the body.

Some SSRIs, specifically fluoxetine, fluvoxamine, and paroxetine, are moderately potent inhibitors of hepatic cytochrome p450 enzymes. SSRI's can interfere with drugs metabolized by CYP-450 and are associated with multiple drug-drug interactions. SSRIs interfere with tamoxifen and its therapeutic effect. Furthermore, SSRIs interfere with the conversion of prodrug opioids, such as codeine, hydrocodone and tramadol, and reduce the analgesic effect and pain relief associated with their administration. SSRI increase intraoperative bleeding up to 2.5× and increase blood transfusions by 2-fold. The risk of bleeding is compounded when combined with NSAIDS, aspirin, warfarin, and other anticoagulants. A preoperative platelet function assay is advocated prior to major spine surgical procedures to protect against significant intraoperative blood loss, as serotonergic antidepressants (e.g., selective serotonin reuptake inhibitors) and bupropion can increase the likelihood of bleeding intraoperatively due to drug-induced platelet dysfunction [8]. SSRIs are contraindicated in patients consuming MAO inhibitors due to the risk of serotonin syndrome. Due to their selective receptor affinity, SSRIs have little effect on other receptors and therefore fewer side effects. However, they still can cause gastrointestinal distress, sexual dysfunction, and weight changes.

Currently one study has reported on perioperative use of SSRI's (escitalopram) as a component in a multimodal pain management regimen.

Antidepressants in Perioperative Settings

Orthopedic surgery: Chronic nociceptive and neuropathic pain are complications of emergency and elective orthopedic surgeries and opioids are the mainstay of perioperative and postoperative pain management. Neuropathic pain is, however, opioid resistant and difficult to treat. SNRI's have demonstrated efficacy in the treatment of chronic pain conditions including neuropathic pain. Several studies have investigated perioperative duloxetine in elective orthopedic spine and joint replacement surgeries (Table 1). In spine surgery, perioperative duloxetine increases time to rescue analgesia, decreases pain, decreases total opioid consumption, and decreases time to ambulation/maintains function [9–13]. No significant side effects were seen with duloxetine [11, 12]. Duloxetine is associated with superior quality of recovery in joint replacement surgery. TKA patients treated with duloxetine and opioid had similar outcomes in terms of pain control, function, and side effects [14, 15] Duloxetine may or may not influence persistent pain in TKA patients with central sensitization: Koh reported reductions in persistent pain following TKA [16], while Rienstra found duloxetine did not reduce postoperative chronic residual pain after TKA/THA [17]. In rotator cuff repairs, the duloxetine treated group did not experience any clinically meaningful pain reduction or reduced opioid consumption [18]. Escitalopram did not reduce pain upon ambulation 24 h after TKA in high pain catastrophizing patients [19]. In summary, duloxetine may be used as an adjunct treatment for postoperative analgesia and reducing opioid consumption.

Table 1 Summary of antidepressant administration in the setting of orthopedic surgery [9, 11, 19]

Name/Year/Study	Number of subjects	Drug/Dose	Pain diagnosis intended to treat	Outcomes
Govil, N. 2020 [9] Randomized double blind placebo controlled trial	96	Duloxetine: 30 mg daily for 2 days preoperatively, 60 mg on the day of surgery and for 2 days post-op, POD 3 and 4 30 mg daily (7 days total)	Postoperative pain after lumbar canal stenosis decompression	Significantly less overall morphine consumption, decreased time to ambulation, and increased time to rescue analgesia in duloxetine group
Branton, M. 2021 [11] Systematic review and meta-analysis of 5 randomized control trials	314	Duloxetine: 60 mg preoperatively and postoperatively; variable dosing	Postoperative pain after elective orthopedic surgeries (lumbar disc repair, laminectomy, fusion, TKA)	Decreased pain scores and significantly lower MME consumption in duloxetine groups
Lunn, T. H. 2015 [19] Randomized double blind placebo controlled trial	120	Escitalopram 10 mg or placebo daily from preanesthesia to postoperative day 6 in addition to a standardized analgesic regime	High pain catastrophizing TKA patients	Pain on ambulation 24 hours after TKA did not decrease but overall pain on ambulation and at rest was reduced from days 2–6 in escitalopram versus placebo group

Gynecologic surgery: At least four randomized controlled trials studied duloxetine in laparoscopic or abdominal gynecologic surgeries [20–22, 24]. Castro-Alves and Kassim reported duloxetine significantly improved postoperative pain, improved recovery, and reduced opioid use [20, 21]. A systematic review and met-analysis of 4 RCT suggests perioperative duloxetine significantly reduces post-op pain, decreases total analgesic consumption, and increases time to first analgesia request in patients undergoing laparoscopic gynecologic surgeries [23]. It is possible that the antidepressant effects of duloxetine may contribute to patient's perception of comfort and emotional wellbeing, thus resulting in improved pain control and quality of life peri-operatively. In contrast, two RCT [22, 24] found duloxetine did not reduce pain or need for opioid analgesia after laparoscopic or abdominal hysterectomy and there were significant adverse effects in the duloxetine treated group. The main adverse events associated with duloxetine treatment included nausea, vomiting, dry mouth, headache, and dizziness. A previous study determined that a preoperative combination of *dexamethasone* with duloxetine significantly reduced nausea and vomiting after surgery in comparison with duloxetine alone as a result of the anti-emetic effect of dexamethasone [21]. Current evidence on the efficacy of duloxetine in gynecologic surgeries is limited (Table 2) and large multicenter RCTs are needed to establish the efficacy and safety profile of duloxetine.

Thoracic surgery: Severe pain after thoracotomy results from activation of nociceptors (rib fractures, costovertebral joint dislocation, pleura irritation) and nerve damage (disruption of intercostal, phrenic and vagus nerves). Patients with post-thoracotomy pain take shallow breaths due to pain and are at a greater risk of atelectasis, hypoxemia, hypercapnia, and respiratory failure. There is one randomized, placebo controlled study that showed duloxetine administered 2 hours before and 24 hours after thoracotomy significantly reduced pain at rest and with activity, and

Table 2 Summary of antidepressant administration in the setting of gynecologic surgery [20–24]

Name/Year/Study	Number of subjects	Drug/Dose	Pain diagnosis intended to treat	Outcomes
Baradwan, S. 2022 [23] Systematic review and meta-analysis of 4 randomized control trials	244	Duloxetine (variable dosing) or placebo	Postoperative pain after laparoscopic gynecologic surgeries	Duloxetine group reported lower VAS pain scores, increased time to first analgesic request and decreased total analgesic consumption. No change in length of stay or side effects
Castro_Alves, I. J. 2016 [20] Randomized double blind placebo controlled	63	Duloxetine: 60 mg 2 hrs prior and 24 hrs postop	Perioperative pain after abdominal hysterectomy	Duloxetine group reported significantly better quality of recovery, less opioid use (1 mg versus 5.5 mg) No difference in nausea, vomiting or time to PACU discharge
Kassim, D. Y. 2018 [21] Randomized clinical trial	75	Duloxetine 60 mg + IV saline Duloxetine 60 mg + IV dexamethasone Placebo capsule + IV saline	Postop pain s/p laparoscopic gynecologic surgeries	Duloxetine 60 mg + IV Dexamethasone 0.1 mg/kg is more effective than Duloxetine 60 mg alone, 2 hrs preop, for improving pain, reducing rescue analgesia and PONV
Bastanhagh, E. 2020 [24] Randomized double blind placebo controlled	76	Duloxetine 60 mg prior to surgery (single dose)	Postoperative pain after abdominal hysterectomy	No significant differences in time to first opioid request or the number of opioids administered between groups. Increased side effects (nausea, vomiting) in duloxetine group
Takamaz, O. 2019 [22] Randomized control trial	80	Duloxetine: 2 doses of 60 mg or placebo 2 hours before and 24 hours after surgery	Postoperative pain and opioid use after laparoscopic hysterectomy	Perioperative duloxetine did not reduce pain, need for opioid analgesia, or hospital length of stay

Table 3 Summary of antidepressant administration in the setting of abdominal surgery [26–28]

Name/Year	Number of subjects	Drug/Dose	Pain diagnosis intended to treat	Outcome (pain levels decrease, opioid use decrease, etc.)
Abdominal surgery Nath, S. 2022 [26] Randomized control trial	60	Duloxetine 60 mg 2 hrs preoperatively	Postoperative pain after laparoscopic cholecystecomy	Duloxetine treated group had decreased total requirement for first and second rescue analgesics; decreased pain upto 12 hrs postoperatively
Abdominal surgery Hetta, D. F. 2021 [27] Randomized control trial	62	Duloxetine 60 mg 2 hrs preoperatively	Postoperative pain after major abdominal cancer surgery	Morphine consumption was reduced 48 hrs postop; Pain reduced during the first 24 hrs; Improved postop quality of recovery scores
Colorectal surgery Erdmann, T. 2022 [28] Randomized control trial	60	Duloxetine 60mg 2 hrs preop and 24 hrs postop	Postoperative pain after major colorectal surgery	Short-term duloxetine did not reduce total opioid consumption or VAS pain scores during the initial 48 hrs

reduced total opioid consumption in the first 48 hours [25]. There was no increase in the frequency of side effects, including nausea, vomiting, dizziness, headache, somnolence in the duloxetine treated group.

Abdominal surgery: Multimodal postoperative pain regimens and diminished reliance on opioid analgesics following abdominopelvic surgery have the potential benefit of better pain control, earlier oral diet initiation, reduced risk of developing postoperative ileus, improved activity tolerance, reduced postoperative complications, and/or reduced hospital length of stay. Perioperative duloxetine following colorectal and gastrointestinal surgeries was effective in 2 studies [26, 27] and no better than placebo in 1 study [28]. Overall, duloxetine is relatively safe following abdominopelvic surgeries and without significant immediate adverse effects (Table 3).

Mastectomy: Chronic post-mastectomy pain occurs in 20–68% women after radical mastectomy. It manifests as hyperalgesia and neuropathic pain around the surgical incision site. One study reported duloxetine 60 mg, 2 hours prior to mastectomy significantly reduced pain and postoperative morphine consumption [29] (Table 4).

Table 4 Summary of antidepressant administration in the setting of mastectomy surgery [29]

Name/Year	Number of subjects	Drug/Dose	Pain diagnosis intended to treat	Outcome (pain levels decrease, opioid use decrease, etc.)
Mastectomy Hetta, D. F 2020 [29] Randomized, placebo controlled trial	88	Duloxetine 30 mg, 60 mg or 90 mg 2 hrs preoperatively versus placebo	Postoperative pain after modified radical mastectomy	Decreased morphine consumption 24 hrs postoperatively, decreased pain at rest and with movement up to 8 hrs in 60 mg and 90 mg duloxetine cohorts; Longer recovery from anesthesia and sedation in 90 mg duloxetine group

3 Conclusion

Optimizing acute pain after surgery is essential for faster recovery, reducing complication in the immediate postoperative period, preventing chronic postsurgical pain and limiting long term opioid use. There is a high prevalence of persistent pain after surgery, especially in surgeries such as mastectomies, thoracotomies, and orthopedic procedures that have a high risk of evolving into chronic pain. Neuropathic pain from nerve injury may play a role in persistent postsurgical pain. Many patients who develop opioid use disorder, start with opioids prescribed to treat postsurgical pain. Post-surgical pain is the most prominent patient concern, and a high number of patients report high/very high anxiety levels about pain before surgery.

Antidepressants have a well-established role in chronic pain management. TCAs have sodium channel activity in addition to inhibiting serotonin and noradrenaline. Several studies have demonstrated the efficacy of amitriptyline and to lesser extent other TCA's in chronic pain and a variety of neuropathic pain conditions. TCA's, like amitriptyline, are associated with multiple significant adverse effects, including hypotension, tachycardia, urinary retention, and QT prolongation, which make TCA's a poor choice for perioperative pain management. SSRIs lack analgesic activity but have antidepressant action and may decrease the perception of pain by improving pain coping while reducing anxiety and depression. There is only one study by Lunn et al. [19] that demonstrated escitalopram was superior to placebo in decreasing overall postoperative pain with ambulation and at rest. A major disadvantage with SSRI's is a 2.5X elevated risk of intraoperative bleeding and a concurrent 2X increased risk of perioperative blood transfusion. SNRIs, including duloxetine and venlafaxine, have demonstrated efficacy in a variety of chronic pain conditions, including neuropathic pain. The efficacy of SNRIs in treating neuropathic pain is independent of antidepressant effects and the analgesic action occurs at lower doses. The majority of studies have demonstrated encouraging results with duloxetine in a variety of acute surgical pain scenarios. Duloxetine reduced pain at rest and with activity, reduced opioid consumption and quality of recovery. One study compared duloxetine to opioids and showed no difference in pain control, function, and side effects. There are a few studies that did not find duloxetine superior to placebo in acute postop pain. The most common side-effects associated with duloxetine are nausea, dry mouth, headache, constipation, dizziness, fatigue, insomnia, diarrhea, somnolence, and hyperhidrosis. However, at doses used peri-operatively, these side effects are rare.

Large multicenter randomized controlled trials are needed to establish the efficacy of duloxetine as an adjunct in acute postoperative pain. Future clinical trials should study opioid sparing effects of duloxetine in acute pain and its potential to prevent persistent postsurgical pain. Additionally future studies are needed to study other SNRI's in acute postoperative pain.

Key Takeaway Points

1. Duloxetine, an SNRI, has shown efficacy in the treatment of acute postoperative pain following a variety of surgical procedures. Several studies report that duloxetine reduces pain and opioid use while improving the quality of recovery. Duloxetine use may prevent the evolution of acute pain to persistent postsurgical pain, but this potential modality requires further investigation. Caution is advised in patients with hepatic and renal impairment.
2. TCA's are effective as antidepressants and analgesics in chronic pain. They are considered poor choices for the treatment of acute postsurgical pain due to significant and multiple adverse effects.
3. SSRI's may improve acute pain by improving mood and coping but are limited by an increased risk of bleeding due to their action on platelet function.

References

1. Neuman MD, Bateman BT, Wunsch H. Inappropriate opioid prescription after surgery. Lancet. 2019;393(10180):1547–57. https://doi.org/10.1016/S0140-6736(19)30428-3. PMID: 30983590; PMCID: PMC6556783.
2. Alam A, Gomes T, Zheng H, Mamdani MM, Juurlink DN, Bell CM. Long-term analgesic use after low-risk surgery: a retrospective cohort study. Arch Intern Med. 2012;172(5):425–30. https://doi.org/10.1001/archinternmed.2011.1827. PMID: 22412106.
3. Hollmann MW, Rathmell JP, Lirk P. Optimal postoperative pain management: redefining the role for opioids. Lancet. 2019;393(10180):1483–5. https://doi.org/10.1016/S0140-6736(19)30854-2. PMID: 30983573. (? Reject).
4. Hyland SJ, Brockhaus KK, Vincent WR, Spence NZ, Lucki MM, Howkins MJ, Cleary RK. Perioperative pain management and opioid stewardship: a practical guide. Healthcare (Basel). 2021;9(3):333. https://doi.org/10.3390/healthcare9030333. PMID: 33809571; PMCID: PMC8001960.
5. Gan TJ, Habib AS, Miller TE, White W, Apfelbaum JL. Incidence, patient satisfaction, and perceptions of post-surgical pain: results from a US national survey. Curr Med Res Opin. 2014;30(1):149–60. https://doi.org/10.1185/03007995.2013.860019. Epub 2013 Nov 15. PMID: 24237004.

6. Glare P, Aubrey KR, Myles PS. Transition from acute to chronic pain after surgery. Lancet. 2019;393(10180):1537–46. https://doi.org/10.1016/S0140-6736(19)30352-6. PMID: 30983589.
7. Finnerup NB, Kuner R, Jensen TS. Neuropathic Pain: From Mechanisms to Treatment. Physiol Rev. 2021;101(1):259–301. https://doi.org/10.1152/physrev.00045.2019. Epub 2020 Jun 25. PMID: 32584191.
8. Bayoumi AB, Ikizgul O, Karaali CN, Bozkurt S, Konya D, Toktas ZO. Antidepressants in Spine Surgery: A Systematic Review to Determine Benefits and Risks. Asian Spine J. 2019;13(6):1036–46. https://doi.org/10.31616/asj.2018.0237. Epub 2019 Aug 20. PMID: 31422644; PMCID: PMC6894961.
9. Govil N, Parag K, Arora P, Khandelwal H, Singh A; Ruchi. Perioperative duloxetine as part of a multimodal analgesia regime reduces postoperative pain in lumbar canal stenosis surgery: a randomized, triple blind, and placebo-controlled trial. Korean J Pain. 2020;33(1):40–47. https://doi.org/10.3344/kjp.2020.33.1.40. PMID: 31888316; PMCID: PMC6944370.
10. Hyer L, Scott C, Mullen CM, McKenzie LC, Robinson JS. Randomized double-blind placebo trial of duloxetine in perioperative spine patients. J Opioid Manag. 2015;11(2):147–55. https://doi.org/10.5055/jom.2015.0264. PMID: 25901480.
11. Branton MW, Hopkins TJ, Nemec EC. Duloxetine for the reduction of opioid use in elective orthopedic surgery: a systematic review and meta-analysis. Int J Clin Pharm. 2021;43(2):394–403. https://doi.org/10.1007/s11096-020-01216-9. Epub 2021 Jan 18. PMID: 33459948.
12. Bedin A, Caldart Bedin RA, Vieira JE, Ashmawi HA. Duloxetine as an analgesic reduces opioid consumption after spine surgery: a randomized, double-blind, controlled study. Clin J Pain. 2017;33(10):865–9. https://doi.org/10.1097/AJP.0000000000000471. PMID: 28002096.
13. Attia JZ, Mansour HS. Perioperative duloxetine and etoricoxibto improve postoperative pain after lumbar laminectomy: a randomized, double-blind, controlled study. BMC Anesthesiol. 2017;17(1):162. https://doi.org/10.1186/s12871-017-0450-z. PMID: 29197345; PMCID: PMC5712123.
14. Kim MS, Koh IJ, Sung YG, Park DC, Na JW, In Y. Preemptive duloxetine relieves postoperative pain and lowers wound temperature in centrally sensitized patients undergoing total knee arthroplasty: a randomized, double-blind, placebo-controlled trial. J Clin Med. 2021;10(13):2809. https://doi.org/10.3390/jcm10132809. PMID: 34202314; PMCID: PMC8269433.
15. Kim MS, Koh IJ, Choi KY, Yang SC, In Y. Efficacy of duloxetine compared with opioid for postoperative pain control following total knee arthroplasty. PLoS One. 2021;16(7):e0253641. https://doi.org/10.1371/journal.pone.0253641. PMID: 34214098; PMCID: PMC8253394.
16. Koh IJ, Kim MS, Sohn S, Song KY, Choi NY, In Y. Duloxetine reduces pain and improves quality of recovery following total knee arthroplasty in centrally sensitized patients: a prospective, randomized controlled study. J Bone Joint Surg Am. 2019;101(1):64–73. https://doi.org/10.2106/JBJS.18.00347. PMID: 30601417.
17. Rienstra W, Blikman T, Dijkstra B, Stewart R, Zijlstra W, van Raaij T, Ten Hagen A, Bulstra S, Stevens M, van den Akker-Scheek I. Effect of preoperative duloxetine treatment on postoperative chronic residual pain after total hip or knee arthroplasty: a randomised controlled trial. BMJ Open. 2021;11(11):e052944. https://doi.org/10.1136/bmjopen-2021-052944. PMID: 34732491; PMCID: PMC8572398.
18. Su P, Pang L, Li S, Sun W, Zhao Y, Fu W, Li J, Tang X. Evaluation of analgesic efficacy and opioid-sparing effect of duloxetine after arthroscopic rotator cuff repair: a randomized clinical trial. Clin J Pain. 2022;38(5):328–333. https://doi.org/10.1097/AJP.0000000000001032. PMID: 35413023.
19. Lunn TH, Frokjaer VG, Hansen TB, Kristensen PW, Lind T, Kehlet H. Analgesic effect of perioperative escitalopram in high pain catastrophizing patients after total knee arthroplasty: a randomized, double-blind, placebo-controlled trial. Anesthesiology. 2015;122(4):884–94. https://doi.org/10.1097/ALN.0000000000000597. PMID: 25782644.
20. Castro-Alves LJ, Oliveira de Medeiros AC, Neves SP, Carneiro de Albuquerque CL, Modolo NS, De Azevedo VL, De Oliveira GS Jr. Perioperative duloxetine to improve postoperative

recovery after abdominal hysterectomy: a prospective, randomized, double-blinded, placebo-controlled study. Anesth Analg. 2016;122(1):98–104. https://doi.org/10.1213/ANE.0000000000000971. PMID: 26421810.

21. Kassim DY, Esmat IM, Elgendy MA. Impact of duloxetine and dexamethasone for improving postoperative pain after laparoscopic gynecological surgeries: a randomized clinical trial. Saudi J Anaesth. 2018;12(1):95–102. https://doi.org/10.4103/sja.SJA_519_17. PMID: 29416464; PMCID: PMC5789514.
22. Takmaz O, Bastu E, Ozbasli E, Gundogan S, Karabuk E, Kocyigit M, Dede S, Naki M, Kose F, Gungor M. Perioperative duloxetine for pain management after laparoscopic hysterectomy: a randomized placebo-controlled trial. J Minim Invasive Gynecol. 2020;27(3):665–72. https://doi.org/10.1016/j.jmig.2019.04.028. Epub 2019 Aug 30. PMID: 31476481.
23. Baradwan S, Alshahrani MS, Alkhamis WH, Allam HS, AlSghan R, Ghazi A, Ragab B, Elmazzaly SMM, Aboshama RA, Ismail RA, Dahshan SA, Al-Touny AA, Daghash NH, Abdelhakim AM, Abbas AM, Fouda AA, Ezzat Abdelfattah L. Preoperative duloxetine on postoperative pain after laparoscopic gynecological surgeries: a systematic review and meta-analysis of randomized controlled trials. J Gynecol Obstet Hum Reprod. 2022;51(3):102305. https://doi.org/10.1016/j.jogoh.2021.102305. Epub 2021 Dec 31. PMID: 34974147.
24. Bastanhagh E, Zamiri F, Samimi Sadeh S, Adabi K, Pourfakhr P. Effect of preoperative duloxetine on opioid consumption in women undergoing abdominal hysterectomy: a randomized, double-blinded, placebo-controlled trial. Anesth Pain Med. 2020;10(5):e103729. https://doi.org/10.5812/aapm.103729. PMID: 34150561; PMCID: PMC8207876.
25. Abdelghafar EM, Othman AH, Elrawas MM, Kilany AM, Shaker EH. The role of duloxetine in reducing opioid consumption after thoracotomy: a prospective, randomized, double-blinded, placebo-controlled pilot trial. Minerva Anestesiol. 2022;88(10):780–8. https://doi.org/10.23736/S0375-9393.22.16277-2. Epub 2022 Apr 5. PMID: 35381839.
26. Nath S, Saha A, Srivastava A. Evaluating the effect of duloxetine premedication on postoperative analgesic requirement in patients undergoing laparoscopic cholecystectomies: a prospective, randomized, double-blinded, placebo-controlled study. Clin J Pain. 2022;38(8):528–35. https://doi.org/10.1097/AJP.0000000000001052. PMID: 35696698.
27. Hetta DF, Elgalaly NA, Mohammad MAF. The efficacy of preoperative duloxetine in patients undergoing major abdominal cancer surgery: a randomized controlled trial. Clin J Pain. 2021;37(12):908–13. https://doi.org/10.1097/AJP.0000000000000983. PMID: 34757343.
28. Erdmann TR, Gerber MT, Gaspareto PB, de Oliveira Filho GR. The effects of a short-term perioperative duloxetine treatment on post-colectomy pain: a randomized, controlled clinical trial. J Clin Anesth. 2022;82:110948. https://doi.org/10.1016/j.jclinane.2022.110948. Epub 2022 Aug 11. PMID: 35963028.
29. Hetta DF, Elgalaly NA, Hetta HF, Fattah Mohammad MA. Preoperative duloxetine to improve acute pain and quality of recovery in patients undergoing modified radical mastectomy: a dose-ranging randomized controlled trial. J Clin Anesth. 2020;67:110007. https://doi.org/10.1016/j.jclinane.2020.110007. Epub 2020 Aug 22. PMID: 32847776.

NMDA-Receptor Antagonists in Perioperative Pain Management

Jeffrey J. Mojica, Deepti Harshavardhana, Aaron Ocker, Kevin Min, and Eric S. Schwenk

Abstract The N-methyl-D-aspartate (NMDA)-receptor plays a central role in the establishment of chronic pain, central sensitization, and other detrimental pain-related processes. As a result, NMDA-receptor antagonists, such as ketamine, magnesium, and methadone, have garnered significant attention for their therapeutic potential. These medications have been shown to produce profound analgesia and reduce opioid consumption following surgery. In this chapter, we discuss the unique pharmacologic properties of NMDA-receptor antagonists and how they can be best utilized for perioperative pain management.

Keywords Perioperative pain management · Central sensitization · Ketamine · Magnesium · Methadone · Opioid-sparing analgesia

1 Introduction

Despite advances in perioperative care over the past several decades, poorly controlled pain remains a challenge. In a survey of surgical patients, 86% of patients reported postoperative pain and close to 75% rated the pain as moderate or extreme [1]. Alternatives to opioids, particularly in the setting of the opioid epidemic, are

J. J. Mojica · D. Harshavardhana · A. Ocker · K. Min · E. S. Schwenk (✉)
Department of Anesthesiology and Perioperative Medicine, Sidney Kimmel Medical College at Thomas Jefferson University, Philadelphia, PA, USA
e-mail: eric.schwenk@jefferson.edu

J. J. Mojica
e-mail: Jeffrey.mojica@jefferson.edu

D. Harshavardhana
e-mail: deepti.harshavardhana@jefferson.edu

A. Ocker
e-mail: aaronocker84@gmail.com

K. Min
e-mail: kevin.min@jefferson.edu

A. Abd-Elsayed and K. Schroeder (eds.), *Perioperative Pain Management*,
https://doi.org/10.1007/978-3-031-67648-2_39

desirable and N-methyl-D-aspartate (NMDA)-receptor antagonists represent one such class of medications. From a conceptual standpoint, NMDA-receptor antagonists are a logical selection given the evidence that the NMDA receptor appears to be involved in opioid-induced hyperalgesia [2] and central as well as peripheral sensitization, all of which can contribute to increased perioperative pain levels. Indeed, drugs that interact with the NMDA receptor have been the subject of focus in recent years, with ketamine [3, 4], magnesium, and methadone having received the bulk of the attention. In this chapter we summarize the current state of evidence supporting NMDA receptor antagonists in the management of perioperative pain with particular emphasis on recently published studies and we also share our experience using these agents.

2 NMDA Receptor Overview

The NMDA receptor plays a critical role in the induction and maintenance of chronic pain as well as the development of opioid-induced hyperalgesia and opioid tolerance [5–7]. These processes occur because of NMDA-receptor-mediated synaptic plasticity at peripheral, central, and supraspinal locations [5, 7].

In its resting state, the NMDA receptor ion channel is blocked by magnesium ions and requires both glutamate binding and persistent neuronal depolarization to become activated. Persistent depolarization occurs in states of inflammation, tissue injury, or nerve damage. Following its activation, an influx of calcium activates intracellular pathways that lead to central sensitization [8]. Central sensitization is a neuroplastic phenomenon that results in an increased responsiveness of nociceptive neurons in the CNS to normal or subthreshold input [8]. Clinically, these cellular changes manifest as allodynia, hyperalgesia, and secondary hyperalgesia [8].

3 Subanesthetic Ketamine

Background

Ketamine is a general anesthetic and potent analgesic that was first synthesized in the 1960s and marketed as a safer alternative to phencyclidine [9]. Ketamine is described as a dissociative anesthetic because it produces a unique state of consciousness where patients appear to be "disconnected from their environment" [9]. Yet, despite having a favorable cardiovascular and respiratory profile, its use as an anesthetic is limited by its unpleasant psychomimetic effects, particularly vivid hallucinations and emergence delirium. In recent years, intravenous ketamine has seen a resurgence in popularity as a non-opioid analgesic for perioperative pain medicine when used at subanesthetic doses. A 2018 Cochrane review on perioperative ketamine use showed that ketamine reduced morphine consumption and patients experienced less pain and less side effects like nausea and vomiting [10]. Recent national guidelines have recommended subanesthetic ketamine for several acute and chronic pain conditions [11, 12].

Pharmacology

Ketamine interacts with a wide range of receptors and cell signaling pathways to produce analgesia, anesthesia, antidepressant and psychomimetic effects [13]. In acute pain, its mechanism of action is thought to be related to its reversible, non-competitive antagonism of the NMDA receptor [14]. Conversely, reversal of central sensitization and modulation of descending pain pathways is believed to be its mechanism of action in the treatment of chronic pain [9]. Ketamine also exerts antinociceptive effects via non-NMDA receptors, including opioid, nicotinic, muscarinic cholinergic, and γ-aminobutyric acid A (GABA-A) receptors [13]. Ketamine's half-life is about 2.3 hours and it is metabolized to norketamine, hydroxynorketamine, and dehydronorketamine by the P450 system in the liver. It is excreted renally [15].

Dosing and Administration

Ketamine is available in a variety of formulations but has most commonly been administered as an intravenous (IV) bolus and/or continuous infusion in the perioperative setting. The analgesic effects of ketamine occur at plasma concentrations between 100 and 200 ng/mL, which is well below the plasma concentrations of 9000–2,5000 ng/mL that occur following an anesthetic induction dose of ketamine [16, 17]. "Subanesthetic ketamine" is used to describe the dosing range used in acute pain management. Recent consensus guidelines on the use of ketamine in acute pain management has defined subanesthetic ketamine as bolus doses that do not exceed 0.35 mg/kg and infusions that does not exceed 1 mg/kg/hr (Table 1) [11].

At our institution, ketamine is usually administered as a pre-incision, intraoperative bolus between 0.1 and 0.3 mg/kg, followed by a continuous infusion starting at 10–20 mg/hr. Patients who may benefit from the continuation of ketamine for postoperative analgesia are followed by our acute pain management service and slowly titrated to a maximum dosage of 1 mg/kg/hr based on analgesic response and adverse effects. Boluses are minimized because of the risk of adverse effects in awake patients. A clonidine transdermal patch or oral clonidine is given to all patients receiving ketamine whose blood pressure will tolerate it in order to minimize the frequency and severity of adverse effects [18]. Patients who only receive intraoperative ketamine do not receive clonidine.

Table 1 Perioperative indications, contraindications, and suggested dosing for subanesthetic ketamine in acute pain

Indications	1. Surgical procedures associated with moderate to severe pain 2. Opioid-tolerant surgical patients 3. Opioid-tolerant non-surgical patients experiencing an acute on chronic pain exacerbation 4. Patients at risk for opioid-related adverse effects or those with obstructive sleep apnea
Dosing	Bolus: 0.35–0.5 mg/kg Infusion: $\leq$ 1 mg/kg/hr
Relative contraindications	1. Poorly controlled cardiovascular disease 2. Poorly controlled psychiatric disease 3. Moderate to severe liver disease 4. Elevated intracranial pressure or intraocular pressure 5. Pregnancy

IV: intravenous; NMDA: N-methyl-D-aspartate

Perioperative Use

Subanesthetic ketamine has profound analgesic effects and is recommended in patients undergoing surgeries in which the severity of postoperative pain is expected to range from moderate to severe [11]. This includes upper abdominal surgery, thoracic surgery, and major orthopedic surgeries (spine and limb). In a meta-analysis of 70 randomized controlled trials (RCTs), Laskowski et. al. found that patients who received intravenous ketamine experienced less pain and consumed fewer opioids [19]. These effects were independent of the timing of administration (preemptively, intraoperatively, or postoperatively) and method of administration (bolus, infusion or patient-controlled analgesia) [19].

The opioid-sparing and analgesic benefits of ketamine have been observed in opioid-tolerant surgical patients, although more studies are needed. Loftus and colleagues found that a pre-incision bolus of 0.5 mg/kg followed by an intraoperative infusion of 0.6 mg/kg/hr improved analgesia and reduced opioid consumption for 48 hours and some improvements were observed up to 6 weeks postoperatively [20]. In another study of 147 opioid-dependent spine surgery patients, Nielsen et al. found that daily opioid usage rates were lower at 1 year postoperatively in the ketamine group [21]. Additional clinical trials are still needed, especially in opioid-tolerant populations. Many trials have excluded these patients and we believe that is why there has been so much inconsistency in ketamine studies. In our experience, opioid-tolerant patients benefit the most from subanesthetic ketamine, mirroring the results of Loftus et al., Nielsen et al., and others who have reached similar conclusions.

Because of the involvement of the NMDA receptor in opioid tolerance and opioid-induced hyperalgesia [22, 23], ketamine may be the closest thing to an ideal analgesic that currently exists for these patients. We frequently employ intra- and postoperative ketamine infusions managed by our acute pain service for major surgery in patients who are opioid tolerant or have an opioid use disorder. A recent case control study found that opioid-tolerant patients experienced fewer infusion-limiting adverse effects of ketamine than opioid-naïve patients, which further reinforces the notion that ketamine works differently in such patients [24]. If possible, we recommend starting the infusion intraoperatively and continuing it postoperatively to maximize benefits. While the study by Loftus et al. found benefits to intraoperative-only use, this strategy is most appropriate when ketamine use outside of the operating room is restricted by the institution [20].

Contraindications, Adverse Effects, and Safety Considerations

Much of the literature regarding ketamine's contraindications is based on its use as a general anesthetic. Whether or not the same contraindications are relevant in the lower, subanesthetic dosing range is less certain [11]. Nevertheless, most experts urge caution in patients with schizophrenia, poorly controlled cardiovascular disease, moderate to severe hepatic dysfunction, and in pregnancy [11].

Ketamine can cause an elevation in liver enzyme levels. Noppers et al. observed that a second exposure 3 weeks following a 100-hours treatment in complex regional pain syndrome type 1 patients caused liver enzymes to triple [25]. Upon termination of the infusion, liver enzymes returned to normal within 3 months [25]. The mechanism of liver injury is not well understood, but possible factors include a decrease in hepatic oxygen delivery, increased lipid peroxidation with the formation of free radicals, and allergic hepatitis [9]. Variable patterns of liver enzyme elevation have been noted, including increases to transaminases, alkaline phosphatase, and bilirubin, and most cases have been reversible upon cessation of ketamine [26, 27].

The most common adverse effects of subanesthetic ketamine include hallucinations, blurry vision, sedation, and nausea and vomiting [11]. The psychomimetic effects of ketamine include hallucinations, visual disturbances, unpleasant dreams, and dysphoria. Reviews of perioperative studies have been inconsistent as to whether these occur more frequently in the ketamine group versus the placebo group [19, 28]. It is interesting to note that while ketamine has been reported to cause nausea and vomiting, reviews have found that the overall incidence of postoperative nausea and vomiting (PONV) was lower in patients who received ketamine [10]. This may be a result of a decrease in opioid use in the ketamine groups. Most adverse effects decrease rapidly after discontinuation and may be attenuated by the use benzodiazepines or alpha-2 agonists such as clonidine [11, 12]. In our practice, patients who have ketamine continued beyond the intraoperative period receive a clonidine patch unless contraindicated to minimize ketamine's psychomimetic effects.

Monitoring outside of the operating room for patients receiving ketamine infusions will vary by institution but may be influenced by patient disease or ketamine dose. Some institutions mandate intensive care unit (ICU) monitoring for all patients receiving ketamine because of its classification as an anesthetic agent but this restriction has eased in some places. The 2018 American Society of Regional Anesthesia and Pain Medicine guidelines for ketamine for chronic pain did not specify exact monitoring requirements for infusions below 1 mg/kg/h but stated that a "monitored setting" with immediate availability of resuscitative personnel and equipment be used for higher doses [12]. We have safely used subanesthetic ketamine with low adverse effect rates for over 20 years through the use of trained acute pain nurses following protocols and in this context ICU-level care is not needed [29]. For institutions just starting a new ketamine program, it may be prudent to use low doses and minimize or restrict titration until staff members gain familiarity and comfort with the drug. An example of introducing ketamine to a hospital was described in a publication by Porter et al [30]. Suggested dosing as well as indications and contraindications for subanesthetic ketamine are shown in Table 1.

4 Methadone

Methadone is a long-acting synthetic opioid with unique pharmacologic properties that make it useful for treating acute postoperative pain in specific settings [31]. It is a potent μ-opioid-receptor agonist, NMDA-receptor antagonist, and serotonin and norepinephrine reuptake inhibitor (SNRI) [32]. At doses greater than 20 mg, a single intraoperative dose of IV methadone has the potential to provide stable levels of analgesia for approximately 24–36 hours [33, 34]. It has a rapid onset of action (8 minutes) that is comparable to the 5–6 minutes onset of fentanyl and sufentanil [34]. Its μ-opioid receptor agonist activity makes it effective for nociceptive postoperative pain. As a NMDA-receptor antagonist, it is effective for treating neuropathic pain and may also protect against the development of opioid tolerance, opioid-induced hyperalgesia, and chronic postsurgical pain [31]. As a SNRI, it can also improve mood and the emotional-affective dimension of pain [35, 36]. As a result of these properties, it has been extensively studied in the perioperative period for various types of surgical procedures. The intraoperative use of methadone has been shown to reduce postoperative pain, opioid consumption, and improve patient satisfaction without increasing the risk of opioid-related adverse effects [37]. There is also evidence that methadone may reduce hyperalgesia and central sensitization [38].

Pharmacologic Considerations

Methadone undergoes substantial and rapid distribution to the peripheral compartment due to its lipophilic properties [39]. As a result, a single IV dose of methadone undergoes a rapid decrease in blood plasma concentration after peak concentration is reached. At doses $\leq$ 10 mg, redistribution is responsible for the short duration of analgesia, and would only be expected to last approximately 30 minutes [34]. At doses $\geq$ 20 mg, however, the elimination half-life determines the duration of analgesia, which is much greater than with 10 mg. At these higher doses, the redistribution phase is followed by a slow elimination phase, where the blood plasma concentration of methadone slowly decreases. As a result, 20 and 30 mg of methadone would be expected to produce approximately 24 and 36 hours of analgesia, respectively [33]. The minimum effective analgesic methadone concentration is approximately 30 ng/ml [33, 34]. The threshold for respiratory depression is concentration of approximately 100 ng/ml [33].

The cytochrome P450 system (CYP), specifically CYP2B6, is responsible for metabolizing methadone into the inactive metabolite, 2-ethyl-1,5-dimethyl-3,3-diphenylpyrrolidine (EDDP). There are significant genetic polymorphisms for the CYP2B6 gene, and these variations may explain interindividual variability in methadone's plasma concentrations, clearance, and metabolism [40].

Dosing and Administration

The effectiveness of intraoperative methadone has been studied as a single intraoperative bolus and typical perioperative doses have ranged from 0.1 to 0.3 mg/kg [37]. Most studies involving major inpatient surgery used a single IV dose of 0.2 mg/kg or a fixed dose of 20 mg that was given during induction. Doses of 0.1 to 0.15 mg/kg are commonly used for ambulatory surgery. A single intraoperative dose of methadone provides stable levels of blood methadone concentration for both intraoperative and postoperative analgesia and without the fluctuations in blood plasma concentrations that occur with bolus dosing or from patient-controlled analgesia.

Perioperative Use

Cardiac Surgery

The pain from cardiac surgery is complex and includes somatic, visceral, neuropathic, and mixed forms of pain [41, 42]. The diverse analgesic mechanisms of methadone may therefore confer additional analgesic benefits compared to other more traditional opioids.

In the largest study of intraoperative methadone in cardiac surgery, 156 patients were randomized to receive 0.3 mg/kg of methadone or fentanyl 12 μg/kg [43]. Patients in both groups received half of the study drug at induction (0.15 mg/kg methadone or 6 μg/kg fentanyl), and the other half via an infusion over the next 2 hours. All patients received IV morphine for postoperative analgesia. Patients in the methadone group reported lower pain scores, consumed less morphine, and reported greater satisfaction with postoperative pain management. The time to first morphine request was also greater in patients that received methadone. Perhaps equally impressive was the lack of difference in opioid-related adverse effects, time to extubation, duration of intensive care stay, and hospital length of stay between the two study groups [43].

A systematic review of intraoperative methadone use in cardiac surgery found that single-dose intraoperative methadone can decrease postoperative opioid consumption in the first 24 hours without increasing adverse events, such as PONV, respiratory failure, or time to tracheal extubation [44].

Complex Spine Surgery

Patients undergoing complex spine surgery frequently experience severe postoperative pain. Patients following posterior spinal fusion have reported severe postoperative pain up to three days following surgery [45]. Compared to 2 mg intravenous hydromorphone at the conclusion of surgery, 0.2 mg/kg of methadone at the start of surgery has been shown to significantly reduce postoperative opioid consumption on postoperative days 1–3, improve resting and dynamic pain scores, and lead to improved patient satisfaction without increasing complications [46]. Combining methadone with ketamine may further improve analgesia [4]. A single intraoperative dose of methadone improved analgesia up to 3 months postoperatively after spine surgery in one RCT [47].

Ambulatory Same-Day Surgery

Compared to complex inpatient surgical procedures, the use of intraoperative methadone for ambulatory same-day surgery has not been extensively studied. In a dose-finding study of ambulatory patients undergoing laparoscopic general surgical and gynecologic procedures, patients were randomized to receive either 0.1 mg/kg (ideal body weight) of IV methadone, 0.15 mg/kg (ideal body weight) of IV methadone, or conventional analgesia with short-acting opioids (control group) [48]. Both methadone groups reported less pain and consumed less intraoperative and postoperative opioids compared to patients in the control group. Only the 0.15 mg/kg methadone group had less pain at rest and consumed less post-discharge opioids during the first 30 postoperative days compared to controls. There was no difference in adverse effects including sedation, respiratory events, PONV, or time to readiness for postoperative anesthesia care unit (PACU) discharge amongst the 3 study groups [48].

Safety Considerations

Concerns that the long half-life of methadone may result in prolonged and/or delayed respiratory depression is a major reason for hesitation for many anesthesiologists.

The published evidence suggests that these risks are low. Several studies looking at single-dose perioperative methadone have not found an increased incidence of respiratory depression when compared to more typical perioperative opioid regimens [4, 44, 46]. Pharmacokinetic studies indicate that respiratory depression would most likely occur in the first 30–45 minutes following a single dose of 20 or 30 mg of IV methadone [33, 34]. This is because methadone is a lipophilic opioid that rapidly redistributes from the central nervous system (CNS) to the blood plasma. Nevertheless, if methadone-induced respiratory depression were suspected, a naloxone infusion should be administered because naloxone has a shorter duration of action than methadone. One noteworthy case report from 1976 described an 81 year old (43.7 kg) patient who received 30 mg of methadone (0.69 mg/kg) for mitral valve replacement surgery [49]. The patient required 1 mg of naloxone prior to tracheal extubation and subsequent doses of naloxone every 2 to 4 hours for the next 8 days for persistent respiratory depression [49]. It is likely that the patient's advanced age and high dose of methadone combined contributed to the prolonged respiratory depressant effects.

It is well established that methadone can prolong the QT interval and produce life-threatening arrhythmias such as torsades de pointes and sudden cardiac death. However, these adverse effects appear to be dose related and are more likely to occur in patients on chronic methadone maintenance therapy for opioid use disorder. To date, there have been no reports of adverse cardiac events following a single intraoperative dose of methadone. However, existing clinical trials were not powered to assess for cardiac-related adverse events [31].

5 Magnesium

Background

Magnesium is the fourth most common mineral in the human body and plays a vital role in numerous cellular and physiologic processes relevant to anesthesiology and perioperative medicine. It is a potent vasodilator, bronchodilator, antiarrhythmic, neuroprotectant, and potentiates the effects of nondepolarizing neuromuscular blockers [50, 51]. Like ketamine, it is a NMDA-receptor antagonist that has been shown to decrease the severity of postoperative pain and reduce opioid consumption for a variety of surgical procedures [52, 53].

Clinical Evidence

Magnesium has been shown to be an effective analgesic adjunct for intraoperative and postoperative pain management. It decreases 24-h analgesic requirements and time to first analgesic request for a wide range of surgical procedures [52–54]. These procedures included the specialties of otolaryngology, orthopedic surgery, general surgery, gynecology, urology, thoracic surgery, transplant surgery, and plastic surgery. A 2021 umbrella review of systematic reviews found that there was sufficient evidence to show that magnesium improved pain scores for up to 24 hours and decreased analgesic consumption, but there was significant heterogeneity in the methodology and reporting outcomes in the individual studies reviewed [54]. In the perioperative setting, IV magnesium has been most commonly administered with a loading dose of 30–50 mg/kg followed by a continuous infusion of 8–20 mg/kg/hr [52, 53].

In addition to IV formulations, intrathecal, epidural and intraarticular magnesium have been shown to be effective as part of a multimodal analgesic regimen [52, 54]. The addition of intrathecal magnesium sulfate to a subarachnoid block has been shown to prolong the sensory and motor blockade and reduce postoperative analgesic requirements even 36 hours after the operation. However, intrathecal magnesium also prolonged the onset of both the sensory and motor blockade [55] For arthroscopic knee surgery, intraarticular magnesium improved pain at rest and with movement up to 24 hours after the operation [56, 57].

Safety Considerations

In standard therapeutic doses, magnesium has minimal side effects due to its wide therapeutic index. Some patients report minor facial flushing and a warm sensation during drug administration. If given rapidly or in high doses, magnesium can cause transient hypotension because of vascular smooth muscle dilation, and it may precipitate nausea and vomiting in susceptible individuals [51]. Similarly, magnesium infusions may cause fatigue and sedation in high doses [51].

Hypermagnesemia is relatively uncommon and usually occurs as an iatrogenic event in patients receiving supplemental magnesium or in patients with preexisting kidney disease. Loss of deep tendon reflexes occurs at serum magnesium levels of around 12 mg/dL and reflex testing can be useful in screening for hypermagnesemia [51]. If left untreated, hypermagnesemia can progress to respiratory failure, heart block and complete cardiovascular collapse. Severe magnesium toxicity is treated with IV calcium gluconate, and if necessary, mechanical ventilation and hemodialysis.

Since magnesium can induce weakness and potentiate the effects of neuromuscular blocking agents, all patients receiving intraoperative magnesium should be monitored for residual neuromuscular blockade. Patients with preexisting neuromuscular disease receiving supplemental magnesium should be closely monitored for worsening weakness, obstruction, and respiratory decompensation [50, 51]. Dosing and safety considerations for methadone and magnesium are shown in Table 2.

Table 2 Perioperative dosing and treatment considerations for methadone and magnesium

	Methadone	Magnesium
Dosing	Inpatient Surgery: 0.2–0.3 mg/kg IV Ambulatory Surgery: 0.1–0.15 mg/kg IV	Loading Dose: 30–50 mg/kg IV Continuous Infusion: 8–20 mg/kg/hr
Safety considerations	Consider dose reduction in patients ≥ 65 years old and those with morbid obesity, obstructive sleep apnea, severe hepatic or cardiovascular disease	– Consider dose reduction in patients with renal failure and pre-existing neuromuscular disorders or weakness – Potentiates neuromuscular blockade
Treatment for overdose	Naloxone	– IV fluids – Diuretics – IV calcium gluconate – Hemodialysis for refractory or severe cases

IV: Intravenous

6 Conclusions

NMDA-receptor activation is a critical step in the development of chronic pain, opioid tolerance, hyperalgesia, and other pain-related processes. In the perioperative setting, these processes can greatly affect the patient experience and if not addressed can contribute to persistent postoperative pain or chronic opioid use. NMDA-receptor antagonists, such as ketamine, methadone, and magnesium, have garnered significant interest for their therapeutic potential, particularly in the current opioid crisis where opioid-sparing strategies are both popular and beneficial. While the level of evidence and specific surgical settings vary for each of the agents, they all hold potential to reduce acute pain, reset the central nervous system, and possibly even prevent or at least decrease the severity of chronic pain. Future studies should examine long-term effects of these agents, individually and combined, and additional research is needed to help identify which patient populations are most at risk and which patient characteristics might help predict positive response to NMDA antagonists.

Key Takeaway Points

1. NMDA-receptor antagonists are used for perioperative pain management because of their profound analgesic effects, and for their potential to reduce opioid consumption and opioid-related adverse effects.
2. Ketamine is the prototypical NMDA-receptor antagonist and has the greatest level of evidence for perioperative pain management.
3. A single intraoperative dose of intravenous methadone is safe and effective for managing postoperative pain in patients undergoing major inpatient surgeries. More data is needed to guide dosing and safety for ambulatory surgery.
4. Magnesium has multiple physiologic functions and can be a useful analgesic adjunct for perioperative pain management.

References

1. Gan TJ, Habib AS, Miller TE, White W, Apfelbaum JL. Incidence, patient satisfaction, and perceptions of post-surgical pain: results from a US national survey. Curr Med Res Opin. 2014;30(1):149–60.
2. Lee M, Silverman SM, Hansen H, Patel VB, Manchikanti L. A comprehensive review of opioid-induced hyperalgesia. Pain Physician. 2011;14(2):145–61.
3. Avidan MS, Maybrier HR, Abdallah AB, Jacobsohn E, Vlisides PE, Pryor KO, et al. Intraoperative ketamine for prevention of postoperative delirium or pain after major surgery in older adults: an international, multicentre, double-blind, randomised clinical trial. Lancet. 2017;390(10091):267–75.
4. Murphy GS, Avram MJ, Greenberg SB, Benson J, Bilimoria S, Maher CE, et al. Perioperative methadone and ketamine for postoperative pain control in spinal surgical patients: a randomized, double-blind. Placebo-controlled Trial Anesthesiol. 2021;134(5):697–708.
5. Bennett GJ. Update on the neurophysiology of pain transmission and modulation: focus on the NMDA-receptor. J Pain Symptom Manage. 2000;19(1 Suppl):S2-6.
6. Dacher M, Nugent FS. Opiates and plasticity. Neuropharmacology. 2011;61(7):1088–96.
7. Petrenko AB, Yamakura T, Baba H, Shimoji K. The role of N-methyl-D-aspartate (NMDA) receptors in pain: a review. Anesth Analg. 2003;97(4):1108–16.
8. Latremoliere A, Woolf CJ. Central sensitization: a generator of pain hypersensitivity by central neural plasticity. J Pain. 2009;10(9):895–926.
9. Niesters M, Martini C, Dahan A. Ketamine for chronic pain: risks and benefits. Br J Clin Pharmacol. 2014;77(2):357–67.
10. Brinck EC, Tiippana E, Heesen M, Bell RF, Straube S, Moore RA, et al. Perioperative intravenous ketamine for acute postoperative pain in adults. Cochrane Database Syst Rev. 2018;12(12):Cd012033.
11. Schwenk ES, Viscusi ER, Buvanendran A, Hurley RW, Wasan AD, Narouze S, et al. Consensus guidelines on the use of intravenous ketamine infusions for acute pain management from the American society of regional anesthesia and pain medicine, the American academy of pain medicine, and the American society of anesthesiologists. Reg Anesth Pain Med. 2018;43(5):456–66.
12. Cohen SP, Bhatia A, Buvanendran A, Schwenk ES, Wasan AD, Hurley RW, et al. Consensus guidelines on the use of intravenous ketamine infusions for chronic pain from the American society of regional anesthesia and pain medicine, the American academy of pain medicine, and the American society of anesthesiologists. Reg Anesth Pain Med. 2018;43(5):521–46.
13. Zanos P, Moaddel R, Morris PJ, Riggs LM, Highland JN, Georgiou P, et al. Ketamine and ketamine metabolite pharmacology: insights into therapeutic mechanisms. Pharmacol Rev. 2018;70(3):621–60.
14. Sigtermans MJ, van Hilten JJ, Bauer MCR, Arbous SM, Marinus J, Sarton EY, et al. Ketamine produces effective and long-term pain relief in patients with complex regional pain syndrome type 1. Pain. 2009;145(3):304–11.
15. Desta Z, Moaddel R, Ogburn ET, Xu C, Ramamoorthy A, Venkata SL, et al. Stereoselective and regiospecific hydroxylation of ketamine and norketamine. Xenobiotica. 2012;42(11):1076–87.
16. Clements JA, Nimmo WS, Grant IS. Bioavailability, pharmacokinetics, and analgesic activity of ketamine in humans. J Pharm Sci. 1982;71(5):539–42.
17. Domino EF, Zsigmond EK, Domino LE, Domino KE, Kothary SP, Domino SE. Plasma levels of ketamine and two of its metabolites in surgical patients using a gas chromatographic mass fragmentographic assay. Anesth Analg. 1982;61(2):87–92.
18. Handa F, Tanaka M, Nishikawa T, Toyooka H. Effects of oral clonidine premedication on side effects of intravenous ketamine anesthesia: a randomized, double-blind, placebo-controlled study. J Clin Anesth. 2000;12(1):19–24.
19. Laskowski K, Stirling A, Mckay WP, Lim HJ. A systematic review of intravenous ketamine for postoperative analgesia. Canadian J Anesthesia/J canadien d'anesthésie. 2011;58(10):911–23.

20. Loftus RW, Yeager MP, Clark JA, Brown JR, Abdu WA, Sengupta DK, et al. Intraoperative ketamine reduces perioperative opiate consumption in opiate-dependent patients with chronic back pain undergoing back surgery. Anesthesiology. 2010;113(3):639–46.
21. Nielsen RV, Fomsgaard JS, Nikolajsen L, Dahl JB, Mathiesen O. Intraoperative S-ketamine for the reduction of opioid consumption and pain one year after spine surgery: a randomized clinical trial of opioid-dependent patients. Eur J Pain. 2019;23(3):455–60.
22. Bespalov AY, Zvartau EE, Beardsley PM. Opioid-NMDA receptor interactions may clarify conditioned (associative) components of opioid analgesic tolerance. Neurosci Biobehav Rev. 2001;25(4):343–53.
23. Colvin LA, Bull F, Hales TG. Perioperative opioid analgesia-when is enough too much? a review of opioid-induced tolerance and hyperalgesia. Lancet. 2019;393(10180):1558–68.
24. Gil LV, Mazzeffi MA, Cai Y, McLeod WW, Porter SB. Reasons for discontinuation of acute postoperative pain ketamine infusions: a retrospective case-control study. Pain Pract. 2021;21(7):759–65.
25. Noppers IM, Niesters M, Aarts L, Bauer MCR, Drewes AM, Dahan A, et al. Drug-induced liver injury following a repeated course of ketamine treatment for chronic pain in CRPS type 1 patients: a report of 3 cases. Pain. 2011;152(9):2173–8.
26. Mendelson AM, Kohan L, Okai J, Wanees M, Gonnella JC, Torjman MC, et al. Adverse drug effects related to multiday ketamine infusions: multicenter study. Reg Anesth Pain Med. 2020.
27. Yu WL, Cho CC, Lung PF, Hung EH, Hui JW, Chau HH, et al. Ketamine-related cholangiopathy: a retrospective study on clinical and imaging findings. Abdom Imaging. 2014;39(6):1241–6.
28. Elia N, Tramer MR. Ketamine and postoperative pain–a quantitative systematic review of randomised trials. Pain. 2005;113(1–2):61–70.
29. Schwenk ES, Goldberg SF, Patel RD, Zhou J, Adams DR, Baratta JL, et al. Adverse drug effects and preoperative medication factors related to perioperative low-dose ketamine infusions. Reg Anesth Pain Med. 2016;41(4):482–7.
30. Porter SB, McClain RL, Howe BL, Ardon AE, Mazer LS, Knestrick BM, et al. Perioperative ketamine for acute postoperative analgesia: the mayo clinic-florida experience. J Perianesth Nurs. 2015;30(3):189–95.
31. Murphy GS, Szokol JW. Intraoperative methadone in surgical patients: a review of clinical investigations. Anesthesiology. 2019;131(3):678–92.
32. Trescot AM, Datta S, Lee M, Hansen H. Opioid pharmacology. Pain Physic. 2008;11(2 Suppl):S133–53.
33. Gourlay GK, Wilson PR, Glynn CJ. Pharmacodynamics and pharmacokinetics of methadone during the perioperative period. Anesthesiology. 1982;57(6):458–67.
34. Kharasch ED. Intraoperative methadone: rediscovery, reappraisal, and reinvigoration? Anesth Analg. 2011;112(1):13–6.
35. Ong WY, Stohler CS, Herr DR. Role of the prefrontal cortex in pain processing. Mol Neurobiol. 2019;56(2):1137–66.
36. Thompson JM, Neugebauer V. Cortico-limbic pain mechanisms. Neurosci Lett. 2019;702:15–23.
37. Machado FC, Vieira JE, de Orange FA, Ashmawi HA. Intraoperative methadone reduces pain and opioid consumption in acute postoperative pain: a systematic review and meta-analysis. Anesth Analg. 2019;129(6):1723–32.
38. Tognoli E, Proto PL, Motta G, Galeone C, Mariani L, Valenza F. Methadone for postoperative analgesia: contribution of N-methyl-D-aspartate receptor antagonism: a randomised controlled trial. Eur J Anaesthesiol. 2020;37(10):934–43.
39. Brown R, Kraus C, Fleming M, Reddy S. Methadone: applied pharmacology and use as adjunctive treatment in chronic pain. Postgrad Med J. 2004;80(949):654–9.
40. Kharasch ED, Regina KJ, Blood J, Friedel C. Methadone pharmacogenetics: CYP2B6 polymorphisms determine plasma concentrations, clearance, and metabolism. Anesthesiology. 2015;123(5):1142–53.
41. Jayakumar S, Borrelli M, Milan Z, Kunst G, Whitaker D. Optimising pain management protocols following cardiac surgery: a protocol for a national quality improvement study. Int J Surg Protoc. 2019;14:1–8.

42. Zubrzycki M, Liebold A, Skrabal C, Reinelt H, Ziegler M, Perdas E, et al. Assessment and pathophysiology of pain in cardiac surgery. J Pain Res. 2018;11:1599–611.
43. Murphy GS, Szokol JW, Avram MJ, Greenberg SB, Marymont JH, Shear T, et al. Intraoperative methadone for the prevention of postoperative pain: a randomized, double-blinded clinical trial in cardiac surgical patients. Anesthesiology. 2015;122(5):1112–22.
44. Lobova VA, Roll JM, Roll MLC. Intraoperative methadone use in cardiac surgery: a systematic review. Pain Med. 2021;22(12):2827–34.
45. Bianconi M, Ferraro L, Ricci R, Zanoli G, Antonelli T, Giulia B, et al. The pharmacokinetics and efficacy of ropivacaine continuous wound instillation after spine fusion surgery. Anesth Analg. 2004;98(1):166–72.
46. Murphy GS, Szokol JW, Avram MJ, Greenberg SB, Shear TD, Deshur MA, et al. Clinical effectiveness and safety of intraoperative methadone in patients undergoing posterior spinal fusion surgery: a randomized, double-blinded. Controlled Trial Anesthesiol. 2017;126(5):822–33.
47. Murphy GS, Avram MJ, Greenberg SB, Shear TD, Deshur MA, Dickerson D, et al. Postoperative pain and analgesic requirements in the first year after intraoperative methadone for complex spine and cardiac surgery. Anesthesiology. 2020;132(2):330–42.
48. Komen H, Brunt LM, Deych E, Blood J, Kharasch ED. Intraoperative methadone in same-day ambulatory surgery: a randomized, double-blinded dose-finding pilot study. Anesth Analg. 2019;128(4):802–10.
49. Norris JV, Don HF. Prolonged depression of respiratory rate following methadone analgesia. Anesthesiology. 1976;45(3):361–2.
50. Do SH. Magnesium: a versatile drug for anesthesiologists. Korean J Anesthesiol. 2013;65(1):4–8.
51. Herroeder S, Schonherr ME, De Hert SG, Hollmann MW. Magnesium–essentials for anesthesiologists. Anesthesiology. 2011;114(4):971–93.
52. Albrecht E, Kirkham KR, Liu SS, Brull R. Peri-operative intravenous administration of magnesium sulphate and postoperative pain: a meta-analysis. Anaesthesia. 2013;68(1):79–90.
53. De Oliveira GS, Jr., Castro-Alves LJ, Khan JH, McCarthy RJ. Perioperative systemic magnesium to minimize postoperative pain: a meta-analysis of randomized controlled trials. Anesthesiology. 2013;119(1):178–90.
54. Choi GJ, Kim YI, Koo YH, Oh HC, Kang H. Perioperative magnesium for postoperative analgesia: an umbrella review of systematic reviews and updated meta-analysis of randomized controlled trials. J Pers Med. 2021;11(12).
55. Pascual-Ramirez J, Gil-Trujillo S, Alcantarilla C. Intrathecal magnesium as analgesic adjuvant for spinal anesthesia: a meta-analysis of randomized trials. Minerva Anestesiol. 2013;79(6):667–78.
56. Shi L, Zhu H, Ma J, Shi LL, Gao F, Sun W. Intra-articular magnesium to alleviate postoperative pain after arthroscopic knee surgery: a meta-analysis of randomized controlled trials. J Orthop Surg Res. 2021;16(1):111.
57. Zeng C, Li YS, Wei J, Xie DX, Xie X, Li LJ, et al. Analgesic effect and safety of single-dose intra-articular magnesium after arthroscopic surgery: a systematic review and meta-analysis. Sci Rep. 2016;6:38024.

Perioperative Use of Acetaminophen and Non-steroidal Anti-inflammatory Agents

Beth A. VanderWielen and Shelly B. Borden

Abstract Multimodal analgesia and Enhanced Recovery After Surgery (ERAS) pathways are employed in the perioperative setting worldwide to control pain and achieve improvements in several recovery characteristics including patient satisfaction, reductions in hospital length of stay, and reductions in hospital readmission rates. This chapter explores the mechanism, perioperative indications, adverse effects, and clinical pearls associated with both acetaminophen and NSAIDS (nonsteroidal anti-inflammatory drugs). Specifically, the literature is thoroughly reviewed to highlight the most efficacious use of these medications in the perioperative setting. Special attention is given to common surgical concerns regarding risks associated with NSAIDS, including perioperative bleeding risk, bone healing, and anastomotic leak. The literature reviewed in this chapter is current and was chosen based on availability in PubMed featuring meta-analyses, randomized controlled trials and systematic reviews published in the range of 2012–2022. This chapter explores subsets of surgical types, patient populations, and dosing routes; the implications of both NSAIDS and acetaminophen are reviewed so the provider can use their discretion to guide clinical administration.

Keywords Acetaminophen · Non-steroidal anti-inflammatory agents · Perioperative use · Efficacy data

B. A. VanderWielen (✉)
Mayo Clinic, 200 1st Street SW, Rochester, MN 55905, USA
e-mail: vanderwielen.beth@mayo.edu

S. B. Borden
William S. Middleton Memorial Veterans' Hospital, 2500 Overlook Terrace, Madison, WI 53705, USA
e-mail: Shalini.borden@va.gov

A. Abd-Elsayed and K. Schroeder (eds.), *Perioperative Pain Management*,
https://doi.org/10.1007/978-3-031-67648-2_40

1 Introduction

Multimodal analgesic strategies are increasingly employed in an effort to hasten surgical recovery, improve analgesia, and curtail the opioid epidemic. This chapter will focus on the use of acetaminophen and nonsteroidal anti-inflammatory drugs (NSAIDS) with particular attention to surgical considerations in the perioperative period. Due to the broad scope of surgeries that increasingly utilize both classes of medications, this chapter is not exhaustive or all-inclusive but rather focuses on several of the more common surgical considerations faced in daily practice. In addition, basic pharmacology, dosing considerations, contraindications and cautions associated with the administration of the most used medications in the United States will be outlined as a practical reference for practitioners.

2 Acetaminophen

Introduction

Acetaminophen (N-acetyl para-aminophenol or paracetamol) is frequently utilized in the perioperative period to assist with postoperative analgesia in both adult and pediatric patients.

While Enhanced Recovery After Surgery (ERAS) pathways commonly include the use of perioperative acetaminophen, meta-analyses and systematic reviews focusing solely on the effect of acetaminophen in the reduction of perioperative pain are more limited as, in practice, acetaminophen is frequently used in combination with other analgesics as part of a multimodal regimen.

Pharmacodynamics/Pharmacokinetics

The complete mechanism of action of acetaminophen remains to be elucidated. Current conjecture is that acetaminophen functions via reductions in the activity of the cyclooxygenase (COX) pathway, but unlike NSAIDS, it does not bind to the active site of either the COX-1 or COX-2 enzyme. It is thought to inhibit the synthesis of prostaglandins in the central nervous system (CNS), resulting in analgesic and antipyretic effects. It has also been suggested to stimulate the descending serotonergic pathways in the CNS as well as activating the cannabinoid receptor system which may augment analgesic effects [1]. Please refer to Table 1 for hepatic reductions, renal reductions, cautions, pregnancy considerations, and dosing information.

Table 1 Perioperative considerations for acetaminophen use

Dosing						Renal reductions	Hepatic reductions	Pregnancy	Cautions
Pediatric			Adult						
IV	PO	PR	IV	PO	PR				
< 2 yrs: 7.5–15 mg/kg q6h; max daily dose 60 mg/kg[∍] $\geq$2 yrs: < 50 kg 15 mg/kg q6h PRN or 12.5 mg/kg q4h PRN, max single dose 750 mg, max daily dose 75 mg/kg/day or 3750 mg/day $\geq$50 kg: 15 mg/kg q6h PRN or 12.5 mg/kg q4h PRN, max single dose 1000 mg, max daily dose 75 mg/kg/day or 4000 mg/day ∵Infuse over 15 min	10–15 mg/kg q4-6h PRN, do not exceed 5 doses in 24 h; max dose 75 mg/kg/day, max daily dose 4000 mg/day Fixed kg interval dosing schedules are also established on specific formulations and will not be further discussed here as these regimens have been established to simplify home/ parental administration	Loading dose 40 mg/kg for 1 dose; maintenance dose 20–25 mg/kg q6h for 2–3 days, max dose is 100 mg/ kg/day, or 4000 mg/day; duration > 5 days has not been studied	$\geq$50 kg 650 mg q4h or 1000 mgq6h; max single dose 1000 mg, max daily dose 4000 mg/day < 50 kg 12.5 mg/kg q4h or 15 mg/ kgq6h; max single dose 15 mg/kg/dose ∵Infuse over 15 min ∵Nausea reported in $\geq$ 30% of adults	325—650 mg q4-6h PRN or 1000 mg q5h PRN; max dose 4000 mg/day	325—650 mg q4-6h PRN, max daily dose 3900 mg/day *Absorption is irregular; bioavailability reduced by 10–20%	Pediatric patients with CrCl < 30 mL/ min nonspecific reduced dosing and additional caution advised for intravenous administration	∵Limit to 2000–3000 mg/day in chronic liver disease/cirrhosis; avoid in active EtOH users with significant liver impairment ∵Avoid use in severe alcoholic hepatitis or acute liver injury ∵Hepatotoxicity occurs through formation of toxic metabolite NAPQI; overdoses treated with NAC within 8h typically do not develop hepatotoxicity	Category C	∵ Acetaminophen-induced hepatotoxicity associated with doses > 4 g/day; there have been some cases reported in patients taking 4g/day and thus, if duration of therapy is > 7 days, dose reduction considerations to 3g/day have been suggested ∵Dose reductions to 2g/ day in the setting of heavy EtOH use, advanced age, liver disease, low body weight, malnutrition have been suggested ∵Use with caution in patients with G6PD deficiency ∵Not well understood mechanism of action[ϕ]

[∍]Manufacturing guidelines note intravenous acetaminophen (Ofirmev®) for the treatment of fever or acute pain has not been studied in patients < 2years old (https://www.accessdata.fda.gov/drugsatfda_docs/label/2010/022450lbl.pdf).
[ϕ]Mechanism of action not well understood- thought to be due to activation of descending serotonergic inhibitor pathways in the CNS; antipyresis from inhibition of hypothalamic heat-regulating center (Lexicomp)
Abbreviations mos, months; yrs, years; mg, milligram; kg, kilogram; d, day; h, hour; q, quaque (every/each); prn, pro re nata (as needed); CrCl, creatine clearance; PO, per os (by mouth); IV, intravenous; EtOH, ethanol; NAPQI, N-acetyl-p-benzoquinoneimine; NAC, n-acetylcysteine
References [∍] Food and Drug Administration (FDA) [2], Lexicomp [3].

Dosing and Route of Administration

Intravenous (IV) versus oral (PO) dosing of acetaminophen has been a topic of keen interest amongst pharmacists and hospital administrators. This interest is in large part due to the cost difference between the two dosing regimens with intravenous dosing formulations costing significantly more than oral dosing regimens. Lexi-Comp® data lists 325–500 mg acetaminophen tablets costing between \$0.01 to \$0.08 per tablet (standard adult 1000 mg dosing approximating \$0.04 to \$0.16/dose) versus intravenous dosing costing \$0.09 to \$0.45 per mL (standard adult 1000 mg dosing approximating \$9 to \$45.00/dose). Recent systematic reviews and meta-analyses that compare IV versus PO dosing routes regardless of surgical intervention demonstrate mixed perioperative outcomes data. Pettersson et al. [4] reported a reduction in opioid use with IV versus PO administration after patient's awoke from coronary artery bypass grafting but this did not translate into a reduction in pain scores. In contrast, Brett et al. [5], found equivalent opioid use in the IV and PO groups in patients who had undergone a knee arthroscopy but a notable reduction in pain scale scores when acetaminophen was given intravenously at 50 min post-operatively. However, 33 percent of patients were discharged by this time mark, biasing the data. Fenlon et al. [6] conducted a non-inferiority study in patients undergoing third molar extraction and found no difference in proportions of VAS score differences between dosing routes (−0.039, 90% CI −0.17 to 0.09). Teng et al. [7] reviewed the literature regarding IV versus PO acetaminophen in the total knee arthroplasty (TKA) literature and similarly found no differences in VAS pain scores at 24 or 48 hours nor in opioid consumption at 24 hours. However, patients receiving IVA did have a slight but significant decreased hospital length of stay (SDM = −0.02, 95% CI −0.03 to −0.01; p = 0.004). Likewise, Stagg [8] conducted a systematic review (9 studies, 2456 patients) also comparing IV vs PO acetaminophen in the perioperative setting from gynecology obstetric, orthopedics, dental and general surgery. The IV formulation was found to have a small but perhaps not clinically relevant reduction in pain scores (0.5 VAS points, 95% CI 0.17 to 0.82) and opioid requirements (MD 5.6 mg, CI 4.38 to 6.83). While most studies demonstrate increased bioavailability of the IV formulation, there is not clear evidence that this translates into increased efficacy compared to the PO formulation as concentration–response relationships have not been clearly established [9].

Rectal acetaminophen is an alternative and available dosing route. Due to the blood supply of the rectum, peak drug levels have been shown to have a ninefold variability, with peak drug levels not reliability achieving therapeutic antipyretic levels [10]. Bioavailability may also be reduced by 10–20 percent compared to oral dosing [11–18]. This variance in drug levels and bioavailability is surmised due to the variable rectal blood supply; the proximal rectum has venous drainage directly into the portal system by which metabolism by the liver takes place [10, 19]. The distal rectum venous beds bypass the portal system, thereby eliminating liver first pass metabolism. Due to the variable pharmacokinetics and pharmacodynamics of the rectal dosing route, the American Academy of Pediatrics currently recommends to refrain from rectal acetaminophen in children due to risk of toxicity. However, this recommendation has been recently challenged by Goldstein et al. [10], who published a metanalysis which included four studies that found no difference in fever reduction between oral versus rectal dosing. However, there was no standardization in the dose and only one study attempted to investigate analgesic effects, of which oral dosing was superior. Rectal versus PO dosing literature again highlights the lack thereof an established concentration–response relationship which further muddles decision making when selecting the optimal route of administration. Rectal suppository cost ranges between \$0.66–0.88 depending on the dosage which ranges from 80 to 650 mg/suppository) [11–18].

Perioperative Uses

Here, we review relevant articles that examine the use of acetaminophen in clinical practice. Maund et al. [20] conducted a systematic review analyzing 60 trials of paracetamol (12 studies), non-selective NSAID (38 studies) and COX-2 selective use (16 studies) on perioperative opioid reduction. Patients underwent a variety of surgeries including thoracic (2 studies), orthopedic (23 studies), gynecological (17 studies), obstetric (5 studies) and general surgery (13 studies). Overall, this study concluded that paracetamol is less effective at reducing morphine use (mean difference MD −6.34 mg, 95% CI −9.02 to −3.65) as compared to non-selective NSAIDS (MD −10.18, CI −11.65 to −8.72) or COX-2 inhibitors (MD −10.92, 95% CI −12.77 to −9.08). Non-selective NSAIDS compared to paracetamol reduced morphine consumption by −3.85 (95% CI −6.80 to 0.89) and COX-2 selective drugs (−4.58, 95% CI −7.83 to −1.35).

Bailey et al. [21] performed a Cochrane systematic review analyzing the effect of ibuprofen and/or paracetamol after wisdom tooth extraction. Only RCTs were included (7 studies, 2241 patients), and the study concluded that 400 mg of ibuprofen provided superior pain relief than 1000 mg of acetaminophen with a risk ratio of 50% pain reduction at 6 hours of 1.47 (95% CI 1.28 to 1.69). When both medications were utilized in a combination tablet, the risk ratio was 1.77 (95% CI 1.32 to 2.39).

Other studies have specifically reviewed outcomes within the pediatric population. Wong et al. [22] evaluated the opioid sparing benefits of NSAIDS and/or paracetamol in pediatric patients (8 overlapping studies with [23]). This review included 31 RCTs and found opioid dose requirements were reduced by 31.6% (95% CI: 16.5% to 46.6%) across all studies. There was significant variability in duration of NSAID/paracetamol duration ranging from $\leq$ 6 hours to $\geq$ 24 hours as well as heterogeneity in comparison groups ranging from continuous IV opioid infusions to intermittent bolus dosing. Oral, rectal and IV administration routes for NSAIDS and paracetamol were included. In addition, various surgical procedures were included which limits the applicability of results. Further, grouping acetaminophen and NSAID administration data complicates any efforts to assign therapeutic efficacy to either analgesic modality.

Archer et al. [24] evaluated the effect of post-operative IV acetaminophen dosing in children who underwent open abdominal and thoracic surgery. Randomized controlled trials (RCTs) were included if they compared IV acetaminophen with opioids to opioids alone. A total of five studies (443 patients) were included and found equivalent pain scores between groups (−0.23, 95% CI −0.88 to 0.40, $p = 0.47$) and a small reduction in opioid use (−1.95 MMEs/kg/48 h, 95% CI −3.95 to 0.05, $p = 0.06$). The stark contrast of these results compared to those reported by Wong et al. [22] demonstrates the need for further studies that seek to evaluate the possible synergistic effects of concurrent acetaminophen and NSAID administration as well as optimal route of administration.

Adverse Effects

Please refer to Table 1 for hepatic dosing and cautions. The risk of hepatoxicity with overdosing cannot be overstated as it is the most common cause of acute liver failure in the United States. This risk may be compounded through the inclusion of acetaminophen in a variety of compounded and readily available/over-the-counter medications that complicates safe dosing regimens. It is estimated that approximately 25 percent of patients with hepatoxicity resulting from acetaminophen overdose require a liver transplant [25, 26], and approximately half of acetaminophen overdoses are thought to be nonintentional and attributed to confusion with proper dosing and/or unfamiliarly with acetaminophen's toxic side effect profile [25]. Risk factors for toxicity beyond dosing in addition to the treatment with N-acetylcysteine are discussed in Table 1.

Conclusion

Acetaminophen can reduce perioperative pain, but the magnitude of effect is smaller than for NSAIDS. Acetaminophen is associated with an elevated risk of hepatotoxicity, while NSAIDS carry other theoretical risks (bleeding, renal dysfunction, etc.) that will later be discussed in further detail. There remains a paucity of systematic reviews and meta-analyses regarding the synergistic effects of acetaminophen and NSAIDS that limit the scope of recommendations that might be made to support this common practice. Acetaminophen use in adult versus pediatric populations may be associated with differences in opioid reduction potential, though high-quality data directly comparing efficacy by age group is currently lacking. Route of dosing does not appear to have a significant effect on clinical outcomes, though studies often do not consider the nuances of clinical practice such as sedation, dysphagia and delirium and a clear concentration–response relationship has yet to be established. With the booming obesity epidemic, research on post-operative apneas and discharge times comparing opioid sparing vs opioid-based pain control regimens may be a topic of future study affecting conclusions above. Much remains unknown regarding the perioperative use of acetaminophen as isolating the drug's effect is often not clinically practical.

3 Non-steroidal Anti-inflammatory Drugs (NSAIDS)

Introduction

Multimodal analgesia with increased use of NSAIDS is gaining popularity in the operating room in an effort to curb opioid use. Under the NSAID mechanism umbrella, there exists significant variability between each NSAID type regarding dosing regimens due to differences in chemical structure and selectivity (Table 2). Clinical apprehensions regarding use during the perioperative period will be discussed below by way of review of systematic reviews and meta-analyses published between 2012 and 2022, with rare additions of literature outside of this timeframe when necessary for dosing or reference context.

Pharmacodynamics/Pharmacokinetics

NSAIDS inhibit the COX enzyme responsible for the conversion of arachidonic acid to thromboxanes, prostaglandins and prostacyclins [36]. When COX is inhibited, the formation of thromboxane A2 is also impaired which thereby can inhibit platelet aggregation [37] (see below for further discussion pertaining to clinical evidence for perioperative bleeding risk). Prostaglandins assist in vasodilation, play a role in temperature regulation in the hypothalamus as well as affect anti-nociception. There are two COX enzymes referred to as COX-1 and COX-2. COX-1 assists with the production of prostaglandins that protect the gastrointestinal mucosa and kidneys as well as play a role in platelet aggregation. On the other hand, COX-2 is expressed locally during an inflammatory response and this expression pattern clarifies how COX-2 selective inhibitors were designed to avoid impairment to the gastric mucosa. NSAIDS are categorized based on chemical structure and selectivity; those included in Table 2 are propionic acids (ibuprofen, ketorolac, ketoprofen, naproxen) acetic acids (diclofenac, indomethacin), enolic acids (meloxicam, piroxicam) and selective COX-2 inhibitors (celecoxib) [36].

Table 2 Perioperative considerations for NSAID use

Non-selective NSAIDS$^{\ominus}$ (COX 1&2 inhibitors)

Drug	Dosing$^{\bullet}$				Renal Reductions	Hepatic Reductions	Pregnancy	Comments	Cautions
	Pediatric		Adult						
	IV	PO	IV	PO					
Ibuprofen (PO) Caldolor (IV)	≥ 6 mos to < 12 yrs: 10 mg/kg/dose q4–6h prn (max dose: 400 mg/ dose); max daily dose: 40 mg/kg/d or 2400 mg/d; whichever is less ≥ 12yrs to ≤ 17 yrs: 400mg q4-6 h prn; max 2400 mg/day Infuse IV dose over ≥ 10 min	4 to 10 mg/ kg/dose q6-8h prn; max dose: 600 mg/ dose; max daily dose: 2400 mg/d	200–400 mg q4-6h prn or 600 -800 mg q6-8h; max dose 3200 mg/d (2400 mg/d suggested for chronic use) infuse IV dose over ≥ 30 min	200–400 mg q4-6h prn or 600–800 mg q6-8h prn; max dose 3200 mg/d (2400 mg/d suggested for chronic use)	AVOID in CrCl ≤ 30 mL/min	None	AVOID NSAIDS ≥ 20 wks GA♣	- Use lowest effective dose for shortest duration to minimize side effects - Avoid in AKI - Avoid in pts ≤ 6 months old (*unless being utilized for tx of PDA; IV ibuprofen as effective as IV indomethacin)	∵Increased risk of MI/CVA/CHF; PRECISION Trial showed no difference of risk between naproxen, ibuprofen, celecoxib$^{\partial}$; FDA concludes insufficient data to denote risk for any specific NSAID compared to another$^{\wp}$ ∵Avoid NSAIDS in patients with aspirin triad (bronchial asthma, aspirin intolerance, rhinitis) ∵Avoid NSAIDS with PUD, recent GI bleeding or perforation ∵CAUTION/AVOID in advanced CKD (see individual comments) ∵Do not combine multiple NSAIDS together or with other anticoagulants ♣AVOID NSAIDS ≥ 20 wks GA as may lead to oligo d/t fetal renal impairment, can cause premature PDA closure ♣May increase risk of miscarriage if taken around time to conception as there is interference with implantation

(continued)

Table 2 (continued)

Non-selective NSAIDS[⊖] (COX 1&2 inhibitors)

Drug	Dosing[•]				Renal Reductions	Hepatic Reductions	Pregnancy	Comments	Cautions
	Pediatric		Adult						
	IV	PO	IV	PO					
Ketorolac	< 6 months: 0.5mg/kg/dose q6h limited to 48 h; postnatal age ≥ 21 days and ≥ PCA 37 wks; normal renal function; UOP ≥ 1 mL/kg/hr; plts ≥ 10,0000/μL; no postop bleeding, daily monitoring of sCr and UOP, plts, hgb/hct at baseline, avoid concurrent nephrotoxic/antiplatelet agents∇ ≥ 6 months to 2yrs: < 0.25–0.5 mg/kg/dose q6-8h, not to exceed 48 to 72 h ≥ 2yo to ≤ 16 yo:- 0.5mg/kg/dose, max 30 mg/dose × 48–72 h; do not exceed 5 days	≥ 2yo to ≤ 16 yo 10 mg/dose; max daily dose 40 mg/day ≥ 17 yo & ≤ 50 kg: 10 mgx1 followed by q4-6 h; max 40 mg/day ≥ 17 yo & ≥ 50 kg: 20 mg × 1 followed by 10 mgq4-6h, max 40 mg qday PO dosing to follow IV dosing (not initial therapy)	< 50 kg or ≥ 65 yo: reduce single dosing to 15 mg × 1 followed by 15mg6h PRN, max dose 120 mg/day ≥ 50 kg and ≤ 65 yo: up to 30 mg/dose × 1 dose followed by 15–30 mg q6h prn, max dose 60 mg/day; limit to 5 days eGFR > 30 to < 60 ml/min/1.73m^2: 7.5–15 mgq6h *Possible analgesic ceiling < 15 mg IV[ϑ]	10 mg q4-6h, max 50 mg qday PO dosing to follow IV dosing (not initial therapy) Use limited to 5 days total (including IV use)	AVOID in CrCl ≤ 30 mL/min	No hepatic dosing reduction recommendations; of note, > 10% incidence of increased LFTs by ≤ 15% (highly protein bound; metabolized hepatically via hydroxylation and glucuronide conjugation)∇	∴BLACK BOX warning of use during L&D as it may affect fetal circulation, inhibit uterine contractions, increase risk of uterine hemorrhage ∴AVOID NSAIDS ≥ 20 wks GA♣ ∴15–30 mg IV after peritoneum closed post C/S delivery recommended per SOAP ERAS Consensus Statementɸ	∴Can also administer IM ∴PO dosing to follow initial IV dosing ∴10% incidence of abdominal pain, dyspepsia, nausea, headache ∴Moderate recommendation for intra-articular injection for TKA/THA (15–30 mg utilized, off label)[∞]	

(continued)

Table 2 (continued)

Non-selective NSAIDS[⊖] (COX 1&2 inhibitors)									
Drug	Dosing[♦]				Renal Reductions	Hepatic Reductions	Pregnancy	Comments	Cautions
	Pediatric		Adult						
	IV	PO	IV	PO					
Keto-profen	—	—	25–50 mg q6-8h, max 300 mg qday	—	AVOID in CrCl ≤ 30 mL/min	Hx of hepatic impairment and serum albumin < 3.5g/dL, max initial dose limited to 100 mg/day; > 10% incidence of increased LFTs by ≤ 15%	AVOID NSAIDS ≥ 20 wks GA[♣]	Enteric coated and ER formulations not recommendation for acute pain and will not be discussed further here	
Naproxen	—	< 60 kg: 5–7 mg/kg/dose q8-12h; max daily dose 1000 mg/d ≥ 60 kg: 5–7 mg/kg/dose q8-12h, max daily 1000 mg/d	—	Immediate release: 500 mg × 1; followed by 250–500 mg q12h or 250 mg q6-8h; max dose 1250 mg day 1, then 1000 mg qday Extended release: 1000 mg/day, can increase up to 1500 mg/day for acute pain	AVOID in CrCl ≤ 30 mL/min	None	∴AVOID NSAIDS ≥ 20 wks GA[♣] ∴ > 10% incidence of dyspepsia and headaches		

(continued)

Table 2 (continued)

Non-selective NSAIDS$^{\Theta}$ (COX 1&2 inhibitors)									
Drug	Dosing•				Renal Reductions	Hepatic Reductions	Pregnancy	Comments	Cautions
	Pediatric		Adult						
	IV	PO	IV	PO					
Diclofenac	–	≥12 yo: 25 mg QID for Immediate release formulation only; PR formulation for postop pain available, 1–2 mg/kg/dose followed by 1 mg/kg/dose TID, max single dose 50mg/dose, max daily dose 3 mg/kg/day, not to exceed 4 days		Diclofenac potassium or sodium: 100-150mg/d divided (suggested 50 mg PO q6-12 hr$^{\Psi}$); Diclofenac acid 18 mg or 35 mg TID; max dose 105 mg/d	AVOID in CrCl ≤ 30 mL/min	None	AVOID NSAIDS ≥ 20 wks GA♣	US max dose 150 to 200 mg/day; Health Canada recommends max dose 100 mg/day to limit risk of vascular events	
Meloxicam	–	Indicated for JIA (not acute pain); ≥ 2 yo: 0.125 mg/kg/day, max dose 7.5 mg/dose ≥60 kg: 7.5 mg/d	30 mg IV/d	Capsule: 5–10 mg/d, max 10mg/d Tablet/suspension: 7.5–15 mg/d, max dose 15 mg/d *Oral dosing is off label	∴AVOID IV in CrCl ≤ 60 mL/min; ∴AVOID PO in CrCl ≤ 30 mL/min	None	AVOID NSAIDS ≥ 20 wks GA♣	Slow onset; not recommended for acute pain; Canadian labeling includes contraindication in children < 18 years of age	

(continued)

Table 2 (continued)

Drug	Dosing[•]				Renal Reductions	Hepatic Reductions	Pregnancy	Comments	Cautions
	Pediatric		Adult						
	IV	PO	IV	PO					
Non-selective NSAIDS[Θ] (COX 1&2 inhibitors)									
Pirox-icam	—	—	—	Indicated for AS at 10-20mg/day or RA at 20mg/day (not indicated for acute pain)	AVOID in CrCl ≤ 60 mL/min	Discontinue if hepatotoxicity occurs during treatment	AVOID NSAIDS ≥ 20 wks GA♣	Canadian labeling includes contraindication in children < 16 years of age	
COX-2[Θ] selective inhibitors									
Celecoxib	—	Indicated for JIA (not acute pain); ≥ 2 yo: ≥ 10 to ≤ 25 kg: 50 mg BID > 25 kg: 100 mg BID	—	400 mg once followed by 200 mg q12h later; followed by 100–200 mg BID; max dose 400 mg/day	AVOID in CrCl ≤ 30 mL/min	Moderate impairment (Child–Pugh class B), reduce dose by 50%; do not use in severe impairment (Child–Pugh class C)	AVOID NSAIDS ≥ 20 wks GA♣	FDA-approved product labeling contradicted in setting of allergy to any sulfonamide chemical group; though reaction is thought to be unlikely between antibiotic sulfonamides reactions and nonantibiotic sulfonamides. Sulfonamide antibiotics are chemically distinct as they contain a arylamine group. Evidence suggests there is no cross-reactivity between arylamine sulfonamides and non-arylamine sulfonamides; Recommend avoiding in patients with a hx of severe reaction to sulfonamides such as SJS/TEN[ξ]	

[Θ]Medications listed only if available within the United States

[•]Acute pain dosing recommendations unless otherwise notated

Abbreviations mos, Months; yrs, Years; mg, Milligram; kg, Kilogram; d, Day; h, Hour; q, Quaque (every/each); wks, Weeks; prn, Pro re nata (as needed); CrCl, Creatine clearance; AKI, Acute kidney injury; tx, Treatment; PDA, Patent ductus arteriosus; MI, Myocardial infarction; CVA, Cerebral vascular accident; CHF, Congestive heart failure; PUD, Peptic ulcer disease; CKD, Chronic kidney disease; PCA, Post conceptual age; UOP, Urine output; plts, Platlet count; µL, Microliter; sCr, Serum creatine; Hgb, Hemoglobin; Hct, Hemocrit; PO, Per os (by mouth); IV, Intravenous; eGFR, Estimated glomerular filtration rate; L&D, Labor and delivery; C/S, C-section; SOAP, Society for Obstetric Anesthesia and Perinatology; ERAS, Enhanced Recovery After Surgery; TKA, Total knee; arthroplasty; THA, Total hip arthroplasty; LFTs, Liver function tests; ER, Extended release; QID, Quarter in die (four times per day); TID, Ter in die (three times per day); BID, Bis in die (two times per day dosing), PR, per rectal; hx, History; JIA, Juvenile idiopathic arthritis; AS, Ankylosing spondylitis; RA, Rheumatoid arthritis; SJS, Stevens-Johnsons syndrome; TEN, Toxic epidermal necrolysis

References [Φ]Bollag et al. [27], [∞]Hannon et al. [28], [℘]Food and Drug Administration (FDA) [29], [ξ]Giles et al. [30], [ϑ]Motov et al. [31], [∂]Nissen et al. [32], Lexicomp [11–18], [Ψ]Schwenk [33], [∇]Stone [34], [ξ]Strom et al. [35]

Dosing and Rout of Administration

The dosing of NSAID agents is complicated by the wide array of agents, their clinical targets, and dosing reductions/clinical considerations. Please refer to Table 2 for renal reductions, hepatic reductions, cautions, pregnancy considerations, and dosing information.

Perioperative Uses

Due to marked differences in various surgical interventions including various amounts of noxious stimulus, it is challenging to decipher the overall perioperative analgesic benefits of NSAID use. McNicol et al. [38] published a Cochrane Review focused on single-dose intravenous ketorolac use for acute postoperative pain in adults. Data was included from 12 studies (1905 patients) in which patients underwent pelvic/abdominal, dental and orthopedic surgery. Ten of the studies included 30 mg intravenous (IV) dosing, while one included 15 mg IV dosing and another 60 mg IV dosing. Eight studies (658 participants) were sub-analyzed to facilitate a comparison of ketorolac to placebo and demonstrated a risk ratio (RR) of participants with at least 50% pain relief over four hours to be 2.81 (95% CI 1.80 to 4.37; number needed to benefit, NNTB = 2.4 (95% CI 1.8 to 3.7). However, this data was based on low certainty evidence with risk of bias, unexplained heterogeneity ($I^2 > 50\%$) and sample size. The time to rescue analgesia was prolonged by a mean of 167 min with ketorolac compared to placebo (6 studies, 633 participants) with moderate certainty.

McNicol et al. [39] also published a Cochrane Review in 2018 investigating single-dose intravenous diclofenac for acute postoperative pain in adults and included 1756 patients from 8 studies. Heterogenous surgical patients were included and doses ranged from 23.75 to 75 mg. The quality of evidence was low due to bias and sample size. Three studies (277 participants) were sub-analyzed comparing diclofenac to placebo which showed a risk ratio (RR) of number of participants with at least 50% pain relief over four hours was 2.4 (95% CI 1.9 to 3.1); and NNTB was 3.8 (95% CI 2.9 to 5.9).

The pediatric population was analyzed in a study conducted by Michelet et al. [23]. In this study, the opioid sparing effects of NSAIDs in pediatric patients were evaluated in a meta-analysis that included 27 RCTs (985 patients). Opioid requirements were reduced post-operatively in the PACU (Standardized Mean Difference, SMD = −0.66, 95% CI −0.84 to −0.48, $p < 0.00001$; $I^2 = 67\%$) and sustained 24-h postoperatively (SMD = −0.83, 95% CI −1.11 to −0.55, $p < 0.00001$), $I^2 = 80\%$). NSAID administration did not decrease pain intensity during the first post-operative day (SMD = −0.32, 95% CI −0.75 to 0.10, $p < 0.00001$; $I^2 = 56\%$). Of note, 8 studies overlap in this meta-analysis with the [30] studies discussed under the acetaminophen subcategory.

Timing of NSAID administration as well as duration of therapy also remains an area for further investigation. Doleman et al. [40] published a Cochrane review including 71 RCTs that evaluated preemptive (medication taken before surgery only, 45 studies) and preventive NSAIDS (those started before and continued during the perioperative period, 26 studies) for postoperative pain in adults. Studies included patients without restriction to surgery performed and evaluation was based on pain scores rated on a Likert scale, 0–10 ranking. Compared to post-incision administration, pre-emptive NSAID administration was demonstrated to decrease both early acute postoperative pain (<6 h post operatively) (MD –0.69, 95% CI −0.97 to −0.41; studies = 36, (2032 patients); $I^2 = 96\%$) as well as late acute postoperative pain (24–48 h postoperative; MD −0.22; 95% CI −0.44 to 0.00; studies = 28 (1645 patients); $I^2 = 87\%$). Time to first analgesic request was increased with pre-emptive NSAID vs post-incision use (MD 17.04 min; 95% CI 3.77 min to 30.31 min, studies = 18; patients = 975; $I^2 = 95\%$) and 24-h morphine consumption was reduced (MD −5.62 mg, 95% CI −9.00 to −2.24 mg; studies = 16; patients = 854, $I^2 = 99\%$). Pre-emptive NSAID administration had no impact on early acute postoperative pain (MD = −0.14 (95% CI −0.39 to 0.12; studies = 18 (1140 patients); late postoperative pain was reduced slightly (MD −0.33, CI −0.59 to −0.07; studies = 21, patients = 1441; $I^2 = 81\%$) and the reduction in 24-h morphine consumption was small (MD −1.93 mg, 95% CI −3.55 to −0.32 mg, studies = 16, patients = 1323, $I^2 = 49\%$). The impact of pre-emptive NSAID administration on time to first analgesic request is unclear (MD 8.51 min; 95% CI −31.24 to 48.27 min, studies = 8, patients = 410, $I^2 = 98\%$). The clinical relevance of these findings is limited based on the magnitude of pain scale score decreases of < 1 point, morphine reduction by 2–6 mg in 24 h and time to first analgesic increased on average by 8–17 min. Conclusions of this study are limited by low certainty evidence but at this time, preemptive versus preventive NSAID administration does not seem to make a large clinical difference.

Adverse Effects

Perioperative Bleeding

From the authors' personal clinical experience, concerns regarding NSAID-induced perioperative bleeding represent the most commonly cited rationale for limited perioperative administration. Diving into the evidence evaluating this surgical dogma, there are two recently published meta-analyses and systematic reviews that specifically evaluate this concern. These studies reveal that the risk of perioperative bleeding is low and outweighed by the overall analgesic benefit of NSAID use in the perioperative period.

Gobble et al. [41] published a meta-analysis of 27 double-blind RCTs (2314 patients) where they evaluated the perioperative use of ketorolac. Dosages of ketorolac in the studies included ranged from 7.5—60 mg and therapeutic duration was between 24 h—4 days postoperatively. Surgical procedures included a wide range of orthopedic, neurosurgical, urologic, abdominal and endoscopic. Five of the seven studies recorded bleeding time; these studies found a nonsignificant prolongation of lab values. Of the two that did find a notable difference, there was no increase in clinically significant bleeding which was defined by the need for postoperative transfusion, readmission or reoperation. The incidence of postoperative bleeding in the ketorolac group was 2.5 versus 2.1% in those patients not exposed to NSAID therapy (OR 1.1; 95% CI 0.61 to 2.06; $p = 0.72$).

Bongiovanni et al. [42] published a broader systematic review and meta-analysis investigating the relationship between NSAIDS and operative bleeding which included a total of 15,1031 patients from 41 RCTs, 27 cohort, and 6 case control studies from all surgical types who received an NSAID during the preoperative, intraoperative or postoperative period. In most studies, patients received ketorolac, diclofenac and ibuprofen. There was no significant increase in the incidence of hematoma formation (35 studies, $p = 0.492$, $I^2 = 19.5\%$), reoperation (19 studies, $p = 0.792$; $I^2 = 10.6\%$), or blood transfusion (16 studies, $p = 0.492$; $I^2 = 0.0\%$) as compared to non-NSAID groups.

Of note, one study by Kelly et al. [43] contributed the majority of patients to this meta-analysis which included 10,6279 patients undergoing elective plastic surgical procedures including breast reduction and body contouring. Specifically, 4924 patients (4.6%) received ketorolac and there was an absolute increased incidence of overall hematoma formation (2.3% vs 1.7%, $p = 0.002$); NNTH = 172 for these patients. Hematoma formation within 72 h of surgery was also elevated in the ketorolac group (1.2 vs. 0.9%; $p = 0.036$). However, when controlling for age, sex, median income, region, Elixhauser comorbidity score, hypertension, deep venous thrombosis history, pulmonary embolism history, tobacco use, need for postoperative anticoagulation and surgical time, there was no difference seen in hematoma formation (Adj OR 1.20; 95% CI 0.99 to1.46). A sub-analysis of patients who received 15 mg of IV ketorolac versus $\geq$ 30 mg IV ketorolac showed no difference in rate of hematoma formation (2.2% vs 2.9%; $p = 0.30$), reoperation (2.5 vs. 2.1%; $p = 0.52$), need for blood transfusion (0.2% vs 0.2%; $p = 0.61$) or renal complications (0.2 vs. 0.0%; $p = 0.35$). There was an increased incidence of reoperation for any reason within 72 h of surgery in the ketorolac group (2.5% vs 1.8%; $p < 0.001$); NNTH = 262; as well as reoperation due to hematoma formation (0.6% vs 0.4%; $p = 0.009$), though the clinical significance of these findings is questionable based on NNTH calculations. The ketorolac group had a decrease in hospital readmission (3.1% vs 5.0%; $p < 0.001$) and a decreased readmission length of stay (3.2 vs. 4.4 days) leading to a notable cost savings. Overall, the authors of this study concluded that the benefits of ketorolac likely outweigh the risks and advocate for postoperative use.

Tonsillectomy, Perioperative Bleeding Risk

Attention has been paid specifically to the bleeding risk with NSAID use after tonsillectomy given that the risk of bleeding may result in respiratory compromise. A 2013 meta-analysis and systematic review by Riggin et al. [44] included only RCTs and analyzed 1747 children and 1446 adults undergoing a tonsillectomy; this study concluded that there was no increased risk of bleeding with NSAID use (adults and children OR 1.30, CI 0.90 to 1.88; $p = 0.16$, children OR 1.06; CI 0.65–1.74; $p = 0.81$). Sub-meta-analyses based on individual NSAIDS demonstrated no increased risk for bleeding for any drug studied including aspirin (n = 1610 [adults only]; OR 4.23, CI 0.64 to 27.66; $p = 0.13$), diclofenac (n = 823; OR 0.98, CI 0.51 to 1.89; $p = 0.95$), ibuprofen (n = 612 [children only]; OR 1.06, CI 0.49 to 2.30; $p = 0.89$), ketoprofen (n = 376; OR 0.89, CI 0.22 to 3.55; $p = 0.87$), ketorolac (n = 579; OR 2.01, CI 0.62 to 6.54, $p = 0.24$) or lornoxicam (n = 120, OR 0.72, CI 0.13 to 4.12; $p = 0.71$). Outcomes measured included bleeding requiring reoperation (n = 1181; OR 1.32, CI 0.59 to 2.95; $p = 0.50$), secondary hemorrhage (n = 584, OR 0.90, CI 0.40 to 2.01; $p = 0.80$), and bleeding requiring readmission (n = 456; OR 1.08, CI 0.54 to 2.15; $p = 0.84$) were all non-significant. Tonsillectomy was performed by electrocautery dissection in 10 studies and cold steel technique in 3 studies. The only significant result regarding bleeding risk was a sub-analysis in which patients were given NSAIDS postoperatively only (n = 2961, OR 2.02, CI 1.25 to 3.27; $p = 0.0042$), but there was no difference in bleeding for NSAID use administered both before, during and/or after surgery (n = 391; OR 0.44, CI 0.12 to 1.65; $p = 0.22$).

Chan and Parikh [45] performed a systematic review and meta-analysis specific to ketorolac use in the tonsillectomy population and concluded that adults are at five times increased risk for post-tonsillectomy hemorrhage with ketorolac use (RR 5.64, CI 2.08 to 15.27, $p < 0.001$); in children (<18 years old) there was no increased risk of bleeding despite use (RR 1.39, CI 0.84 to 2.30; $p = 0.20$). Dosages were not assessed (rather a binary outcome of ketorolac use Y/N) was utilized.

A cochrane review originally published in 2005 and updated in 2012 by Lewis et al. included 1,1011 children (n = 15 studies) concluded there was insufficient evidence to exclude an increased risk of bleeding with NSAID use. A non-significant increase in the risk of bleeding requiring surgical intervention (OR 1.69, CI 0.71 to 4.01) or non-surgical intervention (OR 0.99, CI 0.41 to 2.4) was demonstrated; a reduction in postoperative vomiting with NSAID use was found (RR 0.72, CI 0.61 to 0.85). In comparing ketorolac with other NSAIDS, there was an increased risk of bleeding that required surgical intervention (n = 359; OR 3.82, CI 1.03 to 14.10) [46].

Stokes et al. [47] analyzed 12 RCTs and cohort studies in the tonsillectomy pediatric population that utilized 5–10 mg/kg ibuprofen for postoperative pain control and revealed a non-significant increased tendency for post tonsillar hemorrhage (n = 31,9305; OR = 1.38, CI 1.11 to 1.72; $p = 0.239$).

The American Academy of Otolaryngology Head and Neck Surgery 2019 guidelines state that ketorolac use with tonsillectomy is dependent on provider preference, and it is recognized that there is an increased risk of bleeding in adults which has not been found in children. The society recommends both ibuprofen and acetaminophen for pain control after tonsillectomy and to avoid the use of opioids [48].

We would like to specifically highlight the dosage of ketorolac of included studies in the meta-analysis by Riggin et al. [44] discussed above. A dose of 1 mg/kg IV was utilized in 6 of the included pediatric studies (459 children) and two adult studies utilized dosing regimens of 30 mg IV (80 patients) and 30 mg IM (80 patients).

Current standard pediatric dosing is 0.5 mg/kg (Table 2) and adult dosing ranges from 15- 30 mg IV. Increasingly, 15 mg (vs 30 mg) IV is utilized in adults based on the study by Motov et al. [31] which demonstrated an analgesic ceiling at 10 mg IV based on numeric rating pain scores for patients in the emergency room (Table 2). Ruben et al. (1998), suggested an even lower efficacious dose of 7.5 mg IV q6 hours in spine surgery patients. Experience of the authors (BV and SB) relate that the commonly used dose of 15–30 mg IV in adults is somewhat based on convenience dosing as the dosing vial widely available in the United States contains a concentration of 30 mg/1 mL. According to the manufacture guidelines, patients < 65 years of age are recommended to receive 30 mg IV every 6 hours; in patients ≥ 65 yo, history of renal impairment or < 110 lbs should receive 15 mg IV q6h; labeling includes the caution "not indicated for use in pediatric patients" [49] despite other pharmacy databases including Lexicomp® providing dosing guidelines (Table 2). Dosing as it pertains to clinical bleeding risk, remains a topic for further study.

Plastic Surgery, Perioperative Bleeding

Kelly et al. [50] investigated the effect of ibuprofen on plastic surgery patients. Double-blinded RCTs were included if they had greater than twenty patients; in total 443 patients were included between four studies. All four studies utilized 400 mg PO ibuprofen every four hours, with one study beginning administration preoperatively and the other three starting postoperatively, all continuing at least 1 week postoperatively. Postoperative bleeding was noted in 3.5% of the ibuprofen group and 4.1% in control (RR 0.47; 95% CI 0.10 to 2.09; $p = 0.32$). See above for review of ketorolac in plastic surgery patients also published by Kelley et al. [43].

Walker et al. [51] included 3064 patients from retrospective chart reviews, systematic reviews or RCTs (1679 perioperative NSAID use, 1385 control) and found no difference in bleeding or hematoma formation with overall NSAID use (OR 1.20; 95% CI 0.73 to 1.92; $p = 0.48$) nor when ketorolac (OR 1.48; CI 0.86 to 2.56; $p = 0.57$), ibuprofen (OR 0.55, CI 0.14 to 2.14; $p = 0.87$), or celecoxib (OR 0.22, CI 0.02 to 2.52; $p = 0.39$) were analyzed individually. Of note, the Kelley et al. [50] study was included in this meta-analysis.

Breast Surgery, Perioperative Bleeding

Klifto et al. [52] published a Cochrane Review on the use of NSAIDs for all types of breast surgery. Twelve RCTs were included (1596 patients), of which two studies including 230 patients found no difference in breast hematoma formation within 90 days of surgery as compared to placebo (RR 0.33, 95% CI 0.05 to 2.02, I2 = 0%). Little to no difference was seen in bleeding from any location or need for blood transfusion with NSAID use, yet quality of the evidence was low, limiting confidence in the conclusions.

Aspirin Only Studies-Spine and Cardiac

Two meta-analyses and systematic reviews met our criteria for inclusion for review in this chapter. They are included separately here as aspirin is not typically utilized for pain control. As the only irreversible inhibitor of both cyclooxygenase 1 and 2 enzymes, these studies are reviewed for their benefit in discussing NSAID implications regarding bleeding risk.

Goes et al. [53] published a systematic review and meta-analysis in 2017 investigating aspirin use in spine surgery which found no difference in mean perioperative blood loss compared with placebo. Likewise, no differences were found between groups for cardiac events or stroke. However, only three case series were included, totaling 370 patients, and significant heterogeneity exists between the three studies included by Cuellar et al. [54], Soleman et al. [55] and Park et al. [56]. The study by Cuellar et al. [54] which included 200 patients, found no significant difference in estimated blood loss (642 $\pm$ 905 mLs control vs. 697 $\pm$ 1187 mLs ASA), the amount of blood products transfused, overall intra- and postoperative complication rate (8 vs. 11%), or 30-day hospital readmission rate (5 vs. 5%). However, there was no standardization of surgical types, including cervical through lumbar procedures regardless of the number of segments that required surgical intervention. Further, there was no standardization of aspirin dose with ranges between 81–325 mg reported; 23 of 100 patients who had their aspirin discontinued prior to surgery were taking an unknown dose. Soleman et al. [55] included 102 patients and similarly found no significant difference in estimated blood loss (140 mL control vs 221 ml ASA; $p = 0.08$), postoperative blood loss (168 ml control vs 146 mL ASA; $p = 0.76$), blood transfusion requirements or morbidity and mortality. The third study included was by Park et al. [56] which included 106 patients who underwent a two level or greater segment lumbar fusion. Patients were divided into three groups of which Group 1 (38 patients) did not receive aspirin; group 2 (38 patients) was a chronic aspirin user with instructions to discontinue aspirin one week prior to surgery, while group 3 (30 patients) continued their home use. Similar to the [54, 55] studies, this study also included no difference in intraoperative blood loss (Group 1: 582.8 $\pm$ 259.6 mLs, Group 2: 597.1 $\pm$ 336.0 mLs, and Group 3: 668.1 $\pm$ 453.7 mLs, $p = 0.763$) or total blood loss (Group 1: 1186.5 $\pm$ 383.7, Group 2: 1281.7 $\pm$ 393.6, and Group 3: 1332.8 $\pm$ 464.8 cc; $p = 0.192$). Of note, this study performed platelet function testing on all patients and resulted in Group 1 = 162.7 $\pm$ 65.0, Group 2 = 221.1 $\pm$ 89.4, and Group 3 = 216.1 $\pm$ 92.6 s. These results revealed no statistical difference between groups 2 and 3 ($p = 0.761$), suggesting that the standard recommendations of withholding aspirin for one week prior to surgery may be insufficient for return to normal platelet function. There was a second analysis that was conducted which found a statistical difference in increased blood loss for patients in group 1 who were taking preoperative NSAIDs (1390.1 $\pm$ 370.3 cc vs. 960.3 $\pm$ 260.1 cc; $p = 0.010$), though there was no standardization in specific NSAID medication nor dose and conclusions were also limited by the small sample size.

Hastings et al. [57] investigated perioperative use of aspirin in patients undergoing cardiac surgery and reviewed 13 studies (2399 patients). They concluded that preoperative aspirin reduced the risk of myocardial infarction (OR 0.56; 95% CI 0.33–0.96; $p = 0.03$) but increased postoperative chest tube drainage (mean difference 168 ml; 95% CI, 39–297 ml; P = 0.01), red blood cell transfusion (mean difference 141 ml; 95% CI, 55–226; P = 0.001) and need for surgical re-exploration (OR, 1.85, 95% CI, 1.15 to 2.96; P = 0.01). However, included studies were of low quality and significant heterogeneity, including patients with and without concomitant valve procedures, those undergoing surgery both with and without cardiopulmonary bypass, aspirin dosing ranging from 80 mg—2600 mg daily with no standardization of duration preoperatively, and no standardization of use of antifibrinolytic agents such as aprotinin, tranexamic acid or e-aminocaproic acid.

COX-2 Inhibitors and Perioperative Bleeding

One systematic review and meta-analysis by Teerawattananon et al. [58] was published within the last decade discussing the risks of perioperative bleeding exclusive to cyclooxygenase-2 (COX-2) inhibitors. The sixteen studies (1704 patients) analyzed had treatment groups receiving celecoxib, parecoxib or etoricoxib. Five of the 16 studies (377 patients) reported intraoperative blood loss and found no increase as compared to placebo (weighted mean difference, WMD = −4.96; 95% CI: −17.06 to 7.14; $p = 0.42$), non-selective NSAIDS (WMD = −3.00; 95% CI: −26.3 to 20.3; $p = 0.80$) nor overall combined data (WMD = −4.38; 95% CI: −14.69 to 5.92; $p = 0.4$; $I^2 = 52\%$). Four studies with a total of 324 participants reported postoperative blood loss (mL ± SD) as compared to placebo concluding that COX-2 inhibitors did not significantly increase postoperative blood loss (mL) (WMD = −13.89; 95% CI: −30.24 to 2.47; $p = 0.10$; $I^2 = 13\%$). Four RCTs (430 patients) reported no difference in incidence of blood transfusion between COX-2 inhibitors and placebo or diclofenac in patients undergoing total knee arthroplasty, major abdominal and open prostatectomy surgery. Thirteen RCTs (434 patients) measured serum thromboxane B2 levels; of these, 11 studies found no significant decrease in levels. Two studies with high-dose celecoxib (800 mg single dose) and etoricoxib (90 mg/day) plus aspirin found a significant decrease in platelet dysfunction. Three RCTs (203 patients) found no significant prolongation in bleeding time for patients taking parecoxib and celecoxib when compared to non-selective NSAIDS or placebo. Conclusions are limited by the heterogeneity of surgical type, sample size and COX-2 dosage and duration.

Summary

Regarding bleeding and NSAID use, there is some data to support increase bleeding risk in certain patient populations, such as adult patients undergoing a tonsillectomy with concurrent ketorolac use, that requires the discretion and attention from the provider. However, there is abundant data that suggests safety in the general surgical patient population, as clinically meaningful bleeding has not been demonstrated consistently in the setting of perioperative use of both non-selective and selective COX-2 inhibitors. While data is limited by the broad spectrum of surgical procedures and specific NSAIDs investigated, the consistent findings suggest that more widespread use of NSAID medications during the perioperative period may lead to increased surgical bleeding but not in a clinically meaningful way such as requiring blood transfusions, return to the operating room for hematoma evacuation or an increase in hospital readmissions.

Anastomotic Leak (AL)

There is concern in the colorectal literature for increased risk of anastomotic leak (AL) with NSAID use. While the exact mechanism of AL is unknown, it is thought that NSAIDS reduce the production of hyaluronic acid that is necessary for collagen formation and anastomotic healing [59]. The incidence of AL has been cited between 2–15% and varies based on site of anastomosis and presence of risk factors including advanced age, comorbidities, malnutrition, alcohol and tobacco abuse, surgical indications, operative duration, intraoperative blood loss, adequacy of blood supply to the anastomosis, perioperative hypoxemia and volume deficits [59]. The Enhanced Recovery After Surgery (ERAS) Society for Colorectal Surgery updated their recommendations in 2018 and concluded there was insufficient evidence to avoid NSAID use in this patient population, especially considering the benefits of decreased opioid use and minimized risk of postoperative ileus [60]. In addition, the American Society of Colon and Rectal Surgeons (ASCRS) and Endoscopic Surgeons (SAGES) also supports the use of multimodal analgesia including the short-term use of NSAIDs [61]. The outlined literature below was chosen based on availability on PubMed featuring meta-analyses, randomized controlled trials and systematic reviews published in the last 10 years (2012–2022).

Burton et al. [62] published a systematic review and meta-analysis of RCTs and found no significant difference in the incidence of anastomotic dehiscence in NSAID users as compared to controls, six trials with a total of 480 patients were included. A year later, Bhangu et al. [63] published a meta-analysis which included RCTs and cohort studies with the primary endpoint being anastomotic leak in NSAID exposed humans and animals. In humans, nonselective NSAIDS were found to be associated with an increased risk of anastomotic leak (6 studies, 3074 patients, OR 2.37; $p < 0.001$), while COX-2 inhibitors were not (4 studies, 1223 patients, OR 2.32; $p = 0.170$). Most patients included in this analysis underwent either a colocolic or colorectal anastomosis. In a subgroup analysis by NSAID type, patients receiving diclofenac had a significantly elevated occurrence of anastomotic leak (three studies, 2869 patients, OR 2.32, 95% CI 1.66 to 3.25; $p < 0.001$), but this finding was not found in patients receiving ketorolac (3 studies, 205 patients, OR 3.10, 95% CI 0.81 to 11.82; $p = 0.100$). An increased risk of anastomotic leak with nonselective NSAIDS has been subsequently reiterated in systematic reviews and meta-analyses by Peng et al. [64], Smith et al. [65], Modasi et al. [66], Huang et al. [67], which encompass significant patient overlap and thus are not discussed separately.

Kastora et al. [68] published a systematic review and meta-analysis including 2,5395 colorectal oncology patients from RCTs and cohort studies which found no overall increased incidence of AL in NSAID-exposed patients compared to controls (OR 1.07 (0.82–1.40, $p = 0.62$). In a subgroup analysis examining the site of anastomosis, colocolic anastomoses were found to be more prone to AL in the non-specific NSAID exposed population (OR 1.55, CI 0.93–2.59; $p = 0.10$) in comparison to ileocolic (OR 0.98, CI 0.72 to 1.32; $p = 0.87$) or colorectal anastomoses (OR 0.97, CI 0.76 to 1.23; $p = 0.79$), though notably none of these subgroups were statistically significant. Of the colocolic patients' subgroup only, the rate of AL was increased with nonselective NSAID use (OR 3.25, CI 0.98 to 10.72; $p = 0.054$). This finding did not persist when ketorolac use was analyzed separately from other nonselective NSAIDS (OR 2.11, CI 0.28 to 16.14, $p = 0.47$) nor when exclusive COX-2 inhibitor use was sub-analyzed (OR 1.82, CI 0.51 to 6.52, $p = 0.36$). Overall, male gender was found to be an independent confounder of increased anastomotic leak in the NSAID exposed groups.

Summary

While further investigation with randomized and blinded controlled trials are needed, at this time, the data suggests safety of NSAID use in the perioperative period. The optimal NSAID (selective or non-selective) and dosing regimen that limits the risk of AL remains to be determined, though current evidence is most supportive of COX-2 selective drugs as well as the non-selective agent ketorolac. Diclofenac is avoided due to evidence for increased anastomotic leak. Use should be curtailed to patients without significant comorbidities that may contribute to NSAID morbidity as outlined above and specific anastomotic site may play a role.

Bone Healing

The concern of NSAID impairment of bone healing resulting in fracture nonunion in orthopedic and spine surgery has resulted in understandable hesitancy to utilize these medications despite the desire for opioid alternatives. The mechanism proposed for nonunion is by NSAID inhibition of COX-1 and COX-2 enzymes thereby decreasing prostaglandin E2 (PGE2) and inhibiting osteoblastic expression of receptor activator of nuclear factor kappa-B ligand and osteoprotegerin [69, 70]. While animal studies have signaled concern for this deleterious effect on bone healing, there remains a paucity of prospective randomized controlled trials in humans to confirm this finding [71]. To stay within the scope of this chapter and to focus on current evidence, the studies outlined below are limited to meta-analyses, systematic reviews and randomized controlled trials published within the last decade [2012–2022], indexed on PubMed and focused on the oral (PO or intravenous (IV NSAID administration route in patients sustaining bone fractures or undergoing spine surgery. Tendon and cartilage healing implications are outside the scope of this chapter.

Wheatley et al. [72] conducted a meta-analysis including patients with and without NSAID exposure who had the presence of healing bone from fracture, osteotomy, and/or fusion surgery. Results concluded an increased risk of delayed or nonunion in the NSAID-exposed population (a total of 512 cases of delayed or nonunion were reported of which 226 had been exposed to NSAIDS; OR 2.07; CI 1.19 to 3.61). Further, this finding was more pronounced in a sub-analysis of adult long bone fractures (n = 6 studies; OR 2.34; CI 1.12 to 4.90) and spine fusion surgeries (OR 4.90; CI 1.45 to 16.58). A separate analysis of studies utilizing low-dose NSAID use only (defined as < 125 mg/d of diclofenac, 150 mg/d of indomethacin, or 120 mg/d of ketorolac) or short-duration (<2 weeks of treatment) showed no increased risk of delayed union (at 6 months or more) or nonunion (OR, 1.68; CI, 0.63 to 4.46; 510 cases exposed to NSAIDS vs 599 cases not exposed; total 1109 cases) which included patients undergoing spinal fusion surgery or with femoral or tibial fractures. In the pediatric population (age < 18 years old), there was no increased risk of nonunion; 1181 exposed/836 not exposed (OR, 0.58; CI, 0.27 to 1.21) [72]. Likewise, [73] performed a prospective, randomized, single-blinded study in pediatric patients that also concluded no difference in occurrence of delayed union or nonunion in 102 long bone fractures, again suggesting that age may contribute to risk.

A follow-up study [74] reported a systematic review and meta-analysis including 111 studies which pooled 4,1429 patients exclusively with tibial fractures and assessed risk factors for nonunion; NSAID use was one of fifteen factors identified. In this NSAID-exposed subpopulation, a significant increase in nonunion was found with [p = 0.018, OR 1.536; CI 1.076–2.194] as compared to no NSAID exposure. Of note, this outcome was analyzed as a binary outcome (Y/N) and did not consider the frequency or dose of drug exposure. This study focused on tibial fractures exclusively, and it is recognized that the tibia's long subcutaneous boundary and thereby poorer blood supply independently elevates the risk of nonunion as compared to other long bones.

When considering DEXA-scanning, bone markers and histological changes evaluated at baseline and compared to 1, 2, 6 weeks, 3 months and 1 year follow-up, Aliuskevicus et al. [75], found no difference in patients treated with 600 mg ibuprofen three times a day up to 7 days after Colles' fractures that required external fixation. Likewise, no difference in radiological migration including changes in radius tilt, length and inclination or wrist function measured by differences in motion between the injured and non-injured wrist and DASH score at 3 and 12 months were found in the ibuprofen group [76]. Colle's fracture patients treated without surgical intervention and the same ibuprofen regimen demonstrated no differences in fragment migration or wrist range of motion at 5 week follow-up [77].

Focusing on spinal fusion outcomes, [78] published a systematic review of 68 studies which included biochemical, animal and human studies and concluded that NSAIDS have a dose and duration dependent effect on spinal fusion rate. Specific to humans, using NSAIDs for less than two-weeks postoperatively may be safe and similarly utilizing the lowest effective dose seems most reasonable. Borgeat et al. [79] published a systematic review including only studies specific to humans undergoing a spinal fusion. A total of 1,2895 patients were included and likewise concluded that a short perioperative course of < 14 days, is likely safe. Again, this study highlighted the need for future randomized controlled trials for more definitive conclusions.

Summary

In conclusion, specific dosing regimens, NSAID selection, duration of use, location of fracture or fusion, and age of patient are major factors implicated in modifying bone healing risk with NSAID use. It is challenging to compare pediatric to adult data as the standard of care is to utilize weight-based dosing in pediatric patients, while adult dosing must consider dose reductions for renal impairment but generally does not consider weight as a factor. Further studies are needed to provide additional clarity and solidify recommendations.

4 Conclusion

Acetaminophen and NSAIDs equip the provider with an adjunct or an alternative to the opioid medications commonly given to patients in the perioperative setting. These agents may play a pivotal analgesic role in patients with a history of chronic opioid use, tolerance, dependence, or misuse. In patients treated with opioid receptor antagonists or partial agonists, acetaminophen and NSAID analgesics can help alleviate pain via pathways not already substantially impaired via other therapeutics. In addition, the use of these agents may represent vital components of enhanced recovery pathways as they limit opioid-related side effects including ileus and respiratory depression.

Acetaminophen, via a nebulous mechanism including reduction of the COX pathway and inhibition of prostaglandins in the CNS, results in analgesic effects that are lower than for NSAIDs. Route of administration does not appear to impact clinical effect, but the use of acetaminophen in patients does appear to reduce pain scores in adult and pediatric populations. Further RCTs that evaluate acetaminophen with and without opioid consumption as part of a multimodal perioperative acute pain regimen would offer further clarity on its use without adjuncts.

NSAIDs, by inhibiting COX enzyme and halting production to thromboxanes, prostaglandins and prostacyclins from arachidonic acid, remain a meaningful component of postoperative analgesic regimens. In the clinical setting, conversations discussing administration limitations are common between anesthesia and surgical colleagues; reservations about NSAID-induced clinical bleeding risk and impaired bone healing are common. Based on a literature review, apart from adult patients undergoing a tonsillectomy with concurrent ketorolac, several studies minimize the risk of bleeding by addressing clinically meaningful endpoints including blood transfusion requirement, incidence of return to the operating room for hematoma evacuation or an increased risk of hospital readmissions. The risk of surgical bleeding from NSAIDs, in most circumstances, is not high enough to prevent its use. Surgeons also voice concerns, understandably, about bone healing with the use of NSAIDs due to NSAID inhibition of COX-1 and COX-2 enzymes thereby decreasing prostaglandin E2 (PGE2) and inhibiting osteoblastic expression of receptor activator of nuclear factor kappa-B ligand and osteoprotegerin. There are no solid randomized controlled trials that strictly preclude the use of NSAIDs in orthopedic long bone or spine surgery, but metanalyses have demonstrated that specific dosing regimens and NSAID drug, duration of use, location of fracture or fusion, and age of patient are major identified factors in bone healing risk with NSAID use.

Overall, evidence-based medicine is supportive of the use of acetaminophen and NSAIDs as components of multimodal analgesic plans; this chapter reviews the pertinent literature to allow for prudent decision-making by the provider in terms of dose, route of administration, and perioperative risk estimation.

References

1. Gerriets V, Anderson J, Nappe TM. Acetaminophen. In: Aboubakar S, Abu-Ghosh A, Acharya AB, Adibi Sedeh, P, Aeby TC, et al. Editorial Board. StatPearls [e-book]. Treasure Island (FL): StatPearls Publishing. Available from: https://www.ncbi.nlm.nih.gov/books/NBK482369/ (2022). Cited 18 Sept 2022.
2. Food and Drug Administration (FDA) 2010 Cadence Pharmaceuticals, Inc. Ofirmev (Acetaminophen) Injection. https://www.accessdata.fda.gov/drugsatfda_docs/label/2010/022450lbl.pdf. Accessed 28 Jan 2023.
3. Lexicomp. Acetaminophen: Drug information. UpToDate. https://www-uptodate-com.libproxy.csudh.edu/contents/acetaminophen-drug-information (n.d). Cited 18 Jan 2023.
4. Pettersson PH, Jakobsson J, Öwall A. Intravenous acetaminophen reduced the use of opioids compared with oral administration after coronary artery bypass grafting. J Cardiothorac Vasc Anesth. 2005;19(3):306–9. https://doi.org/10.1053/j.jvca.2005.03.006.
5. Brett CN, Barnett SG, Pearson J. Postoperative plasma paracetamol levels following oral or intravenous paracetamol administration: a double-blind randomised controlled trial. Anaesth Intensive Care. 2012;31(1):166–71. https://doi.org/10.1177/0310057X1204000121.
6. Fenlon S, Collyer J, Giles J, Bidd H, Lees M, Nicholson J, et al. Oral vs intravenous paracetamol for lower third molar extractions under general anaesthesia: is oral administration inferior? Br J Anaesth. 2013;110(3):432–7. https://doi.org/10.1093/bja/aes387.
7. Teng Y, Zhang Y, Li B. Intravenous versus oral acetaminophen as an adjunct on pain and recovery after total knee arthroplasty: a systematic review and meta-analysis. Medicine (Baltimore). 2020;99(50): e23515. https://doi.org/10.1097/MD.0000000000023515.
8. Stagg K. Intravenous versus oral paracetamol for postoperative analgesia: a systematic review. J Perioper Pract. 2021;31(10):373–8. https://doi.org/10.1177/1750458920950652.

9. Jibril F, Sharaby S, Mohamed A, Wilby KJ. Intravenous versus oral acetaminophen for pain: systematic review of current evidence to support clinical decision-making. Can J Hosp Pharm. 2015;68(3):238–47. https://doi.org/10.4212/cjhp.v68i3.1458.
10. Goldstein LH, Berlin M, Berkovitch M, Kozer E. Effectiveness of oral vs rectal acetaminophen: a meta-analysis. Arch Pediatr Adolesc Med. 2008;162(11):1042–6. https://doi.org/10.1001/archpedi.162.11.1042.
11. Lexicomp. Ibuprofen: Drug information. UpToDate. Retrieved January 23, 2023, from https://www-uptodate-com.libproxy.csudh.edu/contents/ibuprofen-drug-information (n.d). Cited 23 Jan 2023.
12. Lexicomp. Ketorolac: Drug information. UpToDate. https://www-uptodate-com.libproxy.csudh.edu/contents/ketorolac-drug-information (n.d). Cited 23 Jan 2023.
13. Lexicomp. Ketoprofen: Drug information. UpToDate. https://www-uptodate-com.libproxy.csudh.edu/contents/ketoprofen-drug-information (n.d). Cited 23 Jan 2023.
14. Lexicomp. Diclofenac: Drug information. UpToDate. https://www.uptodate.com/contents/diclofenac-systemic-drug-information?search=diclofenac:&source=panel_search_result&selectedTitle=1%7E110&usage_type=panel&showDrugLabel=true&display_rank=1 (n.d). Cited 23 Jan 2023.
15. Lexicomp. Naproxen: Drug information. UpToDate. https://www.uptodate.com/contents/naproxen-drug-information?search=naproxen&source=panel_search_result&selectedTitle=1%7E150&usage_type=panel&kp_tab=drug_general&display_rank=1 (n.d). Cited 23 Jan 2023.
16. Lexicomp. Meloxicam: Drug information. UpToDate. https://www.uptodate.com/contents/meloxicam-drug-information?search=meloxicam&source=panel_search_result&selectedTitle=1%7E27&usage_type=panel&kp_tab=drug_general&display_rank=1 (n.d). Cited 23 Jan 2023.
17. Lexicomp. Piroxicam: Drug information. UpToDate. https://www.uptodate.com/contents/piroxicam-drug-information?source=auto_suggest&selectedTitle=1~1---1~4---piroxicam&search=piroxicam (n.d). Cited 23 Jan 2023.
18. Lexicomp. Celecoxib. Drug information. UpToDate. https://www.uptodate.com/contents/celecoxib-drug-information?search=Celecoxib&source=panel_search_result&selectedTitle=1%7E114&usage_type=panel&kp_tab=drug_general&display_rank=1 (n.d). Cited 23 Jan 2023.
19. Birmingham PK, Tobin MJ, Henthorn TK, Fisher DM, Berkelhamer MC, Smith FA, Fanta KB, Coté CJ. Twenty-four-hour pharmacokinetics of rectal acetaminophen in children: an old drug with new recommendations. Anesthesiology. 1997;87(2):244–52. https://doi.org/10.1097/00000542-199708000-00010.
20. Maund E, McDaid C, Rice S, Wright K, Jenkins B, Woolacott N. Paracetamol and selective and non-selective non-steroidal anti-inflammatory drugs for the reduction in morphine-related side-effects after major surgery: a systematic review. Br J Anaesth. 2011;106(3):292–7. https://doi.org/10.1093/bja/aeq406.
21. Bailey E, Worthington H, Coulthard P. Ibuprofen and/or paracetamol (acetaminophen) for pain relief after surgical removal of lower wisdom teeth, a Cochrane systematic review. Br Dent J. 2014;216(8):451–5. https://doi.org/10.1038/sj.bdj.2014.330.
22. Wong I, St John-Green C, Walker SM. Opioid-sparing effects of perioperative paracetamol and nonsteroidal anti-inflammatory drugs (NSAIDs) in children. Paediatr Anaesth. 2013;23(6):475–95. https://doi.org/10.1111/pan.12163.
23. Michelet D, Andreu-Gallien J, Bensalah T, Hilly J, Wood C, Nivoche Y, et al. A meta-analysis of the use of nonsteroidal antiinflammatory drugs for pediatric postoperative pain. Anesth Analg. 2012;114(2):393–406. https://doi.org/10.1213/ANE.0b013e31823d0b45.
24. Archer V, Cloutier Z, Park L, Briatico D, Walton JM. Intravenous acetaminophen for postoperative pain control after open abdominal and thoracic surgery in pediatric patients: a systematic review and meta-analysis. Pediatr Surg Int. 2022;39(1):7. https://doi.org/10.1007/s00383-022-05282-0.
25. Agrawal S, Khazaeni B. Acetaminophen Toxicity. In: Aboubakar S, Abu-Ghosh A, Acharya AB, Adibi Sedeh P, Aeby TC, et al. Editorial Board. StatPearls [e-book]. Treasure Island (FL): StatPearls Publishing. Available from: https://www.ncbi.nlm.nih.gov/books/NBK441917/. (2022). Cited 1 Aug 2022

26. Fontana RJ. Acute liver failure including acetaminophen overdose. Med Clin North Am. 2008;92(4): 761–viii. https://doi.org/10.1016/j.mcna.2008.03.005
27. Bollag L, Lim G, Sultan P, Habib AS, Landau R, Zakowski M, Tiouririne M, Bhambhani S, Carvalho B. Society for obstetric anesthesia and perinatology: consensus statement and recommendations for enhanced recovery after cesarean. Anesth Analg. 2021;132(5):1362–77. https://doi.org/10.1213/ANE.0000000000005257. PMID: 33177330.
28. Hannon CP, Fillingham YA, Spangehl MJ, Karas V, Kamath AF, Hamilton WG, Della Valle CJ; AAHKS Anesthesia & Analgesia Clinical Practice Guideline Workgroup. Periarticular injection in total joint arthroplasty: the clinical practice guidelines of the American association of hip and knee surgeons, American society of regional anesthesia and pain medicine, American academy of orthopaedic surgeons, hip society, and knee society. J Arthroplasty. 2022;37(9):1701–1707. https://doi.org/10.1016/j.arth.2022.03.048. PMID: 35970572.
29. Food and Drug Administration (FDA). FDA Drug Safety Communication: FDA strengthens warning that non-aspirin nonsteroidal anti-inflammatory drugs (NSAIDs) can cause heart attacks or strokes. 2015. https://www.fda.gov/drugs/drug-safety-and-availability/fda-drug-safety-communication-fda-strengthens-warning-non-aspirin-nonsteroidal-anti-inflammatory [PubMed FDA.1]
30. Giles A, Foushee J, Lantz E, Gumina G. Sulfonamide allergies. Pharmacy (Basel). 2019;7(3):132. https://doi.org/10.3390/pharmacy7030132.
31. Motov S, Yasavolian M, Likourezos A, Pushkar I, Hossain R, Drapkin J, et al. Comparison of intravenous ketorolac at three single-dose regimens for treating acute pain in the emergency department: a randomized controlled trial. Ann Emerg Med. 2017;70(2):177–84. https://doi.org/10.1016/j.annemergmed.2016.10.014.
32. Nissen SE, Yeomans ND, Solomon DH, et al. Cardiovascular safety of celecoxib, naproxen, or ibuprofen for arthritis. N Engl J Med. 2016;375(26):2519–29. https://doi.org/10.1056/NEJMoa1611593. [PubMed 27959716].
33. Schwenk ES. Nonopioid pharmacotherapy for acute pain in adults: Table: Nonopioid analgesics commonly used for periop pain. Post TW, ed. UpTo.Date. Waltham, MA: UpToDate INC. http://www.uptodate.com. accessed 23 Jan 2023.
34. Stone SB. Ketorolac in postoperative neonates and infants: a systematic review. J Pediatr Pharmacol Ther. 2021;26(3):240–47. https://doi.org/10.5863/1551-6776-26.3.240. Epub 2021 Mar 31. PMID: 33833624; PMCID: PMC8021237.
35. Strom BL, Schinnar R, Apter AJ, Margolis DJ, Lautenbach E, Hennessy S, Bilker WB, Pettitt D. Absence of cross-reactivity between sulfonamide antibiotics and sulfonamide nonantibiotics. N Engl J Med. 2003;349(17):1628–35. https://doi.org/10.1056/NEJMoa022963. PMID: 14573734.
36. Ghlichloo I, Gerriets V. Nonsteroidal Anti-inflammatory Drugs (NSAIDs). In: Aboubakar S, Abu-Ghosh A, Acharya AB, Adibi Sedeh P, Aeby TC, et al. Editorial Board. StatPearls [e-book]. Treasure Island (FL): StatPearls Publishing. Available from:" https://www.ncbi.nlm.nih.gov/books/NBK547742/ (2022). Cited 18 May 2022.
37. Schafer AI. Effects of nonsteroidal antiinflammatory drugs on platelet function and systemic hemostasis. J Clin Pharmacol. 1995 Mar;35(3):209–19. https://doi.org/10.1002/j.1552-4604.1995.tb04050.x. PMID: 7608308.
38. McNicol ED, Ferguson MC, Schumann R. Single-dose intravenous ketorolac for acute postoperative pain in adults. Cochrane Database Syst Rev. 2021;5(5):CD013263. https://doi.org/10.1002/14651858.CD013263.pub2
39. McNicol ED, Ferguson MC, Schumann R. Single-dose intravenous diclofenac for acute postoperative pain in adults. Cochrane Database Syst Rev. 2018;8(8):CD012498. https://doi.org/10.1002/14651858.CD012498.pub2
40. Doleman B, Leonardi-Bee J, Heinink TP, Boyd-Carson H, Carrick L, Mandalia R, et al. Pre-emptive and preventive NSAIDs for postoperative pain in adults undergoing all types of surgery. Cochrane Database Syst Rev. 2021;6(6):CD012978. https://doi.org/10.1002/14651858.CD012978.pub2

41. Gobble RM, Hoang HLT, Kachniarz B, Orgill DP. Ketorolac does not increase perioperative bleeding: a meta-analysis of randomized controlled trials. Plast Reconstr Surg. 2014;133(3):741–55. https://doi.org/10.1097/01.prs.0000438459.60474.b5.
42. Bongiovanni T, Lancaster E, Ledesma Y, Whitaker E, Steinman MA, Allen IE, et al. Systematic review and meta-analysis of the association between non-steroidal anti-inflammatory drugs and operative bleeding in the perioperative period. J Am Coll Surg. 2021;232(5):765-790.e1. https://doi.org/10.1016/j.jamcollsurg.2021.01.005.
43. Kelley BP, Chung KC, Chung TT, Bennett KG, Sacks G, Sears ED, Waljee JF. Postoperative ketorolac in breast and body contouring procedures: a nationwide claims analysis. Plast Reconstr Surg. 2018;142(4):472e-e480. https://doi.org/10.1097/PRS.0000000000004806.
44. Riggin L, Ramakrishna J, Sommer DD, Koren G. A 2013 updated systematic review & meta-analysis of 36 randomized controlled trials; no apparent effects of non steroidal anti-inflammatory agents on the risk of bleeding after tonsillectomy. Clinical Otolaryngol. 2013;38(2):115–29. https://doi.org/10.1111/coa.12106.
45. Chan DK, Parikh SR. Perioperative ketorolac increases post-tonsillectomy hemorrhage in adults but not children. Laryngoscope. 2014;124(8):1789–93. https://doi.org/10.1002/lary.24555.
46. Lewis SR, Nicholson A, Cardwell ME, Siviter G, Smith AF. Nonsteroidal anti-inflammatory drugs and perioperative bleeding in paediatric tonsillectomy. Cochrane Database Syst Rev. 2013(7):CD003591. https://doi.org/10.1002/14651858.CD003591.pub3
47. Stokes W, Swanson RT, Schubart J, Carr MM. Postoperative bleeding associated with ibuprofen use after tonsillectomy: a meta-analysis. Otolaryngol Head Neck Surg. 2019;161(5):734–41. https://doi.org/10.1177/0194599819852328.
48. Mitchell RB, Archer SM, Ishman SL, Rosenfeld RM, Coles S, Finestone SA et al. Clinical practice guideline: tonsillectomy in children (Update). Otolaryngol Head Neck Surg. 2019;160(1_suppl):S1–S42. https://doi.org/10.1177/0194599818801757.
49. Hospira, Inc. Ketorolac Tromethamine Injection. https://www.accessdata.fda.gov/drugsatfda_docs/label/2014/074802s038lbl.pdf. (2014). Cited 25 Feb 2022.
50. Kelley BP, Bennett KG, Chung KC, Kozlow JH. Ibuprofen may not increase bleeding risk in plastic surgery: a systematic review and meta-analysis. Plast Reconstr Surg. 2016;137(4):1309–16. https://doi.org/10.1097/PRS.0000000000002027.
51. Walker NJ, Jones VM, Kratky L, Chen H, Runyan CM. Hematoma risks of nonsteroidal anti-inflammatory drugs used in plastic surgery procedures: a systematic review and meta-analysis. Ann Plast Surg. 2019;82(6S Suppl 5): S437–S445. https://doi.org/10.1097/SAP.0000000000001898
52. Klifto KM, Elhelali A, Payne RM, Cooney CM, Manahan MA, Rosson GD. Perioperative systemic nonsteroidal anti-inflammatory drugs (NSAIDs) in women undergoing breast surgery. Cochrane Database Syst Rev. 2021;11(11):CD013290. https://doi.org/10.1002/14651858.CD013290.pub2
53. Goes R, Muskens IS, Smith TR, Mekary RA, Broekman MLD, Moojen WA. Risk of aspirin continuation in spinal surgery: a systematic review and meta-analysis. Spine J. 2017;17(12):1939–46. https://doi.org/10.1016/j.spinee.2017.08.238.
54. Cuellar JM, Petrizzo A, Vaswani R, Goldstein JA, Bendo, JA. Does aspirin administration increase perioperative morbidity in patients with cardiac stents undergoing spinal surgery? Spine (Phila Pa 1976). 2015;40(9):629–35. https://doi.org/10.1097/BRS.0000000000000695.
55. Soleman J, Baumgarten P, Perrig WN, Fandino J, Fathi AR. Non-instrumented extradural lumbar spine surgery under low-dose acetylsalicylic acid: a comparative risk analysis study. Eur Spine J. 2015;25(3):732–9. https://doi.org/10.1007/s00586-015-3864-7.
56. Park HJ, Kwon KY, Woo JH. Comparison of blood loss according to use of aspirin in lumbar fusion patients. Eur Spine J. 2014;23(8):1777–82. https://doi.org/10.1007/s00586-014-3294-y.
57. Hastings S, Myles P, McIlroy D. Aspirin and coronary artery surgery: a systematic review and meta-analysis. Br J Anaesth. 2015;115(3):376–85. https://doi.org/10.1093/bja/aev164.

58. Teerawattananon C, Tantayakom P, Suwanawiboon B, Katchamart W. Risk of perioperative bleeding related to highly selective cyclooxygenase-2 inhibitors: a systematic review and meta-analysis. Semin Arthritis Rheum. 2017;46(4):520–8. https://doi.org/10.1016/j.semarthrit.2016.07.008.
59. Slim K, Joris J, Beloeil H, Groupe Francophone de Réhabilitation Améliorée après Chirurgie (GRACE). Colonic anastomoses and non-steroidal anti-inflammatory drugs. J Visc Surg. 2016;153(4):269–75. https://doi.org/10.1016/j.jviscsurg.2016.06.011
60. Gustafsson UO, Scott MJ, Hubner M, Nygren J, Demartines N, Francis N, et al. Guidelines for perioperative care in elective colorectal surgery: enhanced recovery after surgery (eras®) society recommendations: 2018. World J Surg. 2019;43(3):659–95. https://doi.org/10.1007/s00268-018-4844-y.
61. Irani JL, Hedrick TL, Miller TE, Lee L, Steinhagen E, Shogan BD, Goldberg JE, Feingold DL, Lightner AL, Paquette IM. Clinical practice guidelines for enhanced recovery after colon and rectal surgery from the American society of colon and rectal surgeons and the society of American gastrointestinal and endoscopic surgeons. Surg Endosc. 2023;37(1):5–30. https://doi.org/10.1007/s00464-022-09758-x. Epub 2022 Dec 14.
62. Burton TP, Mittal A, Soop M. Nonsteroidal anti-inflammatory drugs and anastomotic dehiscence in bowel surgery: systematic review and meta-analysis of randomized, controlled trials. Dis Colon Rectum. 2013;56(1):126–34. https://doi.org/10.1097/DCR.0b013e31825fe927.
63. Bhangu A, Singh P, Fitzgerald JE, Slesser A, Tekkis P. Postoperative nonsteroidal anti-inflammatory drugs and risk of anastomotic leak: meta-analysis of clinical and experimental studies. World J Surg. 2014;38(9):2247–57. https://doi.org/10.1007/s00268-014-2531-1.
64. Peng F, Liu S, Hu Y, Yu M, Chen J, Liu C. Influence of perioperative nonsteroidal anti-inflammatory drugs on complications after gastrointestinal surgery: a meta-analysis. Acta Anaesthesiol Taiwan. 2016;54(4):121–8. https://doi.org/10.1016/j.aat.2016.11.002.
65. Smith SA, Roberts DJ, Lipson ME, Buie WD, MacLean AR. Postoperative nonsteroidal anti-inflammatory drug use and intestinal anastomotic dehiscence: a systematic review and meta-analysis. Dis Colon Rectum. 2016;59(11):1087–97.
66. Modasi A, Pace D, Godwin M, Smith C, Curtis B. NSAID administration post colorectal surgery increases anastomotic leak rate: systematic review/meta-analysis. Surg Endosc. 2019;33(3):879–85. https://doi.org/10.1007/s00464-018-6355-1.
67. Huang Y, Tang SR, Young CJ. Nonsteroidal anti-inflammatory drugs and anastomotic dehiscence after colorectal surgery: a meta-analysis. ANZ J Surg. 2018;88(10):959–65. https://doi.org/10.1111/ans.14322.
68. Kastora SL, Osborne LL, Jardine R, Kounidas G, Carter B, Myint PK. Non-steroidal anti-inflammatory agents and anastomotic leak rates across colorectal cancer operations and anastomotic sites: a systematic review and meta-analysis of anastomosis specific leak rate and confounding factors. Eur J Surg Oncol. 2021;47(11):2841–8. https://doi.org/10.1016/j.ejso.2021.05.040.
69. Kidd LJ, Cowling NR, Wu AC, Kelly WL, Forwood MR. Selective and non-selective cyclooxygenase inhibitors delay stress fracture healing in the rat ulna. J Orthop Res. 2013;31(2):235–42. https://doi.org/10.1002/jor.22203.
70. Ramirez-Yanez GO, Symons AL. Prostaglandin E2 affects osteoblast biology in a dose-dependent manner: an in vitro study. Arch Oral Biol. 2012;57(9):1274–81. https://doi.org/10.1016/j.archoralbio.2012.03.003.
71. Marquez-Lara A, Hutchinson ID, Nuñez F Jr, Smith TL, Miller AN. Nonsteroidal anti-inflammatory drugs and bone-healing: a systematic review of research quality. JBJS Rev. 2016;4(3): e4. https://doi.org/10.2106/JBJS.RVW.O.00055.
72. Wheatley BM, Nappo KE, Christensen DL, Holman AM, Brooks DI, Potter BK. Effect of NSAIDs on bone healing rates: a meta-analysis. J Am Acad Orthop Surg. 2019;27(7):e330-36. https://doi.org/10.5435/JAAOS-D-17-00727.
73. Nuelle JAV, Coe KM, Oliver HA, Cook JL, Hoernschemeyer DG, Gupta SK. Effect of NSAID use on bone healing in pediatric fractures: a preliminary, prospective, randomized blinded study. J Pediatr Orthop. 2020;40(8):e683–9. https://doi.org/10.1097/BPO.0000000000001603.

74. Tian R, Zheng F, Zhao W, Zhang Y, Yuan J, Zhang B et al. Prevalence and influencing factors of nonunion in patients with tibial fracture: systematic review and meta-analysis. J Orthop Surg Res. 2020;15(1):377. https://doi.org/10.1186/s13018-020-01904-2
75. Aliuskevicius M, Østgaard SE, Hauge EM, Vestergaard P, Rasmussen S. Influence of Ibuprofen on Bone Healing After Colles' fracture: a randomized controlled clinical trial. J Orthop Res. 2020;38(3):545–54. https://doi.org/10.1002/jor.24498.
76. Aliuskevicius M, Østgaard SE, Rasmussen S. No influence of ibuprofen on bone healing after colles' fracture—a randomized controlled clinical trial. Injury. 2019;50(7):1309–17. https://doi.org/10.1016/j.injury.2019.06.011.
77. Aliuskevicius M, Østgaard SE, Vestergaard P, Rasmussen S. The influence of ibuprofen on the healing of nonsurgically treated colles' fractures. Orthopedics. 2021;44(2):105–10. https://doi.org/10.3928/01477447-20201216-04.
78. Sivaganesan A, Chotai S, White-Dzuro G, McGirt MJ, Devin CJ. The effect of NSAIDs on spinal fusion: a cross-disciplinary review of biochemical, animal, and human studies. Eur Spine J. 2017;26(11):2719–28. https://doi.org/10.1007/s00586-017-5021-y.
79. Borgeat A, Ofner C, Saporito A, Farshad M, Aguirre J. The effect of nonsteroidal anti-inflammatory drugs on bone healing in humans: a qualitative, systematic review. J Clin Anesth. 2018;49:92–100. https://doi.org/10.1016/j.jclinane.2018.06.020.
80. American Academy of Pediatrics. Committee on drugs. acetaminophen toxicity in children. Pediatrics. 2001;108(4):1020–4. https://doi.org/10.1542/peds.108.4.1020

Skeletal Muscle Relaxants and Acute Pain

John Silva, Daniel Todorovic, and Kenneth Fiala

Abstract Skeletal muscle relaxants (SMRs) are a mainstay in pain management. The drug class of SMRs represents a heterogenous class of chemically distinct medications that are used in the management of acute and chronic musculoskeletal conditions associated with pain and discomfort. There are variations in the mechanism of action, pharmacokinetics, pharmacodynamics, routes of administration, side effect profile and antispastic versus antispasmodic properties of these agents which largely guide their clinical utilization. This chapter provides a profile of the most commonly prescribed SMRs, their indications, advantages, disadvantages and the evidence supporting their efficacy.

Keywords Skeletal muscle relaxants · Antispastic · Antispasmodic · Pain · Acute pain · Perioperative · Cyclobenzaprine · Methocarbamol · Diazepam · Tizanidine · Clonidine · Baclofen · Dantrolene

1 Introduction

Skeletal muscle relaxants (SMRs) are a heterogenous class of medications used in the management of acute and chronic musculoskeletal conditions associated with pain and discomfort [1, 2]. The mechanisms of these agents are varied and their comparative efficacy is poorly understood, however in general they work to improve musculoskeletal pain either by directly affecting muscles or indirectly by modulating neurotransmitter activity in the brain, spinal cord and peripheral nerves. Certain

J. Silva (✉) · D. Todorovic · K. Fiala
Department of Anesthesiology, University of Wisconsin School of Medicine and Public Health, B6/319 CSC, 600 Highland Avenue, Madison, WI 53792, USA
e-mail: jbsilva@wisc.edu

D. Todorovic
e-mail: dtodorovic@uwhealth.org

K. Fiala
e-mail: kfiala2@wisc.edu

A. Abd-Elsayed and K. Schroeder (eds.), *Perioperative Pain Management*,
https://doi.org/10.1007/978-3-031-67648-2_41

muscle relaxers have established themselves as mainstays in the treatment of pain, however, there is a lack of clarity on individual agent indications or comparative efficacy.

2 Antispasticity Versus Antispasmodic

SMRs in the realm of acute pain generally treat two underlying conditions—muscular pain or spasms from peripheral musculoskeletal conditions and spasticity from upper motor neuron syndromes. Members of this class of drugs differ in their ability to treat one, the other or both and are generally subdivided into antispasmodics, antispastics or both.

Antispasmodic Medications

A muscle spasm, sometimes called a cramp, occurs when a muscle involuntarily and forcibly contracts. These motor activities can involve part or all of a muscle group and can occur anywhere in the body. Severe contractions are painful and can lead to tears in tendons and ligaments. Spasms can be caused by overloading or overuse of a muscle as well as ion imbalances that can result from dehydration or other conditions such as renal failure or diabetes. A subtype of spasm is colic, which is episodic pain caused by a spasm of smooth muscle in a particular organ (e.g. bile duct), that can lead to nausea or vomiting. Medications that are thought to primarily deal with muscle spasm are baclofen and dantrolene.

Antispastic Medications

Spasticity is a condition where there is an abnormal increase in muscle tone leading to stiffness of the muscle. Unlike a muscle spasm, there is not a period of atony whether voluntary or not. Spasticity is usually caused by damage to nerve pathways in the brain or spinal cord responsible for movement and can interfere with movement, speech and often cause discomfort or pain. Examples of conditions that cause spasticity include spinal cord injury, stroke, cerebral palsy, and brain or head trauma. Skeletal muscle relaxers are a mainstay of treatment for these conditions and are frequently used in concert with physical therapy, botulinum injections and surgery. Antispastic agents include cyclobenzaprine, methocarbamol, orphenadrine.

3 Cyclobenzaprine HCL (Flexeril)

Introduction

Cyclobenzaprine is FDA approved for the short-term relief of muscle spasms associated with acute, painful musculoskeletal conditions, such as muscle strains and sprains, and primarily used as an adjunct to rest and physical therapy. Chronic use is rarely warranted given the self-limited nature of its' indications and poor evidence of benefit associated with prolonged administration. Cyclobenzaprine is used in an off-label fashion for the treatment of insomnia associated with conditions such as fibromyalgia [3] and PTSD [4].

Pharmacodynamics/Pharmacokinetics

Cyclobenzaprine is a centrally acting antispasmodic skeletal muscle relaxant that is structurally related to tricyclic antidepressants (TCA) [5]. Cyclobenzaprine is thought to lead to a decline in tonic somatic motor activity through depression of monosynaptic reflexes in the spinal cord between Ia sensory fibers and alpha-motor neurons which relieves muscle spasms without interfering with muscle function [6]. Serotonergic (5-HT2) antagonism may also play a role in the producing the clinical effects observed following cyclobenzaprine administration [6].

Cyclobenzaprine is administered via the oral route and primarily absorbed via the gastrointestinal system. Peak concentration occurs 7–8 hours after extended-release formulation and 4 hours after immediate release formulation administration with steady state achieved within 3–4 days [5]. Cyclobenzaprine is metabolized in the liver by the CYP 450 enzymes (CYP 3A4, CYP 31A2, CYP2D6) and excreted by the kidneys.

Dosing and Route of Administration

Cyclobenzaprine is administered via the oral route and is available in immediate-release tablets (5, 7.5, 10 mg and extended release of 15, 30 mg) and is usually given three times daily [5].

Adverse Effects

Cyclobenzaprine has adverse effects such as drowsiness, hallucinations, urinary retention, dry mouth and confusion that are associated with its' anticholinergic activity and severely limit the ability to use this agent in elderly patients. Secondary to hepatic metabolism and renal excretion, cyclobenzaprine should be used cautiously in patients with moderate to severe hepatic or renal impairment. Chronic use of the drug may be associated with an increase in ALT and measurement of hepatic enzymes may be considered following prolonged administration. Cyclobenzaprine also possesses cardiac effects including a theoretical risk of QT-prolongation associated with TCA-like mechanism of action. Cyclobenzaprine additionally antagonizes alpha-1-adrenergic receptors causing a vasodilatory effect which can contribute to reflex tachycardia.

Perioperative Use

Cyclobenzaprine has repeatedly been shown to provide superior pain relief relative to placebo in relieving the signs and symptoms of acute skeletal muscle spasm. This agent is also generally cost effective and associated with few serious adverse effects [7, 8]. Cyclobenzaprine is often used in the treatment of back pain [9–11], and found to be particularly useful for acute pain management with the greatest effect in the first 4 days of treatment [10]. Cyclobenzaprine has been used successfully perioperatively in the treatment of pain for spine surgery with an associated decrease in opioid use [12], however with a notably increased risk of delirium in patients greater than 65 years old [13]. Cyclobenzaprine has demonstrated mixed results in the treatment of post-surgical pain with no difference found in RCTs assessing its' role in third molar extraction [14] or breast reconstruction [15].

4 Methocarbamol (Robaxin)

Introduction

Methocarbamol is frequently administered in a hospital setting secondary to a relatively forgiving side effect profile, low abuse potential, and efficacy across multiple routes of administration. Methocarbamol was initially approved for use in the treatment of muscle spasms in 1957 [16] where it was found to produce decreased muscle tone without concurrent depression of motor activity [17]. It has since continued to remain in use as an antispasmodic in the treatment of acute musculoskeletal pain. Methocarbamol was initially observed as an effective treatment in patients with spine lesions, such as those caused by herniated intervertebral discs [18]. Methocarbamol has been described as effective when used in an off-label fashion for a variety of pain conditions including acute and chronic low-back pain, fibromyalgia, myofascial pain, trauma and perioperative pain control and tetanus. Notably, Methocarbamol does not treat contracture, rigidity or spasticity believed to originate from upper motor neuron injury [19].

Pharmacokinetics/Pharmacodynamics

Methocarbamol is a centrally active antispasmodic agent with sedative and musculoskeletal relaxant properties. It is a carbamate derivative of guaifenesin and is in the same class of medications as metaloxone, carisoprodol, and chlorzaxone. At this time, methocarbamol's exact mechanism of action is unknown with no direct action seen on the motor nerve fiber, motor nerve endplate or skeletal muscle contractility [18].

Onset of action for methocarbamol is usually 30 minutes with peak plasma concentrations at 2 hours [19]. The half-life is variable ranging from one to two hours, and it is metabolized by the liver and excreted by the kidneys as an inactive metabolite [19].

Dosing and Route of Administration

Methocarbamol is commonly administered via the oral route, but the ability to also deliver this agent intravenously and intramuscularly improves utility in the post-operative phase of care.

Oral tablets are available in 500 mg and 750 mg doses and 6 g is considered the recommended daily maximum dose. Additionally, there is injectable solution of 100 mg/mL concentration that is generally limited to 3 g per day when used for greater than three consecutive days.

Adverse Effects

Oral methocarbamol is associated with GI side effects such as nausea, dyspepsia, emesis and metallic taste. Despite being metabolized by the liver and excreted by the kidney, methocarbamol has been shown to be safe for use in cirrhotic patients [20] and patients on dialysis [21]. Methocarbamol has additive effects to alcohol and other central nervous system depressants and can precipitate withdrawal. It also has anticholinergic properties that can lead to ataxia and confusion in the elderly. Severe effects documented in the methocarbamol package include seizure, leukopenia and cholestatic jaundice however there appears to be difficulty finding reports of these side effects [19].

Therapeutic Utility

Methocarbamol has shown benefit in the treatment of chronic low back pain with greater efficacy when compared with long term opioid administration, and with fewer side effects [22, 23]. When compared to diazepam, methocarbamol was found to be less effective but associated with fewer side effects [24].

Using methocarbamol in the setting of acute back pain has shown benefits [24, 25] over placebo including an improvement in mobility. Methocarbamol has been used in the treatment of trauma pain with mixed results. Aljuhani et al. found that methocarbamol did not improve pain control in the first three days after traumatic injury [26], however studies have found an opioid sparing effect and decreased hospital length of stay in trauma patients with closed rib fractures [27, 28]. Methocarbamol was found to have opioid sparing effects during traumatic brain injury rehabilitation [29].

Perioperatively, methocarbamol has been found to be associated with decreased opioid use in studies evaluating hip and knee replacement [30], posterior spinal arthrodesis [12], and craniotomy [31]. Decreased length of stay was found following methocarbamol administration in the setting of pectus excavatum surgery [32]. An RCT evaluating methocarbamol use following breast augmentation also found significantly lower VAS pain scores in the first hours after surgery [33].

5 Diazepam (Valium)

Introduction

Diazepam is part of the benzodiazepine class of medications that are used as anxiolytics, sedatives, hypnotics, anticonvulsants and/or skeletal muscle relaxants. Much like the other members of the benzodiazepine class, diazepam is fast acting, long-lasting, and associated with significant adverse side effects. One important feature of benzodiazepines is reversibility with the drug flumazenil which increases the safety of drugs in this class and confers significant benefits relative to similar barbiturate agents.

Pharmacokinetics/Pharmacodynamics

Diazepam is a centrally acting antispasmodic that relies on GABA agonism. Specifically, benzodiazepines bind the allosteric site between the alpha and gamma subunits of GABA-A receptor chloride ion channels. Binding causes increased frequency of chloride channel opening which hyperpolarizes the neuronal membrane and reduces neuron activation. This effect occurs across the CNS, causing anxiolysis and sedation in the brain, as well as myorelaxant effects when binding on motor neurons of the spinal cord [34].

Overall, diazepam has a short onset of action and a long terminal elimination half-life that extends the observed duration of effect. Diazepam is primarily given orally, however it can be administered either IM, IV or intranasally. Oral onset of action occurs within 30 minutes, with IV administration resulting in onset of action within 1–3 minutes [34]. IM administration results in variable onsets and is not used outside of specific scenarios such as active epilepsy. Peak plasma concentrations occur 1–1.5 hours following oral administration [34]. Intravenous administration results in peak plasma concentrations within 1–3 minutes. Diazepam is largely metabolized in the liver and excreted renally with several active metabolites including desmethyl-diazepam and minor metabolites oxazepam and temazepam [34]. Diazepam is known to accumulate after several dosages with the average half-life of oral diazepam and its' metabolites extending up to 100 hours following chronic use [34].

Dosing and Route of Administration

Oral dosages of diazepam include 2, 5, 10 mg tablets, 1 or 5 mg/mL oral solution. Concentrated formulations of 5 mg/mL may be given via either IV or IM routes. There is also an intranasal spray that is available in various concentrations.

Adverse Effects

Diazepam has a plethora of side effects that limit wider utilization of the drug. GABA channel activation causes CNS depression which at low doses leads to anxiolysis, anterograde amnesia, disinhibition, but at higher doses causes sedation, delirium, imbalance and finally respiratory depression. Diazepam pharmacology leads to both accumulation following sustained administration and withdrawal after prolonged use. Additionally, diazepam is associated with a variety of medication interactions including synergy with opioids, alcohol and potentiation of barbiturates and MAO-Is. Caution must be exercised when this agent is administered to patients with hepatic and renal impairment. Prescriptions should be avoided in the elderly secondary to particular susceptibility to adverse events. Diazepam should also be avoided in pregnant patients as it is able to pass through breast milk and the placental membrane and may lead to "floppy baby syndrome". Finally, diazepam has a high dependency and abuse potential and therefore this risk should be discussed with patients while prescriptions should be closely monitored, for a limited duration, and specifically avoided in patients with a history of substance abuse.

Therapeutic Utility

Diazepam is FDA approved for the management of anxiety disorders, spasticity associated with upper motor neuron disorders, adjunct therapy for muscle spasms, management of certain refractory epilepsy patients, and in the treatment of symptoms associated with alcohol withdrawal. Diazepam is used in an off-label fashion to provide sedation in the ICU and in the short-term treatment of spasticity in children with cerebral palsy.

In chronic pain, the administration of benzodiazepines is common practice despite the absence of class I or class II evidence [35]. A meta-analysis performed by Richards et al. evaluated the use of diazepam in the treatment of rheumatoid arthritis and found that it did not appear to improve pain over 24 hours or one week and was associated with significant adverse events including drowsiness and dizziness [36].

In the realm of acute pain, specifically in the treatment of acute low back pain, the efficacy of diazepam has been nuanced. In a double-blinded RCT performed by Sharifi et al., diazepam was found to provide pain reduction after 60 minutes, however with a high rate (29.4%) of drowsiness [24]. A similarly structured study performed by Friedman et al. evaluated the use of diazepam and naproxen in the treatment of acute lower back pain in the Emergency Department. This study failed to find improvements in functional outcomes or pain at 1 week or 3 months after ED discharge [37].

Perioperatively, diazepam is associated with significant adverse effects that severely limit widespread utilization. An investigation of postoperative delirium after major orthopedic surgery found diazepam to be an independent risk factor for post-operative delirium (for THA, OR = 5.05, 95%CI: 1.5–16.97, $P = 0.009$; for TKA, OR = 4.40, 95%CI: 1.52–12.75, $P = 0.007$; for spine fusion, OR = 2.17, 95%CI: 1.19–3.97, $P = 0.01$) [38]. Replacement of benzodiazepines in the pain control regimen for single-level transforaminal lumbar interbody fusions was associated with decreased opioid use, reductions in trigger medications and shorter hospitalizations [39]. Despite these issues, diazepam does maintain reasonable clinical utility in specific populations. For example, pediatric patients receiving back surgery for idiopathic scoliosis appear to benefit from the administration of postoperative diazepam and do not appear to suffer from an unacceptably high rate of complications [40].

6 Baclofen

Introduction

The analgesic properties of baclofen have been reported in multiple studies and have demonstrable and dose dependent anti-nociceptive properties [41–43]. This effect was found to be synergistic with opioid administration and additive when combined with buspirone. Though baclofen is primarily utilized in the treatment of spasticity, it is often used as an adjunct in the treatment of a variety of pain conditions.

Pharmacokinetics/Pharmacodynamics

Baclofen is an antispasmodic, centrally acting gamma-aminobutyric acid derivative in the benzodiazepine class that disrupts polysynaptic and monosynaptic reflexes at the level of the spinal cord and brain. Baclofen functions via antagonism at GABA-B receptors thought to inhibit the release of excitatory neurotransmitters [44]. Baclofen possesses an additional affinity for voltage-gated calcium channels [45], however it is unclear if this effect has any clinical significance.

Baclofen is highly bioavailable (70–85%) and rapidly absorbed through the GI tract following oral administration [44]. It has a short half-life of 2–6 hours so frequent administration is required to achieve optimal effect [44]. Baclofen is not hepatically metabolized and is excreted unchanged primarily through the renal system [46].

Dosing and Route of Administration

Baclofen is available for administration via oral, transdermal, and intrathecal routes. Baclofen is notably not recommended for intravenous, subcutaneous, intramuscular or epidural administration [44]. Oral tablets are available in 5, 10 and 20 mg strength, with oral solutions available in 5 mg/5 mL bottles [44]. Intrathecal administration is employed in patients with severe pathology requiring chronic use. Intrathecal solutions are available in a variety of preservative free concentrations (10 mg/20 mL, 20 mg/20 ML, and 40 mg/20 mL) [44]. Initiating intrathecal baclofen administration requires screening, where a patient receives a small intrathecal dose and is monitored for 4–8 hours to ensure efficacy. If there is a positive response, an implantable pump can facilitate drug delivery via an intrathecal catheter [44].

Adverse Effects

The side effect profile of baclofen is similar to that of diazepam. Most commonly, patients experience drowsiness and dizziness with an incidence varying between 10–65% [47]. A significant baclofen overdose may lead to CNS depression, altered mental status and severe overdoses may result in coma and respiratory depression. A major concern in patients maintained on baclofen therapy is an increased risk of falls in the elderly. An evaluation of fall risk following baclofen administration in the elderly found that falls occurred at a rate of 108.4 per 1000 person years (a risk equivalent to cyclobenzaprine, but less than that of tizanidine) [48].

Baclofen does induce tolerance and therefore requires dose escalation with continued administration and occasional drug holidays. Acute withdrawal may result in seizure activity [44]. Due to the lack of hepatic metabolism, baclofen is useful in patients with a high concern for CYP mediated drug interactions or hepatic failure, however should be avoided in patients in renal failure. A retrospective cohort study evaluating complications associated with intrathecal baclofen pumps found an overall complication rate of 37.5% with the most common cause being catheter related complications, with loss of efficacy (16.7%) and baclofen withdrawal (14.5%) being the next most common [49].

Therapeutic Utility

Baclofen is a mainstay in the treatment of spasticity resulting from conditions such as cerebral palsy and multiple sclerosis [8]. What is less established is the role of baclofen in the treatment of pain associated with those conditions. Animal studies have shown a decrease in nociception that occurred in a dose dependent fashion [50], however this has not been seen in humans. Instead, experience has shown that there appear to be responders and non-responders to intrathecal baclofen administration. A study evaluating intrathecal baclofen administration in a small cohort of pediatric cerebral palsy patients found that patients demonstrating a differentiated sensory reactivity profile, characterized by greater behavioral reactivity to acute nociceptive stimuli, experienced a > 50% maximum pain intensity decrease [51]. What this suggests is that there may be subgroups within this patient population who experience pain from spasticity and who many benefit from intrathecal baclofen administration.

In the realm of acute pain, studies generally agree that baclofen does not provide significant analgesia, despite being the most popular adjuvant analgesic administered in some settings [52].

An RCT performed by Friedman et al. evaluated the addition of baclofen to ibuprofen in the treatment of acute low back pain 1 week post ED visit and found no difference in functional or pain outcomes [53]. An analysis of baclofen's effect on pain scores when used in the treatment of lower extremity fracture found little to no benefit [52].

Perioperatively, there are limited studies suggesting a substantial beneficial effect.

Intrathecal baclofen administration as an adjuvant to spinal anesthesia for total knee arthroplasty demonstrated less postoperative opioid usage and less chronic pain at three months [54]. However, this potential benefit has to be weighed against the increased risk of delirium associated with baclofen administration [13].

7 Tizanidine (Zanaflex)

Introduction

Tizanidine was FDA approved for the use of muscle spasticity in 1996 but can be used as both an antispastic and antispasmodic. Tizanidine is used to treat spasticity associated with upper motor neuron injuries that occur with damage to the brain, spine or diffuse degenerative neuronal diseases as well as musculoskeletal pain syndromes, neck and low back pain. The sedating effects of tizanidine are also used in an off-label fashion to mitigate headaches, insomnia, and opioid withdrawal.

Pharmacokinetics/Pharmacodynamics

Tizanidine is an imidazoline derivative that shares many similarities to its sister drug clonidine. Tizanidine functions centrally by activating alpha-2 receptors within the spinal cord that cause presynaptic inhibition of excitatory neurotransmitters such as glutamate and aspartate [55]. Much like clonidine, tizanidine possesses alpha-1 receptor activity.

Tizanidine undergoes extensive first-pass hepatic metabolism through CYP1A2 into inactive compounds and mainly excreted by the kidneys. Tizanidine requires considerable time (24–48 hours) to reach steady-state concentration following dosing initiation [56].

Administration

Tizanidine is only available via the oral route in ascending doses (2, 4, 6 mg capsules or 2 and 4 mg tablets) [55]. Doses are given every 6–8 hours and are increased by 2 mg until there is a significant decrease in the frequency and intensity of muscle spasms.

Adverse Effects

Tizanidine is generally well-tolerated but does share similar side effects with other muscle relaxant agents such as sedation and asthenia. Co-administration of tizanidine with other depressants should be limited or avoided due to additive effects. Due to its alpha agonistic properties, tizanidine has been shown to result in cardiac depression manifesting as hypotension and bradycardia. However, these symptoms are significantly milder than what might be encountered following clonidine administration

[57]. Notably, when given in high doses or over a prolonged period of time, tizanidine needs to be tapered slowly so as not to precipitate tachycardia, hypertension and rebound spasticity [58].

Tizanidine's adverse effect profile is also related to its metabolism and excretion and the drug should be used with caution in patients with hepatic impairment. Additionally, hepatoxicity is a known side effect and requires baseline liver function tests and frequent monitoring in chronic use [55]. In acute liver failure, tizanidine administration may cause significant worsening of side effects such as hypotension and bradycardia [59].

Therapeutic Utility

Tizanidine is increasingly utilized as an adjunct in the treatment of chronic pain where it appears to be effective in the treatment of musculoskeletal conditions [8], chronic pain back pain [60] and neuropathic pain [61, 62]. In the setting of neuropathic pain, tizanidine administration was shown to decrease overall patient pain scores and the severity and quality of neuropathic pain. In other double blinded studies, tizanidine was noted to be as effective as baclofen in decreasing the pain associated with trigeminal neuralgia.

The efficacy of tizanidine as a treatment for acute pain is limited and mixed. When compared to placebo with ibuprofen, tizanidine in combination with ibuprofen was associated with a decrease in the intensity of acute low back pain and a faster recovery [63]. However, a larger study with similar methods performed in an Emergency Department setting noted no improvement after one week of therapy [53].

Perioperatively, tizanidine has also shown some promise in decreasing pain. When evaluated in the treatment of post-operative pain for lumbar fusion surgery in a double-blinded RCT, preoperative treatment with tizanidine was found to be associated with reductions in pain scores that were limited to six hours of duration following surgery [64]. A meta-analysis performed by Abhijit et al. found that tizanidine reduced intraoperative opioid consumption, but was not associated with statistically improved pain scores until 24 hours following surgery. Other studies have found that tizanidine decreased pain scores and opioid requirements in various post-operative settings such as thyroidectomy, hernia repairs and laparoscopic cholecystectomies [65–67].

Ultimately, tizanidine is frequently utilized as a multimodal adjunct in the setting of chronic and acute surgical pain.

8 Orphenadrine

Introduction

Orphenadrine is a centrally acting muscarinic antagonist that has found clinical use in the treatment of acute and chronic musculoskeletal pain. It has been used as an adjunct medication for pain relief in muscle spasm, acute pain accompanying physical therapy and in the treatment of Parkinson's disease symptoms [68].

Pharmacokinetics/Pharmacodynamics

Orphenadrine is a methyl derivative of diphenhydramine, with notable anticholinergic activity [68]. With further research, it was proven that orphenadrine affected NMDA receptors further describing its effect on nociception [69].

Orphenadrine is entirely absorbed by the gastrointestinal tract. It displays large amounts of plasma protein binding and undergoes hepatic metabolism. It is mainly eliminated by the kidneys [70]. While largely metabolized by the liver, it has been noted to be administered safely in cirrhotic patients and has no documented causes of liver toxicity [71].

Administration

Orphenadrine is available in 50 mg short-acting oral tablets as well as 100 mg extended-release versions. There is also a parental version available, however, has been linked with many incidents of anticholinergic toxicity [70].

Adverse Effects

Orphenadrine's adverse effects are similar to other central anticholinergic medications. Notable side effects with over-administration of the medication are tachycardia, palpitations, urinary retention and blurred vision [72]. Cautious prescription of orphenadrine in the elderly and those with a history of cognitive issues is required as the drug may cause significant confusion and anxiety [70]. Concomitant propoxyphene administration should be avoided secondary to additive effects that may increase the risk of altered mental status, anxiety, and tremors [72]. Due to its significant anticholinergic profile, use should be limited in patients with pre-existing neuromuscular diseases (myasthenia gravis) and cardio spasm as it may worsen these conditions [70, 72].

Therapeutic Utility

Early randomized control studies have noted improvements in pain related to musculoskeletal spasm when comparing orphenadrine to placebo [73–76]. Recent research has noted some improvement in post-operative pain control when orphenadrine is used as an adjunct to typical anti-inflammatory medications. Zeiner et al. performed a double blinded study that concluded orphenadrine did not significantly improve pain control relative to diclofenac administration. However, the authors did note a small decrease in PCA usage 24 hours post-operatively with the use of orphenadrine [77]. On the contrary, Dabour et al. conducted a similar study evaluating post-operative opioid consumption in women undergoing mastectomy. They compared combinations of ketorolac/orphenadrine, diclofenac/orphenadrine along with placebo infusions and noted a significant reduction in opioid consumption and pain scores in the ketorolac/orphenadrine group compared to others [78]. Other successful niche uses of orphenadrine have been noted in treating muscle cramps in cirrhotic patients. Abd-Elsalam et al. noted improvements in severity, frequency and overall pain scores related to muscle cramps in cirrhotic patients receiving orphenadrine when compared to placebo [79]. Unfortunately, despite positive results, orphenadrine's therapeutic utility is severely limited by its anticholinergic properties and resulting side effect profile making it rarely used in clinical practice.

9 Clonidine

Introduction

Clonidine was originally developed to be used as an anti-hypertensive. Unlike tizanidine, clonidine functions primarily along the nucleus tractus solaris within the CNS and decreases the stimulatory effects of cardiovascular neurotransmitters [80]. The role of clonidine in the treatment of acute pain is thought to be related to activation of alpha-2 receptors within the dorsal spinal cord effectively inhibiting pain transmission. Clonidine administration has been described in the treatment of cancer related pain, opioid and benzodiazepine withdrawal, and as a neuraxial anesthesia adjunct [80].

Pharmacokinetics/Pharmacodynamics

Clonidine is imidazole derivative, like tizanidine, however, its metabolism is not well understood. It undergoes hydroxylation to inactive metabolites by the CYP enzyme family. Clonidine is largely excreted unchanged by the kidneys [80–82].

Administration

Clonidine is available in transdermal, oral, and injectable solution formulations. Immediate release oral tablets are typically seen for use in hypertensive syndromes. Extended oral release and transdermal forms are available in similar dosages. The injectable form is available in 100 or 500 mcg/ml and is typically added as an adjunct to local anesthetics formulations to achieve a dose of 30 mcg/hr [80].

Adverse Effects

Clonidine is generally tolerated well. The majority of clonidine-related side effects are a direct result of alpha agonism leading to sedation and dry mouth [80, 82]. Secondary to an elevated affinity for central nervous brain centers, clonidine overdoses have been seen at higher rates compared to other imidazole derivatives such as tizanidine [82]. Symptoms of overdose include somnolence, miosis, and eventually, cardiovascular effects including hypotension and bradycardia which may require intensive level care [80, 82].

Therapeutic Utility

Clonidine's role in treating hypertension has been long studied, but its role in treating acute pain remains debated. A meta-analysis noted that the effectiveness of clonidine within acute pain has been limited due to unwanted systemic effects. Of note, clonidine has safely been used within the world of chronic cancer pain and as an effective adjunct in neuraxial anesthetics where it has demonstrated a unique ability to decrease the development of hyperalgesia [80, 83, 84].

There are also promising reports that the use of intrathecal clonidine improved overall pain scores within cancer patients and patients with neuropathic pain that experienced continued pain despite the use of traditional opioid regimens [85, 86]. Clonidine has also been successfully administered via the epidural route and a study by Levand and De'Kock noted a decrease in reported patient chronic pain scores with the addition of epidural clonidine following major abdominal surgery [87].

Systemic clonidine administration in the perioperative and acute pain setting has been limited by its various side effects. However, clonidine does show some promise as an adjunct for post-operative pain control, non-surgical acute pain management, and as a neuraxial anesthetic adjunct. Esmaliane et al. reported that the addition of oral clonidine to standard analgesic regimens resulted in improvements in pain scores and decreased opioid requirements for patients with renal colic [88]. Hsu et al. noted that clonidine administration resulted in improvements in analgesic scores, decreased opioid requirements, and a decreased incidence of post-operative nausea and vomiting following pediatric ophthalmic surgery [89].

Clonidine's role as an adjunct within regional anesthesia has been well researched. Reuban et al. noted sustained analgesia and an increase in the time to first request for additional opioids in patients who had an intravenous regional anesthetic (Bier Block) that included clonidine for hand surgery [90]. A large meta-analysis performed by Popping noted a similar increase in local anesthetic effects in patients undergoing regional anesthesia with various single shot peripheral nerve blocks. However, notable increases in hypotension and sedation remain possible with the use of perineural clonidine and the use of these agents should be considered carefully in patients with limited cardiovascular reserve. When used as a sole adjunct in epidural and spinal anesthetics, Sathesa noted that neuraxial clonidine resulted in a significantly faster onset of sensory and motor blocks and prolonged duration of analgesia for infraumbilical surgery [91].

10 Dantrolene

Introduction

Dantrolene was first described in 1967 by Synder et al. where it was found to have muscle relaxant properties in animals [68]. Most commonly known for its use in the treatment of malignant hyperthermia, dantrolene has multiple uses in chronic skeletal muscle spasticity disorders such as spinal cord injury, multiple sclerosis, stroke, and cerebral palsy [69].

Pharmacokinetics/Pharmacodynamics

Dantrolene is a peripherally acting skeletal muscle relaxant. Although the exact molecular mechanism underlying dantrolene's mechanism of action is not completely understood—it is believed to be a direct-acting skeletal muscle relaxant blocking the release of calcium from the intracellular stores in the sarcoplasmic reticulum [70]. Dantrolene is believed to affect the excitation–contraction coupling process, raising the rheobasic potential and increasing the steepness of the strength-duration curve for mechanical threshold [71]. Morgan et al. found that dantrolene raises the rheobase by directly decreasing the release of calcium from the sarcoplasmic reticulum, proposing that dantrolene inhibits the movement of natural calcium ionophore [71].

The primary site of dantrolene absorption in animals is in the small intestines, with humans absorbing approximately 70% of an oral dose [72]. 4–8 hours following ingestion, peak blood concentrations occur. The dose–response curve appears to be linear with a mean drug half-life of 8.7 hours and steady-state plasma levels being maintained with 3 or 4 administrations of the drug [73]. In Flewellen et al.'s study assessing the dose response of dantrolene in awake patients, it was found that the cumulative dantrolene dose to reach maximal twitch depression was 2.4 mg/kg which resulted in approximately 75% twitch depression with no difference between men and women. The maximal decrease in grip strength found in this study was found to be 42% [74]. It is important to note that dantrolene cannot cause complete paralysis, even if it is used in supra-therapeutic doses [75].

Dosing and Route of Administration

Dantrolene is available as both an oral capsule and as an intravenous injection. Dantrolene has a relatively complex dosing routine compared to other SMRs. For the treatment of chronic muscle spasticity, dantrolene is given three to four times daily starting at 25 mg for 7 days and then titrated with increasing dosages, generally in 25 mg increments, to a maximum dose of 400 mg/day until the desired effect is achieved [69].

Adverse Effects

Oral dantrolene administration can be associated with rare, but serious, side effects. One of the most important of these potential complications is highlighted in a black box warning that describes a rare but serious risk of hepatotoxicity and overt hepatitis [8]. Therefore, liver function tests should be monitored and the discontinuation of dantrolene is recommended if symptoms or signs of liver injury appear. Further, treatment initiation may result in transient drowsiness, weakness, general malaise, fatigue, and diarrhea. It is important to monitor for the appearance of these symptoms in patients who may already have respiratory weakness [76]. In a report of dantrolene related complications from 1987–2006, Brandom et al. found the most common complication to be muscle weakness (21.7%), phlebitis (9%), gastrointestinal upset (4.1%), and respiratory failure (3.8%) [77]. Further, this work showed that the risk of these complications increased by 29% when the dantrolene dose doubled [77].

Therapeutic Utility

Dantrolene is FDA approved in the treatment of chronic skeletal muscle spasticity resulting from upper motor neuron damage that occurs due to spinal cord injury, multiple sclerosis, stroke, and cerebral palsy [69, 78]. Since dantrolene is primarily peripherally acting, it has the advantage of causing less sedation relative to other medications such as baclofen and diazepam [79]. Much of the evidence supporting the use of dantrolene for this indication is somewhat dated. Initial studies, such as those performed by Joynt and Leonard 1980, were able to find that the drug significantly reduced the force of muscle contraction, though with irregular objective functional improvement [92]. More recent studies have found weak to no evidence to support this indication [8, 93]. One potential reason for the minimal improvement observed with dantrolene administration may be related to difficult dosing regimens and adherence struggles. Additionally, this difficult dosing regimen and potential for rare, but severe side effects, significantly preclude dantrolene's use for acute pain. There are a very limited number of studies describing the use of dantrolene in the treatment of acute pain. However, one double blind RCT study evaluated oral dantrolene for tonsillectomy pain and found no difference [94].

11 Conclusion

Early analysis found muscle relaxants to be effective in the management of acute non-specific low back pain [95]. However, many of the studies evaluating the effectiveness of skeletal muscle relaxants are hampered by poor methodologic design. Further analysis, has not been able to establish clinically significant results and have called into question the entire premise of using SMRs for LBP. A review performed by Cashin et al. in 2021 found very low and low certainty evidence that non-benzodiazepine antispasmodics might provide small but clinically insignificant reductions in pain intensity at or before two weeks with an increased risk of adverse events in acute low back pain [96]. Moreover, there was no discernable reduction in disability in the immediate term compared with controls. A more recent analysis by Cashin et al. involving seven Cochrane reviews that included 103 studies (22,238 participants) assessing pharmacological treatments of non-specific low back pain in adults found moderate-certainty evidence for a small between-group difference favoring muscle relaxants (RR 0.55, 95% CI 0.4–0.77) however at the cost of an increased risk of adverse events (RR 1.50, 95% CI 1.14—1.19) [97]. An evaluation of SMRs on acute back pain in the ED specifically found that SMRs lead to no improved outcomes compared to placebo [98].

Overall, skeletal muscle relaxants as a whole have a paucity of large, high quality, placebo-controlled trials to legitimize their use [96]. Additionally, efficacy data from comparator trials do not particularly favor one skeletal muscle relaxant versus another. An evaluation of European clinical practice guidelines on their recommendations for muscle relaxants for lower back pain found that most advocated strongly against prescription with only one guideline recommending it as 2nd line medication where other non-drug and non-opioid treatments are ineffective [99]. Despite this, SMRs represent a mainstay of therapy in the United States. Further research is required to fully crystalize the role of SMRs in acute pain, and despite their limited clinical utility, there may yet be specific subgroups and patient populations that can find therapy with one or more of the members within the drug class.

Key Points

1. Skeletal Muscle relaxant medications are a heterogenous class of medications that may be useful in the setting of clinically significant spasmodic pain.
2. Caution should be exercised in the setting of coadministration of opioids with skeletal muscle relaxant medications as sedation and respiratory depression may develop.
3. Skeletal muscle relaxant administration efficacy data continues to emerge and future evaluations may better elucidate appropriate dosing pathways and indications.

References

1. Waldman HJ. Centrally acting skeletal muscle relaxants and associated drugs. J Pain Symptom Manage. 1994;9(7):434–41. https://doi.org/10.1016/0885-3924(94)90199-6.
2. See S, Ginzburg R. Skeletal muscle relaxants. Pharmacotherapy: J Hum Pharmacol Drug Therap. 2008;28(2):207–13. https://doi.org/10.1592/phco.28.2.207
3. Macfarlane GJ, Kronisch C, Dean LE, et al. EULAR revised recommendations for the management of fibromyalgia. Ann Rheum Dis. 2017;76(2):318–28. https://doi.org/10.1136/annrheumdis-2016-209724.
4. Sullivan GM, Gendreau RM, Gendreau J, et al. Randomized clinical trial of bedtime sublingual cyclobenzaprine (TNX-102 SL) in military-related PTSD and the role of sleep quality in treatment response. Psychiatry Res. 2021;301: 113974. https://doi.org/10.1016/j.psychres.2021.113974.
5. Khan I, Kahwaji CI. *Cyclobenzaprine*. 2023.
6. Kobayashi H, Hasegawa Y, Ono H. Cyclobenzaprine, a centrally acting muscle relaxant, acts on descending serotonergic systems. Eur J Pharmacol. 1996;311(1):29–35. https://doi.org/10.1016/0014-2999(96)00402-5.
7. Katz WA, Dube J. Cyclobenzaprine in the treatment of acute muscle spasm: review of a decade of clinical experience. Clin Ther. 1988;10(2):216–28.
8. Chou R, Peterson K, Helfand M. Comparative efficacy and safety of skeletal muscle relaxants for spasticity and musculoskeletal conditions: a systematic review. J Pain Symptom Manage. 2004;28(2):140–75. https://doi.org/10.1016/j.jpainsymman.2004.05.002.
9. Borenstein DG, Korn S. Efficacy of a low-dose regimen of cyclobenzaprine hydrochloride in acute skeletal muscle spasm: results of two placebo-controlled trials. Clin Ther. 2003;25(4):1056–73. https://doi.org/10.1016/S0149-2918(03)80067-X.
10. Browning R, Jackson JL, O'Malley PG. Cyclobenzaprine and back pain. Arch Intern Med. 2001;161(13):1613. https://doi.org/10.1001/archinte.161.13.1613.
11. Malanga GA, Ruoff GE, Weil AJ, Altman CA, Xie F, Borenstein DG. Cyclobenzaprine ER for muscle spasm associated with low back and neck pain: two randomized, double-blind, placebo-controlled studies of identical design. Curr Med Res Opin. 2009;25(5):1179–96. https://doi.org/10.1185/03007990902851753.
12. Harris AB, Puvanesarajah V, Marrache M, et al. Opioid prescribing practices after posterior spinal arthrodesis for adolescent idiopathic scoliosis. Spine Deform. 2020;8(5):965–73. https://doi.org/10.1007/s43390-020-00127-z.
13. Perez EA, Ray E, Gold CJ, et al. Postoperative use of the muscle relaxants baclofen and/or cyclobenzaprine associated with an increased risk of delirium following lumbar fusion. Spine (Phila Pa 1976). 2023;48(24):1733–40. https://doi.org/10.1097/BRS.0000000000004606

14. de Santana Santos T, Calazans ACM, Martins-Filho PRS, Silva LCF da, de Oliveira e Silva ED, Gomes ACA. Evaluation of the muscle relaxant cyclobenzaprine after third-molar extraction. J Am Dent Assoc. 2011;142(10):1154–62. https://doi.org/10.14219/jada.archive.2011.0084
15. Al Yafi MN, ElHawary H, Al-Halabi B, Alnaeem H, Xu L, Fouda-Neel O. Pain control following alloplastic breast reconstruction with muscle relaxant: a randomized controlled trial. J Plast Reconstr Aesthet Surg. 2021;74(2):407–47. https://doi.org/10.1016/j.bjps.2020.08.053.
16. Sibrack J, Patel P, Hammer R. Methocarbamol. In: StatPearls [Internet]. Treasure Island (FL): StatPearls Publishing; 2024 Jan [Updated 2024 May 2]. Available from: https://www.ncbi.nlm.nih.gov/books/NBK565868/
17. Truitt EB, Patterson RB. Comparative hemolytic activity of mephenesin, guaiacol glycerol ether and methocarbamol in vitro and in vivo. Exp Biol Med. 1957;95(3):422–4. https://doi.org/10.3181/00379727-95-23240.
18. O'Doherty DS. Methocarbamol-new agent in treatment of neurological and neuromuscular diseases. J Am Med Assoc. 1958;167(2):160. https://doi.org/10.1001/jama.1958.02990190014003.
19. Sibrack J, Hammer R. Methocarbamol. 2023.
20. Abd-Elsalam S, Arafa M, Elkadeem M, et al. Randomized-controlled trial of methocarbamol as a novel treatment for muscle cramps in cirrhotic patients. Eur J Gastroenterol Hepatol. 2019;31(4):499–502. https://doi.org/10.1097/MEG.0000000000001310.
21. Sica DA, Comstock TJ, Davis J, et al. Pharmacokinetics and protein binding of methocarbamol in renal insufficiency and normals. Eur J Clin Pharmacol. 1990;39(2):193–4. https://doi.org/10.1007/BF00280060.
22. Ueberall MA, Mueller-Schwefe G. COMET—effectiveness and tolerability of methocarbamol versus oral opioid-analgesics as add-on measure in patients with non-specific low back pain refractory to recommended 1st line treatments. a retrospective analysis of depersonalized propensity score matched open-label real-world 4-week data from the German Pain e-Registry. Curr Med Res Opin. 2022;38(2):237–53. https://doi.org/10.1080/03007995.2021.2003105
23. Überall MA, Emrich OMD, Müller-Schwefe GHH. Wirksamkeit und Verträglichkeit von Methocarbamol bei muskulär bedingten subakuten Kreuz-/Rückenschmerzen. MMW Fortschr Med. 2017;159(S7):6–17. https://doi.org/10.1007/s15006-017-0339-2.
24. Sharifi M, Abdorazzaghnejad A, Yazdchi M, Bahreini M. Methocarbamol versus diazepam in acute low back pain in the emergency department: a randomised double-blind clinical trial. Emerg Med J. 2023;40(7):493–8. https://doi.org/10.1136/emermed-2021-211485.
25. Emrich OMD, Milachowski KA, Strohmeier M. Methocarbamol bei akuten Rückenschmerzen. MMW Fortschr Med. 2015;157(S5):9–16. https://doi.org/10.1007/s15006-015-3307-x.
26. Aljuhani O, Kopp BJ, Patanwala AE. Effect of methocarbamol on acute pain after traumatic injury. Am J Ther. 2017;24(2):e202–6. https://doi.org/10.1097/MJT.0000000000000364.
27. Patanwala AE, Aljuhani O, Kopp BJ, Erstad BL. Methocarbamol use is associated with decreased hospital length of stay in trauma patients with closed rib fractures. Am J Surg. 2017;214(4):738–42. https://doi.org/10.1016/j.amjsurg.2017.01.003.
28. Deloney LP, Smith Condeni M, Carter C, Privette A, Leon S, Eriksson EA. Efficacy of methocarbamol for acute pain management in young adults with traumatic rib fractures. Ann Pharmacother. 2021;55(6):705–10. https://doi.org/10.1177/1060028020964796.
29. King JD, Cautivar K, Tran DA, et al. The impact of non-opioid analgesic usage on total opioid load during traumatic brain injury rehabilitation: a retrospective study. Cureus. 2023;15(10):e46872. https://doi.org/10.7759/cureus.46872.
30. Looke TD, Kluth CT. Effect of preoperative intravenous methocarbamol and intravenous acetaminophen on opioid use after primary total hip and knee replacement. Orthopedics. 2013;36(2):25–32. https://doi.org/10.3928/01477447-20130122-54.
31. Ban VS, Bhoja R, McDonagh DL. Multimodal analgesia for craniotomy. Curr Opin Anaesthesiol. 2019;32(5):592–9. https://doi.org/10.1097/ACO.0000000000000766.
32. Inge TH, Owings E, Blewett CJ, et al. Reduced hospitalization cost for patients with pectus excavatum treated using minimally invasive surgery. Surg Endosc. 2003;17(10):1609–13. https://doi.org/10.1007/s00464-002-8767-0.

33. Hidalgo D, Pusic A. The role of methocarbamol and intercostal nerve blocks for pain management in breast augmentation. Aesthet Surg J. 2005;25(6):571–5. https://doi.org/10.1016/j.asj.2005.09.003.
34. Dhaliwal JS, Rosani A, Saadabadi A. Diazepam. 2023.
35. Brötz D, Maschke E, Burkard S, et al. Is there a role for benzodiazepines in the management of lumbar disc prolapse with acute sciatica? Pain. 2010;149(3):470–5. https://doi.org/10.1016/j.pain.2010.02.015.
36. Richards BL, Whittle SL, Buchbinder R. Muscle relaxants for pain management in rheumatoid arthritis. Cochr Database Systemat Rev. Published online January 18, 2012. https://doi.org/10.1002/14651858.CD008922.pub2
37. Friedman BW, Irizarry E, Solorzano C, et al. Diazepam is no better than placebo when added to naproxen for acute low back pain. Ann Emerg Med. 2017;70(2):169-176.e1. https://doi.org/10.1016/j.annemergmed.2016.10.002.
38. Urban MK, Sasaki M, Schmucker AM, Magid SK. Postoperative delirium after major orthopedic surgery. World J Orthop. 2020;11(2):90–106. https://doi.org/10.5312/wjo.v11.i2.90.
39. Boulter JH, Curry BP, Szuflita NS, et al. Protocolization of post-transforaminal lumbar interbody fusion pain control with elimination of benzodiazepines and long-acting opioids. Neurosurgery. 2020;86(5):717–23. https://doi.org/10.1093/neuros/nyz232.
40. Gornitzky AL, Flynn JM, Muhly WT, Sankar WN. A rapid recovery pathway for adolescent idiopathic scoliosis that improves pain control and reduces time to inpatient recovery after posterior spinal fusion. Spine Deform. 2016;4(4):288–95. https://doi.org/10.1016/j.jspd.2016.01.001.
41. Cutting DA, Jordan CC. Alternative approaches to analgesia: baclofen as a model compound. Br J Pharmacol. 1975;54(2):171–9. https://doi.org/10.1111/j.1476-5381.1975.tb06926.x.
42. Levy RA, Proudfit HK. The analgesic action of baclofen [beta-(4-chlorophenyl)-gamma-aminobutyric acid]. J Pharmacol Exp Ther. 1977;202(2):437–45.
43. Wilkerson JL, Felix JS, Restrepo LF, Ansari MI, Coop A, McMahon LR. The effects of morphine, baclofen, and buspirone alone and in combination on schedule-controlled responding and hot plate antinociception in rats. J Pharmacol Exp Ther. 2019;370(3):380–9. https://doi.org/10.1124/jpet.118.255844.
44. Ghanavatian S, Derian A. Baclofen. 2023.
45. Zvejniece L, Vavers E, Svalbe B, et al. R-phenibut binds to the α2-δ subunit of voltage-dependent calcium channels and exerts gabapentin-like anti-nociceptive effects. Pharmacol Biochem Behav. 2015;137:23–9. https://doi.org/10.1016/j.pbb.2015.07.014.
46. Wuis EW, Dirks MJ, Termond EF, Vree TB, Van der Kleijn E. Plasma and urinary excretion kinetics of oral baclofen in healthy subjects. Eur J Clin Pharmacol. 1989;37(2):181–4. https://doi.org/10.1007/BF00558228.
47. Dease NM, Kershner EK, Wills BK. Baclofen Toxicity. 2023.
48. Hwang YJ, Chang AR, Brotman DJ, Inker LA, Grams ME, Shin JI. Baclofen and the risk of fall and fracture in older adults: a real-world cohort study. J Am Geriatr Soc. Published online November 7, 2023. https://doi.org/10.1111/jgs.18665
49. Qureshi AZ, Shacfe H, Ilyas A, et al. Complications of intrathecal baclofen pump therapy: an institutional experience from Saudi Arabia. Healthcare (Basel). 2023;11(21). https://doi.org/10.3390/healthcare11212820
50. Dirig DM, Yaksh TL. Intrathecal baclofen and muscimol, but not midazolam, are antinociceptive using the rat-formalin model. J Pharmacol Exp Ther. 1995;275(1):219–27.
51. Barney CC, Merbler AM, Simone DA, Walk D, Symons FJ. Investigating the feasibility of a modified quantitative sensory testing approach to profile sensory function and predict pain outcomes following intrathecal baclofen implant surgery in cerebral palsy. Pain Med. 2020;21(1):109–17. https://doi.org/10.1093/pm/pnz114.
52. Griffioen MA, Ziegler ML, O'Toole RV, Dorsey SG, Renn CL. Change in pain score after administration of analgesics for lower extremity fracture pain during hospitalization. Pain Manag Nurs. 2019;20(2):158–63. https://doi.org/10.1016/j.pmn.2018.09.008.

53. Friedman BW, Irizarry E, Solorzano C, et al. A randomized, placebo-controlled trial of ibuprofen plus metaxalone, tizanidine, or baclofen for acute low back pain. Ann Emerg Med. 2019;74(4):512–20. https://doi.org/10.1016/j.annemergmed.2019.02.017.
54. Sanders JC, Gerstein N, Torgeson E, Abram S. Intrathecal baclofen for postoperative analgesia after total knee arthroplasty. J Clin Anesth. 2009;21(7):486–92. https://doi.org/10.1016/j.jclinane.2008.12.019.
55. Ghanavatian S, Derian A. Tizanidine. 2023.
56. Tse FLS, Jaffe JM, Bhuta S. Pharmacokinetics, of orally administered tizanidine in healthy volunteers. Fundam Clin Pharmacol. 1987;1(6):479–88. https://doi.org/10.1111/j.1472-8206.1987.tb00581.x.
57. Coward DM. Tizanidine: neuropharmacology and mechanism of action. Neurology. 1994;44(11 Suppl 9):S6–10; discussion S10–1.
58. Suárez-Lledó A, Padullés A, Lozano T, Cobo-Sacristán S, Colls M, Jódar R. Management of tizanidine withdrawal syndrome: a case report. Clin Med Insights Case Rep. 2018;11:1179547618758022. https://doi.org/10.1177/1179547618758022.
59. Spiller HA, Bosse GM, Adamson LA. Retrospective review of tizanidine (Zanaflex®) overdose. J Toxicol Clin Toxicol. 2004;42(5):593–6. https://doi.org/10.1081/CLT-200026978.
60. Berry H, Hutchinson DR. Tizanidine and ibuprofen in acute low-back pain: results of a double-blind multicentre study in general practice. J Int Med Res. 1988;16(2):83–91. https://doi.org/10.1177/030006058801600202.
61. Fromm GH, Aumentado D, Terrence CF. A clinical and experimental investigation of the effects of tizanidine in trigeminal neuralgia. Pain. 1993;53(3):265–71. https://doi.org/10.1016/0304-3959(93)90222-B.
62. Semenchuk MR, Sherman S. Effectiveness of tizanidine in neuropathic pain: an open-label study. J Pain. 2000;1(4):285–92. https://doi.org/10.1054/jpai.2000.9435.
63. Berry H, Hutchinson DR. A multicentre placebo-controlled study in general practice to evaluate the efficacy and safety of tizanidine in acute low-back pain. J Int Med Res. 1988;16(2):75–82. https://doi.org/10.1177/030006058801600201.
64. Aezi G, Shafizad M, Firouzian A, Mirani A, Kiabi FH. Effects of tizanidine and clonidine on postoperative pain after lumbar fusion surgery. Interdisciplin Neurosurg. 2023;31: 101680. https://doi.org/10.1016/j.inat.2022.101680.
65. Talakoub R, Abbasi S, Maghami E, Zavareh SMHT. The effect of oral tizanidine on postoperative pain relief after elective laparoscopic cholecystectomy. Adv Biomed Res. 2016;5:19. https://doi.org/10.4103/2277-9175.175905.
66. Ahiskalioglu A, Yayik AM, Oral Ahiskalioglu E, et al. Ultrasound-guided bilateral superficial cervical block and preemptive single-dose oral tizanidine for post-thyroidectomy pain: a randomized-controlled double-blind study. J Anesth. 2018;32(2):219–26. https://doi.org/10.1007/s00540-018-2468-x.
67. Yazicioğlu D, Caparlar C, Akkaya T, Mercan U, Kulaçoğlu H. Tizanidine for the management of acute postoperative pain after inguinal hernia repair. Eur J Anaesthesiol. 2016;33(3):215–22. https://doi.org/10.1097/EJA.0000000000000371.
68. Snyder HR, Davis CS, Bickerton RK, Halliday RP. 1-[(5-arylfurfurylidene)amino]hydantoins. A new class of muscle relaxants. J Med Chem. 1967;10(5):807–10. https://doi.org/10.1021/jm00317a011
69. Ratto D, Joyner RW. Dantrolene. 2023.
70. Krause T, Gerbershagen MU, Fiege M, Weisshorn R, Wappler F. Dantrolene–a review of its pharmacology, therapeutic use and new developments. Anaesthesia. 2004;59(4):364–73. https://doi.org/10.1111/j.1365-2044.2004.03658.x.
71. Morgan KG, Bryant SH. The mechanism of action of dantrolene sodium. J Pharmacol Exp Ther. 1977;201(1):138–47.
72. Benson BE. Dantrolene. Critical care toxicology. Springer International Publishing; 2017:2757–2770. https://doi.org/10.1007/978-3-319-17900-1_162
73. Dykes MH. Evaluation of a muscle relaxant: dantrolene sodium (Dantrium). JAMA. 1975;231(8):862–4.

74. Flewellen EH, Nelson TE, Jones WP, Arens JF, Wagner DL. Dantrolene dose response in awake man: implications for management of malignant hyperthermia. Anesthesiology. 1983;59(4):275–80. https://doi.org/10.1097/00000542-198310000-00002.
75. C K, MD P, MD RH, Montenegro MD H. Oral dantrolene causing a decrease in vital capacity, recurrent lung collapse, and respiratory failure in a spinal cord injury patient: a case report. J Lung Dis Treat. 2017;03(01). https://doi.org/10.4172/2472-1018.1000117
76. Pinder RM, Brogden RN, Speight TM, Avery GS. Dantrolene sodium: a review of its pharmacological properties and therapeutic efficacy in spasticity. Drugs. 1977;13(1):3–23. https://doi.org/10.2165/00003495-197713010-00002.
77. Brandom BW, Larach MG, Chen MSA, Young MC. Complications associated with the administration of dantrolene 1987 to 2006: a report from the North American malignant hyperthermia registry of the malignant hyperthermia association of the United States. Anesth Analg. 2011;112(5):1115–23. https://doi.org/10.1213/ANE.0b013e31820b5f1f.
78. Yang HS, Choi JM, In J, Sung TY, Kim YB, Sultana S. Current clinical application of dantrolene sodium. Anesth Pain Med (Seoul). 2023;18(3):220–32. https://doi.org/10.17085/apm.22260.
79. Peck J, Urits I, Crane J, et al. Oral muscle relaxants for the treatment of chronic pain associated with cerebral palsy. Psychopharmacol Bull. 2020;50(4 Suppl 1):142–62
80. Yasaei R, Saadabadi A. Clonidine. 2023.
81. Keränen A, Nykänen S, Taskinen J. Pharmacokinetics and side-effects of clonidine. Eur J Clin Pharmacol. 1978;13(2):97–101. https://doi.org/10.1007/BF00609752.
82. Manzon L, Nappe TM, DelMaestro C, Maguire NJ. Clonidine Toxicity. 2023.
83. Neil MJ. Clonidine: clinical pharmacology and therapeutic use in pain management. Curr Clin Pharmacol. 2011;6(4):280–7. https://doi.org/10.2174/157488411798375886.
84. Eisenach JC, Hood DD, Curry R. Intrathecal, but not intravenous, clonidine reduces experimental thermal or capsaicin-induced pain and hyperalgesia in normal volunteers. Anesth Analg. 1998;87(3):591–6. https://doi.org/10.1097/00000539-199809000-00018.
85. Siddall PJ, Molloy AR, Walker S, Mather LE, Rutkowski SB, Cousins MJ. The efficacy of intrathecal morphine and clonidine in the treatment of pain after spinal cord injury. Anesth Analg. 2000;91(6):1493–8. https://doi.org/10.1097/00000539-200012000-00037.
86. Ackerman LL, Follett KA, Rosenquist RW. Long-term outcomes during treatment of chronic pain with intrathecal clonidine or clonidine/opioid combinations. J Pain Symptom Manage. 2003;26(1):668–77. https://doi.org/10.1016/S0885-3924(03)00144-1.
87. Lavand'homme P, De Kock M. The use of intraoperative epidural or spinal analgesia modulates postoperative hyperalgesia and reduces residual pain after major abdominal surgery. Acta Anaesthesiol Belg. 2006;57(4):373–9.
88. Esmailian M, Golshani K, Tavakolifard N, Amiri A. Effects of adding oral clonidine to standard treatments on pain intensity of patients with acute renal colic: a randomized clinical trial. Adv Biomed Res. 2022;11:28. https://doi.org/10.4103/abr.abr_2_21.
89. Hsu YP, Chu KCW, Bai CH, Huang CJ, Chen C, Hsu CW. Safety and efficacy of clonidine on postoperative vomiting and pain in pediatric ophthalmic surgery: a systematic review and meta-analysis. Paediatr Anaesth. 2019;29(10):1011–23. https://doi.org/10.1111/pan.13712.
90. Reuben SS, Steinberg RB, Klatt JL, Klatt ML. Intravenous regional anesthesia using lidocaine and clonidine. Anesthesiology. 1999;91(3):654–8. https://doi.org/10.1097/00000542-199909000-00015.
91. Sathesha M, Raghavendra Rao RS, Hassan SJ, Sudheesh K. Clonidine as a sole epidural adjuvant in combined spinal-epidural: clinical study. Anesth Essays Res. 2018;12(2):309–12. https://doi.org/10.4103/aer.AER_18_17.
92. Joynt RL, Leonard JA. Dantrolene sodium suspension in treatment of spastic cerebral palsy. Dev Med Child Neurol. 1980;22(6):755–67. https://doi.org/10.1111/j.1469-8749.1980.tb03742.x.
93. Paisley S, Beard S, Hunn A, Wight J. Clinical effectiveness of oral treatments for spasticity in multiple sclerosis: a systematic review. Mult Scler. 2002;8(4):319–29. https://doi.org/10.1191/1352458502ms795rr.
94. Salassa JR, Seaman SL, Ruff T, Lenis A, Bellens EE, Brown AK. Oral dantrolene sodium for tonsillectomy pain: a double-blind study. Otolaryngol Head Neck Surg. 1988;98(1):26–33. https://doi.org/10.1177/019459988809800106.

95. van Tulder MW, Touray T, Furlan AD, Solway S, Bouter LM. Muscle relaxants for non-specific low back pain. Cochrane Database Syst Rev. 2003;2003(2):CD004252. https://doi.org/10.1002/14651858.CD004252
96. Cashin AG, Folly T, Bagg MK, et al. Efficacy, acceptability, and safety of muscle relaxants for adults with non-specific low back pain: systematic review and meta-analysis. BMJ. 2021;374:n1446. https://doi.org/10.1136/bmj.n1446.
97. Cashin AG, Wand BM, O'Connell NE, et al. Pharmacological treatments for low back pain in adults: an overview of Cochrane Reviews. Cochrane Database Syst Rev. 2023;4(4):CD013815. https://doi.org/10.1002/14651858.CD013815.pub2
98. Abril L, Zamora C, Cordero M, Williams AR, Friedman BW. The relative efficacy of seven skeletal muscle relaxants. an analysis of data from randomized studies. J Emerg Med. 2022;62(4):455–61. https://doi.org/10.1016/j.jemermed.2021.09.025
99. Corp N, Mansell G, Stynes S, et al. Evidence-based treatment recommendations for neck and low back pain across Europe: a systematic review of guidelines. Eur J Pain. 2021;25(2):275–95. https://doi.org/10.1002/ejp.1679.

Methadone

Sarah N. Saenz and Marcus Wilson

Keywords Methadone · Perioperative analgesia · Chronic pain management · Opioids

1 Introduction

Methadone is a synthetic, long-acting opioid, with parenteral and oral routes of administration. It is commonly used by physicians for treatment of opioid dependency, perioperative pain management, and chronic pain. Synthesized during World War II to relieve shortages of morphine, methadone was introduced into the United States in 1947 [1]. Its early use was noted in the treatment of opioid withdrawal and maintenance therapy for opioid dependence.

2 Pharmacodynamics/Pharmacokinetics

Methadone is primarily a μ-receptor agonist, *N*-methyl-D-aspartate (NMDA) receptor antagonist, and serotonin and norepinephrine reuptake inhibitor [2]. It can be used orally, intramuscularly, intravenously, subcutaneously, epidurally, and intrathecally. The elimination half-life of 24–36 h allows stable blood concentrations following a single dose compared to the shorter-acting opioids that can result

S. N. Saenz · M. Wilson (✉)
Department of Anesthesiology, University of Wisconsin School of Medicine and Public Health, 750 Highland Avenue, Madison, WI 53726, USA
e-mail: mwilson6@wisc.edu

S. N. Saenz
e-mail: ssaenz@uwhealth.org

A. Abd-Elsayed and K. Schroeder (eds.), *Perioperative Pain Management*,
https://doi.org/10.1007/978-3-031-67648-2_42

in fluctuating blood concentrations after intermittent intravenous boluses. With larger doses, the clinical analgesic effect of 36 hours is similar to the elimination half-life [3].

Methadone has high oral bioavailability (70–80%) with minimal first pass effect (less than 10%) [3]. Oral administration results in the onset of clinical effects within 30 minutes to 1 hours compared to intravenous administration, which has onset time of approximately 8 minutes. The lipophilic properties of methadone cause rapid absorption and tissue distribution, which is responsible for its relatively quick onset [2]. The slow redistribution back into the blood stream causes its long duration of action.

Methadone is metabolized by CYP450 enzyme within the liver to produced inactive byproducts [2]. These byproducts are then eliminated via the bile or urine [2].

3 Dosing and Route of Administration

Perioperative Use in the Opioid Naïve Patient

Recently, the efficacy of methadone in perioperative pain management has gained traction. 20 mg or 0.2 mg/kg of methadone administered at the induction of general anesthesia caused significant reductions in post-operative pain scores in surgeries such as posterior spinal fusions or major abdominal surgeries [3]. Additionally, a study performed by Kharasch et. al., demonstrated less post-operative opioids and reported less pain at home in patients given a single dose of intraoperative methadone (0.25 mg/kg) compared to those patients who received only short acting opioids for next day discharge surgical procedures [4]. A study by Komen et al. demonstrated similar results following the administration of 0.15 mg/kg of methadone in patients presenting for surgery with same day discharge [3, 5].

Care should be taken when methadone is combined with other agents with known sedative properties (i.e. gabapentin) that may be used as components of enhanced recovery after surgery protocols (ERAS). However, isolated methadone administration appears to result in a low incidence of respiratory depression or hypopnea.

Methadone in Opioid Use Disorder

With methadone's good oral bioavailability, low cost, and long half-life, it is suitable for once-a-day dosing, facilitating the management of opioid use disorder through methadone clinics. Single dose administration allows for repeat administration at the same time of day, each day. Synergistic NMDA antagonism and inhibition of serotonin and norepinephrine reuptake provide mechanisms through which methadone can prevent the development of hyperalgesia and improve a patient's mood [6]. The initial methadone dose in patients with low or uncertain opioid tolerance is typically 10–15 mg orally daily [7]. In patients with a high tolerance to opioid analgesics, initial methadone dosing is typically 15–20 mg with dosing rarely going as high as 30 mg daily [7]. This dose is titrated up daily by 5–10 mg, with dose escalation not exceeding 20 mg per week, until maintenance dosing is achieved at 60–120 mg per week [7]. Using these or similar dosing strategies, the treatment of opioid use disorders with methadone has demonstrated an ability to decrease the use of heroin and other drugs. Additionally, methadone maintenance therapy has reduced the transmission of HIV, hepatitis B and C [8].

Due to the high incidence of opioid addiction treatment with concurrent HIV/AIDS therapy, consideration of antiretrovirals effects on the CYP family of enzymes is needed. According to Kharasch et al, despite significant inhibition of CYP3A4 observed with protease inhibitor administration, there appears to be either an increase in methadone metabolism or no effect. CYP2B6 appears to not only participate in but is primary determinant in the metabolism of methadone [3, 9].

Perioperative Use in the Opioid Tolerant Patient

Patients with chronic pain and maintained on chronic opioid therapy can experience difficulties in perioperative pain management. These patients will likely have some form of opioid tolerance from their baseline opioid therapy that requires increasing doses to achieve analgesic effects [9]. As with opioid naive patients, nonpharmacological and nonopioid analgesic options should be added to the multimodal pain regimen. For patients maintained on chronic opioid therapies (including methadone), opioid maintenance dosing should be continued throughout the perioperative phase of care with additional short acting opioids available to treat acute pain that is not well managed with baseline opioid dosing and multimodal analgesics [9]. If possible, continuing the patients baseline methadone administration via the oral route is preferred. However, if oral intake is contraindicated, methadone dosing can be converted to intravenous dosing. Assistance with this transition to intravenous is best facilitated by a dedicated pain management team.

4 Adverse Effects

Methadone is known to prolong the QT-interval, which can predispose patients to the development of a potentially fatal arrythmias including torsades de pointes. The effects of methadone on QT-interval prolongation are more likely at doses greater than 150 mg per day [10]. However, adverse cardiac events have not been observed in the perioperative methadone studies. This risk for QT-interval prolongation appears to be related to not only the dose, but also the chronicity of treatment. As a result, patients maintained on long term methadone therapy and those undergoing active dose titration should have frequent EKG follow-ups.

Since methadone is metabolized in the liver via CYP enzymes, medications that induce or inhibit these enzymes can result in significant alterations of plasma concentrations. These drug interactions may predispose patients to opioid overdose and, specifically, respiratory depression. Common CYP3A4 inhibitors are erythromycin, diltiazem, and verapamil. Common CYP3A4 inducers are phenytoin, carbamazepine, and dexamethasone [10].

As methadone is an opioid, it carries with it the risk of respiratory depression especially in patients who concomitantly use benzodiazepines and other sedative medications, or patients with respiratory diseases such as obstructive sleep apnea or severe asthma. Rapid titration of methadone can result in an increased risk of respiratory depression and possibly death. Close monitoring and careful titration during the dose escalation period is crucial for patient safety.

Other common side-effects as with other opioids are constipation and drowsiness. Elderly patients are at higher risk for adverse effects for opioid induced complications.

5 Conclusion

Methadone has a long history of use in the management of opioid dependency and is starting to gain traction as an agent worthy of consideration for treatment of perioperative pain [1, 3]. Its long half-life allows for a single dose at the time of induction that can help to significantly reduce post-operative pain and opioid consumption [3]. Patients that are receiving methadone as treatment for opioid dependence would benefit from continuing their home dosing through the peri-operative period due to their risk for increased tolerance to opioid medications and difficulty with post-operative pain control [9]. Care should be taken in patients that receive methadone due to the potential for synergistic effects with other sedating medications that may be present in ERAS protocols.

Key Takeaway Points

1. Methadone may be helpful in the peri-operative period for opioid tolerant patients that are more likely to have difficulty with pain control.
2. A long half-life allows for once-a-day dosing or single dosing with the induction of anesthesia.
3. Patients maintained on chronic methadone therapy should continue taking it as prescribed in the peri-operative period if there are concerns with adequate pain control.

4. Care should be taken with additional sedating medications as there may be a synergistic effects with concurrent methadone dosing.

References

1. Payte JT. A brief history of methadone in the treatment of opioid dependence: a personal perspective. J Psychoactive Drugs. 1991;23(2):103–7. https://doi.org/10.1080/02791072.1991.10472226.
2. Hanna V, Senderovich H. Methadone in pain management: a systematic review. J Pain. 2021;22(3):233–45. https://doi.org/10.1016/j.jpain.2020.04.004.
3. Murphy GS, Szokol JW. Intraoperative methadone in surgical patients: a review of clinical investigations. Anesthesiology. 2019;131(3):678–92. https://doi.org/10.1097/ALN.0000000000002755.
4. Kharasch ED, Brunt LM, Blood J, Komen H. Intraoperative methadone in next-day discharge outpatient surgery: a randomized, double-blinded, dose-finding pilot study. Anesthesiology. 2023;139(4):405–19. https://doi.org/10.1097/ALN.0000000000004663. PMID: 37350677; PMCID: PMC10527477.
5. Komen H, Brunt LM, Deych E, Blood J, Kharasch ED. Intraoperative methadone in same-day ambulatory surgery: a randomized, double-blinded, dose-finding pilot study. Anesth Analg. 2019;128(4):802–10. https://doi.org/10.1213/ANE.0000000000003464. PMID: 29847382; PMCID: PMC6995343.
6. Anderson IB, Kearney TE. Use of methadone. West J Med. 2000;172(1):43–6. https://doi.org/10.1136/ewjm.172.1.43.
7. Guidelines for the Psychosocially Assisted Pharmacological Treatment of Opioid Dependence. Geneva: World Health Organization; 2009. Annex 12, Prescribing guidelines. Available from: https://www.ncbi.nlm.nih.gov/books/NBK143167/
8. Brown R, Kraus C, Fleming M, Reddy S. Methadone: applied pharmacology and use as adjunctive treatment in chronic pain. Postgrad Med J. 2004;80(949):654–9. https://doi.org/10.1136/pgmj.2004.022988.
9. Alford DP, Compton P, Samet JH. Acute pain management for patients receiving maintenance methadone or buprenorphine therapy [published correction appears in Ann Intern Med. 2006;144(6):460]. Ann Intern Med. 2006;144(2):127–34. https://doi.org/10.7326/0003-4819-144-2-200601170-00010
10. Kharasch ED. Current concepts in methadone metabolism and transport. Clin Pharmacol Drug Dev. 2017;6(2):125–34. https://doi.org/10.1002/cpdd.326. PMID: 28263461; PMCID: PMC6339814.

Non-pharmacological Adjuncts in the Perioperative Period

Adeeb Oweidat, Nada Sadek, Elie Geara, Mohamad Ayoub, and Rakesh Sondekoppam Vijayashankar

Keywords Nonpharmacological analgesia · Postoperative pain · Adjuncts

Pain represents a significant burden for patients following surgery and can impact their short- and long-term outcomes. While pharmacotherapy is considered the primary forms the main modality associated with perioperative analgesic management of controlling pain, managing pain without medications, otherwise called non-pharmacological adjuncts are recently gaining traction and assuming a substantial contributing role in pain management in the perioperative period. Rightfully so, these modalities are considered adjuncts as they may not be effective as the sole for the treatment for of moderate-to-severe acute pain alone and are hence considered supplementary to the analgesic techniques described in earlier chapters. Many clinicians and patients prefer a combination of pharmacotherapy and non-pharmacologic methods to control post-operative pain. The common practice of utilizing non-pharmacologic

A. Oweidat (✉) · N. Sadek · R. S. Vijayashankar
Clinics Department of Anesthesia, University of Iowa Hospitals, Iowa City, IA, USA
e-mail: adeeb.oweidat@gmail.com

N. Sadek
e-mail: Nada-sadek@uiowa.edu

R. S. Vijayashankar
e-mail: rakesh6282@gmail.com

E. Geara · M. Ayoub
Department of Anesthesiology, Perioperative Care, and Pain Medicine at NYU Grossman School of Medicine, New York, NY, USA
e-mail: Elie.Geara@nyulangone.org

M. Ayoub
e-mail: Mohamad.IbrahimAyoub@nyulangone.org

A. Abd-Elsayed and K. Schroeder (eds.), *Perioperative Pain Management*,
https://doi.org/10.1007/978-3-031-67648-2_43

adjuncts is common in clinical practice. However, these treatments are scarcely translated into the literature and there remains little data describing their is still limited on its efficacy in the context of acute surgical pain.

Several categories of non-pharmacologic techniques exist in clinical practice, and they include a variety of methods. We describe below these techniques and this chapter expands on select methods that are widely prescribed as adjunct pain regimens. These techniques, along with standard pharmacological regimens, can complement the management of post-surgical acute pain. Broadly, they can be classified as:

- Physical measures such as Heat/cold therapy, massage, acupuncture/electroacupuncture, Transcutaneous electric nerve stimulation (TENS) therapy, cryoanalgesia.
- Physical therapy measures such as pre-habilitation, exercise, deep breathing, biofeedback.
- Psychological approaches such as meditation, imagery, visualization, distraction therapies, cognitive behavioral therapy to name a few.

1 Heat and Cold Therapy

Heat and cold therapy modalities are often used to treat acute musculoskeletal injuries despite prevalent confusion about which modality (heat versus cold) to use and when to use it. Most recommendations for the use of heat and cold therapy are based on empirical experience.

Cold Therapy

The application of cold is a popular and established method for treating acute soft tissue injuries. Local cooling of skin induces numerous physiological responses by the reduction of skin surface and subjacent tissue temperature. During a 20-min ice pack application, the muscle temperature and the subcutaneous temperature decrease by 7 °C and 17 °C, respectively [1]. Thus, ice cooling can be applied only for a few minutes on the affected structure and produces the desired effect.

The theoretical mechanisms of cold therapy were based on the positive physiologic effects of cold therapy for tissue recovery after trauma, such as pain relief, decrease of nerve conduction, and decrease of edema by slowing down blood flow with vasoconstriction [2].

In the literature, there are plenty of papers that mentioned the effectiveness of the cold therapy after soft tissue and sports injuries [3, 4]. After any surgery, especially orthopedics surgeries, the control of swelling and pain is crucial to fasten recovery. Several studies have shown that applying ice in the perioperative period can decrease opioid consumption and reduce pain [5, 6]. Cryotherapy can be applied easily and safely by the caregiver of the patient or by a nurse without skin irritations and wound healing problems [5, 6]. Nevertheless, the literature is still scant regarding the effects of perioperative cold therapy.

Cold therapy appears to be effective and harmless, and few complications or side effects have been reported after its use. Prolonged application at very low temperatures should, however, be avoided, as this may cause serious side effects, such as frostbite, allergic reactions, burns, intolerance/pain, and nerve injuries [7]. Cold therapy should not be used in patients with cold hypersensitivity, cold intolerance, or Raynaud's disease, or over areas of vascular compromise [8].

Practical applications, indications, and contraindications are poorly known, and randomized clinical trials have not been performed on the efficacy of cold therapy for patients with soft tissue injuries [9].

Heat Therapy

Heat therapy is the application of heat to the body resulting in increased tissue temperature. Superficial modes of heat therapy include hot water bottles, heat pads, electric heat pads, heat wraps, heated stones, soft heated packs filled with grain, poultices, hot towels, hot baths, sauna, paraffin, steam, and infrared heat lamps [8]. An alternative mode of heat therapy is deep-heat therapy, which involves conversion of another form of energy to heat (e.g., Diathermy and ultrasound) [8, 10].

Physiological effects of heat therapy include pain relief, increases in blood flow and metabolism, and increased elasticity of connective tissue [11]. Increasing tissue temperature enhances vasodilation and increases tissue blood flow, which is thought to promote healing by increasing the supply of nutrients and oxygen to the site of injury while improving metabolism at the cellular level and improving tissue healing [11–13]. Heat-induced changes in the viscoelastic properties of collagenous tissues may underlie the demonstrated efficacy of heat therapy for improving range of movement [14, 15].

Precautions should be taken during the use of heat therapy in patients with multiple sclerosis [11, 16], poor circulation, spinal cord injuries, diabetes mellitus [11], and rheumatoid arthritis, where heat may cause disease progression, burns, skin ulceration, and increased inflammation [11, 16]. Skin should be protected when using heat therapy in heat-sensitive or high-risk patients, especially over regions with decreased sensory function [11].

As with cold therapy, more randomized clinical trials of heat therapy would enhance the body of literature.

2 TENS

Introduction

Transcutaneous electric nerve stimulation (TENS) is an inexpensive and simple tool used internationally as an adjunct treatment to different kinds of acute and chronic pain ranging from musculoskeletal to cancer pain. TENS is delivered through a battery powered device that sends electric impulses to the skin via electrode pads. The area targeted by conventional TENS can either be the skin overlying the painful source or proximally at the site of the nerve. A variant of TENS called acupuncture like TENS delivers these impulses at acupoints. In fact, there are studies that suggest that the application of TENS at acupoints can be more efficacious in reducing pain [17]. The intensity and frequency of TENS impulses is not standardized in clinical practice with multiple studies comparing variations in these parameters and their impact on efficacy [18, 19].

Mechanism of Action

TENS produces analgesia through its action on the central and peripheral nervous system. At the level of the central nervous system, TENS suppresses hyperalgesia through the activation of endogenous inhibitory pathways mediated by opioid, GABA and muscarinic receptors. It has also been proposed to reduce central excitability and sensitization. At the level of the peripheral nervous system, TENS alters the excitability of both nociceptors and adrenergic receptors [20].

Evidence for Its Utility in Perioperative Pain

The efficacy of TENS in treating postoperative pain in different surgical specialties has been explored with promising results. Several studies support the added role of TENS in alleviating post-operative pain and facilitating rehabilitation after total knee arthroplasty [21–23]. Multiple studies demonstrated that TENS, as part of a multimodal analgesic regimen, alleviates post thoracotomy pain and enhances patient recovery [24–26]. One study revealed that this effect is limited to mild to moderate pain [27]. Another study that evaluated Transcutaneous Electrical Acupoint stimulation (TEAS) for VATS lobectomy concluded that it can reduce opioid requirements and pain scores [28]. A pilot study comparing the effect of high frequency TENS compared to sham in weaning from epidural analgesia after open colectomy showed a significant reduction in pain scores reflecting the potential benefit of the TENS in post-operative pain management [29]. Another study highlighted the potential of TENS in relieving pain associated with physical therapy after abdominal surgery

[30]. A study evaluating the postoperative pain experienced by patients undergoing lower abdominal surgery showed that TENS application reduced postoperative opioid requirements and opioid related adverse events [19]. A general trend among published evaluations of TENS therapy is a strong potential benefit of this modality as an adjunct analgesic in the perioperative setting. Standardization of practice may ultimately facilitate pooling of data in order to build strong evidence to support the results of these studies.

The efficacy of TENS has been the subject of controversy since 1970 owing to the heterogeneity of clinical practice compromising pooled data that would allow reviews to reach conclusions with strong evidence. The meta-TENS study, a systemic review and meta-analysis on the effect and safety of TENS for acute and chronic pain concluded that there was moderate-certainty evidence that, compared with placebo, pain intensity is lower after TENS [31].

Side Effects

The safety profile of TENS is an attribute that makes it more attractive as an adjunct therapy. Only mild adverse effects have been reported including skin irritation and discomfort [31]. Electrode pad allergy is another side effect that may rarely be encountered. The only contraindications to TENS therapy are the presence of a pacemaker/implanted defibrillator device or need to closely monitor postoperative telemetry.

Acupuncture

Acupuncture is an ancient medical practice originating over 2000 years ago in China. The concept of acupuncture was first described in the book titled The Yellow Emperor's Classic in Internal Medicine [32]. As centuries passed, acupuncture spread into Japan, Korea, and Southeast Asia before reaching Europe and eventually the United States. It didn't gain significant attention in the US until 1971 when a New York Times journalist featured it as a remedy to his own postoperative pain after an appendectomy in China [33]. Acupuncture continues to boast increasing popularity with visits to acupuncturists almost tripling between 1997 and 2007 [34]. Today, acupuncture is internationally recognized as a complementary therapy for the management of acute and chronic pain. It is recommended as part of a comprehensive pain management pathway by the Agency for Healthcare Research and Quality (AHRQ) and Health and Human Services (HHS) agencies [35].

Understanding traditional acupuncture entails knowledge of its background, which is rooted in Confucianism and Taoism philosophy. Three entities constitute the theory of acupuncture: Qi, Yin and Yang. Qi is the vital energy that propagates through meridians. Yin and Yang are the contrasting complementary forces that are in constant dynamic interplay. In addition to the three main entities, five elements—, fire, earth, metal, water, and wood—constitute the physical and emotional processes of the body [36]. Acupuncture aims to restore the balance between yin and yang and the harmony of the entities to reinstate proper function of the body and its optimal health state.

An acupuncture treatment constitutes the insertion of needles at specific landmarks in the body called acupoints. According to traditional Chinese medicine (TCM), these acupoints are connected by meridians through which the Qi flows. Stimulation of these acupoints is responsible for the physiologic effects of acupuncture. Acupoint manipulation can also encompass electrical stimulation, heat, pressure, and other modalities, with physical manipulation and electric stimulation being the most commonly practiced and studied methods. Needles are usually retained in place for a duration of 15–20 minutes and then removed. Acupuncture sessions can vary in duration and frequency depending on the practitioner and diagnosis. It is important to recognize that acupuncture in TCM is one arm of a holistic approach to patient care, one that encompasses herbal medicine and other lifestyle modifications. While traditional acupuncture is still practiced today, a variety of new methodologies have proliferated that incorporate the foundation of TCM and augment these practices with the application of modern medical theories.

Mechanism of Action

Translating the philosophical beliefs of traditional acupuncture into scientifically proven mechanisms has not yet been well established. Evidence-based studies support the physiologic effects of acupuncture, yet a complete picture of the underlying biologic mechanisms is not clear. Current literature supports the physiologic effect of acupuncture on both the central and peripheral nervous systems.

At the level of the central nervous system, studies have shown that acupuncture and electro-acupuncture trigger the release of endorphins responsible for mediating the analgesic effects of acupuncture [37]. This mechanism for acupuncture efficacy is further backed by another study demonstrating how antagonism of opioid receptors by naloxone in animal models reversed the analgesic effect of acupuncture [38]. Other mediators, such as serotonin, norepinephrine, and peripherally released molecules have also been implicated in the modulation of pain perception via acupuncture. Multiple studies have also evaluated the brain response to acupuncture through functional MRI testing, highlighting its impact on brain activity and connectivity, including areas that correspond to pain pathways [39].

Evidence for Its Utility in Perioperative Pain

The NIH consensus panel concluded that there are good data to support the efficacy of acupuncture in postoperative dental procedures [40]. The literature on acupuncture is growing and more and more studies are supporting its potential role in treating perioperative pain. A review on acupuncture and postoperative pain concluded that acupuncture is a method with minimal side effects that can augment perioperative analgesia, reduce opioid consumption, and minimize the side effects of opioid analgesics [41]. Multiple systemic reviews and meta-analyses (SRM) support the role of acupuncture in reducing postoperative pain and opioid requirements and consequently opioid related side effects [42–45]. Studies assessing auricular therapy revealed positive findings supporting its efficacy in reducing postoperative pain [46–48].

Many studies are emerging evaluating the efficacy of acupuncture in the perioperative setting in different kinds of surgical subspecialties. A study evaluating postoperative pain after open mesh inguinal hernia repair concluded that electroacupuncture reduced postoperative pain and anxiety [49]. A SRM evaluating drug free intervention for total knee arthroplasty concluded that acupuncture reduced and delayed opioid use [50]. Another study that utilized transcutaneous electric acupoint stimulation (TEAS) in thoracoscopic pulmonary resection suggests TEAS as a feasible approach for sedation and postoperative analgesia [51]. A prospective, double blinded, randomized, controlled trial found that acupuncture can complement NSAIDs in the management of post tonsillectomy pain [52].

Guidelines neither recommend nor dismiss the role of acupuncture in the management of perioperative pain. This lack of consensus affirmation is partly secondary to a lack of procedural consistency resulting in a range of duration and frequency of treatments. The lack of a standard sham control intervention further compromises the existing evidence and results in concurrent speculations related to placebo effect versus underestimating the true effect of acupuncture.

Side Effects

Acupuncture is a safe practice when executed by professionally trained practitioners. It is tolerated by patients to the extent that it has been frequently described as relaxing. There have been reports, however, of fatigue, headache and pain at acupuncture sites. Side effects such as nausea, syncope, and exacerbation of symptoms have also been mentioned in the literature. Major side effects such as pneumothorax or the transmission of infectious diseases have been linked to improper training [35].

Cryoanalgesia and Ablation

Cold temperatures have been recognized for thousands of years for their analgesic and anti-inflammatory benefits. Records mentioning the use of cold to treat pain date back to the ancient Egyptians and later Hippocrates. In the 1800s, Napoleon's army surgeon performed regional anesthesia with ice to perform amputations for injured soldiers. Over the past 200 years, cold treatments have evolved and expanded to different fields. The modern practice using a cryoprobe was first described by Cooper et al. in 1961 [53]. Later in 1976, Llyod et al. published the first large article that demonstrated the benefits of cryoanalgesia [54]. Today, new equipment has been developed and additional research reestablished cryoanalgesia as a useful tool in acute and perioperative pain management.

Mechanism of Action

Cryoanalgesia refers to the cooling of peripheral nerves to extremely cold temperatures and causing an interruption in conduction of painful stimuli through reversible nerve damage. This interruption in nerve activity is achieved through contact of the nerve and a cryoprobe set at very low temperatures.

The cryoprobe is a hollow tube within a tube system whereby gas travels from the proximal part of a high pressure smaller inner tube distally into a low pressure larger outer tube. This causes the gas to expand rapidly and the temperatures to drop considerably owing to the Joule-Thompson effect. A ball of ice forms at the tip of cryoprobe because of the drop in temperature and this causes direct neuronal injury [55]. A temperature of at least—20 °C must be achieved to produce effective analgesia and must not exceed − 100 °C to be considered safe and not result in permanent structural damage to the affected nerve [56]. With this technique, analgesia can potentially be sustained for a considerable amount of time ranging from weeks to months and this is mainly determined by the length of the lesion created by the ice ball [57].

Evidence for Its Utility in Perioperative Pain

Percutaneous injection of local anesthesia has been used for the past century to treat perioperative pain. Although effective, the duration of action of local anesthetics is limited. A modality that provides relief for weeks or months has not been achieved with local anesthetics; the majority of single injection techniques provide temporary relief of pain unlikely to extend beyond 24 hours whereas continuous catheter infusions can generally extend analgesia for up to a week before factors emerge that limit the safety of further use. Cryoanalgesia conceptually fills the gap in analgesia that may be required for surgical procedures anticipated to require weeks or months of effective pain relief.

Cryoanalgesia, also known as cryoneurolysis, was first performed intraoperatively under direct visualization after surgical exposure. Early applications of cryoanalgesia in the perioperative setting involved cryoanalgesia of surgically exposed intercostal nerves to relieve pain after thoracotomy [58]. The latter method required landmark identification and/or nerve stimulation. However, with recent advances in imaging technology, percutaneous cryoanalgesia allows accurate access to target structures with similar precision and efficacy [59].

The literature has shown contrasting outcomes when it comes to cryoanalgesia for thoracotomies. Several randomized controlled trials have shown strong benefits ranging from analgesia, opioid sparing and consequently decreased opioid related side effects, improved pulmonary function, and decrease in hospital length of stay. Some studies have even shown superiority to regional anesthesia techniques. However, many randomized controlled trials showed no benefit. A similar pattern of inconsistency in findings was observed in studies involving postoperative herniorrhaphy pain. These outcomes can be explained by differing techniques in the application of cryoanalgesia [60].

Cryoanalgesia shows strong evidence for potential benefit in the setting of hernia repair with multiple studies showing superior analgesia [61]. Cryoablation for perineal pain has also been studied with results showing successful relief in symptoms [62]. One randomized double blinded multicenter trial demonstrated significantly improved knee pain control compared to sham [63]. Another study showed that cryoneurolysis of the occipital nerve is an effective therapy for occipital neuralgia [64]. Cryoanalgesia has also been studied in phantom limb pain with one study showing cryoanalgesia as an effective long term treatment [65].

Contraindications and Adverse Effects

Contraindications to percutaneous cryoanalgesia are patient refusal or incapacity to consent for the procedure, anatomical variations that can prove challenging for the safe execution of the procedure, both bleeding diathesis and coagulopathies, preexisting infection, cold urticaria, cryoglobulinemia and Raynaud's syndrome [66]. It is important to note that targeting mixed motor/sensory nerves will result in both a motor and sensory deficit and this should be considered prior to application.

Cryoanalgesia is a relatively safe procedure with a modest complication risk profile. There is no report in the literature to this day of permanent nerve damage [66]. There is one case report of severe adverse effects manifesting as myonecrosis and abscess formation [67], however most of the side effects are mild to moderate. Side effects from cryoneurolysis don't differ from those that might be encountered following any standard procedure that involves percutaneous injection, and these include bruising, infection, and bleeding. It is very important that nontarget ablation be avoided to prevent possible side effects. Also, acute worsening of the pain and allodynia can result if the target is not appropriately targeted [61].

Psychologic Interventions

Psychological therapy is another entity that aims to alter the psychological processes that may contribute to pain through stress reduction, education, relaxation, attentional strategies, and hypnosis. These are all mechanisms that can be used to alter the way in which patients perceive, interpret, and cope with pain.

In the acute pain setting, hypnosis has been effective in managing pain associated with medical procedures such as burn wound care and bone marrow biopsies [68]. Other relaxation strategies such as distraction (for example: listening to music) and virtual reality have promise as adjuvants in acute pain management. As such, music in the preoperative setting can be used either as an adjuvant or as a replacement for anxiolytics. This can be especially beneficial in patients who may be very sensitive to intravenous anxiolytics and for patients who do not report a significant amount of anxiety. In the intraoperative setting, these modalities can be highly desirable for patients undergoing conscious sedation and/or regional anesthesia as they reduce overall sedative requirements, improve patient comfort, and enhance satisfaction [69]. For example, a common reason that patients may refuse regional anesthetics is simply because they do not want to "hear" their surroundings. In scenarios like this, a simple solution to minimize a patient's fear of hearing their surroundings would be to place a pair of headphones and allow the patient to listen to music during the intraoperative setting.

Finally, biofeedback therapy is an instrument-based learning process employing operant conditioning. Autonomic and neuromuscular activity is measured, and visual, acoustic, and verbal feedback is provided to promote the acquisition of self-control over physiological processes, which are otherwise outside awareness or under less voluntary control [70].

Several landmark studies demonstrated the efficacy of biofeedback for pelvic pain and anorectal disorders. For other phenotypes of chronic pelvic pain, there is tentative evidence that biofeedback-assisted training interventions can improve recovery outcomes through improvements in pain control, overall symptoms, and quality of life. Future studies should aim to investigate further the value of biofeedback in the management of pain in well-designed randomized controlled trials.

Key Takeaways

- Evidence based literature supports the use of TENS as an adjunct analgesic in the perioperative setting.
- Guidelines neither recommend nor dismiss the role of acupuncture in the treatment of perioperative pain.

- Cryoanalgesia is a relatively safe procedure with a modest risk profile of complications that may extend procedural analgesia for weeks or months.
- Hypnosis has been effective in managing pain associated with medical procedures such as burn wound care.
- Music is a safe, nonpharmacologic option to enhance a patient's perioperative experience.
- Biofeedback is a modality that seeks to improve self-efficacy and learning based on operant conditioning.

References

1. Myrer JW, Measom G, Durrant E, et al. Cold- and hot-pack contrast therapy: subcutaneous and intramuscular temperature change. J Athl Train. 1997;32:238–41.
2. Kuyucu E, Bülbül M, Kara A, Koçyiğit F, Erdil M. Is cold therapy really efficient after knee arthroplasty? Ann Med Surg (Lond). 2015;4(4):475–8. Published 2015 Nov 11. https://doi.org/10.1016/j.amsu.2015.10.019.
3. Abramson DI, Chu LS, Tuck S Jr, Lee SW, Richardson G, Levin M. Effect of tissue temperatures and blood flow on motor nerve conduction velocity. JAMA. 1966;198(10):1082–8.
4. Matsen FA 3rd, Questad K, Matsen AL. The effect of local cooling on postfracture swelling. A controlled study. Clin Orthop Relat Res. 1975;(109):201–6. https://doi.org/10.1097/00003086-197506000-00029.
5. Scharf HP. CORRInsights®: Does advanced cryotherapy reduce pain and narcotic consumption after knee arthroplasty? Clin Orthopaedics Relat Res. 2014;472(11):3424–5. https://doi.org/10.1007/s11999-014-3879-0.
6. Webb JM, Williams D, Ivory JP, Day S, Williamson DM. The use of cold compression dressings after total knee replacement: a randomized controlled trial. Orthopedics. 1998;21(1):59–61. https://doi.org/10.3928/0147-7447-19980101-14.
7. Drez D, Faust DC, Evans JP. Cryotherapy and nerve palsy. Am J Sports Med. 1981;9(4):256–7. https://doi.org/10.1177/036354658100900414.
8. Malanga GA, Yan N, Stark J. Mechanisms and efficacy of heat and cold therapies for musculoskeletal injury. Postgrad Med. 2015;127(1):57–65. https://doi.org/10.1080/00325481.2015.992719.
9. Airaksinen OV, Kyrklund N, Latvala K, Kouri JP, Grönblad M, Kolari P. Efficacy of cold gel for soft tissue injuries: a prospective randomized double-blinded trial. Am J Sports Med. 2003;31(5):680–4. https://doi.org/10.1177/03635465030310050801.
10. French SD, Cameron M, Walker BF, Reggars JW, Esterman AJ. Superficial heat or cold for low back pain. Cochrane Database Syst Rev. 2006:CD004750.
11. Nadler SF, Weingand K, Kruse RJ. The physiologic basis and clinical applications of cryotherapy and thermotherapy for the pain practitioner. Pain Physician. 2004;7:395–9.
12. Charkoudian N. Mechanisms and modifiers of reflex induced cutaneous vasodilation and vasoconstriction in humans. J Appl Physiol. 2010;109:1221–8.
13. Reid RW, Foley JM, Prior BM, Weingand KW, Meyer RA. Mild topical heat increases popliteal blood flow as measured by MRI [abstract]. Med Sci Sports Exerc. 1999;31:S208.
14. Bleakley CM, Costello JT. Do thermal agents affect range of movement and mechanical properties in soft tissues? A systematic review. Arch Phys Med Rehabil. 2013;94:149–63.
15. Hardy M, Woodall W. Therapeutic effects of heat, cold, and stretch on connective tissue. J Hand Ther. 1998;11:148–56.
16. Berger JR, Sheremata WA. Persistent neurological deficit precipitated by hot bath test in multiple sclerosis. JAMA. 1983;249:1751–3.

17. Chen L, Tang J, White PF, Sloninsky A, Wender RH, Naruse R, Kariger R. The effect of location of transcutaneous electrical nerve stimulation on postoperative opioid analgesic requirement: acupoint versus nonacupoint stimulation. Anesth Analg. 1998;87(5):1129–34. PMID: 9806695.
18. Wang B, Tang J, White PF, Naruse R, Sloninsky A, Kariger R, Gold J, Wender RH. Effect of the intensity of transcutaneous acupoint electrical stimulation on the postoperative analgesic requirement. Anesth Analg. 1997;85(2):406–13. https://doi.org/10.1097/00000539-199708000-00029. PMID: 9249122.
19. Hamza MA, White PF, Ahmed HE, Ghoname EA. Effect of the frequency of transcutaneous electrical nerve stimulation on the postoperative opioid analgesic requirement and recovery profile. Anesthesiology. 1999;91(5):1232–8. https://doi.org/10.1097/00000542-199911000-00012. PMID: 10551571.
20. Vance CG, Dailey DL, Rakel BA, Sluka KA. Using TENS for pain control: the state of the evidence. Pain Manag. 2014;4(3):197–209. https://doi.org/10.2217/pmt.14.13. PMID: 24953072; PMCID: PMC4186747.
21. Chughtai M, Elmallah RD, Mistry JB, Bhave A, Cherian JJ, McGinn TL, Harwin SF, Mont MA. Nonpharmacologic pain management and muscle strengthening following total knee arthroplasty. J Knee Surg. 2016;29(3):194–200. https://doi.org/10.1055/s-0035-1569147. Epub 2015 Dec 18. PMID: 26683980.
22. Zhang Q, Zhang JH, Tong PJ. Application of transcutaneous electrical nerve stimulation to multimodal analgesia after total knee arthroplasty. Zhongguo Gu Shang. 2014;27(4):283–6. Chinese. PMID: 25029833.
23. Zhu Y, Feng Y, Peng L. Effect of transcutaneous electrical nerve stimulation for pain control after total knee arthroplasty: a systematic review and meta-analysis. J Rehabil Med. 2017;49(9):700–4. https://doi.org/10.2340/16501977-2273. PMID: 28933513.
24. Sezen CB, Akboga SA, Celik A, Kalafat CE, Tastepe AI. Transcutaneous electrical nerve stimulation effect on postoperative complications. Asian Cardiovasc Thorac Ann. 2017;25(4):276–80. https://doi.org/10.1177/0218492317703838. Epub 2017 Mar 28. PMID: 28350210.
25. Freynet A, Falcoz PE. Is transcutaneous electrical nerve stimulation effective in relieving postoperative pain after thoracotomy? Interact Cardiovasc Thorac Surg. 2010;10(2):283–8. https://doi.org/10.1510/icvts.2009.219576. Epub 2009 Nov 12. PMID: 19910359.
26. Chandra A, Banavaliker JN, Das PK, Hasti S. Use of transcutaneous electrical nerve stimulation as an adjunctive to epidural analgesia in the management of acute thoracotomy pain. Indian J Anaesth. 2010;54(2):116–20. https://doi.org/10.4103/0019-5049.63648. PMID: 20661348; PMCID: PMC2900733.
27. Benedetti F, Amanzio M, Casadio C, Cavallo A, Cianci R, Giobbe R, Mancuso M, Ruffini E, Maggi G. Control of postoperative pain by transcutaneous electrical nerve stimulation after thoracic operations. Ann Thorac Surg. 1997;63(3):773–6. https://doi.org/10.1016/s0003-4975(96)01249-0. PMID: 9066400.
28. Huang S, Peng W, Tian X, Liang H, Jia Z, Lo T, He M, Feng Y. Effects of transcutaneous electrical acupoint stimulation at different frequencies on perioperative anesthetic dosage, recovery, complications, and prognosis in video-assisted thoracic surgical lobectomy: a randomized, double-blinded, placebo-controlled trial. J Anesth. 2017;31(1):58–65. https://doi.org/10.1007/s00540-015-2057-1. Epub 2015 Sep 8. PMID: 26350110.
29. Bjerså K, Jildenstaal P, Jakobsson J, Egardt M, Fagevik Olsén M. Adjunct high frequency transcutaneous electric stimulation (TENS) for postoperative pain management during weaning from epidural analgesia following colon surgery: results from a controlled pilot study. Pain Manag Nurs. 2015;16(6):944–50. https://doi.org/10.1016/j.pmn.2015.08.006. Epub 2015 Nov 2. PMID: 26541070.
30. Tonella RM, Araújo S, Silva AM. Estimulação elétrica nervosa transcutânea no alívio da dor pós-operatória relacionada com procedimentos fisioterapêuticos em pacientes submetidos a intervenções cirúrgicas abdominais [Transcutaneous electrical nerve stimulation in the relief of pain related to physical therapy after abdominal surgery.]. Rev Bras Anestesiol. 2006;56(6):630–42. Portuguese. https://doi.org/10.1590/s0034-70942006000600007. PMID: 19468607.

31. Johnson MI, Paley CA, Jones G, Mulvey MR, Wittkopf PG. Efficacy and safety of transcutaneous electrical nerve stimulation (TENS) for acute and chronic pain in adults: a systematic review and meta-analysis of 381 studies (the meta-TENS study). BMJ Open. 2022;12(2):e051073. https://doi.org/10.1136/bmjopen-2021-051073. PMID: 35144946; PMCID: PMC8845179.
32. Curran J. The yellow emperor's classic of internal medicine. BMJ. 2008;336(7647):777. https://doi.org/10.1136/bmj.39527.472303.4E. PMCID: PMC2287209.
33. Reston J. Now about my operation in Peking. NY Times. 1971;1:6.
34. Nahin RL, Barnes PM, Stussman BJ, et al. Costs of complementary and alternative medicine (CAM) and frequency of visits to CAM practitioners: United States, 2007. Natl Health Stat Report. 2009;18:1–14.
35. Nielsen A, Dusek JA, Taylor-Swanson L, Tick H. Acupuncture therapy as an evidence-based nonpharmacologic strategy for comprehensive acute pain care: the academic consortium pain task force white paper update. Pain Med. 2022;23(9):1582–612. https://doi.org/10.1093/pm/pnac056. PMID: 35380733; PMCID: PMC9434305.
36. https://www.uptodate.com/contents/acupuncture?search=acupuncture&source=search_result&selectedTitle=1~150&usage_type=default&display_rank=1#references
37. Han JS. Acupuncture and endorphins. Neurosci Lett. 2004;361(1–3):258–61. https://doi.org/10.1016/j.neulet.2003.12.019. PMID: 15135942.
38. Mayer DJ, Price DD, Rafii A. Antagonism of acupuncture analgesia in man by the narcotic antagonist naloxone. Brain Res. 1977;121:368–72.
39. He T, Zhu W, Du SQ, Yang JW, Li F, Yang BF, Shi GX, Liu CZ. Neural mechanisms of acupuncture as revealed by fMRI studies. Auton Neurosci. 2015;190:1–9. https://doi.org/10.1016/j.autneu.2015.03.006. Epub 2015 Apr 2. PMID: 25900479.
40. NIH Consensus Conference. Acupuncture. JAMA. 1998;280(17):1518–24. PMID: 9809733.
41. Shah S, Godhardt L, Spofford C. Acupuncture and postoperative pain reduction. Curr Pain Headache Rep. 2022;26(6):453–8. https://doi.org/10.1007/s11916-022-01048-4. Epub 2022 Apr 28. PMID: 35482244.
42. Liu XL, Tan JY, Molassiotis A, Suen LK, Shi Y. Acupuncture-point stimulation for postoperative pain control: a systematic review and meta-analysis of randomized controlled trials. Evid Based Complement Alternat Med. 2015;2015:657809. https://doi.org/10.1155/2015/657809. Epub 2015 Oct 12. PMID: 26568767; PMCID: PMC4620376.
43. Wu MS, Chen KH, Chen IF, Huang SK, Tzeng PC, Yeh ML, Lee FP, Lin JG, Chen C. The efficacy of acupuncture in post-operative pain management: a systematic review and meta-analysis. PLoS One. 2016;11(3):e0150367. https://doi.org/10.1371/journal.pone.0150367. PMID: 26959661; PMCID: PMC4784927.
44. Sun Y, Gan TJ, Dubose JW, Habib AS. Acupuncture and related techniques for postoperative pain: a systematic review of randomized controlled trials. Br J Anaesth. 2008;101(2):151–60. https://doi.org/10.1093/bja/aen146. Epub 2008 Jun 2. PMID: 18522936.
45. Zhu J, Xu Q, Zou R, Wu W, Wang X, Wang Y, Ji F, Zheng Z, Zheng M. Distal acupoint stimulation versus peri-incisional stimulation for postoperative pain in open abdominal surgery: a systematic review and implications for clinical practice. BMC Complement Altern Med. 2019;19(1):192. https://doi.org/10.1186/s12906-019-2583-8. PMID: 31362730; PMCID: PMC6668193.
46. Asher GN, Jonas DE, Coeytaux RR, Reilly AC, Loh YL, Motsinger-Reif AA, Winham SJ. Auriculotherapy for pain management: a systematic review and meta-analysis of randomized controlled trials. J Altern Complement Med. 2010;16(10):1097–108. https://doi.org/10.1089/acm.2009.0451. PMID: 20954963; PMCID: PMC3110838.
47. Ye XX, Gao YZ, Xu ZB, Liu QX, Zhan CJ. Effectiveness of perioperative auricular therapy on postoperative pain after total hip arthroplasty: a systematic review and meta-analysis of randomised controlled trials. Evid Based Complement Alternat Med. 2019;2019:2979780. https://doi.org/10.1155/2019/2979780. PMID: 30941191; PMCID: PMC6420993.
48. Murakami M, Fox L, Dijkers MP. Ear acupuncture for immediate pain relief-a systematic review and meta-analysis of randomized controlled trials. Pain Med. 2017;18(3):551–64. https://doi.org/10.1093/pm/pnw215. PMID: 28395101.

49. Dalamagka M, Mavrommatis C, Grosomanidis V, Karakoulas K, Vasilakos D. Postoperative analgesia after low-frequency electroacupuncture as adjunctive treatment in inguinal hernia surgery with abdominal wall mesh reconstruction. Acupunct Med. 2015;33(5):360–7. https://doi.org/10.1136/acupmed-2014-010689. Epub 2015 Jun 3. PMID: 26040491.
50. Tedesco D, Gori D, Desai KR, Asch S, Carroll IR, Curtin C, McDonald KM, Fantini MP, Hernandez-Boussard T. Drug-free interventions to reduce pain or opioid consumption after total knee arthroplasty: a systematic review and meta-analysis. JAMA Surg. 2017;152(10):e172872. https://doi.org/10.1001/jamasurg.2017.2872. Epub 2017 Oct 18. Erratum in: JAMA Surg. 2018;153(4):396. PMID: 28813550; PMCID: PMC5831469.
51. Chen J, Zhang Y, Li X, Wan Y, Ji X, Wang W, Kang X, Yan W, Fan Z. Efficacy of transcutaneous electrical acupoint stimulation combined with general anesthesia for sedation and postoperative analgesia in minimally invasive lung cancer surgery: a randomized, double-blind, placebo-controlled trial. Thorac Cancer. 2020;11(4):928–934. https://doi.org/10.1111/1759-7714.13343. Epub 2020 Feb 16. PMID: 32062864; PMCID: PMC7113057.
52. Dingemann J, Plewig B, Baumann I, Plinkert PK, Sertel S. Acupuncture in posttonsillectomy pain: a prospective, double-blinded, randomized, controlled trial. HNO. 2017;65(Suppl 1):73–9. English. https://doi.org/10.1007/s00106-016-0289-5. PMID: 28070602.
53. Cooper SM, Dawber RP. The history of cryosurgery. J R Soc Med. 2001;94(4):196–201. https://doi.org/10.1177/014107680109400416.
54. Lloyd JW, Barnard JD, Glynn CJ. Cryoanalgesia. A new approach to pain relief. Lancet (London, England). 1976;2(7992):932–4. https://doi.org/10.1016/s0140-6736(76)90893-x.
55. Trescot AM. Cryoanalgesia in interventional pain management. Pain Physician. 2003;6(3):345–60. PMID: 16880882.
56. Zhou L, Kambin P, Casey KF, Bonner FJ, O'Brien E, Shao Z, Ou S. Mechanism research of cryoanalgesia. Neurol Res. 1995;17(4):307–11. https://doi.org/10.1080/01616412.1995.11740333.
57. Myers RR, Heckman HM, Powell HC. Axonal viability and the persistence of thermal hyperalgesia after partial freeze lesions of nerve. J Neurol Sci. 1996;139(1):28–38. PMID: 8836969.
58. Maiwand O, Makey AR. Cryoanalgesia for relief of pain after thoracotomy. Br Med J (Clin Res Ed). 1981;282:1749–50.
59. Ilfeld BM, Gabriel RA, Trescot AM. Ultrasound-guided percutaneous cryoneurolysis for treatment of acute pain: could cryoanalgesia replace continuous peripheral nerve blocks? Br J Anaesth. 2017;119:703–6.
60. Ilfeld BM, Finneran JJ. Cryoneurolysis and percutaneous peripheral nerve stimulation to treat acute pain. Anesthesiology. 2020;133(5):1127–49. https://doi.org/10.1097/ALN.0000000000003532. PMID: 32898231.
61. Bittman RW, Behbahani K, Gonzalez F, Prologo JD. Interventional cryoneurolysis: what is the same, what is different, what is new? Semin Intervent Radiol. 2019;36(5):374–80. https://doi.org/10.1055/s-0039-1696705. Epub 2019 Dec 2. PMID: 31798210; PMCID: PMC6887526.
62. Evans PJ, Lloyd JW, Jack TM. Cryoanalgesia for intractable perineal pain. J R Soc Med. 1981;74(11):804–9. https://doi.org/10.1177/014107688107401106. PMID: 7299782; PMCID: PMC1439365.
63. Radnovich R, Scott D, Patel AT, Olson R, Dasa V, Segal N, Lane NE, Shrock K, Naranjo J, Darr K, Surowitz R, Choo J, Valadie A, Harrell R, Wei N, Metyas S. Cryoneurolysis to treat the pain and symptoms of knee osteoarthritis: a multicenter, randomized, double-blind, sham-controlled trial. Osteoarthritis Cartilage. 2017;25(8):1247–1256. https://doi.org/10.1016/j.joca.2017.03.006. Epub 2017 Mar 20. PMID: 28336454.
64. Kim CH, Hu W, Gao J, Dragan K, Whealton T, Julian C. Cryoablation for the treatment of occipital neuralgia. Pain Physician. 2015;18(3):E363–8. PMID: 26000683.
65. Moesker AA, Karl HW, Trescot AM. Treatment of phantom limb pain by cryoneurolysis of the amputated nerve. Pain Pract. 2014;14(1):52–6. https://doi.org/10.1111/papr.12020. Epub 2012 Dec 19. PMID: 23279331.

66. Filippiadis D, Efthymiou E, Tsochatzis A, Kelekis A, Prologo JD. Percutaneous cryoanalgesia for pain palliation: current status and future trends. Diagn Interv Imaging. 2021;102(5):273–8. https://doi.org/10.1016/j.diii.2020.11.007. Epub 2020 Dec 3. PMID: 33281081.
67. Cahani D, Chacko J, Hahn B. Myonecrosis: a rare complication of cryoneurolysis. J Emerg Med. 2019;57(3):e73–6. https://doi.org/10.1016/j.jemermed.2019.06.017. Epub 2019 Aug 7. PMID: 31400988.
68. Stoelb BL, Molton IR, Jensen MP, et al. The efficacy of hypnotic analgesia in adults: a review of the literature. Contemp Hypn. 2009;26(1):24–39.
69. Nilsson U, Unosson M, Rawal N. Stress reduction and analgesia in patients exposed to calming music postoperatively: a randomized controlled trial. Eur J Anaesthesiol. 2005;22(2):96–102.
70. Wagner B, Steiner M, Huber DFX, Crevenna R. The effect of biofeedback interventions on pain, overall symptoms, quality of life and physiological parameters in patients with pelvic pain: a systematic review. Wien Klin Wochenschr. 2022;134(Suppl 1):11–48. https://doi.org/10.1007/s00508-021-01827-w.

Closing Remarks

The Future of Perioperative Pain Management

Elizabeth Scholzen and Kristopher Schroeder

Abstract The field of pain management is rapidly expanding as it parallels the significant increase in surgical procedure breadth and volume. As healthcare systems transition to performing a larger percentage of surgical care in the outpatient or ambulatory setting, the field of pain management will need to evolve to ensure efficient discharge readiness with adequate pain control regimens that minimize the risk of opioid related adverse events and need for unplanned readmissions. New pathways within pain management may significantly change the current pain medicine landscape. The use of artificial intelligence (AI) software may help to improve access to and success of regional anesthesia techniques. AI may also be useful in sifting through large amounts of data to determine the best pain management regimen for a specific patient. Genetics may also be a key to the future of pain management. Knowing an individual's specific genetic response to pain stimuli and their response to various medications will be helpful in tailoring a pain regimen that is highly individualized. Finally, the perioperative home model of care can help to identify patients that would benefit from additional prehabilitation or counseling prior to surgery. Patients with a history of frailty or chronic pain who need a more comprehensive pain plan for their postoperative course may benefit greatly from enhanced preoperative planning. There are many changes on the horizon in the field of pain management that will improve access and benefit patients experiencing acute pain.

Keywords Collaboration · Artificial intelligence · Perioperative surgical home · Enhanced recovery · Genetics

---

E. Scholzen · K. Schroeder (✉)
Department of Anesthesiology, University of Wisconsin School of Medicine and Public Health, Madison, WI, USA
e-mail: Kmschro1@wisc.edu

E. Scholzen
e-mail: naab@wisc.edu

A. Abd-Elsayed and K. Schroeder (eds.), *Perioperative Pain Management*,
https://doi.org/10.1007/978-3-031-67648-2_44

1 Introduction

Perioperative pain medicine is continuing to evolve and this evolution will likely only accelerate as increased surgical volumes induce healthcare systems to expedite the care of patients while simultaneously improving outcomes and maximizing profits. In 2020, it was reported that 40–50 million major surgical procedures were performed in the United States annually. In ambulatory centers, which realized a 300% increase in surgical volume between 1996 and 2006, there is an increased emphasis on ensuring that patients experience adequate pain control to ensure efficient and safe discharge readiness [1]. By 2018, the number of annual ambulatory procedures increased to 19.2 million [2]. With the staggering number of cases already being performed in the ambulatory setting, it is worth noting that there are groups predicting that procedures in the ambulatory surgical setting will increase an additional 25% in the next decade [3]. This growth in surgical case volume will require a redesign of existing structures, a massive investment in new surgical centers, and a rethinking of surgical, anesthetic, and pain management paradigms. This realignment of ambulatory procedure management goals is occurring in the setting of an opioid abuse epidemic. Patients now present for surgical procedures with opioid receptors tolerant, occupied, or blocked and it is therefore critical that non-opioid based analgesic treatment strategies are developed and enhanced. Although treatment for this patient population may be challenging, multiple emerging strategies may represent the key to future pain management.

2 Future

Artificial intelligence (AI) represents a technology that seemed like science fiction a short time ago. However, the reality is that AI has already been deployed to aid in the management of a spectrum of activities and workflows that permeate our daily existence. At its core, AI seeks to mimic human intelligence through the use of algorithms that leverage large amounts of data to make predictions and study outcomes. In a variety of perioperative settings, AI may perform tasks such as problem-solving, object/word recognition, and decision-making that can aid healthcare professionals in the delivery of high-quality medical care. Already, AI platforms are being utilized to produce patient-specific risk scores with perioperative predictions that outperform physicians [4–8]. In the perioperative period, AI technologies have been applied to perform a variety of important clinical tasks including depth of anesthesia monitoring, control of anesthesia delivery, and event prediction [9]. In addition to general perioperative management, AI systems have also demonstrated efficacy in the evaluation and management of postoperative pain. AI and machine learning has demonstrated the ability to analyze clinical factors involved in the development of significant rebound pain following block resolution and determine the impact of concomitant selective serotonin reuptake inhibitor administration on perioperative pain control.

One exciting development in AI technologies is the new ability of this technology to assist with ultrasound-based procedures. These technologies can interpret ultrasound images and accurately identify targets of interest. This technology has recently been advanced to such a degree that nerves, muscles, and vessels can be labeled in real time on ultrasound imaging across a wide range of potential regional anesthesia targets [10]. These technology advancements have the potential to improve regional ultrasound performance safety and expand the pool of competent healthcare professionals available to perform regional anesthesia techniques.

AI may also represent the future of meta-analysis and published data review. In a study that compared a traditional meta-analysis evaluation of regional anesthesia for hip and knee arthroplasty, an AI algorithm was able to achieve the same conclusions in only ten minutes time [11]. This technological advance may have arrived just in time to assist healthcare professionals as they attempt to sort through an ever-increasing deluge of published literature.

AI technologies harbor several limitations that require serious consideration. First, this technology should never supplant the patient-healthcare professional interaction as there needs to be oversight to the decisions made by AI. The input of bad data into the decision-making algorithm makes it susceptible to making erroneous judgements and there needs to be oversight to prevent errors in diagnosis and treatment. A common example might be the ECG interference caused by cauterization and how an erroneous diagnosis of ventricular tachycardia may result in inappropriate cardiac rhythm restoration responses. Poorly conducted studies or erroneous/fraudulent data may negatively influence the results of an AI generated recommendation. In addition, the algorithms themselves may be subject to scrutiny if there is a lack of transparency in the generation of these prediction tools [12]. However, many of these AI interfaces have the opportunity to undergo machine learning where they learn from their mistakes, integrate new data, and continuously improve their ability to make accurate predictions. Ultimately, AI is incredibly unlikely to supplant healthcare professionals who are better able to ensure that patients are treated with empathy and compassion. However, it is also likely true that AI will become an increasingly present companion and adjunct in the healthcare arena [13]

While robots and powerful machine learning AI generates tremendous excitement for the advancement and future potential of analgesic management, the most powerful tool may be locked away in the genetic code of each of our patients. Every healthcare professional recognizes that any drug or therapeutic agent has an unknown efficacy and side-effect profile that is likely determined by the genetic makeup of the individual undergoing treatment. In addition, patients seem to have wide variability in their pain experience following similar surgical procedures. There may be a genetic component to some of this encountered variability as polymorphisms in catechol-O-methyl transferase (COMT) may result in accumulations of catecholamines and elevated pain sensitivity [14–16]. Pharmacogenomics studies the uniqueness of each individual and how their genetic profile or polymorphisms influence drug pharmacokinetics and pharmacodynamics. Genetic variability can impact drug elimination, transport, and receptors and impact drug duration, dosing, efficacy, side-effect profile, and safety. This academic pursuit holds the key to improvements in individualized medicine that will facilitate greater efficacy and safety in medication delivery. Perhaps the most well-known genetic polymorphisms known to impact drug metabolism exist in the cytochrome P450 superfamily. These enzymes are known to exist in multiple confirmations that can either diminish or enhance the metabolism of therapeutic agents. Codeine represents a common example of how genetic variability might influence drug effect. Codeine requires metabolism by a cytochrome P450 enzyme for conversion to its active metabolite, morphine. A patient that poorly metabolized codeine would likely experience inadequate analgesia and be at increased risk for readmission. However, patients that metabolized morphine to a greater than anticipated extent would encounter higher serum levels of morphine and an increased risk of perioperative respiratory depression. In addition to codeine, numerous other analgesics including tramadol, hydrocodone, and oxycodone require cytochrome P450 enzyme metabolism for analgesic effect [17].

Beyond metabolism, transporter polymorphisms have been reported in brain capillary endothelial cells that impact the degree to which systemic opioids might induce postoperative respiratory depression [18]. There are also polymorphisms in mu-opioid receptors that might impact opioid dosing paradigms with individual patients demonstrating phenotypic differences in opioid responsiveness. Finally, COMT enzyme polymorphisms may impact the upregulation of opioid receptors and have a significant role in determining subsequent opioid dosing [19–22]. Genetic polymorphisms may also impact the efficacy and side-effect profile of nonsteroidal anti-inflammatory drugs [23–25].

Local anesthetic effect can also be significantly influenced by genetic polymorphisms. There exist mutations in nerve axon sodium channels that may limit the ability of local anesthetics to terminate action potential propagation [26, 27]. The result of these polymorphisms might be regional anesthetic blocks of short duration or limited efficacy. Where these polymorphisms might become critically important are in scenarios where there is a contraindication to general anesthesia. An unexpected need to convert to a general anesthetic might result in adverse intraoperative events or increased need for postoperative admission. In addition, if local anesthetic techniques are of diminished efficacy or duration, patients may require inpatient admission or additional opioids that could increase their risk of an opioid related adverse event.

In the not-too-distant future, preoperative genetic testing offers the promise of individualized and precision medicine and perioperative analgesic guidance. While these genetic polymorphisms will not supplant enhanced recovery profiles or empathetic patient care paradigms, they will better facilitate perioperative planning and individualized treatment pathways. These tests would need to be completed far enough in advance of the planned surgical procedure to allow for formation of an individualized pain management pathway. At some point in the future, this testing may indicate appropriate analgesic agent and dosing selection that maximizes efficacy and minimizes side effects [28]. This preoperative testing may also help predict which patients might be more successfully transitioned to outpatient procedures versus those that will require more prolonged hospitalizations. Genetic testing may also help to better predict which patients will have difficulty weaning from opioids or be more likely to develop chronic pain syndromes. Ultimately, improvements in the efficiency of healthcare administration may result in substantial improvements in patient safety and cost savings.

There are, however, significant barriers that limit routine utilization of pharmacogenomic data. There remain limitations on pharmacogenomic testing availability and testing, when available, requires a significant time investment. Even when testing is completed, there are limitations in data storage within electronic medical record platforms that will allow for only the documentation of highly pertinent or meaningful polymorphisms [29]. Identifying the most clinically relevant targets for genetic evaluation represents one avenue for improving the implementation of perioperative genetic testing. There also remain reimbursement limitations and concerns about healthcare information privacy that may limit patient enthusiasm for preoperative genomic testing. Physicians will certainly require enhanced education relevant to healthcare planning in the presence of genetic data. There are then ethical dilemmas associated with the collection of genetic information and what other predictive data might be collected [30]. Patients should likely be counseled that it is possible that preoperative genetic testing may predict that a genetic predisposition exists for any number of detrimental cancers or degenerative diseases. Prior to more widespread implementation of preoperative genetic testing, counseling and follow-up services are required to help patients acclimate to any newly diagnosed clinical predilection.

While individualized medicine has the potential to revolutionize the care for patients with genetic polymorphisms, widely applying evidence-based best practices has the greatest potential to convey postoperative analgesic benefits to the widest breadth of surgical patients. While the ideal mechanism to deploy these evidence-based strategies is yet to be determined, the perioperative surgical home coupled with enhanced recovery pathways offers the promise of adherence to best practices and continued re-evaluation of outcome variables.

A central tenet of the perioperative surgical home is that there is a centralized group of physicians that help usher patients throughout the perioperative process from the time that they are scheduled for a surgical procedure until they have fully recovered and transitioned off or back to their baseline level of opioid analgesics. Through initiating interactions with patients and their families early in the process, there is an enhanced opportunity for patient education and involvement of patients as active participants in their care.

In many surgical patients, it is incredibly important to consider that pain management is more than a numbers game. For example, frailty represents an increasingly recognized risk factor for perioperative morbidity, mortality, and readmission [31–33]. The etiology of frailty is very frequently multifactorial. Age plays a large contributing role in frailty diagnoses and has been reported to be present in <10% of the population below 65 years of age and >50% of those greater than 85 [34]. Beyond age, mental health, cognition, malnutrition, and physical performance can all substantially contribute to an increased likelihood of patients presenting for surgery with heightened levels of pain and barriers to recovery. Consider the case of a patient presenting for total knee arthroplasty. These patients generally present with long-standing painful arthropathies that have limited their mobility/physical functioning and frequently contribute to declining mental health. Data specific to total joint arthroplasty demonstrates that patients presenting with frailty are at elevated risk for a range of postoperative complications including hematoma/seroma, wound dehiscence, infection, postoperative anemia, and mortality. In addition, frail patients impact medical systems by requiring a longer length of stay, more frequent admissions to rehabilitation facilities and generating higher total hospital charges [35, 36]. While previous research has demonstrated that (in addition to improvements in nutrition and mental health) prescriptions for exercise/strengthening prehabilitation can substantially improve functional outcomes and decrease complication rates, patients presenting for knee arthroplasty are frequently so limited by pain that their ability to engage in these exercises might be limited [37–41]. Exciting new research has demonstrated that there may be pathways and interventions in the preoperative phase of care that can impact recovery in a meaningful way. Multiple studies have demonstrated that patients receiving cryoneurolysis prior to knee arthroplasty surgery encounter decreased pain and opioid requirements, decreased length of hospital admission, and improved functional outcomes [42, 43]. While cryoneurolysis has demonstrated the ability to effectively improve rehabilitation, the application of this therapy well in advance of surgery may also offer the promise of facilitating prehabilitation and improvements in strength and function prior to surgery that will ultimately result in reduced frailty and improved patient outcomes [44].

Beyond the application of therapies that can diminish pain and improve functional status, there is much to be gained from meeting with patients prior to surgery. In meeting with patients prior to their surgical procedure, there exists a unique opportunity to establish care and discuss previous efforts with pain management that have either been successful or proven inadequate. These patients, especially those with a history of chronic pain or opioid use, can be brought in as collaborators in planning their future analgesic management. Ideally, discussing interventional pain management procedures prior to the day of surgery will result in an improved consent process and an enhanced acceptance by patients. This meeting also introduces an opportunity to have patients disclose a history of illicit opioid use, set realistic perioperative analgesic management goals, and establish boundaries for escalations in opioid dosing. While these meetings had historically been a time where discontinuation or down-titration of opioid agonist therapeutics (including buprenorphine) might be considered, it is now most commonly recommended that these medications are continued into the postoperative phase of care and that additional analgesic needs are addressed with multimodal analgesics and regional anesthesia techniques [45].

Enhanced recovery pathways are designed to minimize the physiologic impact on patients presenting for surgery. Improved pain management and strategies to minimize opioid administration, such as regional anesthesia techniques, remain a key tenet of successful enhanced recovery pathways. In many cases, the optimal regional anesthetic regimen has yet to be determined (i.e. epidural vs any number of potential fascial plane blocks) but the use of the regional anesthetic techniques is generally associated with a recovery profile that might include decreased pain, decreased opioid requirements and opioid related adverse events, and decreased hospital lengths of stay. In addition, enhanced recovery pathways are helpful in the delivery codification of non-opioid analgesics including acetaminophen, NSAIDs, gabapentinoids, ketamine, and intravenous lidocaine infusions [46–48]. With enhanced recovery pathways, there remain significant opportunities for protocol refinement that might serve to better define surgical procedures and patient populations most likely to benefit from these interventions. In addition, electronic records and ordering systems may ultimately serve as an effective tool to standardize the delivery of the enhanced recovery profile elements across a range of providers.

As the science of perioperative pain management progresses, remaining up to date on recent advancements will guide future clinical practice improvements. With the rapid description and deployment of advanced fascial plane blocks, future research is required to determine which blocks are more clinically useful versus those that should be relegated to second (or lower) tier status. It may also be possible that the increasing interest in peripheral regional anesthesia, overall skill with ultrasound guidance, and improved teaching modalities will result in a gradual improvement in the delivery of regional anesthesia techniques. While randomized trials represent the pinnacle of data acquisition, increased utilization of collaborative data-set evaluations will facilitate a better understanding of how these procedures are functioning in the real world and help to better guide clinical practice. In addition, feedback from data-sets to local providers may allow for procedure performance feedback and enhancement. At some point, it may become possible to identify areas where additional education and training will improve practice performance. Future therapeutic advancement is difficult to predict but it is certainly possible that major breakthroughs could fundamentally change pain management practice. Already, novel opioids have been developed that offer the promise of analgesia and improved safety with a decreased side-effect profile [49]. While liposomal formulations of local anesthetics offer the promise of 72–96 hours of analgesia, cost considerations and unclear efficacy enhancements have thus far limited more widespread utilization [50, 51]. Future research may provide more clear recommendations regarding when the use of liposomal local anesthetic administration is warranted and when the use of local anesthetic additives may be indicated. Future local anesthetic preparations may also offer an even greater duration of action or selective sensory blockade that could fundamentally alter the practice of perioperative analgesia.

Finally, it is beyond time for healthcare professionals to recognize that much of what we are asked to treat exists on a continuum and that what we do to help patients overlaps significantly with the work of others. For example, the work of acute and chronic/interventional pain providers overlaps to a significant extent as patients with chronic pain and opioid requirements present for surgical procedures. In these patients, baseline pain management optimization through procedural intervention and therapeutic optimization can provide substantial perioperative benefits. In the same regard, the work that is done in the perioperative period may have lasting impacts on opioid induced hyperalgesia and postoperative opioid dose escalation [52]. Newly created transitional pain clinics will become increasingly important as more patients present for surgical intervention with baseline pain and opioid tolerance. Collectively, there needs to be more of an effort to limit opioid analgesics in the community and manage the opioid epidemic that is currently claiming far too many lives [53]. Finally, there is an increased need to adopt multidisciplinary approaches to perioperative pain management and opioid restriction. These efforts should acknowledge that each healthcare professional is essential to the ultimate goal of effective perioperative pain management and improved patient safety.

We now exist at the dawn of an exciting era in perioperative pain management. We have developed less invasive surgical techniques, accumulated the wisdom to know how dangerous our analgesics might be, and developed new analgesic/therapeutic interventions that offer the hope of a diminished need for opioid analgesics. However, now is the time to double-down on our collective commitment to our patients and their perioperative pain needs through continued advancement and support of analgesic programs. Only through this commitment, can we continue in the acceleration of surgical procedural volume growth and ensure the safety of our patients.

3 Conclusion

Healthcare professionals are now armed with advances in therapeutics and regional anesthetic techniques that extend the ability to provide effective perioperative analgesia. However, patients are now presenting with an increasing reliance and tolerance to opioid analgesics that significantly complicates pain management. Healthcare systems are overburdened and efforts to improve analgesia that concurrently hasten inpatient discharges or convert procedures to an outpatient status should be pursued. Novel advancements in genetics and artificial intelligence offer the promise of great advancements in individualized medicine while enhanced recovery pathways are critical to ensuing the delivery of evidence-based best practices. However, the greatest potential for advancements in perioperative analgesia can be found in collaborative efforts made between healthcare professionals throughout a patient's perioperative journey.

References

1. file:///Users/kristopherschroeder/Downloads/surgery_final_report.pdf. Accessed 10/02/2023.
2. https://www.hcup-us.ahrq.gov/reports/statbriefs/sb287-Ambulatory-Surgery-Overview-2019.pdf. Accessed 10/02/2023.
3. https://www.beckersasc.com/asc-transactions-and-valuation-issues/can-ascs-handle-the-boom-in-case-volume.html#:~:text=ASC%20surgery%20volume%20is%20projected,Forecast%20Highlights%2C%22%20June%204. Accessed 10/02/2023.
4. Bihorac A, Ozrazgat-Baslanti T, Ebadi A, et al. MySurgeryRisk: development and validation of a machine-learning risk algorithm for major complications and death after surgery. Ann Surg. 2019;269:652–62.

5. Brennan M, Puri S, Ozrazgat-Baslanti T, et al. Comparing clinical judgment with the MySurgeryRisk algorithm for preoperative risk assessment: a pilot usability study. Surgery. 2019;165:1035–45.
6. Xue B, Li D, Lu C, et al. Use of machine learning to develop and evaluate models using preoperative and intraoperative data to identify risks of postoperative complications. JAMA Netw Open. 2021;4: e212240.
7. Maheshwari K, Ruetzler K, Saugel. Perioperative intelligence: applications of artificial intelligence in preoperative medicine. J Clin Monit Comput. 2020;34:625–8.
8. Yoon HK, Yang HL, Jung CW, Lee HC. Artificial intelligence in perioperative medicine: a narrative review. Korean J Anesthesiol. 2022;75:202–15.
9. Hashimoto DA, Witkowski E, Gao L, Meireles O, Rosman G. Artificial intelligence in anesthesiology. Current techniques, clinical applications, and limitations. Anesthesiology. 2020;132:379–94.
10. https://nerveblox.com/. Accessed 10/02/2023.
11. Myszewski J, Klossowski E, Schroeder KM. Evaluation of language analysis to summarize the literature: a comparison to traditional meta-analysis in primary hip and knee surgery. Reg Anesth Pain Med. 2022;47:151–4.
12. Pasero D, Terragni P. Artificial intelligence and perioperative medicine. Minerva Anestesiol. 2021;87:755–6.
13. Canales C, Lee C, Cannesson M. Science without conscience is but the ruin of the soul: the ethics of big data and artificial intelligence in perioperative medicine. Anesth Analg. 2020;130:1234–43.
14. Diatchenko L, Nackley AG, Slade GD, et al. Catechol-O-methyltransferase gene polymorphisms are associated with multiple pain-evoking stimuli. Pain. 2006;125:216–24.
15. Diatchenko L, Slade GD, Nackley AG, et al. Genetic basis for individual variations in pain perception and the development of a chronic pain condition. Hum Mol Genet. 2005;14:135–43.
16. Packiasabapathy S, Horn N, Sadhasivam S. Genetics of perioperative pain management. Curr Opin Anaesthesiol. 2018;31:749–55.
17. Palmer SN, Giesecke NM, Body SC, et al. Pharmacogenetics of anesthetic and analgesic agents. Anesthesiology. 2005;102(3):663e71.
18. Sadhasivam S, Chidambaran V, Zhang X, et al. Opioid-induced respiratory depression: ABCB1 transporter pharmacogenetics. Pharmacogenomics J. 2015;15(2):119e26.
19. Landau R, Kern C, Columb MO, et al. Genetic variability of the mu-opioid receptor influences intrathecal fentanyl analgesia requirements in laboring women. Pain. 2008;139(1):5e14.
20. Zhang F, Tong J, Hu J, et al. COMT gene haplotypes are closely associated with postoperative fentanyl dose in patients. Anesth Analg. 2015;120(4):933e40.
21. Hwang IC, Park JY, Myung SK, et al. OPRM1 A118G gene variant and postoperative opioid requirement: a systematic review and meta-analysis. Anesthesiology. 2014;121:825–34.
22. Palada V, Kaunisto MA, Kalso E. Genetics and genomics in postoperative pain and analgesia. Curr Opin Anaesthesiol. 2018;31:569–74.
23. Kapur BM, Lala PK, Shaw JLV. Pharmacogenetics of chronic pain management. Clin Biochem. 2014;47:1169e87.
24. Pilotto A, Seripa D, Franceschi M, et al. Genetic susceptibility to nonsteroidal anti-inflammatory drug related gastroduodenal bleeding: role of cytochrome P450 2C9 polymorphisms. Gastroenterology. 2007;133:465e71.
25. Carbonell N, Verstuyft C, Massard J, et al. CYP2C9*3 loss-of-function allele is associated with acute upper gastrointestinal bleeding related to the use of NSAIDs other than aspirin. Clin Pharmacol Ther. 2010;87:693e8.
26. Trescot AM. Genetics and implications in perioperative analgesia. Best Pract Res Clin Anaesthesiol. 2014;28(2):153–66.
27. Cohen M, Sadhasivam S, Vinks AA. Pharmacogenetics in perioperative medicine. Curr Opin Anaesthesiol. 2012;25(4):419–27.
28. Chaturvedi R, Alexander B, A'Court AM, Waterman RS, Burton BN, Urman RD, Gabriel RA. Genomics testing and personalized medicine in the preoperative setting: can it change outcomes in postoperative pain management? Best Pract Res Clin Anaesthesiol. 2020;34:283–95.

29. Kaye AD, Koress CM, Novisch MB, Jung JW, Urets I, Viswanath O, Renschler JS, Alpaugh ES, Cornett EM. Pharmacogenomics, concepts for the future of perioperative medicine and pain management: a review. Best Pract Res Clin Anaesthesiol. 2020;34:651–62.
30. Kaye AD, Mahakian T, Kaye AJ, Pham AA, Hart BM, Genus S, Cornett EM, Gabriel RA, Urman RD. Pharmacogenomics, precision medicine, and implications for anesthesia care. Best Pract Res Clin Anaesthesiol. 2018;32:61–81.
31. Lin HS, Watts JN, Peel NM, Hubbard RE. Frailty and post- operative outcomes in older surgical patients: a systematic review. BMC Geriatr. 2016;16:157.
32. Kim DH, Kim CA, Placide S, Lipsitz LA, Marcantonio ER. Preoperative frailty assessment and outcomes at 6 months or later in older adults undergoing cardiac surgical procedures: a systematic review. Ann Intern Med. 2016;165:650–60.
33. Beggs T, Sepehri A, Szwajcer A, Tangri N, Arora RC. Frailty and perioperative outcomes: a narrative review. Can J Anaesth. 2015;62:143–57.
34. McIsaac DI, MacDonald DB, Aucoin SD. Frailty for perioperative clinicians: a narrative review. Anesth Analg. 2020;130:1450–60.
35. Zalikha AK, Pham L, Keeley J, Hussein IH, El-Othmani MM. Frailty among total hip and knee arthroplasty recipients: epidemiology and propensity score-weighted analysis of effect on in-hospital postoperative outcomes. J Am Acad Orthop Surg. 2022. https://doi.org/10.5435/JAAOS-D-22-00642. Epub ahead of print. PMID: 36728666.
36. Cook MJ, Lunt M, Board T, O'Neill TW. The impact of frailty on short-term mortality following primary total hip and knee arthroplasty due to osteoarthritis. Age Ageing. 2022;51(6):afac118. https://doi.org/10.1093/ageing/afac118. PMID: 35679192; PMCID: PMC9180921.
37. Minnella EM, Awasthi R, Loiselle SE, Agnihotram RV, Ferri LE, Carli F. Effect of exercise and nutrition prehabilitation on functional capacity in esophagogastric cancer surgery: a randomized clinical trial. JAMA Surg. 2018;153:1081–9.
38. Barberan-Garcia A, Ubré M, Roca J, et al. Personalised prehabilitation in high-risk patients undergoing elective major abdominal surgery: a randomized blinded controlled trial. Ann Surg. 2018;267:50–6.
39. Gillis C, Li C, Lee L, et al. Prehabilitation versus rehabilitation: a randomized control trial in patients undergoing colorectal resection for cancer. Anesthesiology. 2014;121:937–47.
40. McIsaac DI, Jen T, Mookerji N, Patel A, Lalu MM. Interventions to improve the outcomes of frail people having surgery: a systematic review. PLoS ONE. 2017;12: e0190071.
41. Vervullens S, Meert L, Baert I, Smeets RJEM, Verdonk P, Rahusen F, Meeus M. Prehabilitation before total knee arthroplasty: a systematic review on the use and efficacy of stratified care. Ann Phys Rehabil Med. 2022;66(4):101705. https://doi.org/10.1016/j.rehab.2022.101705. Epub ahead of print. PMID: 36115573.
42. Mihalko WM, Kerkhof AL, Ford MC, Crockarell JR Jr, Harkess JW, Guyton JL. Cryoneurolysis before total knee arthroplasty in patients with severe osteoarthritis for reduction of postoperative pain and opioid use in a single-center randomized controlled trial. J Arthroplasty. 2021;36(5):1590–8.
43. Urban JA, Dolesh K, Martin E. A multimodal pain management protocol including preoperative cryoneurolysis for total knee arthroplasty to reduce pain, opioid consumption, and length of stay. Arthroplast Today. 2021;12(10):87–92.
44. Lung BE, Karasavvidis T, Sharma AK, Amirhekmat A, Stepanyan H, McMaster W, Yang S, So DH. Cryoneurolysis is a safe, effective modality to improve rehabilitation after total knee arthroplasty. Life (Basel). 2022;12(9):1344.
45. Kohan L, Potru S, Barreveld AM, Sprintz M, Lane O, Aryal A, Emerick T, Dopp A, Chhay S, Viscusi E. Buprenorphine management in the perioperative period: educational review and recommendations from a multisociety expert panel. Reg Anesth Pain Med. 2021;46(10):840–59.
46. Cheung CK, Adeola JO, Beutler SS, Urman RD. Postoperative pain management in enhanced recovery pathways. J Pain Res. 2022;13(15):123–35.
47. Tan M, Law LS, Gan TJ. Optimizing pain management to facilitate enhanced recovery after surgery pathways. Can J Anaesth. 2015;62(2):203–18.

48. Ghai B, Jafra A, Bhatia N, Chanana N, Bansal D, Mehta V. Opioid sparing strategies for perioperative pain management other than regional anaesthesia: a narrative review. J Anaesthesiol Clin Pharmacol. 2022;38(1):3–10.
49. Tan HS, Habib AS. Oliceridine: a novel drug for the management of moderate to severe acute pain—a review of current evidence. J Pain Res. 2021;14(14):969–79.
50. Prabhakar A, Ward CT, Watson M, Sanford J, Fiza B, Moll V, Kaye RJ, Morgan Hall O, Cornett EM, Urman RD, Kaye AD. Liposomal bupivacaine and novel local anesthetic formulations. Best Pract Res Clin Anaesthesiol. 2019;33(4):425–32.
51. Ilfeld BM, Eisenach JC, Gabriel RA. Clinical effectiveness of liposomal bupivacaine administered by infiltration or peripheral nerve block to treat postoperative pain. Anesthesiology. 2021;134(2):283–344.
52. Schroeder KM, Sites BD, Narouze S. ASRA pain medicine: an established society with an updated vision. Reg Anesth Pain Med. 2021;46(12):1029–30.
53. Bedene A, Dahan A, Rosendaal FR, van Dorp ELA. Opioid epidemic: lessons learned and updated recommendations for misuse involving prescription versus non-prescription opioids. Expert Rev Clin Pharmacol. 2022;15(9):1081–94.

Correction to: Perioperative Care of the Opioid-Tolerant Patient

Nathan J. Rudin

Correction to:
Chapter "Perioperative Care of the Opioid-Tolerant Patient" in: A. Abd-Elsayed and K. Schroeder (eds.), *Perioperative Pain Management*, https://doi.org/10.1007/978-3-031-67648-2_20

In the original version of this chapter, the title has been changed from "Perioperative Care of the Opioid-Tolerant Patient: A Complimentary Perspectives" to "Perioperative Care of the Opioid-Tolerant Patient". The chapter has been updated with the change.

The updated version of this chapter can be found at
https://doi.org/10.1007/978-3-031-67648-2_20

A. Abd-Elsayed and K. Schroeder (eds.), *Perioperative Pain Management*,
https://doi.org/10.1007/978-3-031-67648-2_45

Index

A. Abd-Elsayed and K. Schroeder (eds.), *Perioperative Pain Management*, https://doi.org/10.1007/978-3-031-67648-2

B

C

GPSR Compliance

The European Union's (EU) General Product Safety Regulation (GPSR) is a set of rules that requires consumer products to be safe and our obligations to ensure this.

If you have any concerns about our products, you can contact us on ProductSafety@springernature.com

In case Publisher is established outside the EU, the EU authorized representative is:

Springer Nature Customer Service Center GmbH
Europaplatz 3
69115 Heidelberg, Germany

Batch number: 10756373

Printed by Printforce, the Netherlands